Key Advances in the Treatment of the Critically Ill

Key Advances in the Treatment of the Critically Ill

Editor

Spyros D. Mentzelopoulos

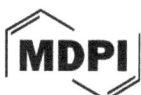

Basel • Beijing • Wuhan • Barcelona • Belgrade • Novi Sad • Cluj • Manchester

Editor
Spyros D. Mentzelopoulos
National and Kapodistrian
University of Athens,
Evaggelismos General
Hospital
Athens
Greece

Editorial Office
MDPI
St. Alban-Anlage 66
4052 Basel, Switzerland

This is a reprint of articles from the Special Issue published online in the open access journal *Journal of Clinical Medicine* (ISSN 2077-0383) (available at: https://www.mdpi.com/journal/jcm/special_issues/critical_ill).

For citation purposes, cite each article independently as indicated on the article page online and as indicated below:

Lastname, A.A.; Lastname, B.B. Article Title. *Journal Name* **Year**, *Volume Number*, Page Range.

ISBN 978-3-7258-0267-8 (Hbk)
ISBN 978-3-7258-0268-5 (PDF)
doi.org/10.3390/books978-3-7258-0268-5

© 2024 by the authors. Articles in this book are Open Access and distributed under the Creative Commons Attribution (CC BY) license. The book as a whole is distributed by MDPI under the terms and conditions of the Creative Commons Attribution-NonCommercial-NoDerivs (CC BY-NC-ND) license.

Contents

Spyros D. Mentzelopoulos and George Adamos
Key Advances in Intensive Care and the Coronavirus Disease-19 Research and Practice Boost
Reprinted from: *J. Clin. Med.* **2022**, *11*, 3370, doi:10.3390/jcm11123370 1

Charlotte Marie Schanke, Anne Kristine Brekka, Stein Arne Rimehaug, Mari Klokkerud and Tiina Maarit Andersen
Norwegian Version of the Chelsea Critical Care Physical Assessment Tool (CPAx-NOR): Translation, Face Validity, Cross-Cultural Adaptation and Inter-Rater Reliability
Reprinted from: *J. Clin. Med.* **2023**, *12*, 5033, doi:10.3390/jcm12155033 6

George Karlis, Despina Markantonaki, Sotirios Kakavas, Dimitra Bakali, Georgia Katsagani, Theodora Katsarou, Christos Kyritsis, and et al.
Prone Position Ventilation in Severe ARDS due to COVID-19: Comparison between Prolonged and Intermittent Strategies
Reprinted from: *J. Clin. Med.* **2023**, *12*, 3526, doi:10.3390/jcm12103526 19

Mark E. Seubert and Marco Goeijenbier
Early Patient-Triggered Pressure Support Breathing in Mechanically Ventilated Patients with COVID-19 May Be Associated with Lower Rates of Acute Kidney Injury
Reprinted from: *J. Clin. Med.* **2023**, *12*, 1859, doi:10.3390/jcm12051859 28

Piotr Smuszkiewicz, Natalia Jawień, Jakub Szrama, Marta Lubarska, Krzysztof Kusza and Przemysław Guzik
Admission Lactate Concentration, Base Excess, and Alactic Base Excess Predict the 28-Day Inward Mortality in Shock Patients
Reprinted from: *J. Clin. Med.* **2022**, *11*, 6125, doi:10.3390/jcm11206125 34

Paolo Formenti, Silvia Coppola, Laura Massironi, Giacomo Annibali, Francesco Mazza, Lisa Gilardi, Tommaso Pozzi, and et al.
Left Ventricular Diastolic Dysfunction in ARDS Patients
Reprinted from: *J. Clin. Med.* **2022**, *11*, 5998, doi:10.3390/jcm11205998 46

Lukas Martin Müller-Wirtz, Dustin Grimm, Frederic Walter Albrecht, Tobias Fink, Thomas Volk and Andreas Meiser
Increased Respiratory Drive after Prolonged Isoflurane Sedation: A Retrospective Cohort Study
Reprinted from: *J. Clin. Med.* **2022**, *11*, 5422, doi:10.3390/jcm11185422 57

Elisabeth Zechendorf, Katharina Schröder, Lara Stiehler, Nadine Frank, Christian Beckers, Sandra Kraemer, Michael Dreher, and et al.
The Potential Impact of Heparanase Activity and Endothelial Damage in COVID-19 Disease
Reprinted from: *J. Clin. Med.* **2022**, *11*, 5261, doi:10.3390/jcm11185261 67

Spyros D. Mentzelopoulos, Keith Couper, Violetta Raffay, Jana Djakow and Leo Bossaert
Evolution of European Resuscitation and End-of-Life Practices from 2015 to 2019: A Survey-Based Comparative Evaluation
Reprinted from: *J. Clin. Med.* **2022**, *11*, 4005, doi:10.3390/jcm11144005 78

Rickard Lagedal, Oskar Eriksson, Anna Sörman, Joram B. Huckriede, Bjarne Kristensen, Stephanie Franzén, Anders Larsson, and et al.
Impaired Antibody Response Is Associated with Histone-Release, Organ Dysfunction and Mortality in Critically Ill COVID-19 Patients
Reprinted from: *J. Clin. Med.* **2022**, *11*, 3419, doi:10.3390/jcm11123419 95

Subin Hwang, Danbee Kang, Hyejeong Park, Youngha Kim, Eliseo Guallar, Junseok Jeon, Jung-Eun Lee, and et al.
Impact of Renal Replacement Therapy on Mortality and Renal Outcomes in Critically Ill Patients with Acute Kidney Injury: A Population-Based Cohort Study in Korea between 2008 and 2015
Reprinted from: *J. Clin. Med.* **2022**, *11*, 2392, doi:10.3390/jcm11092392 . . . . **109**

Giorgio Berlot, Silvia Zanchi, Edoardo Moro, Ariella Tomasini and Mattia Bixio
The Role of the Intravenous IgA and IgM-Enriched Immunoglobulin Preparation in the Treatment of Sepsis and Septic Shock
Reprinted from: *J. Clin. Med.* **2023**, *12*, 4645, doi:10.3390/jcm12144645 . . . . **122**

Athanasios Chalkias, Georgios Adamos and Spyros D. Mentzelopoulos
General Critical Care, Temperature Control, and End-of-Life Decision Making in Patients Resuscitated from Cardiac Arrest
Reprinted from: *J. Clin. Med.* **2023**, *12*, 4118, doi:10.3390/jcm12124118 . . . . **133**

Giorgio Berlot, Ariella Tomasini, Silvia Zanchi and Edoardo Moro
The Techniques of Blood Purification in the Treatment of Sepsis and Other Hyperinflammatory Conditions
Reprinted from: *J. Clin. Med.* **2023**, *12*, 1723, doi:10.3390/jcm12051723 . . . . **164**

John Selickman, Charikleia S. Vrettou, Spyros D. Mentzelopoulos and John J. Marini
COVID-19-Related ARDS: Key Mechanistic Features and Treatments
Reprinted from: *J. Clin. Med.* **2022**, *11*, 4896, doi:10.3390/jcm11164896 . . . . **176**

Charikleia S. Vrettou and Spyros D. Mentzelopoulos
Second- and Third-Tier Therapies for Severe Traumatic Brain Injury
Reprinted from: *J. Clin. Med.* **2022**, *11*, 4790, doi:10.3390/jcm11164790 . . . . **198**

Nikoletta Rovina, Evangelia Koukaki, Vasiliki Romanou, Sevasti Ampelioti, Konstantinos Loverdos, Vasiliki Chantziara, Antonia Koutsoukou, and et al.
Fungal Infections in Critically Ill COVID-19 Patients: Inevitabile Malum
Reprinted from: *J. Clin. Med.* **2022**, *11*, 2017, doi:10.3390/jcm11072017 . . . . **210**

Liliana Mirea, Cristian Cobilinschi, Raluca Ungureanu, Ana-Maria Cotae, Raluca Darie, Radu Tincu, Oana Avram, , and et al.
A Trend towards Diaphragmatic Muscle Waste after Invasive Mechanical Ventilation in Multiple Trauma Patients—What to Expect?
Reprinted from: *J. Clin. Med.* **2023**, *12*, 3338, doi:10.3390/jcm12093338 . . . . **232**

Giorgia Montrucchio, Eleonora Balzani, Davide Lombardo, Alice Giaccone, Anna Vaninetti, Giulia D'Antonio, Francesca Rumbolo, and et al.
Proadrenomedullin in the Management of COVID-19 Critically Ill Patients in Intensive Care Unit: A Systematic Review and Meta-Analysis of Evidence and Uncertainties in Existing Literature
Reprinted from: *J. Clin. Med.* **2022**, *11*, 4543, doi:10.3390/jcm11154543 . . . . **241**

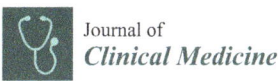

Editorial

Key Advances in Intensive Care and the Coronavirus Disease-19 Research and Practice Boost

Spyros D. Mentzelopoulos * and George Adamos

First Department of Intensive Care Medicine, National and Kapodistrian University of Athens Medical School, Evaggelismos General Hospital, 45-47 Ipsilandou Street, GR-10675 Athens, Greece; george.adamos1983@gmail.com
* Correspondence: sdmentzelopoulos@yahoo.com or sdmentzelopoulos@gmail.com

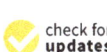

Citation: Mentzelopoulos, S.D.; Adamos, G. Key Advances in Intensive Care and the Coronavirus Disease-19 Research and Practice Boost. *J. Clin. Med.* **2022**, *11*, 3370. https://doi.org/10.3390/jcm11123370

Received: 1 June 2022
Accepted: 9 June 2022
Published: 12 June 2022

Publisher's Note: MDPI stays neutral with regard to jurisdictional claims in published maps and institutional affiliations.

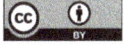

Copyright: © 2022 by the authors. Licensee MDPI, Basel, Switzerland. This article is an open access article distributed under the terms and conditions of the Creative Commons Attribution (CC BY) license (https://creativecommons.org/licenses/by/4.0/).

Components of intensive care include resuscitation, cardiorespiratory stabilization, reversal of organ/system dysfunction or failure, treatment of the underlying pathology, weaning from external support of vital organs, and supportive interventions (e.g., physiotherapy, psychological interventions) aimed at paving the way to an uneventful recovery and rehabilitation. Depending on patient values, goals and preferences, the holistic intensive treatment(s) may be limited or withdrawn and replaced/followed by end-of-life care interventions for the prevention or alleviation of any distressing symptoms (e.g., dyspnea, pain etc.) [1].

Current treatment recommendations for specific subgroups of critically ill patients are based on a systematic and rigorous evaluation of published evidence, including the results of randomized controlled trials (RCTs). When the Grading of Recommendations, Assessment, Development and Evaluation approach is adopted, evidence quality is rated as high, moderate, low, or very low and evidence profiles (summaries) are generated using the online Guideline Development Tool (https://gdt.guidelinedevelopment.org, accessed on 30 May 2022) [2–4].

Over the past decade, and especially over the past 3 years of the coronavirus disease 2019 (COVID-19) pandemic, several potentially beneficial interventions were tested in multicenter RCTs. Relevant published evidence has already been partly systematically reviewed and/or meta-analyzed. Pertinent, prominent examples include (1) noninvasive techniques of respiratory support (e.g., high-flow nasal canula, continuous positive airway pressure), prone positioning (for ≥ 16 consecutive hours per day with lung-protective ventilation) and veno-venous extracorporeal membrane oxygenation (ECMO) in acute respiratory distress syndrome (ARDS) of varying severity [5–10]; (2) use of RCT evidence-supported physiological targets such as ventilator driving pressure of <15 cm H_2O during low-tidal volume ventilation in ARDS [11]; (3) adjunctive hydrocortisone with or without fludrocortisone in septic shock, and dexamethasone in ARDS (of COVID-19 or non-COVID-19 etiology) [12–16]; (4) targeted temperature management (e.g., hypothermia or normothermia with target temperature of 33 or ≤ 37.5 °C, respectively) after cardiac arrest [17–19]; (5) vasopressin, stress-dose steroids, and epinephrine in in-hospital cardiac arrest [20–24]; (6) early inhibition of fibrinolysis by tranexamic acid in acute severe bleeding due to trauma and in postpartum hemorrhage [25–27]; (7) nucleotide inhibition of severe acute respiratory syndrome coronavirus 2 RNA-dependent RNA polymerase [28,29]; and (8) immunomodulating interventions such as interleukin (IL)-6 receptor blockade, Janus kinase inhibition, or IL-1 alpha and IL-1 beta antagonism guided by soluble urokinase plasminogen receptor plasma levels in COVID-19 [30–34].

Beneficial interventions are frequently based on robust physiological, mechanistic data. For example, prior studies have shown that prone position reduces transpulmonary pressure (i.e., lung parenchymal stress) and the tidal volume to end-expiratory lung volume ratio (i.e., lung strain or tidal parenchymal deformation) in severe ARDS [35,36]. In contrast to the supine or semirecumbent position, shape matching of the "cone-like" lung to the "cylinder-like" chest wall and gravitational forces act in opposite directions in the prone position [37]. This attenuates the derecruitment of the dependent ventral lung units, while dorsal and medial lung units are being recruited following the relief of the supine position-associated, external compression of small airways by the abdominal contents and heart, respectively [37,38]. Supine position's transpulmonary pressure gradient is reduced by pronation [37,38]. Whenever dorsal lung recruitment prevails over ventral lung derecruitment, pronation is associated with a lower lung stress distributed more homogenously over an increased number of aerated lung units [35,37,38]. Concurrently, dorsal lung perfusion is maintained, resulting in improved ventilation-perfusion matching, reduced shunt fraction, and improved oxygenation [35,37,38]. Carbon dioxide clearance may also improve following pronation, partly because of reduced overdistention of the dependent, ventral lung, and concurrent sparing from overdistention of the nondependent, dorsal lung [37]. Pronation may result in reduced dead space ventilation and lower $PaCO_2$ [35], and these physiological benefits may translate into improved survival to hospital discharge [39].

During the COVID-19 pandemic, intensive care practice was guided by the prompt issuance of guidelines including recommendations based on both direct and indirect (i.e., extrapolated from other viral pneumonias) evidence [4] and by an abundance of concurrently emerging RCT data [8,28–34]. Furthermore, two simplified models of COVID-19-related ARDS (CARDS) were proposed as opposite extremes of a pathophysiological spectrum that includes "intermediate stages" with overlapping characteristics. The least severe form of CARDS (termed "type L") comprises low lung elastance and weight, and is relatively unresponsive to positive end-expiratory pressure (PEEP). The most severe form (termed "type H") comprises extensive computerized tomographic consolidations, high lung elastance and weight, and is responsive to PEEP [40]. In this context, it was postulated that high lung stress secondary to vigorous, spontaneous inspiratory effort during "type L" CARDS may result in patient's self-inflicted lung injury, thereby expediting transition to "type H" CARDS [40,41]. Accordingly, timely endotracheal intubation of hypoxemic/hypercapnic COVID-19 patients with evidence of high breathing work (e.g., phasic contraction on palpation of the sternomastoid muscle) has been suggested [41,42].

The COVID-19 mass casualty crisis and dismal outcomes of severe CARDS have also prompted the introduction and/or preliminary evaluation of interventions such as awake prone positioning and pronation during ECMO, respectively. Recent physiological data suggest that awake pronation may reduce the respiratory rate and work of breathing in CARDS patients supported by continuous positive airway pressure [43]. However, in a recent RCT of 400 CARDS patients receiving noninvasive respiratory support, awake pronation did not significantly reduce intubation rates or in-hospital mortality, and this mandates further evaluation in larger RCTs [44]. Pronation might also disrupt a potentially vicious cycle of ongoing native lung damage during ECMO [45]. In a recent meta-analysis, pronation during ECMO improved oxygenation, reduced driving pressure, and was associated with a cumulative survival rate of 57%; however, it was also associated with prolonged ECMO runs and ICU length of stay [46].

The COVID-19-associated, compelling need for new and effective life-sustaining and curative interventions in the presence of periodic healthcare systems' saturation has also prompted the issuance of ethical guidelines including evidence-based recommendations about advance care planning, shared decision making, and rationing of resources [47,48]. Ethical, legal, and pandemic-related challenges pertaining to ECMO use in cardiac arrest have also been analyzed [49].

The current special issue on "Key Advances in the Treatment of the Critically Ill" primarily aims to highlight major aspects of the rapidly evolving knowledge of the mechanisms and pathophysiology of critical illness (including COVID-19), and the rapidly accumulating evidence on the efficacy of new life-sustaining and/or therapeutic interventions. Reports on the ethics of end-of-life decisions and practices are also encouraged.

Author Contributions: S.D.M. and G.A. have contributed to the drafting and critical revision of the manuscript. All authors have read and agreed to the published version of the manuscript.

Funding: This research received no external funding.

Conflicts of Interest: The authors declare no conflict of interest.

References

1. Downar, J.; Delaney, J.W.; Hawryluck, L.; Kenny, L. Guidelines for the withdrawal of life-sustaining measures. *Intensive Care Med.* **2016**, *42*, 1003–1017. [CrossRef] [PubMed]
2. Guyatt, G.H.; Oxman, A.D.; Vist, G.E.; Kunz, R.; Falck-Ytter, Y.; Alonso-Coello, P.; Schünemann, H.J.; GRADE Working, Group. GRADE: An emerging consensus on rating quality of evidence and strength of recommendations. *BMJ* **2008**, *336*, 924–926. [CrossRef] [PubMed]
3. Guyatt, G.H.; Oxman, A.D.; Santesso, N.; Helfand, M.; Vist, G.; Kunz, R.; Brozek, J.; Norris, S.; Meerpohl, J.; Djulbegovic, B.; et al. GRADE guidelines: 12. Preparing summary of findings tables-binary outcomes. *J. Clin. Epidemiol.* **2013**, *66*, 158–172. [CrossRef]
4. Alhazzani, W.; Møller, M.H.; Arabi, Y.M.; Loeb, M.; Gong, M.N.; Fan, E.; Oczkowski, S.; Levy, M.M.; Derde, L.; Dzierba, A.; et al. Surviving Sepsis Campaign: Guidelines on the management of critically ill adults with Coronavirus Disease 2019 (COVID-19). *Intensive Care Med.* **2020**, *46*, 854–887. [CrossRef] [PubMed]
5. Azoulay, E.; Lemiale, V.; Mokart, D.; Nseir, S.; Argaud, L.; Pène, F.; Kontar, L.; Bruneel, F.; Klouche, K.; Barbier, F.; et al. Effect of high-flow nasal oxygen vs standard oxygen on 28-day mortality in immunocompromised patients with acute respiratory failure: The High randomized clinical trial. *JAMA* **2018**, *320*, 2099–2107. [CrossRef]
6. Rochwerg, B.; Granton, D.; Wang, D.X.; Helviz, Y.; Einav, S.; Frat, J.P.; Mekontso-Dessap, A.; Schreiber, A.; Azoulay, E.; Mercat, A.; et al. High flow nasal cannula compared with conventional oxygen therapy for acute hypoxemic respiratory failure: A systematic review and meta-analysis. *Intensive Care Med.* **2019**, *45*, 563–572. [CrossRef]
7. Ferreyro, B.L.; Angriman, F.; Munshi, L.; Del Sorbo, L.; Ferguson, N.D.; Rochwerg, B.; Ryu, M.J.; Saskin, R.; Wunsch, H.; da Costa, B.R.; et al. Association of noninvasive oxygenation strategies with all-cause mortality in adults with acute hypoxemic respiratory failure: A systematic review and meta-analysis. *JAMA* **2020**, *324*, 57–67. [CrossRef]
8. Perkins, G.D.; Ji, C.; Connolly, B.A.; Couper, K.; Lall, R.; Baillie, J.K.; Bradley, J.M.; Dark, P.; Dave, C.; De Soyza, A.; et al. Effect of Noninvasive Respiratory Strategies on Intubation or Mortality Among Patients With Acute Hypoxemic Respiratory Failure and COVID-19: The RECOVERY-RS Randomized Clinical Trial. *JAMA* **2022**, *327*, 546–558. [CrossRef]
9. Guérin, C.; Reignier, J.; Richard, J.C.; Beuret, P.; Gacouin, A.; Boulain, T.; Mercier, E.; Badet, M.; Mercat, A.; Baudin, O.; et al. Prone positioning in severe acute respiratory distress syndrome. *N. Engl. J. Med.* **2013**, *368*, 2159–2168. [CrossRef]
10. Combes, A.; Hajage, D.; Capellier, G.; Demoule, A.; Lavoué, S.; Guervilly, C.; Da Silva, D.; Zafrani, L.; Tirot, P.; Veber, B.; et al. Extracorporeal membrane oxygenation for severe acute respiratory distress syndrome. *N. Engl. J. Med.* **2018**, *378*, 1965–1975. [CrossRef]
11. Amato, M.B.; Meade, M.O.; Slutsky, A.S.; Brochard, L.; Costa, E.L.; Schoenfeld, D.A.; Stewart, T.E.; Briel, M.; Talmor, D.; Mercat, A.; et al. Driving pressure and survival in the acute respiratory distress syndrome. *N. Engl. J. Med.* **2015**, *372*, 747–755. [CrossRef] [PubMed]
12. Annane, D.; Renault, A.; Brun-Buisson, C.; Megarbane, B.; Quenot, J.P.; Siami, S.; Cariou, A.; Forceville, X.; Schwebel, C.; Martin, C.; et al. Hydrocortisone plus Fludrocortisone for Adults with Septic Shock. *N. Engl. J. Med.* **2018**, *378*, 809–818. [CrossRef]
13. Venkatesh, B.; Finfer, S.; Cohen, J.; Rajbhandari, D.; Arabi, Y.; Bellomo, R.; Billot, L.; Correa, M.; Glass, P.; Harward, M.; et al. ADRENAL Trial Investigators and the Australian–New Zealand Intensive Care Society Clinical Trials Group. Adjunctive Glucocorticoid Therapy in Patients with Septic Shock. *N. Engl. J. Med.* **2018**, *378*, 797–808. [CrossRef] [PubMed]
14. Villar, J.; Ferrando, C.; Martínez, D.; Ambrós, A.; Muñoz, T.; Soler, J.A.; Aguilar, G.; Alba, F.; González-Higueras, E.; Conesa, L.A.; et al. Dexamethasone treatment for the acute respiratory distress syndrome: A multicentre, randomised controlled trial. *Lancet Respir. Med.* **2020**, *8*, 267–276. [CrossRef]
15. Tomazini, B.M.; Maia, I.S.; Cavalcanti, A.B.; Berwanger, O.; Rosa, R.G.; Veiga, V.C.; Avezum, A.; Lopes, R.D.; Bueno, F.R.; Silva, M.V.A.O.; et al. Effect of dexamethasone on days alive and ventilator-free in patients with moderate or severe acute respiratory distress syndrome and COVID-19: The CoDEX randomized clinical trial. *JAMA* **2020**, *324*, 1307–1316. [CrossRef]
16. RECOVERY Collaborative Group; Horby, P.; Lim, W.S.; Emberson, J.R.; Mafham, M.; Bell, J.L.; Linsell, L.; Staplin, N.; Brightling, C.; Ustianowski, A.; et al. Dexamethasone in hospitalized patients with COVID-19. *N. Engl. J. Med.* **2021**, *384*, 693–704.
17. Lascarrou, J.B.; Merdji, H.; Le Gouge, A.; Colin, G.; Grillet, G.; Girardie, P.; Coupez, E.; Dequin, P.F.; Cariou, A.; Boulain, T.; et al. Targeted temperature management for cardiac arrest with nonshockable rhythm. *N. Engl. J. Med.* **2019**, *381*, 2327–2337. [CrossRef]
18. Dankiewicz, J.; Cronberg, T.; Lilja, G.; Jakobsen, J.C.; Levin, H.; Ullén, S.; Rylander, C.; Wise, M.P.; Oddo, M.; Cariou, A.; et al. Hypothermia versus normothermia after out-of-hospital cardiac arrest. *N. Engl. J. Med.* **2021**, *384*, 2283–2294. [CrossRef]
19. Blanc, A.; Colin, G.; Cariou, A.; Merdji, H.; Grillet, G.; Girardie, P.; Coupez, E.; Dequin, P.F.; Boulain, T.; Frat, J.P.; et al. Targeted Temperature Management After In-Hospital Cardiac Arrest: An Ancillary Analysis of Targeted Temperature Management for Cardiac Arrest With Nonshockable Rhythm Trial Data. *Chest* **2022**, *in press*. [CrossRef]

20. Mentzelopoulos, S.D.; Zakynthinos, S.G.; Tzoufi, M.; Katsios, N.; Papastylianou, A.; Gkisioti, S.; Stathopoulos, A.; Kollintza, A.; Stamataki, E.; Roussos, C. Vasopressin, epinephrine, and corticosteroids for in-hospital cardiac arrest. *Arch. Intern. Med.* **2009**, *169*, 15–24. [CrossRef]
21. Mentzelopoulos, S.D.; Malachias, S.; Chamos, C.; Konstantopoulos, D.; Ntaidou, T.; Papastylianou, A.; Kolliantzaki, I.; Theodoridi, M.; Ischaki, H.; Makris, D.; et al. Vasopressin, steroids, and epinephrine and neurologically favorable survival after in-hospital cardiac arrest: A randomized clinical trial. *JAMA* **2013**, *310*, 270–279. [CrossRef] [PubMed]
22. Andersen, L.W.; Isbye, D.; Kjærgaard, J.; Kristensen, C.M.; Darling, S.; Zwisler, S.T.; Fisker, S.; Schmidt, J.C.; Kirkegaard, H.; Grejs, A.M.; et al. Effect of vasopressin and methylprednisolone vs placebo on return of spontaneous circulation in patients with in-hospital cardiac arrest: A randomized clinical trial. *JAMA* **2021**, *326*, 1586–1594. [CrossRef] [PubMed]
23. Holmberg, M.J.; Granfeldt, A.; Mentzelopoulos, S.D.; Andersen, L.W. Vasopressin and glucocorticoids for in-hospital cardiac arrest: A systematic review and meta-analysis of individual participant data. *Resuscitation* **2022**, *171*, 48–56. [CrossRef] [PubMed]
24. Granfeldt, A.; Sindberg, B.; Isbye, D.; Kjærgaard, J.; Kristensen, C.M.; Darling, S.; Zwisler, S.T.; Fisker, S.; Schmidt, J.C.; Kirkegaard, H.; et al. Effect of vasopressin and methylprednisolone vs. placebo on long-term outcomes in patients with in-hospital cardiac arrest a randomized clinical trial. *Resuscitation* **2022**, *175*, 67–71. [CrossRef]
25. CRASH-3 trial collaborators. Effects of tranexamic acid on death, disability, vascular occlusive events and other morbidities in patients with acute traumatic brain injury (CRASH-3): A randomised, placebo-controlled trial. *Lancet* **2019**, *394*, 1713–1723, Erratum in *Lancet* **2019**, *394*, 1712. [CrossRef]
26. WOMAN Trial Collaborators. Effect of early tranexamic acid administration on mortality, hysterectomy, and other morbidities in women with post-partum haemorrhage (WOMAN): An international, randomised, double-blind, placebo-controlled trial. *Lancet* **2017**, *389*, 2105–2116, Erratum in *Lancet* **2017**, *389*, 2104. [CrossRef]
27. Gayet-Ageron, A.; Prieto-Merino, D.; Ker, K.; Shakur, H.; Ageron, F.X.; Roberts, I.; Antifibrinolytic Trials Collaboration. Effect of treatment delay on the effectiveness and safety of antifibrinolytics in acute severe haemorrhage: A meta-analysis of individual patient-level data from 40,138 bleeding patients. *Lancet* **2018**, *391*, 125–132. [CrossRef]
28. Beigel, J.H.; Tomashek, K.M.; Dodd, L.E.; Mehta, A.K.; Zingman, B.S.; Kalil, A.C.; Hohmann, E.; Chu, H.Y.; Luetkemeyer, A.; Kline, S.; et al. Remdesivir for the Treatment of COVID-19—Final Report. *N. Engl. J. Med.* **2020**, *383*, 1813–1826. [CrossRef]
29. Goldman, J.D.; Lye, D.C.B.; Hui, D.S.; Marks, K.M.; Bruno, R.; Montejano, R.; Spinner, C.D.; Galli, M.; Ahn, M.Y.; Nahass, R.G.; et al. Remdesivir for 5 or 10 days in patients with severe COVID-19. *N. Engl. J. Med.* **2020**, *383*, 1827–1837. [CrossRef]
30. Stone, J.H.; Frigault, M.J.; Serling-Boyd, N.J.; Fernandes, A.D.; Harvey, L.; Foulkes, A.S.; Horick, N.K.; Healy, B.C.; Shah, R.; Bensaci, A.M.; et al. Efficacy of tocilizumab in patients hospitalized with COVID-19. *N. Engl. J. Med.* **2020**, *383*, 2333–2344. [CrossRef]
31. Kalil, A.C.; Patterson, T.F.; Mehta, A.K.; Tomashek, K.M.; Wolfe, C.R.; Ghazaryan, V.; Marconi, V.C.; Ruiz-Palacios, G.M.; Hsieh, L.; Kline, S.; et al. Baricitinib plus remdesivir for hospitalized adults with COVID-19. *N. Engl. J. Med.* **2021**, *384*, 795–807. [CrossRef]
32. Marconi, V.C.; Ramanan, A.V.; de Bono, S.; Kartman, C.E.; Krishnan, V.; Liao, R.; Piruzeli, M.L.B.; Goldman, J.D.; Alatorre-Alexander, J.; de Cassia Pellegrini, R.; et al. Efficacy and safety of baricitinib for the treatment of hospitalised adults with COVID-19 (COV-BARRIER): A randomised, double-blind, parallel-group, placebo-controlled phase 3 trial. *Lancet Respir. Med.* **2021**, *9*, 1407–1418, Erratum in *Lancet Respir. Med.* **2021**, *9*, e102. [CrossRef]
33. Wolfe, C.R.; Tomashek, K.M.; Patterson, T.F.; Gomez, C.A.; Marconi, V.C.; Jain, M.K.; Yang, O.O.; Paules, C.I.; Palacios, G.M.R.; Grossberg, R.; et al. Baricitinib versus dexamethasone for adults hospitalised with COVID-19 (ACTT-4): A randomised, double-blind, double placebo-controlled trial. *Lancet Respir. Med.* **2022**, in press. [CrossRef]
34. Kyriazopoulou, E.; Poulakou, G.; Milionis, H.; Metallidis, S.; Adamis, G.; Tsiakos, K.; Fragkou, A.; Rapti, A.; Damoulari, C.; Fantoni, M.; et al. Early treatment of COVID-19 with anakinra guided by soluble urokinase plasminogen receptor plasma levels: A double-blind, randomized controlled phase 3 trial. *Nat. Med.* **2021**, *27*, 1752–1760. [CrossRef] [PubMed]
35. Mentzelopoulos, S.D.; Roussos, C.; Zakynthinos, S.G. Prone position reduces lung stress and strain in severe acute respiratory distress syndrome. *Eur. Respir. J.* **2005**, *25*, 534–544. [CrossRef] [PubMed]
36. ARDS Definition Task Force; Ranieri, V.M.; Rubenfeld, G.D.; Thompson, B.T.; Ferguson, N.D.; Caldwell, E.; Fan, E.; Camporota, L.; Slutsky, A.S. Acute respiratory distress syndrome: The Berlin Definition. *JAMA* **2012**, *307*, 2526–2533.
37. Gattinoni, L.; Taccone, P.; Carlesso, E.; Marini, J.J. Prone position in acute respiratory distress syndrome. Rationale, indications, and limits. *Am. J. Respir. Crit. Care Med.* **2013**, *188*, 1286–1293. [CrossRef] [PubMed]
38. Chen, L.; Zhang, Y.; Li, Y.; Song, C.; Lin, F.; Pan, P. The Application of Awake-Prone Positioning Among Non-intubated Patients With COVID-19-Related ARDS: A Narrative Review. *Front. Med.* **2022**, *9*, 817689. [CrossRef]
39. Gattinoni, L.; Vagginelli, F.; Carlesso, E.; Taccone, P.; Conte, V.; Chiumello, D.; Valenza, F.; Caironi, P.; Pesenti, A.; Prone-Supine Study Group. Decrease in PaCO$_2$ with prone position is predictive of improved outcome in acute respiratory distress syndrome. *Crit. Care Med.* **2003**, *31*, 2727–2733. [CrossRef]
40. Marini, J.J.; Gattinoni, L. Management of COVID-19 respiratory distress. *JAMA* **2020**, *323*, 2329–2330. [CrossRef]
41. Fan, E.; Beitler, J.R.; Brochard, L.; Calfee, C.S.; Ferguson, N.D.; Slutsky, A.S.; Brodie, D. COVID-19-associated acute respiratory distress syndrome: Is a different approach to management warranted? *Lancet Respir. Med.* **2020**, *8*, 816–821. [CrossRef]
42. Tobin, M.J. Basing respiratory management of COVID-19 on physiological principles. *Am. J. Respir. Crit. Care Med.* **2020**, *201*, 1319–1320. [CrossRef]

43. Chiumello, D.; Chiodaroli, E.; Coppola, S.; Cappio Borlino, S.; Granata, C.; Pitimada, M.; Wendel Garcia, P.D. Awake prone position reduces work of breathing in patients with COVID-19 ARDS supported by CPAP. *Ann. Intensive Care.* **2021**, *11*, 179. [CrossRef] [PubMed]
44. Alhazzani, W.; Parhar, K.K.S.; Weatherald, J.; Al Duhailib, Z.; Alshahrani, M.; Al-Fares, A.; Buabbas, S.; Cherian, S.V.; Munshi, L.; Fan, E.; et al. Effect of Awake Prone Positioning on Endotracheal Intubation in Patients With COVID-19 and Acute Respiratory Failure: A Randomized Clinical Trial. *JAMA* **2022**, *327*, 2104–2113, Epub ahead of print. [CrossRef]
45. Shekar, K.; Ramanathan, K.; Brodie, D. Prone positioning of patients during venovenous extracorporeal membrane oxygenation. *Ann. Am. Thorac. Soc.* **2021**, *18*, 421–423. [CrossRef] [PubMed]
46. Poon, W.H.; Ramanathan, K.; Ling, R.R.; Yang, I.X.; Tan, C.S.; Schmidt, M.; Shekar, K. Prone positioning during venovenous extracorporeal membrane oxygenation for acute respiratory distress syndrome: A systematic review and meta-analysis. *Crit. Care* **2021**, *25*, 292. [CrossRef]
47. Van de Voorde, P.; Bossaert, L.; Mentzelopoulos, S.; Blom, M.T.; Couper, K.; Djakow, J.; Druwé, P.; Lilja, G.; Lulic, I.; Raffay, V.; et al. Ethik der Reanimation und Entscheidungen am Lebensende: COVID-19-Leitlinien des European Resuscitation Council [Ethics of resuscitation and end-of-life decisions]. *Notf. Rett. Med.* **2020**, *23*, 263–267.
48. Mentzelopoulos, S.D.; Couper, K.; Voorde, P.V.; Druwé, P.; Blom, M.; Perkins, G.D.; Lulic, I.; Djakow, J.; Raffay, V.; Lilja, G.; et al. European Resuscitation Council Guidelines 2021: Ethics of resuscitation and end of life decisions. *Resuscitation* **2021**, *161*, 408–432. [CrossRef]
49. Mentzelopoulos, S.D.; Vrettou, C.S.; Sprung, C.L. Extracorporeal cardiopulmonary resuscitation: The need for high-quality research and the associated legal, ethical and pandemic-related challenges. *Resuscitation* **2021**, *169*, 143–145. [CrossRef]

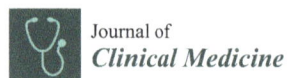

Article

Norwegian Version of the Chelsea Critical Care Physical Assessment Tool (CPAx-NOR): Translation, Face Validity, Cross-Cultural Adaptation and Inter-Rater Reliability

Charlotte Marie Schanke [1,*], Anne Kristine Brekka [2,3], Stein Arne Rimehaug [1], Mari Klokkerud [1,4] and Tiina Maarit Andersen [3,5]

1. Regional Rehabilitation Knowledge Center in South East Norway, 1453 Nesodden, Norway; stein.arne.rimehaug@sunnaas.no (S.A.R.); mariklok@oslomet.no (M.K.)
2. Department of Physiotherapy, Sorlandet Hospital, 4838 Arendal, Norway; anne.kristine.brekka@sshf.no
3. Department of Thoracic Medicine, Haukeland University Hospital, 5021 Bergen, Norway; tiina.maarit.andersen@helse-bergen.no
4. Department of Rehabilitation Science and Health Technology, Oslo Metropolitan University, 0130 Oslo, Norway
5. Faculty of Health and Social Sciences, Bergen University College, 5063 Bergen, Norway
* Correspondence: charlotte.marie.schanke@sunnaas.no

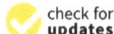

Citation: Schanke, C.M.; Brekka, A.K.; Rimehaug, S.A.; Klokkerud, M.; Andersen, T.M. Norwegian Version of the Chelsea Critical Care Physical Assessment Tool (CPAx-NOR): Translation, Face Validity, Cross-Cultural Adaptation and Inter-Rater Reliability. *J. Clin. Med.* 2023, *12*, 5033. https://doi.org/10.3390/jcm12155033

Academic Editor: Spyros D. Mentzelopoulos

Received: 17 June 2023
Revised: 19 July 2023
Accepted: 24 July 2023
Published: 31 July 2023

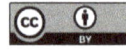

Copyright: © 2023 by the authors. Licensee MDPI, Basel, Switzerland. This article is an open access article distributed under the terms and conditions of the Creative Commons Attribution (CC BY) license (https://creativecommons.org/licenses/by/4.0/).

Abstract: Background: Assessment of physical and respiratory function in the intensive care unit (ICU) is useful for developing an individualized treatment plan and evaluating patient progress. There is a need for measurement tools that are culturally adapted, reliable and easy to use. The Chelsea Critical Care Physical Assessment Tool (CPAx) is a valid measurement tool with strong psychometric properties for the intensive care population. This study aims to translate, adapt and test face validity and inter-rater reliability of the Norwegian version of CPAx (CPAx-NOR) for use in critically ill adult patients receiving prolonged mechanical ventilation. Method: CPAx-NOR was forward backward translated, culturally adapted and tested by experts and patients for face validity. Thereafter tested by 10 physiotherapists in five hospitals for inter-rater reliability. Results: The experts and pilot testers reached consensus on the translation and face validity. Patients were tested at time point A (n = 57) and at time point B (n = 53). The reliability of CPAx-NOR at "A" was 0.990 (0.983–0.994) and at "B" 0.994 (0.990–0.997). Based on A+B combined and adjusted, the ICC was 0.990 (95% CI 0.996–0.998). Standard error of measurement (SEM) was 0.68 and the minimal detectable change (MDC) was 1.89. The Bland–Altman plot showed low bias and no sign of heteroscedasticity. CPAx-NOR changed with a mean score of 14.9, and showed a moderate floor effect at the start of physiotherapy and low ceiling effects at discharge. Conclusion: CPAx-NOR demonstrated good face validity and excellent inter-rater reliability. It can be used as an assessment tool for physical function in critically ill adults receiving prolonged mechanical ventilation in Norway.

Keywords: physiotherapy; physical function; early rehabilitation; measurement tool; critical illness; CPAx; critical care

1. Introduction

Intensive care unit–acquired weakness (ICU-AW) is common, and if patients survive, it negatively affects quality of life [1] and leads to continuing physical, cognitive and mental impairments [2–5]. Early rehabilitation starting in the ICU seems to both prevent ICU-AW and improve rehabilitation outcomes [6]. Assessment of several aspects of physical function is essential when developing a treatment plan and evaluating patient progress, as well as to ensure continuity of care from the ICU to the hospital ward [7–9]. Physiotherapists' main responsibility in the multidisciplinary ICU team is to assess and improve the patients respiratory- and general physical function [7–9]. Many measurement tools with adequate psychometric properties have been developed for use with ICU patients [10]; however, most of these lack important relevant aspects with regards to respiratory and cough function.

The Chelsea Critical Care Physical Assessment Tool (CPAx) is an observation-based measurement tool developed by Dr. Evelyn Corner. The tool is unique as it incorporates assessment of respiratory function and cough, and both functional and specific muscle testing [10–12]. CPAx is valid for the intensive care population and has been translated and tested in different languages, including Danish, Swedish, German and Chinese. It has demonstrated strong psychometric properties and excellent inter-rater reliability in all translations [13–16]. Considering these aspects CPAx-NOR is minding an important gap in early rehabilitation in critically ill patients in Norway.

To make the measurement tool available and ready for implementation in Norway, it is necessary to agree on a translated and adapted Norwegian version and to test its reliability and ability to detect changes in physical function. It is important to investigate systematic and random errors and establish the minimal detectable change to make the Norwegian version a reliable outcome measure in a Norwegian ICU population.

The aims of this study were to translate, cross-culturally adapt and test face validity of the Chelsea Critical Care Physical Assessment Tool into Norwegian (CPAx-NOR) and to test its inter-rater reliability in critically ill adult patients receiving prolonged mechanical ventilation.

2. Materials and Methods

The study had two stages:

Stage I (August 2021–January 2022): Translation, discussions on face validity and cross-cultural adaption of CPAx to Norwegian, and

Stage II (February 2022–September 2022): Evaluation of CPAx-NOR's inter-rater reliability

The reporting of this study has been structured according to the STROBE recommendations for observational studies [17].

2.1. Chelsea Critical Care Physical Assessment—CPAx

CPAx consists of ten different items graded from 0 (unable/dependent) to 5 (independent) on a Guttman scale. The ten items are summarized in an aggregated total score, which indicates the total need for help with a minimum score of 0 (completely dependent) and a maximum score of 50 (independent). The patient is observed and assessed bedside, and the only equipment needed is a handheld dynamometer for measuring grip strength. The use of CPAx is considered feasible in clinical practice, and its visual display makes it easy to understand for both healthcare professionals and patients [11].

2.1.1. Stage I. Translation and Cross-Cultural Adaption

Based on international recommendations [18–20], a step-by-step forward-backward translation including cross-cultural adaptation with a multidisciplinary expert committee was conducted. The CPAx-NOR was completed in agreement with the original developer, Dr. Evelyn Corner. The process is illustrated in Figure 1 (Step 1 to 3).

As rehabilitation is a multidisciplinary process in the ICU, it was important to ensure that CPAx-NOR was easy to understand both for multidisciplinary teams and for patients. The expert committee members, eight persons, were therefore carefully chosen from hospitals in the South-East health region to involve a broad professional environment. The committee consisted of one senior ICU nurse PhD, one anesthesiologist, one former intensive care patient and five physiotherapists. Three of the physiotherapists had long experience in ICU (>10 years), MSc and specialization in ICU physiotherapy (including two of the authors, CMS and AKB). The other physiotherapists had little ICU experience, whereas one was newly educated. The physiotherapists in the expert committee did not participate in the data collection to test reliability.

The preliminary CPAx-NOR (T12) was then tested in a pilot conducted by another three physiotherapists employed at three of the included hospitals. The physiotherapists:

one male and two female with experience ranging from 2–15 years, were not involved in the translation process. They tested one patient each. During a roundtable discussion with the three physiotherapists and CMS and AKB, the final version of CPAx-NOR was agreed upon with one minor change (Figure 1, Step 4).

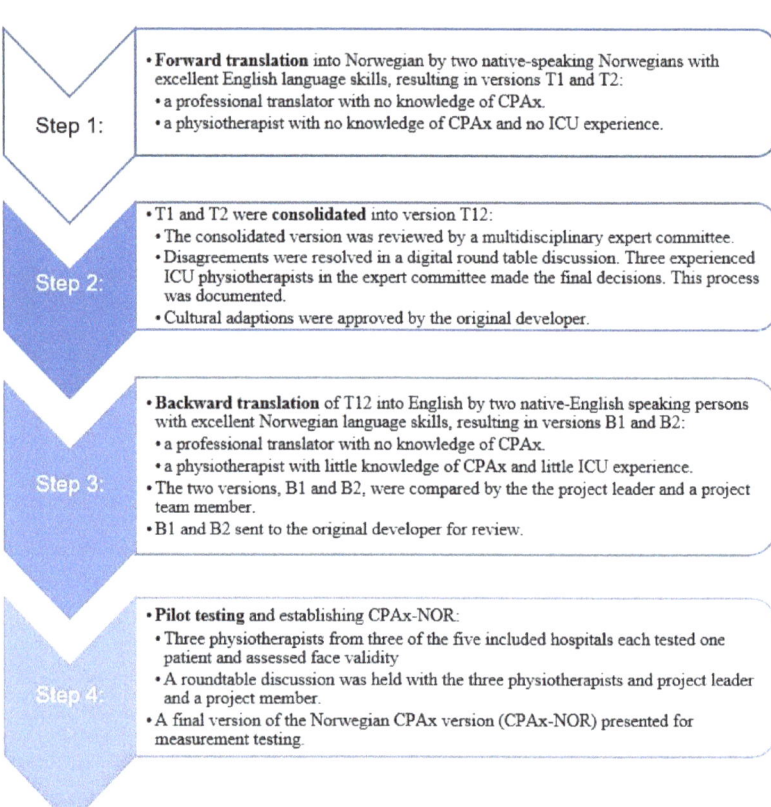

Figure 1. Stage I. The translation process.

2.1.2. Face Validity

Assessment of face validity as described by COSMIN [21] was conducted by considering the relevance, purpose and whether the items reflected the construct to be measured in discussions between physiotherapists, anesthesiologist, nurse and former ICU patient (Figure 1, step 2) and physiotherapists, patients, and the project leader and a project member (Figure 1, Step 4).

2.2. Stage II. Evaluation of CPAx-NOR Inter-Rater Reliability

Design and Setting

A multicentre study with a prospective cross-sectional design was conducted in five hospitals in Norway's South-East health region including both large university hospitals and smaller local hospitals. All the units were general ICUs and included 33 ICU beds at the time of the inclusion period. The study was presented to the Regional Ethics Committee, which concluded that it did not require approval. The Data Inspectorate at all the local hospitals and SIKT (Norwegian Agency for Shared Services in Education and Research, formerly the Norwegian Centre for Research Data), approved the study, project number

777606. The study was conducted according to the Helsinki Declaration, and all participants (physiotherapists and patients) gave informed, written consent before inclusion in the study.

2.3. Participants and Patients

The aim of this part of the study was to investigate inter-rater reliability and therefore the participants of interest were the physiotherapists using CPAx-NOR, and how they used CPAx-NOR to rate patients in clinical practice in the ICU. Ten physiotherapists (one man and nine women), age 28 to 64 years, participated as testers for CPAx-NOR. Six of them were specialists in ICU physiotherapy. They all had more than four years clinical experience from a hospital, and their clinical experience at the ICU ranged from one to more than 30 years. None of the physiotherapists had used CPAx routinely prior to the study.

The median length of stay in Norwegian ICUs is 2.1 days and median time on mechanical ventilation is 1.5 days [22]. Therefor the physiotherapists included and tested patients according to the following criteria: The patients had to be referred to physiotherapy at the ICU. Adults (age > 18 years) who were mechanically ventilated ≥ 48 h during their stay in the ICU were considered at risk of ICU-AW and included. No exclusion criteria were set.

2.4. Data Collection, Procedures and Measurement

The only demographic data collected were age, sex, diagnosis and CPAx-NOR score.

All the participating physiotherapists completed the same education to use CPAx-NOR in clinical practice. The original English eLearning platform used in previous studies was not available, therefore a six-hour digital course in Norwegian was developed and discussed in agreement with the original CPAx developer, Evelyn Corner. It consisted of three parts, (1) a theory part on the use of standardized measurement tools in general, (2) a comprehensive review of the CPAx, (3) an instructional video of a physiotherapy treatment session with a simulated patient to be scored and discussed in a plenary setting. At each hospital, two physiotherapists completed all the assessments at the same time in pairs with separate roles; one conducted the assessment while the other observed. They both scored separately and blinded. The testers decided the roles without further instructions from the project leader. To facilitate patient inclusion and to help with practical problem-solving during testing of CPAx-NOR, monthly digital meetings were arranged for all the participating physiotherapists in combination with an open invitation to correspond via e-mail, and one in-person meeting at each participating hospital.

2.5. Inter-Rater Reliability

Inter-rater reliability was assessed at start of physiotherapy and at discharge from ICU, according to COSMIN criteria [23], and a sample size of at least 50 patient scoring was considered sufficient for inter-rater reliability testing [24]. It is important to establish reliability before measurement instruments can be used in clinical practice as reliability refers to the extent the measurement can be replicated [25]. We hypothesized that CPAx-NOR would show good inter-rater reliability of aggregated scores and individual items with an ICC > 0.80 and weighted kappa values >0.81.

2.6. Change in Scores during Patient Trajectory

Change in scores, understood as CPAx-NOR's ability to detect change in a patient trajectory in the ICU unit over time, was described by effect size (ES) and standard response mean (SRM) [26,27].

2.7. Statistical Analysis

Descriptive and non-parametric statistics were used to describe the demographic characteristics and distribution of scores, expressed as the mean, standard deviation (SD), median, interquartile range (IQR), frequency and percentage of the data. To analyze the inter-rater reliability, we used the intraclass correlation coefficient (ICC) with 95% confidence intervals for aggregated scores. Because this was a multicenter study, and not every patient was rated by each rater, we used a one-way random effects model (single measurement) as described in Koo and Li [25] and Shrout and Fleiss [28] at each of the two time points (A and B) and for both visits. Since CPAx is an ordinal scale and absolute disagreements between raters are investigated, it is important to give different weights to the size of disagreements using quadratic weighted Cohen's kappa for individual items [24,29]. The standard error of measurement (SEM = SD × (sqr 1 − ICC) and minimal detectable change (MDC) (=SEM × 1.96 × $\sqrt{2}$) with limits of agreement (LOA) were calculated as parameters of measurement error for aggregated scores at both measurement points. SEM was considered acceptable if equal to the original, ≤ 3 [30]. Limits of agreement (LOA) were defined as $d \pm 1.96 \times SD\text{diff}$ where d = mean difference between raters and $SD\text{diff}$ = the standard deviation of the differences. A Bland–Altman plot was used to visualize the scores and to look for outliers, systematic bias and heteroscedasticity [31] on each time point and total scores were corrected for repeated measures using the 'true value varies' method [32]. The measurement error for individual items was calculated and displayed as percentage agreement. To calculate effect size (ES) we used the mean of aggregated discharge score minus the mean of aggregated initiation of physiotherapy score divided by the SD of mean initiation score. To calculate the standardized response mean (SRM) we used the mean of aggregated discharge score minus the mean of aggregated initiation of physiotherapy score divided by the SD of mean difference [26]. Floor and ceiling effects are reported as the percentage of patients scoring zero or fifty at the two measurement points and are considered acceptable if <15% [24]. Data were stored and processed in IBM SPSS version 28.0.1 for Windows or Microsoft Excel.

3. Results

3.1. Translation, Cross-Cultural Adaption and Face Validity

The CPAx-NOR was translated in a step-by-step protocol shown in Figure 1. The expert committee discussed several minor cultural and linguistic differences, and the original developer approved all the adjustments. There was a need to clarify the item 'cough'. Deep suction was defined as suction below the cannula. Further, the term 'Yankauer suction' is not used in Norway and was described instead as 'suction in the mouth and upper throat'. Another important clarification was the rating of patients' physical function based on actual performance with the need for 'minimal, moderate or maximal' assistance. After the adjustments, all the participants in the expert committee agreed on the preliminary CPAx-NOR version to be tested in clinical practice. The pilot testing demonstrated that the preliminary CPAx-NOR was feasible for use and valid with one minor adjustment. The Norwegian CPAx was established. Both the expert committee and the physiotherapists and patients in the pilot testing, agreed that the items in CPAx-NOR was relevant and reflected the constructs to be measured in an adult patient population in ICU, thereby demonstrating good face validity. The final version of CPAx-NOR is located in Supplementary Materials.

3.2. Patient Population at Start of Physiotherapy (A) and at Discharge from the ICU (B)

After the CPAx-NOR was established and the education completed, the five hospitals started including patients from their ICUs, see Figure 2. From February 1 until the end of September 2022, 57 patients (23 women), mean age 64 years, were included at time point A—start of physiotherapy. At point B—discharge from ICU—53 patients (20 women), mean age 64 years, were included. See Table 1 for further details. The patients were divided into five diagnostic groups representative of the intensive care population in Norway [22]. No informed consent was withdrawn in this study.

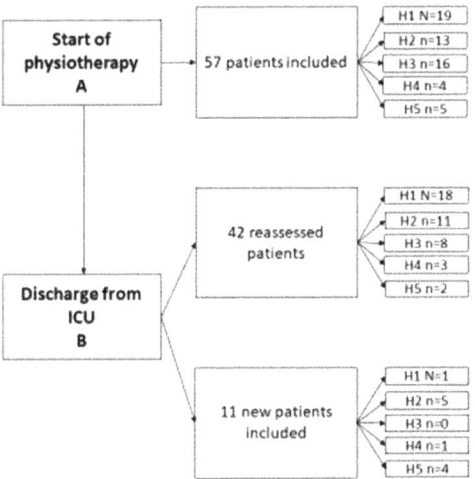

Figure 2. Flow chart showing patient inclusion in the 5 different hospitals (H1-H5) during the study.

Table 1. Characteristics of the included patients at time point A—start of physiotherapy, and at time point B—at discharge from the ICU.

Characteristics of the Patient Population Scored with CPAx-NOR	Start of Physiotherapy n = 57 A	Discharge from ICU n = 53 B
Sex, n (%)	Men 34 (n = 60%) Women 23 (n = 40%)	Men 33 (n = 62%) Women 20 (n = 38%)
Age, yrs Mean (range)	64 (24–84)	64 (24–84)
Type of diagnosis, % (n = men/women):		
Cardiovascular	21.1 (8/4)	20.8 (8/3)
Respiratory	28.1 (11/5)	26.4 (10/4)
Infection	21.1 (7/5)	18.9 (5/5)
Postoperative complications	15.8 (3/6)	17.0 (4/5)
Other *	14.0 (5/3)	17.0 (6/3)

* includes neurological, multitrauma, intox etc.

3.3. Inter-Rater Reliability and Limits of Agreement

The ICC was 0.990 (0.983–0.994) at time point A and 0.994 (0.990–0.997) at time point B. The ICC for both time points combined (A+B) was 0.998, SEM 0.68 and the MDC was 1.89. See Table 2.

Table 2. Inter-rater reliability results of aggregated scores of CPAx-NOR at start of physiotherapy (A), discharge from ICU (B) and A+B.

CPAx-NOR Score	Lead Rater Mean (SD) Min-Max	Observer Rater Mean (SD) Min-Max	ICC (95%CI)	SEM	MDC
Time point A n = 57	9.60 (10.84) 0–50	9.72 (11.00) 0–50	0.990 (0.983–0.994)	0.77	2.12
Time point B n = 53	28.45 (13.24) 1–50	28.06 (13.15) 2–50	0.994 (0.990–0.997)	0.72	2.0
Time point A + B n = 110			0.998 (0.996–0.998)	0.68	1.89

SD: standard deviation; ICC: intraclass correlation coefficient; 95%CI: confidence interval; SEM: standard error of measurement (SEM = SD × (sqr 1 − ICC)); MDC; minimal detectable change (=SEM × 1.96 × √2).

The Bland–Altman plot for the total scores combined shows the mean difference between raters was −0.13 (SD 1.50) and 95% limits of agreement were from −2.82 to 3.07. The limits of agreement are shown in Figure 3.

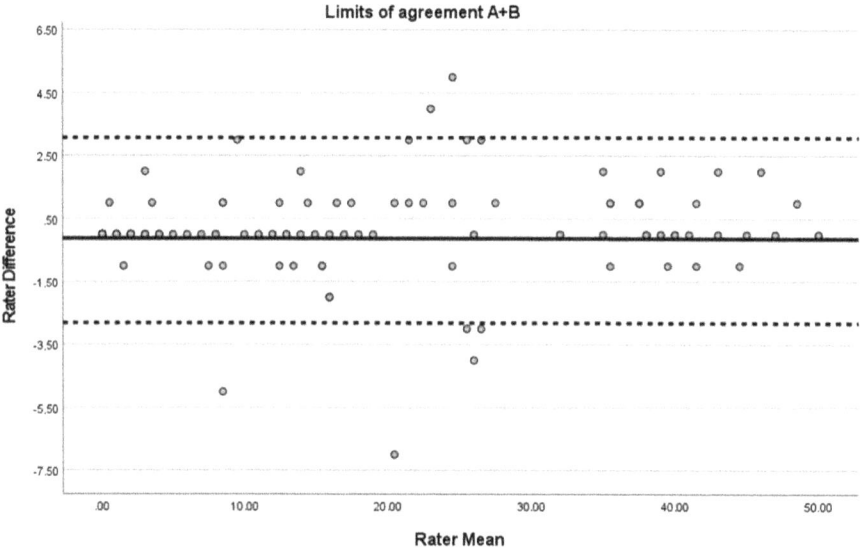

Figure 3. Modified Bland–Altman plot of data adjusted for repeated measurements. Limits of agreement were defined as $d \pm 1.96 \times SD\text{diff}$ where d = mean difference between raters and $SD\text{diff}$ = the standard deviation of the differences. The mean CPAx-NOR score is indicated with a solid line and the upper and lower limits are indicated with dotted lines.

At time point A, the mean difference between raters was −0.12 (SD 1.58) and 95% limits of agreement was −3.22 to 2.98. At time point B, the mean difference between raters was 0.40 (SD 1.38) and 95% limits of agreement was −2.31 to 3.09. The limits of agreement are shown in Figure 4.

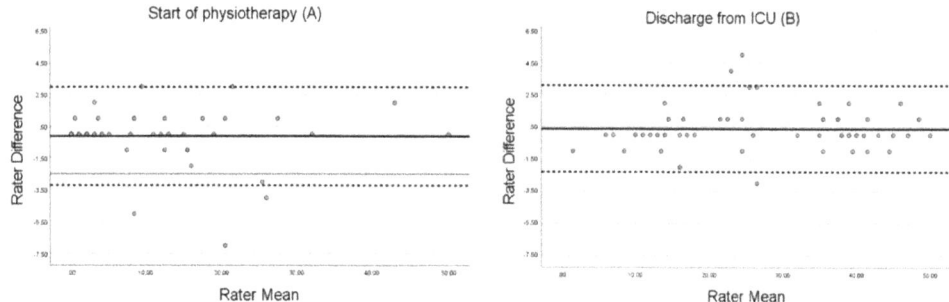

Figure 4. Bland–Altman plot of data from 57 assessments of critically ill patients at time point A and 53 assessments at time point B. The mean is indicated with a solid line and the upper and lower limits are indicated with dotted lines.

The ten individual items showed weighted kappa values between 0.957 and 0.996 at time point A and between 0.925 and 0.980 at time point B. The percentage agreement for individual items, as a parameter for measurement error, ranged from 77.2% to 98.2% at time point A and 73.6% to 98.1% at time point B. Results are presented in Table 3.

Table 3. Inter-rater reliability of individual items of CPAx-NOR in ICU patients at time point A and time point B.

CPAx-NOR Items	Start of Physiotherapy (A) n = 57				Discharge from the ICU (B) n = 53			
	Lead Rater Median (IQR 25–75%)	Observer Rater Median (IQR 25–75%)	Weighted Kappa Values	Absolute Agreement (%)	Lead Rater Median (IQR 25–75%)	Observer Rater Median (IQR 25–75%)	Weighted Kappa Values	Absolute Agreement (%)
Respiratory function	2 (1–4)	2 (1–4)	0.987	93.0	5 (4–5)	5 (4–5)	0.980	98.1
Cough	2 (1–4)	2 (1 4)	0.940	77.2	5 (4–5)	5 (4–5)	0.931	79.2
Moving within the bed	0 (0 1)	0 (0 1)	0.905	86.0	3 (2–4)	3 (1–4)	0.925	73.6
Supine to sitting on the edge of the bed	0 (0–1)	0 (0–1)	0.972	93.0	2 (1–4)	2 (1 4)	0.965	83.0
Dynamic sitting	0 (0–2)	0 (0–2)	0.957	87.7	4 (3–5)	4 (3–5)	0.961	79.2
Standing balance	0 (0–0)	0 (0–0)	0.959	94.7	3 (0–4)	3 (0 4)	0.990	94.3
Sit to stand	0 (0–0)	0 (0–0)	0.967	93.0	2 (0–3)	2 (0–3)	0.980	88.7
Transferring from bed to chair	0 (0–0)	0 (0–0)	0.975	98.2	2 (0–4)	2 (0–4)	0.992	96.2
Stepping	0 (0–0)	0 (0–0)	0.969	96.5	2 (0–4)	2 (0–4)	0.970	88.7
Grip strength	0 (0–2)	0 (0–2)	0.996	98.2	2 (1–3)	2 (1–3)	0.992	96.2

IQR: interquartile range.

3.4. Change in Scores of CPAx-NOR

The mean difference in CPAx-NOR score between time points A and B (n = 42) was 14.9 (95% CI 11.0; 18.7). ES was 1.3 and SRM was calculated as 1.2.

3.5. Floor and Ceiling Effects

Nine patients scored 0 (16%) and one patient scored 50 (1.8%) at the start of physiotherapy (median 5, IQR 2–15.5; range 0–50). At ICU discharge, none of the patients scored 0. One patient scored 50 points (2%) (median 28, IQR 15.5–39.5; range 1–50). These results indicate that problems related to floor effects may be moderate while problems related to ceiling effects are minimal.

4. Discussion

The objective of this study was to translate, adapt, test face validity and the inter-rater reliability of CPAx-NOR in critically ill adult patients undergoing prolonged mechanical ventilation in the ICU. CPAx-NOR was successfully translated in a forward-backward translation, cross-culturally adapted and pilot tested in clinical practice. Face validity was assessed through expert group and patient discussions, and demonstrated good results. CPAx-NOR demonstrated excellent inter-rater reliability for both aggregated score and all ten individual items across the ICU stay. The measurement error was small with a minimal detectable change of two points. CPAx-NOR exhibited a moderate floor effect at start of physiotherapy and low floor and ceiling effects at ICU discharge, as expected. These results indicate that CPAx-NOR is a valid and reliable measurement tool for physical function during the continuum of an ICU stay for adult patients on mechanical ventilation for more than 48 h. Whether the results are generalizable to other ICU patients with shorter time on mechanical ventilation has not been investigated.

4.1. Reliability

The MDC is of great importance when evaluating change in physical function. Previous studies investigating CPAx [13,14,30], have reported the SEM and MDC at only one time point. However, in the German version MDC has been reported on several time points [15]. The present study measured SEM and MDC at the two time points and showed that if two different raters assess the patient early in the ICU stay (at the start of physiotherapy), a change of >3 points indicate a detectable/true change in physical function above the measurement error. Later in the patient trajectory, at measurement point B, when a higher level of functioning is present, a change of >2 points indicated a detectable change in physical function. This is an important consideration when evaluating the patients' rehabilitation process throughout the patient trajectory when not only one, but several physiotherapists perform assessments. These results are similar to the Danish version [13]. When the scores of the time points were combined (A+B), we also found that a change of 2 points indicated a detectable change in physical function, similar to the German version [15]. Different MDC across the measurement tool's scale has also been established in other measurement tools such as the Bergs Balance Scale [33]. The differences in the MDC reported in CPAx studies [13–15,30] may be related to the defined time point for the assessment and the selected method of reporting this psychometric. This needs to be standardized when designing future international studies.

Different MDC's corresponds to the finding that the agreement was somewhat lower for the items 'cough' (77.2% and 79.2%), 'moving within the bed' (86.0% and 73.6%) and 'dynamic sitting' (87.7% and 79.2%). Despite the clarification of the item 'cough' during the translation, disagreements among the raters were still present at both time points. Suctioning is a part of the item 'cough', and in Norway, this task is assigned to nurses, which might have complicated the evaluation. The minimal, moderate and maximal assistance ratings were the subject of several discussions between clinicians during the testing period and may be the reason for the lower agreement on these items, similar to findings from previous publications using CPAx [12–14]. This underpins the need to develop local standardized recommendations prior to the implementation of CPAx-NOR in clinical practice.

Our SEM and MDC at time point A are similar to the original version [27], and the agreement between tester and observer was high in general, both on each time point and in total, as shown in the Bland–Altman plot (Figures 2 and 3). These Bland-Altman Plots showed no bias due to the role of the rater during assessments (tester or observer) and no heteroscedasticity. These results correspond to those of other studies that have used this method to illustrate agreement [12–15].

CPAx-NOR is a clinically useful tool for assessing low-functioning patients receiving prolonged mechanical ventilation in the study population representative of the Norwegian ICU population expressed as the SEM, MDC and LOA throughout the ICU trajectory. The results of previous studies assessing inter-rater reliability, together with the current study, support the claim that CPAx is in general a reliable tool to assess function in the ICU population.

4.2. Change in Scores

Our results showed a mean change of 15 points in scores between the start of physiotherapy and discharge from the ICU. This indicates that the patients' physical function improved during the trajectory, a finding supported by the large ES and SRM. These findings are similar to those in studies of responsiveness of the original and the Danish version [13,30]. Generally, patients had a first visit from a physiotherapist within 72 h, but as as we did not collecta data on this, we can not report median time. Corner [30] established a Minimal Clinical Important Difference (MCID) to be six points, but as this was in a burn population, we cannot directly compare the populations although the change in scores exceeded six points. A specific investigation of both the MCID and the responsiveness of CPAx-NOR including data on length of stay in the ICU needs to be conducted to come to any conclusion on this matter.

4.3. Floor and Ceiling Effects

As with the original version of CPAx [30], the floor effect (patients with a total score of 0) was moderate at the start of physiotherapy (16%); all patients with aggregated score

0 died during the study period and the authors suggested the total score of 0 can predict death [30]. In this study, 55.5% of the patients with total score 0, survived the ICU stay and were discharged to a regular ward. We do not have discharge scores for the remaining 44.5% and are not able to make conclusions regarding survival or death for these patients. Thus, the present study does not indicate that a total score of 0 at the start of physiotherapy in Norway predicts death. However, the patients with a total CPAx-NOR score of 0 at the time point A did score less than 12 points at time point B. This aggregated score is below the mean total score in the present study, indicating poorer physical function requiring a higher level of care. This may be useful in predicting what level of care and what degree of rehabilitation intensive care patients need after discharge from hospitals in Norway but needs to be investigated further. Both patients and the healthcare system have a great interest in starting planning early to ensure a seamless rehabilitation process, and CPAx has already demonstrated these qualities as a predictive measurement tool in the original and German versions [34,35].

At time point B, no patients scored 0 points, and only 2% scored 50 points, meaning no floor effect and a highly acceptable ceiling effect. This corresponds with the results reported in the original [30] and three other translations [13–15]. These results indicate that CPAx-NOR is applicable for clinical use in Norwegian intensive care units from early in the rehabilitation process through the patient trajectory, including discharge from the ICU to a regular ward.

4.4. Perspective, Further Research and Clinical Implications

CPAx-NOR is an important tool in clinical practice to help establish rehabilitation goals for ICU patients, as they fight their way back toward regaining independent respiratory and physical function [11]. Standardized measuring tools are crucial to document the effect of physiotherapy and early rehabilitation, both clinically and in research. Barriers and facilitators to implementing measurement tools should be further investigated, in order to successfully implement the CPAx-NOR and maintain sustainability in clinical practice. Future studies should include also other aspects of validity.

Both the similarities and differences between the original and translated CPAx versions, highlights the importance of a solid translation- and cross-cultural adaptation process that is needed for further standardization when implementing the CPAx versions into clinical practice. These findings are of importance in future research when designing international multicenter studies, with aims to investigate the effect of early rehabilitation at the ICU. Of clinical importance, is how to apply the MDC results of this study. The authors recommend applying the combined result of the two time points A+B (MDC = 2 points) in clinical practice, similar to the Danish and German versions [13,15].

4.5. Strengths and Limitations

The strengths of the present study include the comprehensive translation process with two professional translators and two clinicians involved in both the forward and backwards translations, along with a multidisciplinary expert committee including a former intensive care patient, before further evaluation of inter-rater reliability. Due to the multicentre design of this study, with five hospitals considered representative of Norwegian ICUs in terms of size, organization and patient population, the results can be considered generalizable to other ICUs in Norway. Further, the use of raters with a range of experience as physiotherapists in acute hospital settings supports our confidence that the use of CPAx-NOR is feasible for a wide variety of physiotherapists working in ICUs.

As in the other European translation studies, all the raters completed a digital course to the testing period, but unlike in those studies, the original English eLearning platform was not available. All raters received training before assessing patients, and generalizability for physiotherapists without any training is limited. Another possible limitation of the design was that the assessments were completed in pairs with raters alternating between the roles of leader and observer without structure. This made it difficult to identify systematic between-raters error.

Moreover, we did not have data on median time on time point A or on length of stay (ICU LOS) in the patients that were tested. Therefore we were not able to link CPAx-NOR to a specific time point in the patient trajectory and to make any conclusions regarding responsiveness.

5. Conclusions

CPAx has been successfully translated and cross-culturally adapted into Norwegian, resulting in CPAx-NOR. The adapted tool has been found to show good face validity in clinical practice and has demonstrated excellent inter-rater reliability. CPAx-NOR can be considered an important measurement instrument for physiotherapists working in the ICU for assessing respiratory and physical function and planning and setting goals for early rehabilitation in the multidisciplinary team in intensive care units in Norway. Future studies should focus on an extended validation, establishing MCID and studying responsiveness in order to insure CPAx-NOR as a clinically important and knowledge based robust tool for physiotherapists working in the intensive care unit with critically ill patients.

Supplementary Materials: The following supporting information can be downloaded at: https://www.mdpi.com/article/10.3390/jcm12155033/s1, Norwegian Version of Chelsea Critical Physical Assessment Tool—CPAx NOR. Reference [36] is cited in the supplementary materials.

Author Contributions: Conceptualization, C.M.S., A.K.B., M.K. and T.M.A.; methodology, C.M.S., A.K.B., M.K. and T.M.A.; formal analysis; C.M.S. and S.A.R.; data curation, C.M.S. and S.A.R.; writing—original draft preparation, C.M.S. and A.K.B.; writing—review and editing, C.M.S., A.K.B., S.A.R., M.K. and T.M.A.; visualization, C.M.S., A.K.B. and S.A.R.; project administration, C.M.S.; funding acquisition, C.M.S., A.K.B., M.K. and T.M.A. All authors have read and agreed to the published version of the manuscript.

Funding: The translation process was funded by Regional Rehabilitation Knowledge Center in South East Norway, Sunnaas Rehabilitation Hospital HF. The inter-rater reliability study was funded by The Foundation Dam, (grant number 2022/HE1-394474).

Institutional Review Board Statement: The study was presented to the Regional Ethics Committee which concluded that it did not require approval. The study was approved by ethical committees at all the local hospitals and SIKT (Norwegian Agency for Shared Services in Education and Research, formerly the Norwegian Centre for Research Data); project number 777606.

Informed Consent Statement: Informed consent was obtained from all subjects involved in the study.

Data Availability Statement: The data presented in this study are available on request from the corresponding author. The data are not publicly available due to privacy and ethical restrictions in the statement from SIKT (Norwegian Agency for Shared Services in Education and Research.

Acknowledgments: The authors wish to thank Evelyn Corner for permission to translate the CPAx and for her contribution to the process. The authors wish to thank Stacey Haukeland-Parker for contributing to the translation process. We would like to thank the expert committee for interesting discussions and important contributions: Marit Follsund Viravong, Sander Guttormsen, Hendrik Detlef Gleichmar, Brita Fosser Olsen, Njål Kinne og Tom Rosenvinge. We would also like to thank the three physiotherapists who tested the preliminary version and provided valuable feedback: Ellen Wiersholm, Marianne Smith and Vetle Osenbroch Kallevik. Thank you to Jenni Moore for her contribution to the discussions on clinical value and the use of standardized measurement tools in clinical practice. Finally, our heartfelt thanks to the participating physiotherapists for their dedication and to the patients and their relatives who consented to participate in this study.

Conflicts of Interest: The authors declare no conflict of interest. The funders had no role in the design of the study; in the collection, analyses, or interpretation of data; in the writing of the manuscript; or in the decision to publish the results.

References

1. Fan, E.; Cheek, F.; Chlan, L.; Gosselink, R.; Hart, N.; Herridge, M.S.; Hopkins, R.O.; Hough, C.L.; Kress, J.P.; Latronico, N.; et al. An official American Thoracic Society Clinical Practice guideline: The diagnosis of intensive care unit–acquired weakness in adults. *Am. J. Respir. Crit. Care Med.* **2014**, *190*, 1437–1446. [CrossRef] [PubMed]
2. Herridge, M.S.; Tansey, C.M.; Matte, A.; Tomlinson, G.; Diaz-Granados, N.; Cooper, A.; Guest, C.B.; Mazer, C.D.; Mehta, S.; Stewart, T.E.; et al. Functional disability 5 years after acute respiratory distress syndrome. *N. Engl. J. Med.* **2011**, *364*, 1293–1304. [CrossRef] [PubMed]
3. Ohtake, P.J.; Lee, A.C.; Scott, J.C.; Hinman, R.S.; Ali, N.A.; Hinkson, C.R.; Needham, D.M.; Shutter, L.; Smith-Gabai, H.; Spires, M.C.; et al. Physical Impairments Associated with Post-Intensive Care Syndrome: Systematic Review Based on the World Health Organization's International Classification of Functioning, Disability and Health Framework. *Phys. Ther.* **2018**, *98*, 631–645. [CrossRef]
4. Gandotra, S.; Lovato, J.; Case, D.; Bakhru, R.N.; Gibbs, K.; Berry, M.; Files, D.C.; Morris, P.E. Physical Function Trajectories in Survivors of Acute Respiratory Failure. *Ann. Am. Thorac. Soc.* **2019**, *16*, 471–477. [CrossRef] [PubMed]
5. Kamdar, B.B.; Suri, R.; Suchyta, M.R.; Digrande, K.F.; Sherwood, K.D.; Colantuoni, E.; Dinglas, V.D.; Needham, D.M.; Hopkins, R.O. Return to work after critical illness: A systematic review and meta-analysis. *Thorax* **2020**, *75*, 17–27. [CrossRef] [PubMed]
6. Gosselink, R.; Bott, J.; Johnson, M.; Dean, E.; Nava, S.; Norrenberg, M.; Schönhofer, B.; Stiller, K.; van de Leur, H.; Vincent, J.L. Physiotherapy for adult patients with critical illness: Recommendations of the European Respiratory Society and European Society of Intensive Care Medicine Task Force on Physiotherapy for Critically Ill Patients. *Intensive Care Med.* **2008**, *34*, 1188–1199. [CrossRef]
7. Arias-Fernandez, P.; Romero-Martin, M.; Gomez-Salgado, J.; Fernandez-Garcia, D. Rehabilitation and early mobilization in the critical patient: Systematic review. *J. Phys. Ther. Sci.* **2018**, *30*, 1193–1201. [CrossRef]
8. Sommers, J.; Engelbert, R.H.; Dettling-Ihnenfeldt, D.; Gosselink, R.; Spronk, P.E.; Nollet, F.; van der Schaaf, M. Physiotherapy in the intensive care unit: An evidence-based, expert driven, practical statement and rehabilitation recommendations. *Clin. Rehabil.* **2015**, *29*, 1051–1063. [CrossRef]
9. Stiller, K. Physiotherapy in intensive care: An updated systematic review. *Chest* **2013**, *144*, 825–847. [CrossRef]
10. Parry, S.M.; Huang, M.; Needham, D.M. Evaluating physical functioning in critical care: Considerations for clinical practice and research. *Crit. Care* **2017**, *21*, 249. [CrossRef]
11. Parry, S.M.; Granger, C.L.; Berney, S.; Jones, J.; Beach, L.; El-Ansary, D.; Koopman, R.; Denehy, L. Assessment of impairment and activity limitations in the critically ill: A systematic review of measurement instruments and their clinimetric properties. *Intensive Care Med.* **2015**, *41*, 744–762. [CrossRef] [PubMed]
12. Corner, E.; Wood, H.; Englebretsen, C.; Thomas, A.; Grant, R.; Nikoletou, D.; Soni, N. The Chelsea critical care physical assessment tool (CPAx): Validation of an innovative new tool to measure physical morbidity in the general adult critical care population; an observational proof-of-concept pilot study. *Physiotherapy* **2013**, *99*, 33–41. [CrossRef] [PubMed]
13. Astrup, K.; Corner, E.; Van Tulder, M.; Sorensen, L. Reliability and responsiveness of the Danish version of The Chelsea Critical Care Physical Assessment tool (CPAx). *Physiother. Theory Pract.* **2021**, *39*, 193–199. [CrossRef] [PubMed]
14. Holdar, U.; Eriksson, F.; Siesage, K.; Corner, E.J.; Ledström, V.; Svensson-Raskh, A.; Kierkegaard, M. Cross-cultural adaptation and inter-rater reliability of the Swedish version of the Chelsea critical care assessment tool (CPAX-Swe) in critically ill patients. *Disabil. Rehabil.* **2021**, *43*, 1600–1604. [CrossRef]
15. Eggmann, S.; Verra, M.L.; Stefanicki, V.; Kindler, A.; Seyler, D.; Hilfiker, R.; Schefold, J.C.; Bastiaenen, C.H.G.; Zante, B. German version of the Chelsea Critical Care Physical Assessment Tool (CPAx-GE): Translation, cross-cultural adaptation, validity, and reliability. *Disabil. Rehabil.* **2022**, *44*, 4509–4518. [CrossRef]
16. Zhang, Z.; Wang, G.; Wu, Y.; Guo, J.; Ding, N.; Jiang, B.; Wei, H.; Li, B.; Yue, W.; Tian, J. Chinesisation, adaptation and validation of the Chelsea Critical Care Physical Assessment Tool in critically ill patients: A cross-sectional observational study. *BMJ Open* **2021**, *11*, e045550. [CrossRef]
17. Vandenbroucke, J.P.; von Elm, E.; Altman, D.G.; Gøtzsche, P.C.; Mulrow, C.D.; Pocock, S.J.; Poole, C.; Schlesselman, J.J.; Egger, M.; STROBE initiative. Strengthening the Reporting of Observational Studies in Epidemiology (STROBE): Explanation and elaboration. *Ann. Intern. Med.* **2007**, *147*, W-163–W-194. [CrossRef] [PubMed]
18. Beaton, D.E.; Bombardier, C.; Guillemin, F.; Ferraz, M.B. Guidelines for the process of cross-cultural adaptation of self-report measures. *Spine* **2000**, *25*, 3186–3191. [CrossRef]
19. Wild, D.; Grove, A.; Martin, M.; Eremenco, S.; McElroy, S.; Verjee-Lorenz, A.; Erikson, P.; ISPOR Task Force for Translation and Cultural Adaptation. Principles of Good Practice for the Translation and Cultural Adaptation Process for Patient-Reported Outcomes (PRO) Measures: Report of the ISPOR Task Force for Translation and Cultural Adaptation. *Value Health* **2005**, *8*, 94–104. [CrossRef]
20. Sousa, V.D.; Rojjanasrirat, W. Translation, adaptation and validation of instruments or scales for use in cross-cultural health care research: A clear and user-friendly guideline. *J. Eval. Clin. Pract.* **2011**, *17*, 268–274. [CrossRef]
21. Mokkink, L.B.; Terwee, C.B.; Patrick, D.L.; Alonso, J.; Stratford, P.W.; Knol, D.L.; Bouter, L.M.; de Vet, H.C. The COSMIN checklist for assessing the methodological quality of studies on measurement properties of health status measurement instruments: An international Delphi study. *Qual. Life Res.* **2010**, *19*, 539–549. [CrossRef]

22. Buanes, E.A.; Kristine, R.K.; Helland, F.; Barrat-Due, A. Norsk Intensiv-OG Pandemiregister. Årsrapport for 2021 Med Plan for Forbetringstiltak 2022. Available online: https://helse-bergen.no/seksjon/intensivregister/Documents/%C3%85rsrapporter%20 i%20NIR/NIPaR%20%C3%85rsrapport%202021.pdf (accessed on 23 December 2022).
23. Mokkink, L.B.; Terwee, C.B.; Patrick, D.L.; Alonso, J.; Stratford, P.W.; Knol, D.L.; Bouter, L.M.; de Vet, H.C. The COSMIN study reached international consensus on taxonomy, terminology, and definitions of measurement properties for health-related patient-reported outcomes. *J. Clin. Epidemiol.* **2010**, *63*, 737–745. [CrossRef] [PubMed]
24. Terwee, C.B.; Bot, S.D.M.; de Boer, M.R.; van der Windt, D.A.W.M.; Knol, D.L.; Dekker, J.; Bouter, L.M.; de Vet, H.C.W. Quality criteria were proposed for measurement properties of health status questionnaires. *J. Clin. Epidemiol.* **2007**, *60*, 34–42. [CrossRef]
25. Koo, T.K.; Li, M.Y. A guideline of selecting and reporting intraclass correlation coefficients for reliability research. *J. Chiropr. Med.* **2016**, *15*, 155–163. [CrossRef]
26. Kazis, L.E.; Anderson, J.J.; Meenan, R.F. Effect sizes for interpreting changes in health status. *Med. Care* **1989**, *27*, S178–S189. [CrossRef]
27. Rosenthal, R.; Cooper, H.; Hedges, L. Parametric measures of effect size. In *The Handbook of Research Synthesis*; Russell Sage Foundation: New York, NY, USA, 1994; pp. 231–244.
28. Shrout, P.E.; Fleiss, J.L. Intraclass correlations: Uses in assessing rater reliability. *Psychol. Bull.* **1979**, *86*, 420–428. [CrossRef]
29. Altman, D.G. *Practical Statistics for Medical Research*; Chapman & Hall/CRC: Boca Raton, FL, USA, 1991.
30. Corner, E.J. The responsiveness of the Chelsea Critical Care Physical Assessment tool in measuring functional recovery in the burns critical care population: An observational study. *Burns* **2015**, *41*, 241–247. [CrossRef] [PubMed]
31. Ranganathan, P.; Pramesh, C.S.; Aggarwal, R. Common pitfalls in statistical analysis: Measures of agreement. *Perspect. Clin. Res.* **2017**, *8*, 187–191. [CrossRef] [PubMed]
32. Olofsen, E.; Dahan, A.; Borsboom, G.; Drummond, G. Improvements in the application and reporting of advanced Bland-Altman methods of comparison. *J. Clin. Monit. Comput.* **2015**, *29*, 127–139. [CrossRef]
33. Donoghue, D.; Stokes, E.K. How much change is true change? The minimum detectable change of the Berg Balance Scale in elderly people. *J. Rehabil. Med.* **2009**, *41*, 343–346. [CrossRef]
34. Corner, E.J.; Soni, N.; Handy, J.M.; Brett, S.J. Construct validity of the Chelsea critical care physical assessment tool: An observational study of recovery from critical illness. *Crit. Care* **2014**, *18*, R55. [CrossRef] [PubMed]
35. Eggmann, S.; Verra, M.L.; Stefanicki, V.; Kindler, A.; Schefold, J.C.; Zante, B.; Bastiaenen, C.H.G. Predictive validity of the Chelsea Critical Care Physical Assessment tool (CPAx) in critically ill, mechanically ventilated adults: A prospective clinimetric study. *Disabil. Rehabil.* **2022**, *45*, 111–116. [CrossRef] [PubMed]
36. Gilbertson, L.; Barber-Lomax, S. Power and Pinch Grip Strength Recorded Using the Hand-Held Jamar Dynamometer and B+L Hydraulic Pinch Guage: British Normative Data for Adults. *Br. J. Occup. Ther.* **1994**, *57*, 483–488. [CrossRef]

Disclaimer/Publisher's Note: The statements, opinions and data contained in all publications are solely those of the individual author(s) and contributor(s) and not of MDPI and/or the editor(s). MDPI and/or the editor(s) disclaim responsibility for any injury to people or property resulting from any ideas, methods, instructions or products referred to in the content.

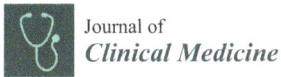

Article

Prone Position Ventilation in Severe ARDS due to COVID-19: Comparison between Prolonged and Intermittent Strategies

George Karlis [1,*], Despina Markantonaki [1], Sotirios Kakavas [2], Dimitra Bakali [1], Georgia Katsagani [1], Theodora Katsarou [1], Christos Kyritsis [1], Vasiliki Karaouli [1], Paraskevi Athanasiou [1] and Mary Daganou [1]

[1] ICU, Thoracic Diseases General Hospital "Sotiria", 115 27 Athens, Greece; despinamark@gmail.com (D.M.); demevbak@gmail.com (D.B.); gkatsagani@hotmail.com (G.K.); katsaroutheo@gmail.com (T.K.); silkarol@yahoo.gr (V.K.); athanasiou.par@hotmail.com (P.A.); mdaganou@hotmail.com (M.D.)
[2] Henry Dunant Hospital Center, 115 26 Athens, Greece; sotikaka@yahoo.com
* Correspondence: georgekarlis@yahoo.com; Tel.: +30-6937582535

Abstract: Ventilation in a prone position (PP) for 12 to 16 h per day improves survival in ARDS. However, the optimal duration of the intervention is unknown. We performed a prospective observational study to compare the efficacy and safety of a prolonged PP protocol with conventional prone ventilation in COVID-19-associated ARDS. Prone position was undertaken if P/F < 150 with FiO_2 > 0.6 and PEEP > 10 cm H_2O. Oxygenation parameters and respiratory mechanics were recorded before the first PP cycle, at the end of the PP cycle and 4 h after supination. We included 63 consecutive intubated patients with a mean age of 63.5 years. Of them, 37 (58.7%) underwent prolonged prone position (PPP group) and 26 (41.3%) standard prone position (SPP group). The median cycle duration for the SPP group was 20 h and for the PPP group 46 h ($p < 0.001$). No significant differences in oxygenation, respiratory mechanics, number of PP cycles and rate of complications were observed between groups. The 28-day survival was 78.4% in the PPP group versus 65.4% in the SPP group ($p = 0.253$). Extending the duration of PP was as safe and efficacious as conventional PP, but did not confer any survival benefit in a cohort of patients with severe ARDS due to COVID-19.

Keywords: ARDS; prone position; COVID-19; mechanical ventilation

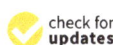

Citation: Karlis, G.; Markantonaki, D.; Kakavas, S.; Bakali, D.; Katsagani, G.; Katsarou, T.; Kyritsis, C.; Karaouli, V.; Athanasiou, P.; Daganou, M. Prone Position Ventilation in Severe ARDS due to COVID-19: Comparison between Prolonged and Intermittent Strategies. *J. Clin. Med.* **2023**, *12*, 3526. https://doi.org/10.3390/jcm12103526

Academic Editor: Andrew Bentley

Received: 7 April 2023
Revised: 11 May 2023
Accepted: 14 May 2023
Published: 17 May 2023

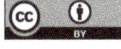

Copyright: © 2023 by the authors. Licensee MDPI, Basel, Switzerland. This article is an open access article distributed under the terms and conditions of the Creative Commons Attribution (CC BY) license (https:// creativecommons.org/licenses/by/ 4.0/).

1. Introduction

The COVID-19 pandemic created unprecedented pressure on healthcare systems worldwide and subsequently provoked significant changes in the organization of healthcare services. Coronavirus disease has a broad spectrum of clinical manifestations ranging from asymptomatic infection to critical illness, most frequently presenting as an acute hypoxemic respiratory failure that meets the Berlin definition of acute respiratory distress syndrome (ARDS). Patients with COVID-19-associated ARDS commonly require intensive care unit (ICU) admission and invasive mechanical ventilation and have high mortality rates [1,2]. Whether ARDS due to COVID-19 and ARDS due to other etiologies are similar has been a matter of debate. It seems that COVID-19 pneumonia is a specific disease with distinct features, namely the dissociation between the severity of the hypoxemia and the maintenance of relatively good respiratory mechanics, as well as the common (micro)thrombosis in the pulmonary vasculature [3].

It is well established that early application of prone-positioning (PP) sessions of at least 12 h improve survival in moderate-to-severe ARDS [4,5]. The beneficial effect of prone ventilation is likely attributed to better ventilation-perfusion matching, lung recruitment and protection from ventilator-induced lung injury (VILI) [6]. Current guidelines on the management of ARDS strongly recommend the use of PP for 12 to 16 h per day in patients with a P/F ratio ≤ 150 mmHg [4,5,7]. However, the optimal duration of the intervention to gain maximum benefit is not known. During COVID-19 pandemic prone ventilation was widely adopted as a prominent therapeutic intervention for patients receiving mechanical ventilation. Retrospective data from this patient population showed that early application of PP is associated with improved oxygenation and reduced hospital mortality [8,9].

One of the challenges of PP is that it can increase the workload for the ICU staff in a period of crisis. To overcome this problem, it was suggested to implement a prolonged pronation protocol, beyond the usual 16 h, aiming to reduce the number of pronation cycles per patient. Nevertheless, the intervention is not without risks. The most severe complications are accidental extubation, airway obstruction, central venous catheter or arterial catheter dislocation, pressure ulcers, peripheral nerve palsies and musculoskeletal injuries [10]. There are reports that prolonged prone ventilation is feasible and relatively safe [11,12], but comparison with standard PP has been scarce.

We sought to examine the efficacy and safety of a prolonged PP protocol compared to the standard of care.

2. Materials and Methods

We conducted a prospective observational study. General Hospital of Thoracic Diseases "Sotiria" is a tertiary public hospital that serves as the main referral center for COVID-19 in Athens, Greece. The study was conducted in a 12-bed COVID-19 ICU during a 6-month period. Patient demographics, clinical and mechanical ventilation (MV) variables were entered into an electronic spreadsheet and cross-validated with source documentation in real-time. The study was approved by the local Institutional Review Board (protocol number 172/24-05-2021). The need for informed consent was waived.

Lung protective ventilation was universally applied to all study patients, namely a tidal volume of 6–8 mL/PBW with PEEP titration to achieve a driving pressure <14 cm H_2O. The level of PEEP was applied and modified by the treating physician. PP was initiated for severe hypoxemia defined as P/F ratio < 150 mmHg with FiO_2 > 0.6 and PEEP > 10 cm H_2O. Patients with severe hemodynamic instability, pregnancy, recent cardiac or abdominal surgery, and unstable fractures were not candidates for prone ventilation in our study. In the prolonged PP (PPP) group patients were proned for more than 24 h whereas the standard PP (SPP) group included patients proned for 24 h or less. The cut-off of 24 h was based on a recent study of ARDS patients which suggested that it is beneficial to prolong PP sessions to 24 h and extend it further if the P/F ratio remains below 150 [13]. We left the decision for the duration of PP solely at the discretion of the treating physician, according to a guiding protocol stating that return to the supine position would be performed after at least 16 h if the P/F ratio was above 150 and if an experienced staff was available. For safety reasons, repositioning during the night shift was avoided, unless it was deemed necessary. Pronation cycles were stopped when the P/F ratio remained >150 mmHg in a supine position. Oxygenation parameters and respiratory mechanics were recorded for the first pronation cycle before PP, at the end of the cycle and 4 h after supine repositioning. We included all the intubated patients > 18 years old, with a positive PCR for SARS-CoV-2, who underwent at least one cycle of PP during the specified time period. Patients proned for less than 4 h were excluded from the analysis.

Prone positioning and repositioning to the supine position were performed manually by experienced ICU staff according to a standardized protocol. Normally, 5 healthcare professionals were involved with the pronation/supination of non-obese patients, while 7 or more were involved if the patient was obese or morbidly obese. Alternating pressure air mattresses were used in all patients. Foam wedges, foam dressings, gel rings and pillows were used for pressure injury prevention. Alternating arm and head repositioning in the "swimming position" were performed every 6–8 h. Sedation and analgesia were titrated to achieve deep sedation (Richmond Sedation Agitation Scale score of 4–5) and neuromuscular blockade was administered to all patients during PP. Pressure wounds and other complications were recorded daily by bedside nurses, until the end of the pronation cycles.

2.1. Outcomes

The primary clinical outcomes were changes in oxygenation and respiratory mechanics during and after PP and the number of PP cycles. The secondary outcome was 28-day survival. A subgroup analysis of obese patients (BMI > 30 kg/m^2) was additionally performed. We also examined the safety and the complications of the procedure.

2.2. Statistical Analysis

Variables were first tested for normality using the Kolmogorov–Smirnov criterion. Quantitative variables were expressed as mean (Standard Deviation) or median (interquartile range). Qualitative variables were expressed as absolute and relative frequencies. Student's *t*-tests and Mann–Whitney tests were used for the comparison of continuous variables between the two groups. For the comparison of proportions chi-square and Fisher's exact tests were used. Pearson correlation coefficients (r) were used to explore the association of two continuous variables. Repeated measurements analysis of variance (ANOVA) was adopted to evaluate the changes observed in respiratory parameters over the follow-up period, between the two groups. Logistic regression analysis in a stepwise method (p for entry 0.05, p for removal 0.10) was used in order to find independent factors associated with 28-day survival. Adjusted odds ratios (OR) with 95% confidence intervals (95% CI) were computed from the results of the logistic regression analysis. All reported p values are two-tailed. Statistical significance was set at $p < 0.05$ and analyses were conducted using SPSS statistical software (version 26.0).

3. Results

From March 2021 to August 2021, we recorded 68 consecutive intubated patients with COVID-19-associated ARDS who underwent prone ventilation. Five patients were excluded because PP was terminated in less than 4 h due to hemodynamic instability or worsening of oxygenation. The final study sample consisted of 63 patients (63.5% males), with a mean age of 63.5 years. Thirty-seven patients (58.7%) underwent prolonged prone position (PPP group) and 26 (41.3%) standard prone position (SPP group). The median PP duration for the SPP group was 20 h (IQR: 20–22) and for the PPP group 46 h (IQR: 40–48), $p < 0.001$. The cumulative duration of pronation was longer for the PPP group. Patients' characteristics by group are presented in Table 1. No significant differences were found between the two groups, except for a higher proportion of obese patients among the PPP group. All patients received corticosteroids while tocilizumab was administered to similar proportions in both groups.

Table 1. Patients' characteristics.

	Group		
	SPP $n = 26$	PPP $n = 37$	p
Gender, n (%)			
Males	15 (57.7)	25 (67.6)	0.42
Females	11 (42.3)	12 (32.4)	
Age, mean (SD)	66.5 (9.7)	61.5 (15.1)	0.14
BMI, mean (SD)	30.5 (5.5)	33.4 (7.0)	0.08
BMI			
Normal (18.5–24.9 kg/m^2)	1 (3.8)	0 (0)	0.049
Overweight (25–29.9 kg/m^2)	15 (57.7)	12 (33.3)	
Obese (>30 kg/m^2)	10 (38.5)	24 (66.7)	

Table 1. Cont.

	Group		p
	SPP n = 26	PPP n = 37	
APACHE II, mean (SD)	19.3 (3.8)	19.5 (7.1)	0.89
Tocilizumab, n (%)	17 (65%)	21 (57%)	0.49
Vt (ml), median (IQR)	425 (375–450)	425 (375–475)	0.59
Vt (ml/PBW), median (IQR)	6.3 (6.2–6.7)	6.3 (6.2–6.7)	0.78
RR, median (IQR)	27.5 (25–32)	30 (27–32)	0.24
Time to proning, h, median (IQR)	22.5 (16–48)	20 (10–48)	0.59
Duration of 1st PP cycle, h, median (IQR)	20 (20–22)	46 (40–48)	<0.001
Cumulative duration of proning, h, mean (SD)	42.42 (22.27)	70.22 (38.29)	0.001

The change in P/F ratio was similar across all time points between SPP and PPP groups, in the total sample and in the subgroup of obese patients. In both groups, the P/F ratio during and after PP was significantly higher compared to the baseline (Table 2).

Table 2. P/F ratio in total sample and in obese patients.

Group		P/F Ratio (mmHg)			p^2			p^3
		Baseline	During			After	After	
		Mean (SD)	Mean (SD)	Mean (SD)	During vs. Baseline	vs. During	vs. Baseline	
Total sample	SPP	103.4 (25.8)	173.6 (59)	150.2 (32)	<0.001	0.09	<0.001	0.13
	PPP	97.6 (27.4)	197.9 (70.1)	162.2 (58.8)	<0.001	<0.001	<0.001	
	p^1	0.39	0.15	0.35				
Obese	SPP	105.1 (29.2)	176.5 (67.9)	152.8 (25.2)	0.002	0.69	0.004	0.43
	PPP	95.8 (27.1)	194.6 (67.8)	156.7 (48.7)	<0.001	0.014	<0.001	
	p^1	0.38	0.48	0.81				

[1] p-value for group effect [2] p-value for time effect after Bonferroni correction [3] p-value from repeated measures ANOVA, regarding time × group effect.

The degree of P/F ratio change from baseline to the end of the first PP cycle to 4 h after supination was similar in both groups (Figure 1). Furthermore, PP duration was not correlated with the P/F ratio (r = 0.18; p = 0.161).

The change in respiratory parameters by the group throughout the follow-up period is presented in Table 3. No significant differences were found between SPP and PPP groups at any time point. Pplat was slightly lower during the maneuver compared to baseline in both groups, while after supination it remained lower than baseline only in the PPP group. However, because PEEP was also lower during and after the maneuver, DP and Cstat were similar throughout time.

Table 3. Changes of respiratory parameters.

	Group	Baseline Mean (SD)	During Mean (SD)	After Mean (SD)	During vs. Baseline	After vs. During	After vs. Baseline	p^3
							p^2	
$PaCO_2$ (mmHg)	SPP	50.9 (8.8)	47.8 (7.5)	48.3 (6.3)	0.22	>0.99	0.46	0.95
	PPP	50.8 (10.6)	47.6 (7.1)	48.5 (7.9)	0.08	>0.99	0.39	
	p^1	0.97	0.89	0.92				
PEEP (cm H_2O)	SPP	12 (2.7)	11.1 (2.8)	11.2 (2.6)	0.012	>0.99	0.02	0.49
	PPP	12.3 (2.4)	11.6 (2.6)	11.2 (2.2)	0.018	0.29	<0.001	
	p^1	0.64	0.49	0.99				
Pplat (cm H_2O)	SPP	25.3 (3.6)	23.6 (3.2)	23.9 (3.3)	0.009	>0.99	0.09	0.65
	PPP	25.5 (3.4)	23.9 (3.5)	23.5 (3.3)	0.003	>0.99	0.002	
	p^1	0.84	0.77	0.68				
DP (cm H_2O)	SPP	13.4 (3.9)	12.2 (2.4)	12.2 (2.8)	0.16	>0.99	0.27	0.82
	PPP	12.9 (3.2)	12.1 (2.4)	12.2 (2.6)	0.25	>0.99	0.50	
	p^1	0.62	0.82	0.92				
Cstat (mL/cm H_2O)	SPP	35.8 (10.2)	36.9 (11.6)	36.8 (10.7)	>0.99	>0.99	>0.99	0.75
	PPP	35.2 (9.5)	37.6 (9.3)	36.4 (8.8)	0.22	0.84	>0.99	
	p^1	0.81	0.77	0.87				

[1] p-value for group effect [2] p-value for time effect after Bonferroni correction [3] p-value from repeated measures ANOVA, regarding time × group effect.

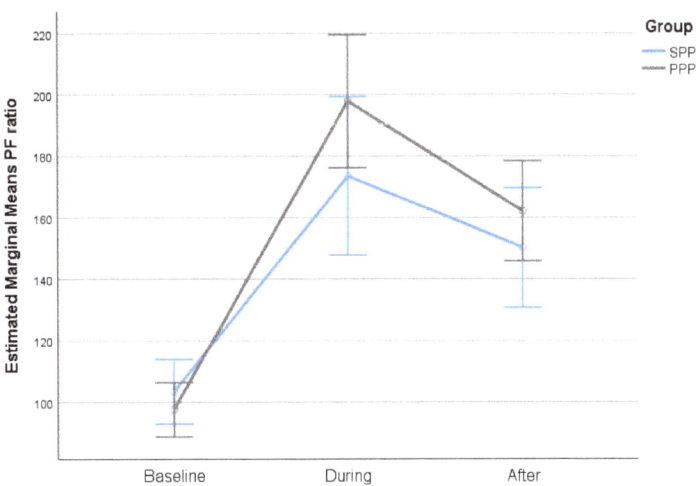

Figure 1. P/F ratio change, by group.

No significant difference was found in 28-day survival between the two groups. The number of pronation cycles was also comparable [median (IQR), 2(1–3) for SPP vs. 1(1–2) for PPP group]. Seven patients (26.9%) in the SPP group and 5 (13.5%) in the PPP group required 3 or more pronation cycles. No major complications were encountered in either group after the completion of the required pronation cycles. Facial edema and pressure injuries in stage I were recorded in six patients during PPP and in four patients during SPP, while one patient in each group developed a stage II facial pressure ulcer and one patient in the PPP group developed a stage III facial injury and periorbital edema (Table 4). Similar results were recorded for obese patients as shown in Table 5.

Table 4. Outcomes and complications.

	Group		p
	SPP n = 26	PPP n = 37	
28-day survival, n (%)			0.25
No	9 (34.6)	8 (21.6)	
Yes	17 (65.4)	29 (78.4)	
Number of cycles, median (IQR)	2 (1–3)	1 (1–2)	0.12
Complications, n (%)			>0.99
No	21 (80.8)	29 (78.4)	
Yes	5 (19.2)	8 (21.6)	

Table 5. Outcomes among obese patients.

		Group		p
		SPP (n = 10)	PPP (n = 24)	
		Median	Median	
28-day survival	No	4 (40)	5 (20.8)	0.39
	Yes	6 (60)	19 (79.2)	
Number of cycles, median (IQR)		2 (2–3)	1 (1–2)	0.19

After conducting multiple logistic regression, in a stepwise method, it was found that the number of PP cycles, APACHE II and $PaCO_2$ at baseline (before pronation) were independently associated with 28-day survival. Specifically, a higher number of cycles, higher APACHE II score and higher $PaCO_2$ at baseline were significantly associated with a lower probability of surviving (Table 6).

Table 6. Logistic regression for 28-day survival.

	OR (95% CI)	p
Number of cycles	0.27 (0.12–0.63)	0.002
APACHE II	0.78 (0.66–0.92)	0.003
$PaCO_2$ baseline (mmHg)	0.92 (0.86–0.99)	0.031

4. Discussion

In a cohort of COVID-19 intubated patients with severe ARDS, in whom protective ventilation was applied, a prolonged prone positioning protocol was not shown to confer any advantage in improving oxygenation and respiratory mechanics compared to the traditional strategy of daily prone ventilation. Furthermore, it was not associated with significantly fewer total pronation cycles. Twenty-eight-day survival was similar between the two groups. The intervention was feasible and safe with only minor observed complications.

Prone position ventilation for at least 16 h has been shown to reduce mortality in patients with ARDS and a P/F ratio of <150 mmHg. This beneficial effect does not depend on gas exchange improvement but is rather attributed to protection from VILI by reducing overdistension of non-dependent and enhancing alveolar recruitment of dependent lung zones, leading to more homogeneous lung expansion and reducing lung stress and strain [4]. Prone ventilation was widely adopted during the COVID-19 pandemic. While the LUNG

SAFE study in 2016 [14] reported the application of prone positioning in only 16.3% of patients with moderate to severe ARDS, the intervention was used in more than 70% of mechanically ventilated patients with COVID-19 [15,16].

Early prone ventilation has been associated with improved survival among COVID-19 patients [9]. However, it is a labor-intensive procedure requiring at least 5 highly trained ICU professionals to execute each pronation and supination maneuver [17]. In conditions of increased workload, as was the case during the pandemic, prolongation of the duration of prone ventilation to more than 24 h seemed an attractive option to reduce the burden of this life-saving intervention. Furthermore, prolonging PP has a physiological rationale as there is data suggesting that the beneficial effects of PP may persist for at least up to 24 h for some patients [13], while supination is often accompanied by de-recruitment events. Prior studies in COVID-19 patients with ARDS showed that prolonged PP is efficacious and safe when performed by experienced staff [12]. However, the efficacy of the maneuver compared to the standard practice of shorter duration daily cycles has not been extensively studied. In a single-center study of patients with pneumonia and ARDS, Jochmans et al. reported that the maximum physiological beneficial effect of PP was obtained between 16 and 19 h in most patients and extending pronation for more than 24 h offered no survival benefit [13]. In patients with COVID-19-related ARDS, improvement of oxygenation with proning has been associated with lower mortality [18].

In a recent retrospective study of intubated COVID-19 patients, Okin et al. [19] reported reduced mortality and fewer pronation-supination cycles for the prolonged PP compared to the standard PP. The authors found no difference in oxygenation improvement between PPP and SPP, measured as the change in P/F ratio within 6 h of pronation. In the present study, we found a similar increase in the P/F ratio between prolonged and intermittent proning during the maneuver and up to 4 h after supination. Furthermore, there was no correlation between PP duration and the P/F ratio. It seems that extending proning beyond 24 h confers little further improvement in oxygenation. Changes in respiratory mechanics were of little clinical significance in both groups. Okin et al., attribute the beneficial effect on survival to the reduced de-recruitment events associated with fewer supination sessions. Despite similar patient characteristics and similar duration of prolonged pronation protocol between the two studies, we did not find a survival advantage of PPP over SPP. However, there are caveats that should be addressed. First, 28-day mortality rates in our cohort are similar to those in Okin's study (21.6% vs. 25.5% for the PPP group and 34,6% vs. 34.9% for the SPP group). Therefore, the lack of significance is probably due to the smaller sample size of our study. Second, although we found no difference in the total number of performed PP cycles between groups, the number of cycles was an independent risk factor for mortality. The more the pronation cycles, the greater the mortality, lending support to the assumption that de-recruitment associated with repeated supination may be injurious to the lung, may worsen VILI and may contribute to mortality. It can be speculated that PPP may reduce mortality when it results in fewer pronation and supination events. Third, in our study, a higher proportion of obese patients were included in PPP than in the SPP group. Since the decision for the duration of PP was solely at the discretion of the treating physicians, we can only assume that obese patients were deemed more appropriate candidates for prolonged pronation to reduce the risk of complications and adverse events from frequent maneuvers. Several meta-analyses have shown that obesity is associated with increased severity and higher mortality among COVID-19 patients [20]. In a previous study, De Jong et al. reported a better response in oxygenation with prone ventilation among morbidly obese compared to non-obese patients with ARDS [21]. However, a subgroup analysis of our cohort showed that obese patients had no additional benefit with PPP compared to SPP.

The number of cycles per se was found to be associated with 28-day survival in our study. It is fair to assume that the sickest ARDS patients require more PP cycles while aiming to improve their oxygenation. Most of the patients in our cohort required 1 or 2 cycles which were akin to the corresponding study of Okin et al. [19] with a median of 2 cycles overall. Moreover, in a non-COVID population with ARDS due to pneumonia [13] a mean of 2.2 cycles per patient was reported, while in the PROSEVA trial which included ARDS from various etiologies, patients required a mean of 4 cycles [4]. It is not clear if there is an association between the etiology of ARDS and the response to PP.

The rate of complications in our study was very low in both groups and almost exclusively consisted of minor facial pressure injuries. Pressure injuries are the most frequent complication of prone ventilation. In a retrospective study of 81 patients with COVID-19 who were ventilated in PP for a median of 39 h, 26% developed pressure injuries stage II and 2.5% stage III and IV. The cumulative duration of PP sessions, but not the duration of each session, was associated with the occurrence of pressure injuries [22]. Okin et al., reported an incidence of pressure sores of about 30%, with no difference between prolonged and intermittent PP. In our study, the prophylactic use of foam pads, foam dressings, gel rings and regular head repositioning, probably contributed to the low incidence of complications, which was also evident in the group of prolonged pronation.

There are several limitations to our study. It was a single-center non-randomized study with a potential risk for selection bias. The sample size was small and the study itself was not powered to detect a mortality difference. We recorded only immediate complications. There was no long-term follow-up and therefore we might have missed late complications such as plexopathy and nerve damage [23]. Moreover, the use of prophylactic measures along with the accumulated experience of our staff, possibly resulted in a low rate of early complications, which might not be generalizable to all ICU settings.

However, the present study confirms the feasibility and safety of prolonged prone ventilation among patients with severe ARDS caused by COVID-19 and highlights the urgent need for multi-center randomized trials comparing the efficacy of this maneuver with the standard technique of daily proning and supination in ARDS patients of various etiology. Should this approach prove to further improve mortality, it could be safely added to lung protective ventilation, which is so far the only lifesaving intervention in this patient population. In any case, this strategy seems to be a useful option in periods of increased ICU workload or for specific groups of patients, such as the obese.

5. Conclusions

Among intubated COVID-19 patients with severe ARDS, prolonging PP to more than 24 h was as safe and efficient as traditional PP, but it was not associated with survival benefits.

Author Contributions: Conceptualization, G.K. (George Karlis) and M.D.; Data curation, D.M.; Investigation, G.K. (George Karlis), D.B., G.K. (Georgia Katsagani), T.K., C.K., V.K. and P.A.; Methodology, S.K.; Supervision, D.M. and M.D.; Writing—original draft, G.K. (George Karlis); Writing—review & editing, D.M. and M.D. All authors have read and agreed to the published version of the manuscript.

Funding: This research received no external funding.

Institutional Review Board Statement: The study was conducted in accordance with the Declaration of Helsinki, and approved by the Institutional Review Board of General Hospital of Thoracic Diseases "Sotiria" (172/24 May 2021).

Informed Consent Statement: Informed consent was waived due to the observational, non-interventional nature of the study.

Data Availability Statement: The data presented in this study are available on request from the corresponding author. The data are not publicly available due to privacy restrictions.

Conflicts of Interest: The authors declare no conflict of interest.

References

1. ARDS Definition Task Force; Ranieri, V.M.; Rubenfeld, G.D.; Thompson, B.T.; Ferguson, N.D.; Caldwell, E.; Fan, E.; Camporota, L.; Slutsky, A.S. Acute respiratory distress syndrome: The Berlin Definition. *JAMA* **2012**, *307*, 2526–2533. [CrossRef] [PubMed]
2. Grasselli, G.; Tonetti, T.; Protti, A.; Langer, T.; Girardis, M.; Bellani, G.; Laffey, J.; Carrafiello, G.; Carsana, L.; Rizzuto, C.; et al. Pathophysiology of COVID-19-associated acute respiratory distress syndrome: A multicentre prospective observational study. *Lancet Respir. Med.* **2020**, *8*, 1201–1208. [CrossRef] [PubMed]

3. Gattinoni, L.; Chiumello, D.; Rossi, S. COVID-19 pneumonia: ARDS or not? *Crit. Care* **2020**, *24*, 154. [CrossRef] [PubMed]
4. Guérin, C.; Reignier, J.; Richard, J.C.; Beuret, P.; Gacouin, A.; Boulain, T.; Mercier, E.; Badet, M.; Mercat, A.; Baudin, O.; et al. Prone positioning in severe acute respiratory distress syndrome. *N. Engl. J. Med.* **2013**, *368*, 2159–2168. [CrossRef] [PubMed]
5. Gattinoni, L.; Taccone, P.; Carlesso, E.; Marini, J.J. Prone position in acute respiratory distress syndrome. Rationale, indications, and limits. *Am. J. Respir. Crit. Care Med.* **2013**, *188*, 1286–1293. [CrossRef] [PubMed]
6. Guérin, C.; Albert, R.K.; Beitler, J.; Gattinoni, L.; Jaber, S.; Marini, J.J.; Munshi, L.; Papazian, L.; Pesenti, A.; Vieillard-Baron, A.; et al. Prone position in ARDS patients: Why, when, how and for whom. *Intensive Care Med.* **2020**, *46*, 2385–2396. [CrossRef]
7. Griffiths, M.J.D.; McAuley, D.F.; Perkins, G.D.; Barrett, N.; Blackwood, B.; Boyle, A.; Chee, N.; Connolly, B.; Dark, P.; Finney, S.; et al. Guidelines on the management of acute respiratory distress syndrome. *BMJ Open Respir. Res.* **2019**, *6*, e000420. [CrossRef]
8. Langer, T.; Brioni, M.; Guzzardella, A.; Carlesso, E.; Cabrini, L.; Castelli, G.; Dalla Corte, F.; De Robertis, E.; Favarato, M.; Forastieri, A.; et al. Prone position in intubated, mechanically ventilated patients with COVID-19: A multi-centric study of more than 1000 patients. *Crit. Care* **2021**, *25*, 128. [CrossRef]
9. Mathews, K.S.; Soh, H.; Shaefi, S.; Wang, W.; Bose, S.; Coca, S.; Gupta, S.; Hayek, S.S.; Srivastava, A.; Brenner, S.K.; et al. Prone Positioning and Survival in Mechanically Ventilated Patients with Coronavirus Disease 2019-Related Respiratory Failure. *Crit. Care Med.* **2021**, *49*, 1026–1037. [CrossRef]
10. Le, M.Q.; Rosales, R.; Shapiro, L.T.; Huang, L.Y. The DownSide of Prone Positioning: The Case of a Coronavirus 2019 Survivor. *Am. J. Phys. Med. Rehabil.* **2020**, *99*, 870–872. [CrossRef]
11. Douglas, I.S.; Rosenthal, C.A.; Swanson, D.D.; Hiller, T.; Oakes, J.; Bach, J.; Whelchel, C.; Pickering, J.; George, T.; Kearns, M.; et al. Safety and Outcomes of Prolonged Usual Care Prone Position Mechanical Ventilation to Treat Acute Coronavirus Disease 2019 Hypoxemic Respiratory Failure. *Crit. Care Med.* **2021**, *49*, 490–502. [CrossRef] [PubMed]
12. Carsetti, A.; Damia Paciarini, A.; Marini, B.; Pantanetti, S.; Adrario, E.; Donati, A. Prolonged prone position ventilation for SARS-CoV-2 patients is feasible and effective. *Crit. Care* **2020**, *24*, 225. [CrossRef] [PubMed]
13. Jochmans, S.; Mazerand, S.; Chelly, J.; Pourcine, F.; Sy, O.; Thieulot-Rolin, N.; Ellrodt, O.; Mercier Des Rochettes, E.; Michaud, G.; Serbource-Goguel, J.; et al. Duration of prone position sessions: A prospective cohort study. *Ann. Intensive Care* **2020**, *10*, 66. [CrossRef]
14. Bellani, G.; Laffey, J.G.; Pham, T.; Fan, E.; Brochard, L.; Esteban, A.; Gattinoni, L.; van Haren, F.; Larsson, A.; McAuley, D.F.; et al. Epidemiology, Patterns of Care, and Mortality for Patients with Acute Respiratory Distress Syndrome in Intensive Care Units in 50 Countries. *JAMA* **2016**, *315*, 788–800. [CrossRef] [PubMed]
15. Ferrando, C.; Suarez-Sipmann, F.; Mellado-Artigas, R.; Hernández, M.; Gea, A.; Arruti, E.; Aldecoa, C.; Martínez-Pallí, G.; Martínez-González, M.A.; Slutsky, A.S.; et al. Clinical features, ventilatory management, and outcome of ARDS caused by COVID-19 are similar to other causes of ARDS. *Intensive Care Med.* **2020**, *46*, 2200–2211. [CrossRef]
16. COVID-ICU Group on behalf of the REVA Network and the COVID-ICU Investigators. Clinical characteristics and day-90 outcomes of 4244 critically ill adults with COVID-19: A prospective cohort study. *Intensive Care Med.* **2021**, *47*, 60–73. [CrossRef]
17. Harcombe, C.J. Nursing patients with ARDS in the prone position. *Nurs. Stand.* **2004**, *18*, 33–39. [CrossRef]
18. Scaramuzzo, G.; Gamberini, L.; Tonetti, T.; Zani, G.; Ottaviani, I.; Mazzoli, C.A.; Capozzi, C.; Giampalma, E.; Bacchi Reggiani, M.L.; Bertellini, E.; et al. Sustained oxygenation improvement after first prone positioning is associated with liberation from mechanical ventilation and mortality in critically ill COVID-19 patients: A cohort study. *Ann. Intensive Care* **2021**, *11*, 63. [CrossRef]
19. Okin, D.; Huang, C.Y.; Alba, G.A.; Jesudasen, S.J.; Dandawate, N.A.; Gavralidis, A.; Chang, L.L.; Moin, E.E.; Ahmad, I.; Witkin, A.S.; et al. Prolonged prone position ventilation is associated with reduced mortality in intubated COVID-19 patients. *Chest* **2022**, *163*, 533–542. [CrossRef]
20. Singh, R.; Rathore, S.S.; Khan, H.; Karale, S.; Chawla, Y.; Iqbal, K.; Bhurwal, A.; Tekin, A.; Jain, N.; Mehra, I.; et al. Association of Obesity with COVID-19 Severity and Mortality: An Updated Systemic Review, Meta-Analysis, and Meta-Regression. *Front. Endocrinol.* **2022**, *13*, 780872. [CrossRef]
21. De Jong, A.; Molinari, N.; Sebbane, M.; Prades, A.; Futier, E.; Jung, B.; Chanques, G.; Jaber, S. Feasibility and effectiveness of prone position in morbidly obese patients with ARDS: A case-control clinical study. *Chest* **2013**, *143*, 1554–1561. [CrossRef] [PubMed]
22. Walter, T.; Zucman, N.; Mullaert, J.; Thiry, I.; Gernez, C.; Roux, D.; Ricard, J.D. Extended prone positioning duration for COVID-19-related ARDS: Benefits and detriments. *Crit. Care* **2022**, *26*, 208. [CrossRef] [PubMed]
23. Brugliera, L.; Filippi, M.; Del Carro, U.; Butera, C.; Bianchi, F.; Castellazzi, P.; Cimino, P.; Capodaglio, P.; Monti, G.; Mortini, P.; et al. Nerve Compression Injuries After Prolonged Prone Position Ventilation in Patients with SARS-CoV-2: A Case Series. *Arch. Phys. Med. Rehabil.* **2021**, *102*, 359–362. [CrossRef] [PubMed]

Disclaimer/Publisher's Note: The statements, opinions and data contained in all publications are solely those of the individual author(s) and contributor(s) and not of MDPI and/or the editor(s). MDPI and/or the editor(s) disclaim responsibility for any injury to people or property resulting from any ideas, methods, instructions or products referred to in the content.

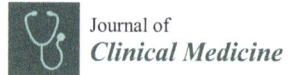

Communication

Early Patient-Triggered Pressure Support Breathing in Mechanically Ventilated Patients with COVID-19 May Be Associated with Lower Rates of Acute Kidney Injury

Mark E. Seubert [1,*] and Marco Goeijenbier [2,3]

1. Intensive Care, The LangeLand Hospital, 2725 NA Zoetermeer, The Netherlands
2. Intensive Care, Spaarne Gasthuis, 2035 RC Haarlem, The Netherlands
3. Intensive Care, Erasmus MC, 3015 GD Rotterdam, The Netherlands
* Correspondence: mark@intensivistnodig.nl

Abstract: Background: Acute respiratory distress syndrome (ARDS) in COVID-19 patients often necessitates mechanical ventilation. Although much has been written regarding intensive care admission and treatment for COVID-19, evidence on specific ventilation strategies for ARDS is limited. Support mode during invasive mechanical ventilation offers potential benefits such as conserving diaphragmatic motility, sidestepping the negative consequences of the longer usage of neuromuscular blockers, and limiting the occurrence of ventilator-induced lung injury (VILI). Methods: In this retrospective cohort study of mechanically ventilated and confirmed non-hyperdynamic SARS-CoV-2 patients, we studied the relation between the occurrence of kidney injury and the decreased ratio of support to controlled ventilation. Results: Total AKI incidence in this cohort was low (5/41). In total, 16 of 41 patients underwent patient-triggered pressure support breathing at least 80% of the time. In this group we observed a lower percentage of AKI (0/16 vs. 5/25), determined as a creatinine level above 177 µmol/L in the first 200 h. There was a negative correlation between time spent on support ventilation and peak creatinine levels (r = −0.35 (−0.6–0.1)). The group predominantly on control ventilation showed significantly higher disease severity scores. Conclusions: Early patient-triggered ventilation in patients with COVID-19 may be associated with lower rates of acute kidney injury.

Keywords: COVID-19; mechanical ventilation; acute kidney injury (AKI); acute respiratory distress syndrome (ARDS); ventilator-induced kidney injury (VIKI)

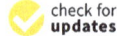

Citation: Seubert, M.E.; Goeijenbier, M. Early Patient-Triggered Pressure Support Breathing in Mechanically Ventilated Patients with COVID-19 May Be Associated with Lower Rates of Acute Kidney Injury. *J. Clin. Med.* 2023, 12, 1859. https://doi.org/10.3390/jcm12051859

Academic Editor: Spyros D. Mentzelopoulos

Received: 29 December 2022
Revised: 19 February 2023
Accepted: 23 February 2023
Published: 26 February 2023

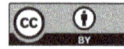

Copyright: © 2023 by the authors. Licensee MDPI, Basel, Switzerland. This article is an open access article distributed under the terms and conditions of the Creative Commons Attribution (CC BY) license (https://creativecommons.org/licenses/by/4.0/).

1. Introduction

Critical care practitioners debate when or whether to allow patient-triggered ventilation in acute respiratory distress syndrome (ARDS) patients. A recent Cochrane intervention review by Hohmann et al. pointed out that there is a lack of data on the benefits and harms of early supported ventilation in invasively ventilated persons with COVID-19 [1].

Invasive mechanical ventilation, in any form, is associated with a threefold increased risk of developing acute kidney injury (AKI), and no direct association is seen between various tidal volume settings or level of positive end-expiratory pressure (PEEP) [2]. As early as 1947, Drury et al. published the first study of the effects of mechanical ventilation on renal function. Studying the effect of varying levels of continuous positive airway pressure on urea clearance in healthy subjects suggested the kidney–lung connection [3]. Although not completely understood and even harder to predict, the systemic effects of mechanical ventilation suggest potential mechanisms of ventilator-induced kidney injury (VIKI) and suggest that these mechanisms might be predicted using biomarkers [4]. Ideas on why ventilator-induced kidney injury can occur include the fact that mechanical ventilation may induce rapid hemodynamic changes, neurohumoral mediated alterations in intrarenal blood flow, and systemic inflammatory cytokines released systemically due to ventilator-induced lung injury [4]. Overall, invasive mechanical ventilation is a proven risk factor for the occurrence of early AKI [5].

Especially in prolonged ICU stays, as seen in severe COVID-19, it is important to differentiate between early AKI that is directly related to the primary pathology and treatment (i.e., within the first 14 days of ICU admittance) versus late AKI, which is predominantly related to other causes such as superinfections and drug toxicity [6,7]. A recent study suggested a relation between the occurrence of AKI and the level of PEEP used. Of specific interest is that nearly all AKI patients in this study were treated with neuromuscular blockade (NMB) (97 vs. 80%, respectively), and thus there were no patient-triggered breathing efforts [8]. We hypothesized that the high incidence of AKI in COVID-19 patients is related to a high percentage of time spent on controlled ventilation in the first 200 h after starting invasive respiratory support. To investigate this, we analyzed the patient data from a single-center intensive care unit in Zoetermeer, the Netherlands.

2. Materials and Methods

We evaluated a retrospective cohort of COVID-19 patients admitted to the intensive care unit between March 2020 and March 2022 in the LangeLand Hospital in Zoetermeer, the Netherlands. The aim of this study was to assess the relation between the incidence of AKI and the ratio of pressure support to control (PS/PC + PS ratio) in invasive mechanical ventilation. The KDIGO (Kidney Disease: Improving Global Outcomes) guidelines are used to define AKI.

Data from the first 200 h of mechanical ventilation were used, and the ratio for each patient was determined by dividing the hours spent on pressure support by the total hours spent on mechanical ventilation (pressure support + pressure control). Graph Pad Prism 9.0 was used for statistical analyses. The ethics committee of the LangeLand Hospital approved the study.

3. Results

In total, 130 patients with COVID-19 were admitted to intensive care during the study period. Of these, 46 patients needed invasive mechanical ventilation, of which 41 were not transferred to another hospital within the investigated timeframe (i.e., were transferred to another hospital within 14 days of intensive care admittance or were admitted from another intensive care and already ventilated for longer than 3 days). Prone positioning was initiated when the pao2/fio2-ratio < 150 (while maintaining pressure support if not previously on pressure control setting). Interleukine-6 inhibitors and dexamethasone were administered as soon as evidence for their beneficial effects was established. Patient characteristics of interest are summarized in Table 1. In total, 16 of 41 patients underwent patient-triggered pressure support breathing at least 80% of the time during invasive mechanical ventilation (meaning a PS to PC ratio of 0.8). Briefly, the significant differences between a PS/PC + PS ratio above 80% versus below 80% were the Apache IV score (50 ± 14.5 vs. 66 (±17.9), SAPS II score (25 ± 0 vs. 31 (±9), and the number of patients with a creatinine level above 177 µmol/L in the first 200 h (0/16 vs. 5/25). Based on current guidelines, three of the forty-one patients required renal replacement therapy. However, this was deemed futile and not started in two cases, based on comorbidity and pre-disease performance.

Table 1. Baseline characteristics of 41 patients undergoing invasive mechanical ventilation due to COVID-19 ARDS. Numbers represent the mean ± standard deviation.

	PS-PC Ratio > 0.8	PS-PC Ratio < 0.8	p Value
n	16	25	
Age	60 (47–73)	62 (54–70)	p = 0.79 NS
Days in ICU	20 ± 18	14 (±8)	p = 0.51 NS
90-day mortality	1/16	5/25	p = 0.2 NS
APACHE IV score	50 (±14.5)	66 (±17.9)	p = 0.008 *
SAPS II	25 (±9)	31 (±9)	p = 0.02 *
APACHE IV, no AKI	47 (±14.5)	62 (±16)	p = 0.009 *
SAPS II, no AKI	24 (±8)	31 (±9)	p = 0.01 *
Peak creatinin in µmol/L	88 (±28)	160 (±150)	p = 0.2
Creatinin > 177 µmol/L in first 200 h	0/16	5/25	p = 0.05 *
PC hours first 200 h	13 (±10)	80 (±35)	p = 0.0001 *
Average PEEP §	14.31	15.25	p = 0.24

§ Set PEEP (cmH2O) with unadjusted setting for at least 4 h to exclude measurements from recruitment procedures, etc. * $p \leq 0.05$.

The group with a higher percentage of controlled mechanical ventilation had a higher incidence of AKI, defined as a creatinine level above 177 µmol/L (5/25 vs. 0/16) within the first 200 h of mechanical ventilation. However, this group also showed higher disease severity based on the increased APACHE IV and SAPS scores. When disease severity scores were corrected for AKI, the difference decreases but remains significant. In the cohort as a whole, the PS/PC + PS ratio was negatively correlated with the peak level of creatinine (r = −0.35 (−0.6–0.1) p 0.03) (see Figure 1), meaning that time spent on supported ventilation was negatively correlated with peak creatinine levels.

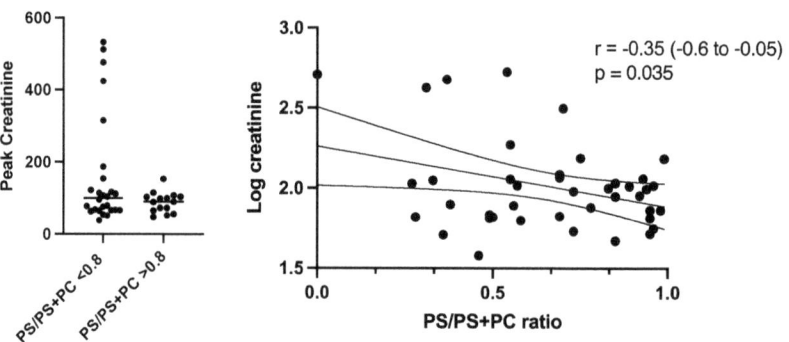

Figure 1. First panel shows the peak creatinine levels in µmol/L during the ICU stay in patients with a ratio (PS/PC + PS) above 80% and below 80%. A trend is seen but is not statistically significant (p = 0.072). In the second panel a significant negative correlation (r = −0.35) is seen between peak creatinine levels and the predominance of controlled ventilation.

4. Discussion

In this retrospective cohort study, a significant negative correlation was observed between peak creatinine levels and the predominance of controlled ventilation. Furthermore, we observed a remarkably low level of AKI compared to other intensive care patients. The occurrence of AKI in the early phase of COVID-19 disease can be the result of many factors. Overall, five patients (12.2%) showed an increase in creatinine above 177 µmol/L within 14 days after intensive care admittance, and only three (7.3%) potentially qualified for renal replacement therapy. However, in two cases RRT was not initiated due to treatment restrictions based on comorbidity and pre-disease performance. If we look at the complete cohort of mechanically ventilated COVID-19 patients, we find a much lower incidence of AKI compared to past data for this relation, i.e., ranging from 20% to as high as 90% [2,9–12].

In this cohort, as in most intensive care settings treating COVID-19 patients, several patients were ventilated with high levels of PEEP, up to 22 cmH$_2$O, and required prone positioning for longer periods of time. We found it possible to also have these patients ventilated on a patient-triggered assisted mode if sedation and analgesics were dosed accordingly. This is done through continuously monitoring end tidal CO$_2$ and performing blood-gas analysis regularly, in addition to assuring patient comfort. Clearly, hyperventilation would be an initial sign of discomfort, and hypoventilation often would result in decreasing the dosage of intravenous opiates.

A retrospective cohort study on an intensive care unit comes with many potential pitfalls and possible alternative explanations. First, a potential reason for the low AKI incidence is that patients in our cohort were less ill compared to the published cohorts. Based on APACHE IV scores (Table 1) and the fact that there was no selection of patients referred to the hospital during the pandemic, this is considered less likely. Another explanation could be that more severely ill patients were selected for transfer to other hospitals, diluting the case severity mix. However, the APACHE scores from patients in our cohort did not differ from national data from a national cohort study [13]. One factor that could influence the potential explanation for the lower AKI incidence could be the high percentage of patient-triggered breathing allowed. We hypothesize that increasing the time spent on support ventilation, more specifically patient-triggered assisted ventilation, could decrease the incidence of ventilator-induced kidney injury. This idea is supported by the significant negative relation between the time spent on assisted ventilation and peak creatinine levels. However, we are aware that our limited data must be interpreted with caution. The biggest shortcoming of this retrospective study is the difference in disease severity within this cohort, of which only a small part can be explained by the change in renal function. One could argue that comparison within this small cohort is not feasible. Alternative explanations such as comorbidities, fluid overload, vasopressor use, and nephrotoxic drugs all contribute to the incidence of AKI on the ICU. Taking this in mind, statistical results from the comparison of two groups in this small cohort might not be very useful and could be prone to bias. However, overall, the low AKI incidence and the significant relation between renal function and time spent on pressure support the idea of a renal–pulmonary interaction.

The association between controlled mechanical ventilation and AKI is of great interest and has been studied before [3,4]. The COVID-19 pandemic gives us more opportunities to compare choices made in mechanical ventilation and their effects on renal function. AKI in COVID-19 shows a relatively high incidence, as much as double that in other viral respiratory diseases such as influenza [14,15]. The suggested pathophysiology of AKI in COVID currently relies on nonspecific mechanisms (hypovolemia, nephrotoxic drugs, high PEEP, right heart failure), direct viral injury, imbalanced renin–angiotensin–aldosterone system (RAAS) activation, elevation of proinflammatory cytokines elicited by viral infection, and a profound procoagulant state [14,16]. In addition to the need for understanding the concept of renal interstitial edema when treating patients in general, limiting intravenous fluids significantly and prioritizing pressure-support modality over pressure or volume control settings could play a pivotal role. COVID-19 patients predominantly present with single-organ failure, and compared to patients with sepsis, exhibit only a limited increase in catabolic state, measured through the necessary respiratory minute volume (MV) when sufficiently sedated and anaesthetized. The MV rarely exceeds 12 L and mostly remains under 10 L without inducing hypercapnia. Therefore, in pathology limited to COVID-19, or perhaps even within other patient groups in a non-hyperdynamic state, the work of breathing is not excessive when ventilated in a pressure support manner. Therefore, it is necessary to titrate sedation and analgesia to this aim. Another contributing explanation could be the effects of neuromuscular blocking agents when used for longer periods of time. Marchiset et al. reported a significant increased risk of the development of AKI during intensive care stay associated with the use of these agents. Naturally, with the use of neuromuscular blocking agents patient-triggered breaths will be nearly absent [17].

Finally, although based on a relatively small number of patients, and even considering the potential alternative explanations for some of the AKI cases, compared with the existing literature our observations support evaluation through future studies to explore the beneficial relation between predominantly supportive ventilation and a decreased incidence in kidney injury. We feel this may be an important contributing factor explaining the increased incidence of AKI in mechanically ventilated patients, especially patients with COVID-19, and possibly even for other patients, after the suggested relation has been confirmed.

Author Contributions: M.E.S. and M.G. analyzed the data and wrote and revised the manuscript. All authors have read and agreed to the published version of the manuscript.

Funding: This research received no external funding.

Institutional Review Board Statement: Ethical review and approval were waived for this study by the LangeLand hospital ethical board. Retrospective data analysis not warranting further ethical approval.

Informed Consent Statement: Not applicable.

Data Availability Statement: The data presented in this study are available on request from the corresponding author.

Conflicts of Interest: The authors declare no conflict of interest.

References

1. Hohmann, F.; Wedekind, L.; Grundeis, F.; Dickel, S.; Frank, J.; Golinski, M.; Griesel, M.; Grimm, C.; Herchenhahn, C.; Kramer, A.; et al. Early spontaneous breathing for acute respiratory distress syndrome in individuals with COVID-19. *Cochrane Database Syst. Rev.* **2022**, *6*, CD015077. [PubMed]
2. Weaver, L.; Das, A.; Saffaran, S.; Yehya, N.; Scott, T.E.; Chikhani, M.; Laffey, J.G.; Hardman, J.G.; Comporota, L.; Batas, D.G. High risk of patient self-inflicted lung injury in COVID-19 with frequently encountered spontaneous breathing patterns: A computational modelling study. *Ann. Intensive Care* **2021**, *11*, 109. [CrossRef] [PubMed]
3. Drury, D.R.; Henry, J.P.; Goodman, J. The effects of continuous pressure breathing on kidney function. *J. Clin. Investig.* **1947**, *26*, 945–951. [CrossRef] [PubMed]
4. Hepokoski, M.L.; Malhotra, A.; Singh, P.; Crotty Alexander, L.E. Ventilator-Induced Kidney Injury: Are Novel Biomarkers the Key to Prevention? *Nephron* **2018**, *140*, 90–93. [CrossRef] [PubMed]
5. van den Akker, J.P.C.; Egal, M.; Groeneveld, A.B.J. Invasive mechanical ventilation as a risk factor for acute kidney injury in the critically ill: A systematic review and meta-analysis. *Crit. Care* **2013**, *17*, R98. [CrossRef] [PubMed]
6. Gupta, S.; Coca, S.G.; Chan, L.; Melamed, M.L.; Brenner, S.K.; Hayek, S.S.; Sutherland, A.; Puri, S.; Srivastava, A.; Leonberg-Yoo, A.; et al. AKI Treated with Renal Replacement Therapy in Critically Ill Patients with COVID-19. *J. Am. Soc. Nephrol.* **2021**, *32*, 161–176. [CrossRef] [PubMed]
7. Contrera Rolón, N.; Varela, C.F.; Ferraris, A.; Rojano, A.; Carboni Bisso, I.; Greloni, G.; Bratti, G.I.; San Román, J.E.; Heras, M.L.; Sinner, J.F.; et al. Characteristics of acute kidney injury in adult patients with severe COVID-19. *Med. (B Aires) Argent.* **2022**, *82*, 172–180.
8. Roger, C.; Collange, O.; Mezzarobba, M.; Abou-Arab, O.; Teule, L.; Garnier, M.; Hoffmann, C.; Muller, L.; Lefrant, J.-Y.; Guinot, P.G.; et al. French multicentre observational study on SARS-CoV-2 infections intensive care initial management: The French Corona study. *Anaesth. Crit. Care Pain Med.* **2021**, *40*, 100931. [CrossRef] [PubMed]
9. Nadim, M.K.; Forni, L.G.; Mehta, R.L.; Connor, M.J., Jr.; Liu, K.D.; Ostermann, M.; Rimmelé, T.; Zarbock, A.; Bell, S.; Bihorac, A.; et al. COVID-19-associated acute kidney injury: Consensus report of the 25th Acute Disease Quality Initiative (ADQI) Workgroup. *Nat. Rev. Nephrol.* **2020**, *16*, 747–764. [CrossRef] [PubMed]
10. Aukland, E.A.; Klepstad, P.; Aukland, S.M.; Ghavidel, F.Z.; Buanes, E.A. Acute kidney injury in patients with COVID-19 in the intensive care unit: Evaluation of risk factors and mortality in a national cohort. *BMJ Open.* **2022**, *12*, e059046. [CrossRef] [PubMed]

11. Arrestier, R.; Gendreau, S.; Mokrani, D.; Bastard, J.-P.; Fellahi, S.; Bagate, F.; Masi, P.; D'Humières, T.; Razazi, K.; Carteaux, G.; et al. Acute Kidney Injury in Critically-Ill COVID-19 Patients. *J. Clin. Med.* **2022**, *11*, 2029. [CrossRef] [PubMed]
12. Passoni, R.; Lordani, T.V.A.; Peres, L.A.B.; Carvalho, A.R.d.S. Occurrence of acute kidney injury in adult patients hospitalized with COVID-19: A systematic review and meta-analysis. *Nefrologia* **2022**, *42*, 404–414. [CrossRef] [PubMed]
13. Dongelmans, D.A.; Termorshuizen, F.; Brinkman, S.; Bakhshi-Raiez, F.; Arbous, M.S.; de Lange, D.W.; van Bussel, B.C.T.; de Keizer, N.F.; Verbiest, D.P.; Velde, L.F.T.; et al. Characteristics and outcome of COVID-19 patients admitted to the ICU: A nationwide cohort study on the comparison between the first and the consecutive upsurges of the second wave of the COVID-19 pandemic in the Netherlands. *Ann. Intensive Care* **2022**, *12*, 5. [CrossRef] [PubMed]
14. Gabarre, P.; Dumas, G.; Dupont, T.; Darmon, M.; Azoulay, E.; Zafrani, L. Acute kidney injury in critically ill patients with COVID-19. *Intensive Care Med.* **2020**, *46*, 1339–1348. [CrossRef] [PubMed]
15. Melero, R.; Mijaylova, A.; Rodríguez-Benítez, P.; García-Prieto, A.; Cedeño, J.; Goicoechea, M. Mortality and renal long-term outcome of critically ill COVID-19 patients with acute kidney failure, continuous renal replacement therapy and invasive mechanical ventilation. *Med. Clin.* **2022**, *159*, 529–535. [CrossRef] [PubMed]
16. Ottolina, D.; Zazzeron, L.; Trevisi, L.; Agarossi, A.; Colombo, R.; Fossali, T.; Passeri, M.; Borghi, B.; Ballone, E.; Rech, R.; et al. Acute kidney injury (AKI) in patients with COVID-19 infection is associated with ventilatory management with elevated positive end-expiratory pressure (PEEP). *J. Nephrol.* **2022**, *35*, 99–111. [CrossRef] [PubMed]
17. Marchiset, A.; Serazin, V.; Salem, O.B.H.; Pichereau, C.; Da Silva, L.L.; Au, S.-M.; Barbier, C.; Loubieres, Y.; Hayon, J.; Gross, J.; et al. Risk Factors of AKI in Acute Respiratory Distress Syndrome: A Time-Dependent Competing Risk Analysis on Severe COVID-19 Patients. *Can. J. Kidney Health Dis.* **2023**, *10*, 20543581221145073. [CrossRef] [PubMed]

Disclaimer/Publisher's Note: The statements, opinions and data contained in all publications are solely those of the individual author(s) and contributor(s) and not of MDPI and/or the editor(s). MDPI and/or the editor(s) disclaim responsibility for any injury to people or property resulting from any ideas, methods, instructions or products referred to in the content.

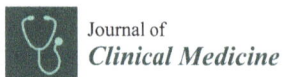

Article

Admission Lactate Concentration, Base Excess, and Alactic Base Excess Predict the 28-Day Inward Mortality in Shock Patients

Piotr Smuszkiewicz [1,†], Natalia Jawień [1,†], Jakub Szrama [1], Marta Lubarska [2], Krzysztof Kusza [1] and Przemysław Guzik [2,*]

1 Department of Anesthesiology, Intensive Therapy and Pain Management, Poznan University of Medical Sciences, 60-355 Poznan, Poland
2 Department of Cardiology—Intensive Therapy, Poznan University of Medical Sciences, 60-355 Poznan, Poland
* Correspondence: pguzik@ptkardio.pl; Tel.: +48-618691391
† These authors contributed equally to this work.

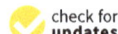

Citation: Smuszkiewicz, P.; Jawień, N.; Szrama, J.; Lubarska, M.; Kusza, K.; Guzik, P. Admission Lactate Concentration, Base Excess, and Alactic Base Excess Predict the 28-Day Inward Mortality in Shock Patients. *J. Clin. Med.* 2022, 11, 6125. https://doi.org/10.3390/jcm11206125

Academic Editor: Spyros D. Mentzelopoulos

Received: 2 September 2022
Accepted: 14 October 2022
Published: 18 October 2022

Publisher's Note: MDPI stays neutral with regard to jurisdictional claims in published maps and institutional affiliations.

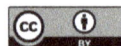

Copyright: © 2022 by the authors. Licensee MDPI, Basel, Switzerland. This article is an open access article distributed under the terms and conditions of the Creative Commons Attribution (CC BY) license (https://creativecommons.org/licenses/by/4.0/).

Abstract: Base excess (BE) and lactate concentration may predict mortality in critically ill patients. However, the predictive values of alactic BE (aBE; the sum of BE and lactate), or a combination of BE and lactate are unknown. The study aimed to investigate whether BE, lactate, and aBE measured on admission to ICU may predict the 28-day mortality for patients undergoing any form of shock. In 143 consecutive adults, arterial BE, lactate, and aBE were measured upon ICU admission. Receiver Operating Curve (ROC) characteristics and Cox proportional hazard regression models (adjusted to age, gender, forms of shock, and presence of severe renal failure) were then used to investigate any association between these parameters and 28-day mortality. aBE < −3.63 mmol/L was found to be associated with a hazard ratio of 3.19 (HR; 95% confidence interval (CI): 1.62–6.27) for mortality. Risk of death was higher for BE < −9.5 mmol/L (HR: 4.22; 95% CI: 2.21–8.05), particularly at lactate concentrations > 4.5 mmol/L (HR: 4.62; 95% CI: 2.56–8.33). A 15.71% mortality rate was found for the combined condition of BE > cut-off and lactate < cut-off. When BE was below but lactate above their respective cut-offs, the mortality rate increased to 78.91%. The Cox regression model demonstrated that the predictive values of BE and lactate were mutually independent and additive. The 28-day mortality in shock patients admitted to ICU can be predicted by aBE, but BE and lactate deliver greater prognostic value, particularly when combined. The clinical value of our findings deserves further prospective evaluation.

Keywords: base excess; alactic base excess; hyperlactatemia; mortality; shock

1. Introduction

Shock is a life-threatening haemodynamic emergency associated with tissue and organ hypoperfusion, leading to severe metabolic changes at the cellular level. Low oxygen delivery, high oxygen consumption, or inadequate utilisation can prompt various metabolic derangements, thus resulting in an acid–base imbalance with or without hyperlactataemia.

Patients in shock are routinely admitted to an intensive care unit (ICU). Mortality is usually high in such patients but varies depending on clinical status, for example, due to metabolic abnormalities. Identifying the most at-risk patients is necessary for successful treatment to prevent further deterioration, to reverse metabolic derangements, and to reduce mortality. In addition to standard risk scores, e.g., Sequential Organ Failure Assessment (SOFA) [1], various parameters have been evaluated in critically ill individuals for assessing mortality risk.

Predictive value has been demonstrated for acid–base balance parameters or lactate concentration and its kinetics in ICU patients [2–8], including those with septic shock, unstable haemodynamics, cardiac arrest, urgency laparotomy, and patients requiring ECMO support during transportation [9–15].

Lactate metabolism in shock patients is very complex. Traditionally, hyperlactataemia is interpreted as an indicator of anaerobic metabolism due to tissue hypoxia [16–18]. It may also reflect abnormal oxygen extraction and utilisation, effects of prolonged excess of catecholamines, presence of veno-arterial shunts in peripheral tissues [19–24], mitochondrial dysfunction [25], liver dysfunction impairing lactate clearance [26], and thiamine depletion due to shock-induced upregulated metabolic processes [27].

Hyperlactataemia may be accompanied by metabolic acidosis or as a separate phenomenon not affecting the acid–base status. In 2019, Gattinoni et al. [28] proposed the term alactic base excess (aBE) to distinguish between metabolic acidosis caused by lactate accumulation and that caused by increased amounts of non-lactate fixed acids (unmeasured strong anions) not eliminated through the lungs, e.g., phosphate and sulphate acids. Conceptually, aBE is a sum of negative values of BE and lactate. Gattinoni et al. [28] studied aBE in septic patients, concluding that it possibly reflects the impact of renal dysfunction on plasma lactate concentration and acid–base balance. They have also demonstrated that increased plasma lactate indicates sepsis severity and that aBE may be used to estimate renal capability to control acid–base balance.

Nevertheless, the predictive value of aBE has not yet been investigated in either septic or non-septic ICU patients. In this study, we aim to investigate a potential prognostic value of aBE and its contributors, i.e., BE and lactate concentration to predicting 28-day mortality in shock patients admitted to ICU. Additionally, we examine whether the prognostic values of BE and lactate are simultaneously independent and additive.

2. Materials and Methods

2.1. Study Design and Population

It is a retrospective observational study using clinical data of patients hospitalized in a teaching hospital's mixed medical–surgical ICU. The study included one hundred forty-three consecutive adult patients (minimum age 18 years) with any form of shock, unconscious at admission, requiring intravenous norepinephrine and mechanical ventilation. All were new patients not hospitalized before at any other ICU or another hospital for the current clinical state. The only exclusion criterion was moribund status. Patients were managed with standard procedures, including treatment of the underlying cause, lung protective mechanical ventilation, hemodynamic monitoring, fluid resuscitation, supply of vasoactive agents, and other clinically justified interventions. In the case of septic shock, patients were treated according to the guidelines of the Surviving Sepsis Campaign, including the appropriate administration of antibiotics [29]. The scientific purpose of this study did not affect any clinical decisions or the duration of inward stay. According to the enrolment criteria, patients were unconscious at the time of admission. Thus, the Bioethics Committee at the Poznan University of Medical Sciences in Poland waived the requirement to obtain informed consent and approved the study protocol. All patients were given unique codes to keep their anonymity in the database. No names or contact details were circulating among researchers involved in the study. In this way, patients' anonymity was preserved. All methods were carried out following relevant guidelines and regulations.

Data Collection

Patient information on demographics, Acute Physiology and Chronic Health Evaluation II's (APACHE II) [30], and SOFA score [1] were collected. The results of standard clinical and laboratory parameters were also collected, including arterial and central venous blood gas analysis measured at the bedside within the first 5–10 min after admission to the ICU (Radiometer ABL 90 Flex Plus). Standard BE and aBE per patient were calculated according to Gattinoni [28] as follows:

$$\text{standard BE (mmol/L)} = [HCO_3 \text{ (mmol/L)} - 24.8 \text{ (mmol/L)}] + 16.2 \text{ mmol/L} \times (pH - 7.4)$$

$$\text{alactic BE (mmol/L)} = \text{standard Base Excess (mmol/L)} + \text{lactate (mmol/L)}$$

2.2. Data Coding and Statistical Analysis

Qualitative data were represented as overall numbers and percentages or by subgroups of survivors and non-survivors. All continuous data were summarised using either mean values with standard deviation (SD), or medians with the 25th and 75th percentiles (IQR) due to normal or non-Gaussian distributions (the D'Agostino-Pearson normality test).

Total mortality during the 28-day hospitalisation at the ICU was used as a primary end-point. Patients discharged earlier were treated as censored without further follow-up, whereas patients who required extended ICU stay were labelled as alive. Those who were re-admitted to the ICU were not considered as separate hospitalisations. The date of death, discharge from ICU, or end of follow-up was recorded for each patient. All patients were divided into categories of those who survived or died during the 28-day ICU stay for comparisons of (1) continuous data (with either the unpaired t-test or Mann–Whitney test, as appropriate); (2) binomial data (with the Fisher exact test). The Receiver Operating Curve (ROC) characteristics test was used to analyse the association of BE, lactate concentration, and aBE with 28-day mortality, using optimal cut-off values for these parameters determined by the Youden criterion. The Cox proportional hazard models were adjusted to the patient's age, gender, type of shock (four categories: septic, cardiac, hypovolemic, and other), and the presence of estimated glomerular filtration rate (eGFR) <30 mL/min/1.73 m^2. The results were then shown as Hazard Ratios (HR) with their 95% Confidence Interval (95% CI). Different Cox Hazard models were built based only on cut-off values of BE, lactate concentration, or aBE. Additional models for BE and lactate concentration cut-off values were built according to the following criteria:

- category 0—if BE was above (less severe or no acidaemia) and lactate concentration was below (non-severe or no hyperlactataemia) their respective cut-off values, i.e., no patient had severe acidaemia and hyperlactataemia;
- category 1—if either BE was below or lactate concentration was above their respective cut-off values, i.e., patients with either severe acidaemia or severe hyperlactataemia;
- category 2—if both BE was below and lactate concentration was above their respective cut-off values, i.e., patients with coexisting severe acidosis and hyperlactataemia.

Finally, both BE and lactate concentration values were entered into the same Cox Hazard model to investigate whether they have independent and additive predictive values.

Mutual associations between indices of renal function, i.e., between creatinine concentration and estimated glomerular filtration rate (eGFR), or between BE, aBE, and lactate concentration, were analysed using the Spearman correlation. The correlation between aBE and either lactate concentration or BE was not analysed since aBE is mathematically related to both.

Statistical differences with $p < 0.05$ were considered to be significant. All statistical analyses were performed using the MedCalc Statistical Software version 19.1 (MedCalc Software bv, Ostend, Belgium) or PQStat version 1.8.2.202 (PQStat Software, Poznan, Poland).

3. Results

Table 1 summarises the comparison of clinical characteristics related to the main hypotheses between survivors and non-survivors. The clinical characteristics of all studied patients are shown in Table S1 for qualitative and Table S2 for quantitative data. The comparisons of other clinical characteristics between survivors and non-survivors are presented in Table S3 for the qualitative and Table S4 for the quantitative data.

Non-survivors were older by six years; had higher APACHE II and SOFA scores, 10 points and 3 points, respectively; and required additional vasoactive drugs more frequently than survivors. Hypovolemic shock was less frequent but $SaO_2 < 94\%$ was present in every second patient from non-survivors. Their pH, standard HCO_3, BE, and aBE were found to be significantly lower (reduced to approximately -7 mmol/L and -4.5 mmol/L for BE and aBE, respectively), whereas lactate concentration was higher (>2.5 mmol/L). Non-survivors had significantly more frequent reduced bicarbonates, acidaemia, and hyperlactatemia. Median values of systolic and diastolic BP were also lower in non-survivors than survivors at the admission to ICU.

Table 1. Summary of comparisons of clinical characteristics in a group of patients with shock divided into survivors and non-survivors of the 28-day stay at ICU.

	Qualitative Data					
	Survivors		Non-Survivors		# p Value
Parameter	N	%	N	%	
Number of patients	90	63	53	37	
Men	65	72.2	30	56.6	0.0677
Cardiogenic shock	18	20.0	18	34.0	0.0743
Hypovolemic shock	23	25.6	5	9.4	0.0278
Septic shock	49	54.4	30	56.6	0.8626
Other shocks	4	4.4	3	5.7	0.7102
Additional catecholamine	23	25.6	27	50.9	0.0034
eGFR < 30 mL/min/1.73 m^2	29	32.2	20	37.7	0.5849
SaO$_2$ < 94%	28	31.1	27	50.9	0.0216
standard HCO$_3^-$ < 22 mmol/L	49	54.4	46	86.8	<0.0001
pH < 7.35	61	67.8	45	84.9	0.0295
BE < −3 mmol/L	60	66.7	46	86.8	0.0098
Lactate concentration > 2 mmol/L	51	56.7	46	86.8	0.0002

	Continuous and Discrete Data									
	Survivors					Non-Survivors				
Parameter	Mean	SD	Median	25 P.	75 P.	Mean	SD	Median	25 P.	75 P.	p Value
Age (years)	58.42	14.54	61	47	69	65.51	11.85	67	59	72	0.0031
APACHE II	21.91	7.49	22	16.25	27	31.55	7.38	32	27	38	<0.0001 *
SOFA	11.67	3.09	12	10	14	14.45	2.76	15	12.75	16	<0.0001 *
Length of ICU stay (days)	9.57	8	6	4	14	5.78	6.41	3	1	10	0.6427 *
HR (beats/min)	108.73	17.99	110	95	120	111.04	22.94	115	100	120	0.3364 *
Systolic BP (mmHg)	123.69	29.60	120.00	105.00	145.00	105.111	31.8764	109.000	82.75	122.00	0.0236 *
Diastolic BP (mmHg)	66.79	15.64	67.00	58.00	80.00	53.556	17.3700	56.000	40.50	64.25	0.0026 *
Creatinine (mg/dL)	2.05	1.66	1.44	0.98	2.7	2.3	1.64	1.68	1.14	2.82	0.162 *
pH	7.29	0.13	7.3	7.23	7.38	7.17	0.16	7.2	7.12	7.29	<0.0001
Standard HCO$_3$ (mmol/L)	21	5.46	20.95	17.7	24.2	16.1	5.79	15.7	13.28	18.25	<0.0001
Standard BE (mmol/L)	−5.65	7.17	−5.46	−9.53	−0.93	−12.37	8.07	−12.26	−16.98	−9.15	<0.0001
Lactate level (mmol/L)	3.36	3.03	2.45	1.3	3.9	6.43	4.85	5	2.58	8.3	<0.0001 *
aBE (mmol/L)	−2.29	6.13	−1.93	−6.24	1.44	−5.93	6.39	−6.46	−10.19	−3.36	0.001

Fisher exact test for binomial data; * Mann–Whitney test. Abbreviations: aBE—alactic base excess; APACHE II—the Acute Physiology and Chronic Health Evaluation II; BE—base excess; BP—blood pressure; HCO$_3$—bicarbonate concentration; HR—heart rate; ICU—intensive care unit; P.—percentile; pH—the power of hydrogen; SOFA—Sequential Organ Failure Assessment.

AUCs from the ROC analysis were observed to be largest for BE and smallest for aBE, with the AUC for BE being larger than that of aBE ($p = 0.0049$). No significant differences in AUCs were observed when comparing lactate concentration with either BE ($p = 0.4946$) or aBE ($p = 0.4355$). ROC analysis results with AUCs and identified cut-off values of BE, lactic concentration, and aBE are shown in Figure 1.

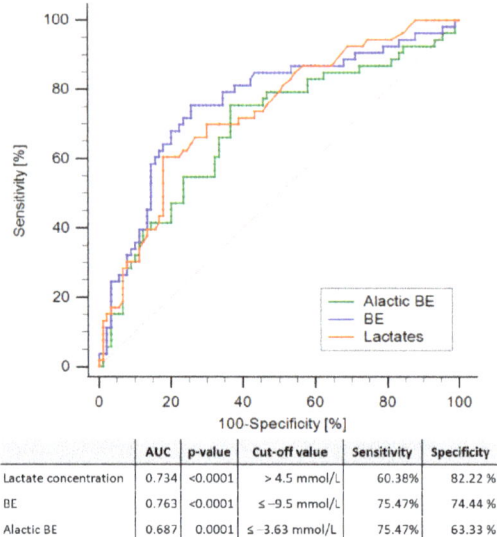

Figure 1. Results of the Receiver Operator Curve characteristics analysis for the prediction of 28-day mortality in shock patients hospitalised in intensive care by aBE (green line), BE (blue line), and lactate concentration (orange line). Median values of areas under the curve (AUC), optimal cut-offs, specificity and sensitivity of BE, lactic concentration, and aBE are shown underneath the graph. Abbreviations: AUC—area under the curve; BE—base excess.

Table 2 summarises mortality rates for specific subgroups of patients stratified according to the defined cut-offs for BE; lactate concentration; aBE; and categories 0, 1, and 2, reflecting various combinations of the cut-offs for BE and lactates. The 28-day ICU mortality in shock patients was found to be lowest for category 0 (15.71%) and highest for category 2 (78.94%).

Table 2. The mortality rate in specific subgroups of patients stratified to cut-off values of BE; lactate concentration; alactic BE; or categories 0, 1, and 2 based on combined cut-offs of BE and lactate concentration.

Stratifying Variable	Non-Survivors	Mortality Rate (%)
BE > −9.5 mmol/L	13	16.25
BE < −9.5 mmol/L	40	63.49
Lactate concentration < 4.5 mmol/L	21	22.11
Lactate concentration > 4.5 mmol/L	32	66.67
aBE > −3.63 mmol/L	13	18.57
aBE < −3.63 mmol/L	40	54.79
Category 0 (BE > −9.5 mmol/L and lactates < 4.5 mmol/L)	11	15.71
Category 1 (either BE < −9.5 mmol/L or lactates > 4.5 mmol/L)	12	21.81
Category 2 (both BE > −9.5 mmol/L and lactates < 4.5 mmol/L)	30	78.94

Abbreviations: aBE—alactic base excess; BE—base excess.

In unadjusted and adjusted Cox regression models, patients with BE < −9.5 mmol/L, lactate concentration > 4.5 mmol/L, or aBE < −3.63 mmol/L had significantly increased risk of premature death during the 28-day ICU stay (Table 3).

In these models, a change in one category from 0 to 1, or from 1 to 2 was also significantly associated with mortality. Figure 2 shows survival curves derived from Cox proportional hazard models for patients stratified by either the cut-off values for BE; lactate concentration; aBE; or categories 0, 1, or 2 (i.e., three combinations of BE and lactate cut-offs).

Table 3. Results of unadjusted and adjusted Cox proportional hazards regression models for the 28-day ICU mortality in patients with shock. Adjustments were made according to patients' age, gender, presence of severe renal failure (eGFR < 30 mL/min/1.73 m^2), and type of shock.

Stratifying Variable	Unadjusted Model			Adjusted Model		
	HR	95% CI	p Value	HR	95% CI	p Value
BE < −9.5 mmol/L	4.26	2.27–7.98	<0.0001	4.22	2.21–8.05	<0.0001
Lactate concentration > 4.5 mmol/L	3.58	2.05–6.23	<0.0001	4.62	2.56–8.33	<0.0001
aBE < −3.63 mmol/L	3.09	1.65–5.78	0.0004	3.19	1.62–6.27	0.0008
Change of one category	2.68	1.88–3.84	<0.0001	2.78	1.94–4.01	<0.0001

Abbreviations: aBE—alactic base excess; BE—base excess; CI—confidence interval; HR—hazard ratio.

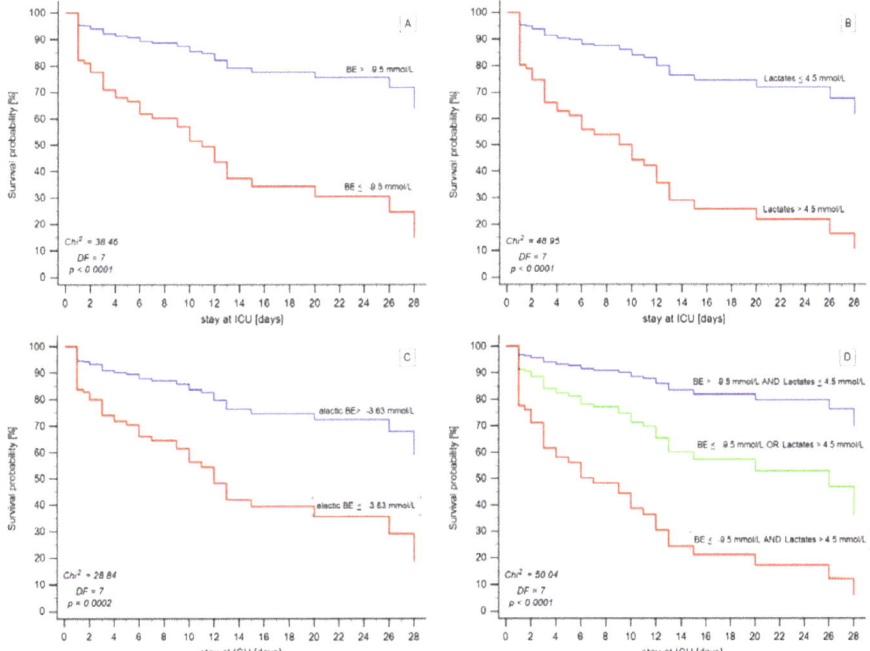

Figure 2. Comparison of survival curves modelled by the Cox proportional hazard regressions for the 28-day ICU mortality in shock patients, stratified according to the admission values of BE (Panel (**A**)), lactate concentration (Panel (**B**)), aBE (Panel (**C**)), and the combination of BE and lactate concentration (Panel (**D**)) based on cut-off values defined by the ROC analysis. Red lines correspond to patients with the highest risk, whereas blue lines correspond to those with the lowest risk. The green line in Panel (**D**) corresponds to the middle-risk group (category 1). Values of chi^2, degrees of freedom (DF), and *p* for the models are shown in the bottom-left corners of each panel. Abbreviations: BE—base excess; aBE—alactic base excess, DF—degrees of freedom; ICU—intensive care unit.

As BE and lactate concentrations (dichotomised according to their cut-off values) have prognostic values both as single covariates or combined into categories, it was also investigated whether they were simultaneously independent of one another and additive. The final adjusted Cox regression model (chi^2 = 50.13; $p < 0.0001$) confirmed these assumptions with a hazard ratio of 2.54 (95% CI 1.25–5.15; $p = 0.0100$) for BE < −9.5 mmol/L and 3.02 (95% CI 1.58–5.78; $p = 0.0008$) for aBE.

From the nonparametric Spearman correlation, it was found that BE values and lactate concentrations were significantly and negatively correlated (rho = −0.58; $p < 0.0001$) (Figure 3). Upon visual inspection, relatively more non-survivors (Figure 3, Panel A) are located in the bottom right quadrant of the graph (patients from category 2 with the most severe acidaemia and hyperlactatemia) than in the remaining quadrants. The upper left quadrant contains the fewest non-survivors (patients from category 0). When severe renal failure was considered, patients from category 2 did not present eGFR < 30 mL/min/1.73 m^2 more often than patients from other categories.

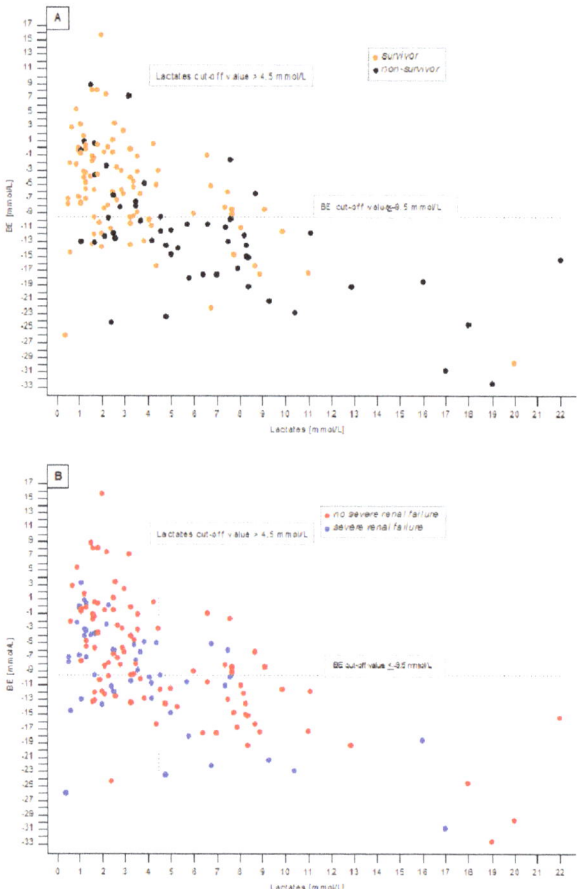

Figure 3. Association between BE value and lactate concentration in all patients, with a horizontal line for the BE cut-off and a vertical line for the lactates cut-off. In this way, four quadrants are presented. Patients in category 0 are in the upper left quadrant, and those from category 2 are in the bottom right quadrant. Individuals from category 1 are either in the upper right or bottom left quadrants. The same association is shown in both panels (**A**,**B**). However, in panel (**A**), patients are marked according to their ICU survival status at the end of the 28-day follow-up, whereas in panel (**B**), patients are marked according to the presence of severe renal failure, i.e., eGFR < 30 mL/min/1.73 m^2.

Associations between creatinine concentration or eGFR and BE, aBE, and lactate concentration are shown in Table 4. Lactate concentration was found not to correlate with either creatinine or eGFR, whereas BE and aBE were significant, although weakly related. Worsening of renal function was associated with deteriorating acidosis, regardless of whether BE or aBE was considered.

Table 4. Spearman correlation between renal function indices and BE, aBE, and lactate concentration.

Parameters	Creatinine Concentration		eGFR	
	Rho	p Value	rho	p Value
BE	−0.29	0.0004	0.31	0.0002
Lactate concentration	0.02	0.7952	−0.03	0.7216
aBE	−0.36	0.0000	0.37	0.0000

Abbreviations: BE—base excess; aBE—alactic BE; eGFR—estimated glomerular filtration rate; rho—coefficient of nonparametric Spearman correlation.

4. Discussion

We report that lactate concentration, standard BE, and alactic BE measured on admission to the ICU in patients with shock can have prognostic values for determining 28-day ICU mortality. The prognostic value of these parameters is significant regardless of the effects of age, gender, type of shock, and presence of eGFR < 30 mL/min/1.73 m^2. Moreover, the prognostic value of standard BE and lactate concentration are independent and additive, with their combined values allowing for the classification of shock patients into low, moderate, and high-risk categories of mortality.

A direct comparison of our findings with other studies is problematic. Lactate and BE are routinely measured in critically ill patients suffering from various diseases, and both serve as mortality predictors in ICU (for example, in post-cardiac surgery patients or those with cardiogenic shock, ruptured abdominal aortic aneurysms, or trauma) [4,31–41]. Whether BE or lactate concentrations serve as better predictors of mortality in critical care patients has not yet been determined [4,33–36], with no studies reporting with certainty whether these predictors are both independent and/or additive.

All studies focus on critically ill patients. However, substantial differences in clinical features still exist (e.g., the cause and severity of specific clinical conditions, treatment methods, and length of stay or follow-up).

Smith et al. [42] found that both BE and lactate correlated with mortality for 148 patients admitted to ICU for different reasons. However, upon admission, the SOFA score for all patients was ≤5, with approximately 70% needing mechanical ventilation and 35% requiring an intravenous infusion of catecholamines. In contrast, the median SOFA for patients enrolled in this study was 13 points, with all patients requiring mechanical ventilation and infusion of at least norepinephrine.

Similarly, Schork et al. reported a relationship between lactate, BE, and pH and mortality in 4067 intensive care unit patients [40]. The predicted mortality by SAPS II was 29%, and only 47% of them required mechanical ventilation. For admission to ICU, the cut-off values for mortality were 2.1 mmol/L for lactate and −3.8 mmol/L for BE [40]. Compared with that study, all our patients were mechanically ventilated, their predicted mortality assessed by the SOFA score was around 55%, and the cut-offs for lactate and BE were 4.5 mmol/L and −9.5 mmol/L, respectively.

Wernly et al. [43] studied approximately 5600 septic patients. They found simultaneous acidosis and hyperlactataemia to be stronger predictors of mortality than either acidosis or lactate concentration (>2.3 mmol/L) alone. Similarly to our study, all patients were categorised into three groups according to acidosis with BE ≤6 and hyperlactataemia with lactate concentration >2.3 mmol/L. The cut-off values of BE and lactate concentrations for a higher risk of 28-day ICU mortality suggest that the patients in our study had even more advanced acidaemia (−6 vs. <−9.5 mmol/L for BE) and hyperlactataemia (>2.3 vs. >4.5 mmol/L for lactates) than those in Wernly et al.'s study [43]. Additionally, the patients in our study suffered from more severe shock, with all (vs. 76% for Wernly et al. [43]) requiring intubation with mechanical ventilation and intravenous infusion of norepinephrine, with an average SOFA score approximately six points higher (12.7 ± 3.25 vs. 7 ± 4).

It is also worth noting that some parameters, e.g., BE, are computed using different formulas in various studies. For example, Wernly et al. [43] used the Van Slyke equation for BE computation [44], whereas Smith et al. [42] used BE measured directly by a standard ward-based arterial blood gas analyser (Radio-meter ABL system 625/620), providing no formula. We apply the same formula in our practice as Gattinoni [28]. For these reasons, any comparison between various studies becomes difficult.

Both BE and lactate sum up to aBE, which, according to Gattinoni et al. [28], is a marker of a possible accumulation of plasma acids excreted by kidneys. It thus indirectly reflects the renal regulation of acid–base balance. Gattinoni et al. [28] have postulated that aBE measurements should improve the management of critically ill patients. Wernly et al. [43] were the first to demonstrate that aBE has any, although weak, predictive value for ICU mortality in a large group of 5586 septic patients (AUC 0.56, 95% CI 0.54–0.58). We expand upon this, demonstrating that admission aBE may predict the risk of 28-day ICU mortality in shock patients regardless of the impact of several other covariates, including the presence of severe renal failure.

Gattinoni et al. [28] postulated that hyperlactataemia accompanies acidaemia if renal function deteriorates. In our study, Cox regression models adjusted to the presence of eGFR < 30 mL/min/1.73 m^2 confirmed that BE, aBE, and lactate concentration were all predictors of death in patients with and without severely impaired renal function. Table 4 shows that, in contrast to BE and aBE, lactate concentration is not correlated with indices of renal function. It can be seen from Figure 3 that lactate and BE are negatively related. Four quadrants defined by BE and lactate cut-offs illustrate how survivors and non-survivors separate into groups of varying mortality rates. It also aids in visualising how a combination of BE and lactates further stratifies patients in shock into categories of lowest, moderate, and highest mortality. This figure independently confirms the results of Cox regression models and survival curves, separating all patients into three categories according to BE and lactate concentration values. To our knowledge, no other study has reported similar findings. Figure 3 also demonstrates that individuals with severe renal failure are relatively equally scattered across the lactate concentration and BE correlogram.

Similarly to other studies, our investigation confirms that patients in shock with severe acidosis (BE < −9.5 mmol/L) or hyperlactataemia (lactate > 4.5 mmol/L) upon admission are at increased risk of ICU mortality. Novel findings of our study are as follows: firstly, alactic BE has not been shown before to predict mortality in shock patients. We demonstrate that alactic BE measured upon admission (<−3.63 mmol/L) and indicating the presence of severe acidosis originating from non-lactic organic acids may also predict ICU mortality. Second, the predictive value of lactates and BE is independent and additive. When both are combined, three groups of shock patients can be separated, low, medium, and high risk. The coexistence of both severe acidosis and hyperlactatemia (category 2) appeared to be the most vital risk factor for premature death in ICU shock patients. Finally, the cut-off values for BE and lactates indicate that analysed high-risk patients present more profound acidosis and hyperlactataemia than in other studies suggesting that people undergoing more severe acidosis are treatable and can be rescued.

Targeting such metabolic abnormalities is complex, and it is unknown whether such patients will benefit from even more attention and even more aggressive therapy, but it is always worth trying to intensify our management. The risk stratification of shock patients into low, medium, and high-risk categories based on the admission acid-base analysis, allows for a very early selection of patients with the highest risk of dying with the most severe acidosis and hyperlactataemia. Our finding appears to yield interesting clinical and prognostic information and might be used for future planning of a prospective study on such individuals. We also underline that alactic BE may provide predictive information for 28-day mortality. However, the combination of lactates and BE appears to outperform the prognostic information derived from either lactate alone, BE alone, or alactic BE.

Limitations of This Study

It was a single-centre study involving a relatively small number of patients. However, many other similar studies are also single-centred. Included patients were admitted to the ICU at various stages of their acute critical condition, a shock of mixed aetiology. Some were admitted directly from their home due to sudden cardiac arrest, cardiovascular collapse, or out-of-hospital environment after accidents. Other patients were already hospitalised at other departments, e.g., surgery, cardiology, or neurology. Nevertheless, all patients were enrolled consecutively without complex inclusion or exclusion criteria, so the distribution of different forms of shock and the severity of clinical conditions reflect daily ICU practice. However, the rate of different shocks and patient management may not be the same in various hospitals and ICU units. Compared to other studies, a new limitation was introduced by cut-off values for BE and lactates to predict death during hospitalisation in ICU. It appears to be a consequence of distinct clinical features and/or various formulas used for BE calculation. We have deliberately applied the same formula as Gattinoni et al. [28] to overcome this issue partially. Even though the reported cut-offs for BE and lactate concentration in our subjects suggest that they were undergoing more severe acidosis than subjects in other studies [7,8,13,33,40,42,43,45]. It may also suggest that their progression in intensive care shifts the border of severe acidosis from a morbid to treatable zone, giving more high-risk patients hope for survival.

5. Conclusions

We have demonstrated that aBE <-3.63 mmol/L may be associated with an increased risk of 28-day all-cause mortality. Additionally, the predictive value of BE and lactate concentration, which contributes to aBE, is independent and additive. Finally, the combination of BE < -9.5 mmol/L and lactate > 4.5 mmol/L better selects patients at the highest risk of death than BE or lactate concentration alone, or aBE. Notably, the predictive value of these metabolic indices is significant regardless of the influence of patients' age, gender, a form of shock, and the presence of severe renal failure.

Supplementary Materials: The following supporting information can be downloaded at: https://www.mdpi.com/article/10.3390/jcm11206125/s1, Table S1: Summary of additional qualitative clinical characteristics of all studied patients with shock admitted to ICU; Table S2: Summary of additional quantitative and discrete clinical characteristics of all studied patients with shock admitted to ICU; Tables S3 and S4: Comparison of additional qualitative data rates between the 28-day survivors and non-survivors admitted due to shock to ICU.

Author Contributions: Conceptualization, P.S., N.J., P.G.; methodology, N.J., P.S., P.G.; formal analysis, P.S., N.J., P.G.; investigation, N.J., P.S., J.S., K.K., P.G.; resources, P.S., N.J., J.S., M.L., P.G.; data curation, P.S., N.J., P.G.; statistical analysis, P.G.; writing—original draft preparation, N.J., P.S., J.S., K.K., P.G.; writing—review and editing, N.J., P.S., J.S., M.L., K.K., P.G. supervision; P.G., K.K. All authors have read and agreed to the published version of the manuscript.

Funding: This research received no external funding.

Institutional Review Board Statement: The study was conducted in accordance with the Declaration of Helsinki and approved by the Bioethics Committee at the Poznan University of Medical Sciences on 5 April 2019.

Informed Consent Statement: Patient consent was waived by the Bioethics Committee at the Poznan University of Medical Sciences.

Data Availability Statement: The datasets generated and/or analysed for this study are currently not publicly available due to their in other analyses. Selected data, however, are available from the corresponding author upon request.

Conflicts of Interest: The authors declare no conflict of interest.

References

1. Vincent, J.-L.; De Mendonca, A.; Cantraine, F.; Moreno, R.; Takala, J.; Suter, P.M.; Sprung, C.L.; Colardyn, F.; Blecher, S. Use of the SOFA score to assess the incidence of organ dysfunction/failure in intensive care units: Results of a multicenter, prospective study. *Crit. Care Med.* **1988**, *26*, 1793–1800. [CrossRef]
2. Masyuk, M.; Wernly, B.; Lichtenauer, M.; Franz, M.; Kabisch, B.; Muessig, J.M.; Zimmermann, G.; Lauten, A.; Schulze, P.C.; Hoppe, U.C.; et al. Prognostic relevance of serum lactate kinetics in critically ill patients. *Intensiv. Care Med.* **2019**, *45*, 55–61. [CrossRef]
3. Davis, J.W.; Kaups, K.L. Base deficit in the elderly: A marker of severe injury and death. *J. Trauma* **1998**, *45*, 873–877. [CrossRef]
4. Zante, B.; Reichenspurner, H.; Kubik, M.; Kluge, S.; Schefold, J.C.; Pfortmueller, C.A. Base excess is superior to lactate-levels in prediction of ICU mortality after cardiac surgery. *PLoS ONE* **2018**, *5*, e0205309. [CrossRef]
5. Vitek, V.; Cowley, R.A. Blood lactate in the prognosis of various forms of shock. *Ann Surg.* **1971**, *173*, 308–313. [CrossRef]
6. Bakker, J.; Coffernils, M.; Leon, M.; Gris, P.; Vincent, J.L. Blood lactate levels are superior to oxygen-derived variables in predicting outcome in human septic shock. *Chest* **1991**, *99*, 956–962. [CrossRef]
7. Jansen, T.C.; van Bommel, J.; Woodward, R.; Mulder, P.G.; Bakker, J. Association between blood lactate levels, Sequential Organ Failure Assessment subscores, and 28-day mortality during early and late intensive care unit stay: A retrospective observational study. *Crit. Care Med.* **2009**, *37*, 2369–2374. [CrossRef]
8. Vanni, S.; Viviani, G.; Baioni, M.; Pepe, G.; Nazerian, P.; Socci, F.; Bartolucci, M.; Bartolini, M.; Grifoni, S. Prognostic value of plasma lactate levels among patients with acute pulmonary embolism: The thrombo-embolism lactate outcome study. *Ann. Emerg. Med.* **2013**, *61*, 330–338. [CrossRef]
9. Shapiro, N.I.; Howell, M.D.; Talmor, D.; Nathanson, L.A.; Lisbon, A.; Wolfe, R.E.; Weiss, J.W. Serum lactate as a predictor of mortality in emergency department patients with infection. *Ann. Emerg. Med.* **2005**, *45*, 524–548. [CrossRef]
10. Ferreruela, M.; Raurich, J.M.; Ayestarán, I.; Llompart-Pou, J.A. Hyperlactataemia in ICU patients: Incidence, causes and associated mortality. *J. Crit. Care* **2017**, *42*, 200–205. [CrossRef]
11. Chertoff, J.; Chisum, M.; Simmons, L.; King, B.; Walker, M.; Lascano, J. Prognostic utility of plasma lactate measured between 24 and 48 h after initiation of early goal-directed therapy in the management of sepsis, severe sepsis, and septic shock. *J. Intensiv. Care* **2016**, *4*, 13. [CrossRef]
12. Lee, S.G.; Song, J.; Park, D.W.; Moon, S.; Cho, H.J.; Kim, J.Y.; Park, J.; Cha, J.H. Prognostic value of lactate levels and lactate clearance in sepsis and septic shock with initial hyperlactataemia: A retrospective cohort study according to the Sepsis-3 definitions. *Medicine* **2021**, *100*, e24835. [CrossRef]
13. Burstein, B.; Vallabhajosyula, S.; Ternus, B.; Barsness, G.W.; Kashani, K.; Jentzer, J.C. The Prognostic Value of Lactate in Cardiac Intensive Care Unit Patients with Cardiac Arrest and Shock. *Shock* **2021**, *55*, 613–619. [CrossRef]
14. Jobin, S.P.; Maitra, S.; Baidya, D.K.; Subramaniam, R.; Prasad, G.; Seenu, V. Role of serial lactate measurement to predict 28-day mortality in patients undergoing emergency laparotomy for perforation peritonitis: Prospective observational study. *J. Intensiv. Care* **2019**, *7*, 58. [CrossRef]
15. Rypulak, E.; Szczukocka, M.; Zyzak, K.; Piwowarczyk, P.; Borys, M.; Czuczwar, M. Transportation of patients with severe respiratory failure on ECMO support. Four-year experience of a single ECMO center. *Anaesthesiol. Intensiv. Ther.* **2020**, *52*, 91–96. [CrossRef]
16. Rimachi, R.; Bruzzi de Carvahlo, F.; Orellano-Jimenez, C.; Cotton, F.; Vincent, J.L.; De Backer, D. Lactate/pyruvate ratio as a marker of tissue hypoxia in circulatory and septic shock. *Anaesth. Intensiv. Care* **2012**, *40*, 427–432. [CrossRef]
17. Nakane, M. Biological effects of the oxygen molecule in critically ill patients. *J. Intensiv. Care* **2020**, *8*, 95. [CrossRef]
18. Russel, A.; Rivers, E.; Giri, P.; Jaehne, A.; Nguyen, B. A physiologic Approach to Hemodynamic Monitoring and Optimizing Oxygen Delivery in Shock Resuscitation. *J. Clin. Med.* **2020**, *9*, 2052. [CrossRef]
19. Hernandez, G.; Boerma, E.C.; Dubin, A.; Bruhn, A.; Koopmans, M.; Edul, V.K.; Ruiz, C.; Castro, R.; Pozo, M.O.; Pedreros, C.; et al. Severe abnormalities in microvascular perfused vessel density are associated to organ dysfunctions and mortality and can be predicted by hyperlactataemia and norepinephrine requirements in septic shock patients. *J. Crit. Care* **2013**, *28*, e9–e14. [CrossRef]
20. Hernandez, G.; Bellomo, R.; Bakker, J. The ten pitfalls of lactate clearance in sepsis. *Intensiv. Care Med.* **2019**, *45*, 82–85. [CrossRef]
21. Suetrong, B.; Walley, K.R. Lactic Acidosis in Sepsis: It's Not All Anaerobic: Implications for Diagnosis and Management. *Chest* **2016**, *149*, 252–261. [CrossRef]
22. Garcia-Alvarez, M.; Marik, P.; Bellomo, R. Sepsis-associated hyperlactataemia. *Crit. Care* **2014**, *9*, 503. [CrossRef]
23. Marik, P.E.; Bellomo, R. Lactate clearance as a target of therapy in sepsis: A flawed paradigm. *OA Crit. Care* **2013**, *1*, 3. [CrossRef]
24. Ince, C.; Mik, E.G. Microcirculatory and mitochondrial hypoxia in sepsis, shock, and resuscitation. *J. Appl. Physiol.* **2016**, *120*, 226–235. [CrossRef]
25. Brealey, D.; Brand, M.; Hargreaves, I.; Heales, S.; Land, J.; Smolenski, R.; Davies, N.A.; Cooper, C.E.; Singer, M. Association between mitochondrial dysfunction and severity and outcome of septic shock. *Lancet* **2002**, *360*, 219–223. [CrossRef]
26. Sterling, S.A.; Puskarich, M.A.; Jones, A.E. The effect of liver disease on lactate normalisation in severe sepsis and septic shock: A cohort study. *Clin. Exp. Emerg. Med.* **2015**, *2*, 197–202. [CrossRef]
27. Donnino, M.W.; Andersen, L.W.; Chase, M.; Berg, K.M.; Tidswell, M.; Giberson, T.; Wolfe, R.; Moskowitz, A.; Smithline, H.; Ngo, L.; et al. Randomized, Double-Blind, Placebo-Controlled Trial of Thiamine as a Metabolic Resuscitator in Septic Shock: A Pilot Study. *Crit. Care Med.* **2016**, *44*, 360–367. [CrossRef]

28. Gattinoni, L.; Vasques, F.; Camporota, L.; Meessen, J.; Romitti, F.; Pasticci, I.; Duscio, E.; Vassalli, F.; Forni, L.G.; Payen, D.; et al. Understanding Lactataemia in Human Sepsis. Potential Impact for Early Management. *Am. J. Respir. Crit. Care Med.* **2019**, *200*, 582–589. [CrossRef]
29. Rhodes, A.; Evans, L.E.; Alhazzani, W.; Levy, M.M.; Antonelli, M.; Ferrer, R.; Kumar, A.; Sevransky, J.E.; Sprung, C.L.; Nunnally, M.E.; et al. Surviving Sepsis Campaign: International Guidelines for Management of Sepsis and Septic Shock: 2016. *Intensiv. Care Med.* **2017**, *43*, 304–377. [CrossRef]
30. Knaus, W.A.; Draper, E.A.; Wagner, D.P.; Zimmerman, J.E. APACHE II: A severity of disease classification system. *Crit. Care Med.* **1985**, *13*, 818–829. [CrossRef]
31. Jentzer, J.C.; Kashani, K.B.; Wiley, B.M.; Patel, P.C.; Baran, D.A.; Barsness, G.W.; Henry, T.D.; Van Diepen, S. Laboratory Markers of Acidosis and Mortality in Cardiogenic Shock: Developing a Definition of Hemometabolic Shock. *Shock* **2021**, *Epub ahead of print*. [CrossRef] [PubMed]
32. Singhal, R.; Coghill, J.E.; Guy, A.; Bradbury, A.W.; Adam, D.J.; Scriven, J.M. Serum lactate and base deficit as predictors of mortality after ruptured abdominal aortic aneurysm repair. *Eur. J. Vasc. Endovasc. Surg.* **2005**, *30*, 263–266. [CrossRef]
33. Caputo, N.D.; Kanter, M.; Fraser, R.; Simon, R. Comparing biomarkers of traumatic shock: The utility of anion gap, base excess, and serum lactate in the ED. *Am. J. Emerg. Med.* **2015**, *33*, 1134–1139. [CrossRef] [PubMed]
34. Callaway, D.W.; Shapiro, N.I.; Donnino, M.W.; Baker, C.; Rosen, C.L. Serum lactate and base deficit as predictors of mortality in normotensive elderly blunt trauma patients. *J. Trauma* **2009**, *66*, 1040–1044. [CrossRef]
35. Gale, S.C.; Kocik, J.F.; Creath, R.; Crystal, J.S.; Dombrovskiy, V.Y. A comparison of initial lactate and initial base deficit as predictors of mortality after severe blunt trauma. *J. Surg. Res.* **2016**, *205*, 446–455. [CrossRef] [PubMed]
36. Davis, J.W.; Dirks, R.C.; Kaups, K.L.; Tran, P. Base deficit is superior to lactate in trauma. *Am. J. Surg.* **2018**, *215*, 682–685. [CrossRef]
37. Mutschler, M.; Nienaber, U.; Brockamp, T.; Wafaisade, A.; Fabian, T.; Paffrath, T.; Bouillon, B.; Maegele, M.; Trauma Register DGU. Renaissance of base deficit for the initial assessment of trauma patients: A base deficit-based classification for hypovolemic shock developed on data from 16,305 patients derived from the TraumaRegister DGU®. *Crit. Care* **2013**, *17*, R42. [CrossRef]
38. Ibrahim, I.; Chor, W.P.; Chue, K.M.; Tan, C.S.; Tan, H.L.; Siddiqui, F.J.; Hartman, M. Is arterial base deficit still a useful prognostic marker in trauma? A systematic review. *Am. J. Emerg. Med.* **2016**, *34*, 626–635. [CrossRef]
39. Jouffroy, R.; Léguillier, T.; Gilbert, B.; Tourtier, J.P.; Bloch-Laine, E.; Ecollan, P.; Bounes, V.; Boularan, J.; Gueye-Ngalgou, P.; Nivet-Antoine, V.; et al. Pre-Hospital Lactatemia Predicts 30-Day Mortality in Patients with Septic Shock—Preliminary Results from the LAPHSUS Study. *J. Clin. Med.* **2020**, *9*, 3290. [CrossRef]
40. Schork, A.; Moll, K.; Haap, M.; Riessen, R.; Wagner, R. Course of lactate, pH and base excess for prediction of mortality in medical intensive care patients. *PLoS ONE* **2021**, *16*, e0261564. [CrossRef]
41. Hsu, J.-C.; Lee, I.-K.; Huang, W.-C.; Chen, Y.-C.; Tsai, C.-Y. Clinical Characteristics and Predictors of Mortality in Critically Ill Influenza Adult Patients. *J. Clin. Med.* **2020**, *9*, 1073. [CrossRef] [PubMed]
42. Smith, I.; Kumar, P.; Molloy, S.; Rhodes, A.; Newman, P.J.; Grounds, R.M.; Bennett, E.D. Base excess and lactate as prognostic indicators for patients admitted to intensive care. *Intensiv. Care Med.* **2001**, *27*, 74–83. [CrossRef] [PubMed]
43. Wernly, B.; Heramvand, N.; Masyuk, M.; Rezar, R.; Bruno, R.R.; Kelm, M.; Niederseer, D.; Lichtenauer, M.; Hoppe, U.C.; Bakker, J.; et al. Acidosis predicts mortality independently from hyperlactataemia in patients with sepsis. *Eur. J. Intern. Med.* **2020**, *76*, 76–81. [CrossRef] [PubMed]
44. Lang, W.; Zander, R. The accuracy of calculated base excess in blood. *Clin. Chem. Lab. Med.* **2002**, *40*, 404–410. [CrossRef] [PubMed]
45. Ho, K.M.; Lan, N.S.H.; Williams, T.A.; Harahsheh, Y.; Chapman, A.R.; Dobb, G.J.; Magder, S. A comparison of prognostic significance of strong ion gap (SIG) with other acid-base markers in the critically ill: A cohort study. *J. Intensiv. Care* **2016**, *4*, 43. [CrossRef]

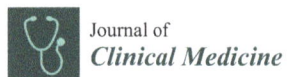

Article

Left Ventricular Diastolic Dysfunction in ARDS Patients

Paolo Formenti [1], Silvia Coppola [1], Laura Massironi [2], Giacomo Annibali [3], Francesco Mazza [3], Lisa Gilardi [3], Tommaso Pozzi [3] and Davide Chiumello [1,3,4,*]

1. Department of Anesthesia and Intensive Care, ASST Santi Paolo e Carlo, San Paolo University Hospital, 20142 Milan, Italy
2. Division of Cardiology, Department of Health Sciences, San Paolo Hospital, University of Milan, 20142 Milan, Italy
3. Department of Health Sciences, University of Milan, 20142 Milan, Italy
4. Coordinated Research Center on Respiratory Failure, University of Milan, 2014 Milan, Italy
* Correspondence: davide.chiumello@unimi.it

Abstract: Background: The aim of this study was to evaluate the possible presence of diastolic dysfunction and its possible effects in terms of respiratory mechanics, gas exchange and lung recruitability in mechanically ventilated ARDS. Methods: Consecutive patients admitted in intensive care unit (ICU) with ARDS were enrolled. Echocardiographic evaluation was acquired at clinical PEEP level. Lung CT-scan was performed at 5 and 45 cmH$_2$O. In the study, 2 levels of PEEP (5 and 15 cmH$_2$O) were randomly applied. Results: A total of 30 patients were enrolled with a mean PaO$_2$/FiO$_2$ and a median PEEP of 137 ± 52 and 10 [9–10] cmH$_2$O, respectively. Of those, 9 patients (30%) had a diastolic dysfunction of grade 1, 2 and 3 in 33%, 45% and 22%, respectively, without any difference in gas exchange and respiratory mechanics. The total lung weight was significantly higher in patients with diastolic dysfunction (1669 [1354–1909] versus 1554 [1146–1942] g) but the lung recruitability was similar between groups (33.3 [27.3–41.4] versus 30.6 [20.0–38.8] %). Left ventricular ejection fraction (57 [39–62] versus 60 [57–60]%) and TAPSE (20.0 [17.0–24.0] versus 24.0 [20.0–27.0] mL) were similar between the two groups. The response to changes of PEEP from 5 to 15 cmH$_2$O in terms of oxygenation and respiratory mechanics was not affected by the presence of diastolic dysfunction. Conclusions: ARDS patients with left ventricular diastolic dysfunction presented a higher amount of lung edema and worse outcome.

Keywords: ARDS; left ventricular diastolic dysfunction; total lung weight

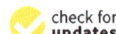

Citation: Formenti, P.; Coppola, S.; Massironi, L.; Annibali, G.; Mazza, F.; Gilardi, L.; Pozzi, T.; Chiumello, D. Left Ventricular Diastolic Dysfunction in ARDS Patients. *J. Clin. Med.* **2022**, *11*, 5998. https://doi.org/10.3390/jcm11205998

Academic Editors: Spyros D. Mentzelopoulos and Juan F. Delgado Jiménez

Received: 26 August 2022
Accepted: 7 October 2022
Published: 11 October 2022

Publisher's Note: MDPI stays neutral with regard to jurisdictional claims in published maps and institutional affiliations.

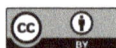

Copyright: © 2022 by the authors. Licensee MDPI, Basel, Switzerland. This article is an open access article distributed under the terms and conditions of the Creative Commons Attribution (CC BY) license (https:// creativecommons.org/licenses/by/ 4.0/).

1. Introduction

The most severe form of acute respiratory failure is ARDS, which is defined by inflammatory edema, increase in vascular permeability and the impairment of gas exchange [1,2]. Although the current ARDS definition excludes any form of hydrostatic pulmonary edema, the absence of invasive pulmonary monitoring can hide a possible cardiac failure (systolic, diastolic dysfunction) or fluid overload [3,4]. Diastolic function is affected by an active relaxation and passive compliance [5–7]. Thus, diastolic dysfunction is defined by the presence of any alteration in the relaxation, distensibility or filling of the left ventricle with a preserved systolic function [8,9]. The common predisposing factors are the presence of obesity, arterial hypertension, or diabetes mellitus, the female sex and ageing [10,11]. In addition, the possible presence of sepsis, hypoxemia, inflammation activation and cytokine release can promote a systolic/diastolic dysfunction [11,12]. The diastolic dysfunction in sepsis/septic shock ranged from 20% to 67% according to the definition applied and was reversible in patients who survived [11]. Moreover, in septic shock, the diastolic dysfunction was the strongest independent predictor of early mortality, better than cardiac biomarkers, even after adjusting for the severity of the disease, stroke volume and arterial hypoxemia [11,13,14]. In ARDS patients, the requirement of positive mechanical ventilation, fluid load and vasopressor in the early phase and during the weaning phase, leading to a possible increase in the venous return and afterload, can increase the risk of diastolic dysfunction and pulmonary edema [3,4]. Several studies including meta-analyses reported that patients who failed the weaning process presented a higher incidence of diastolic dysfunction [15–19]. Echocardiography has been recommended as the primary noninvasive clinical examination for evaluating the presence of diastolic dysfunction [20,21]. Several echocardiographic measurements for categorizing the diastolic dysfunction have been previously recommended; however, these measurements could not be applied in critically ill patients due to the presence of tachycardia or atrial fibrillation [21]. A more simplified definition based on Doppler echocardiography, which computes the ratio between the early diastolic velocity of mitral inflow to mitral annular velocity (E/e'), has been suggested [22]. This parameter showed a strong association with the left atrial pressure and with the categorization of patients with diastolic dysfunction according to the previous American Society of Echocardiography guidelines [22]. Although the diastolic dysfunction has been described since 1998 and accounted for more than 50% of the total heart failure, its role in ARDS patients is not well known. The aim of this study was to evaluate the possible presence of diastolic dysfunction by a simplified approach with echocardiography in the early phase of ARDS patients receiving mechanical ventilation. The secondary aim was to detect differences between patients with and without diastolic dysfunction in terms of respiratory mechanics, gas exchange and lung recruitability.

2. Materials and Methods

2.1. Study Design

This was a prospective observational study conducted between October 2017 and September 2019 at intensive care unit of San Paolo Hospital, Milan, Italy. The protocol was approved by the institutional review board and written consent was obtained according to the regulation applied (n. 7185/2019).

2.2. Patients

All consecutive patients admitted with ARDS according to the Berlin definition were enrolled. Exclusion criteria were absence of a sinus rhythm, a moribund status and a poor-quality echocardiographic images and measurements and a known history of diastolic dysfunction. At baseline patients were sedated, paralyzed and managed according to a lung protective ventilation strategy (tidal volume between 6–8 mL/Kg of ideal body weight) with a PEEP set to achieve an arterial saturation between 93–97%. Briefly, after a recruitment maneuver, a PEEP trial, (at two different levels of PEEP, 5 and 15 cmH$_2$O randomly applied) by maintaining constant the tidal volume and oxygen fraction, was performed. At each PEEP level, blood gas analysis and partitioned respiratory mechanics measurements were performed. After the PEEP trial, patients underwent a lung CT scan performed in 2 different static conditions at 5 cmH$_2$O of PEEP and at 45 cmH$_2$O of airway plateau pressure [23] (Figure 1). A quantitative CT scan lung analysis using dedicated software (Maluna) was applied to compute the total lung gas, volume, weight and its amount of the different compartments (not inflated, poorly inflated, well inflated and overinflated tissue) [24]. The lung recruitability was computed as the difference between not-inflated lung tissue at 5 cmH$_2$O and 45 cmH$_2$O of airway plateau pressure to the total lung tissue at 5 cmH$_2$O of PEEP [23].

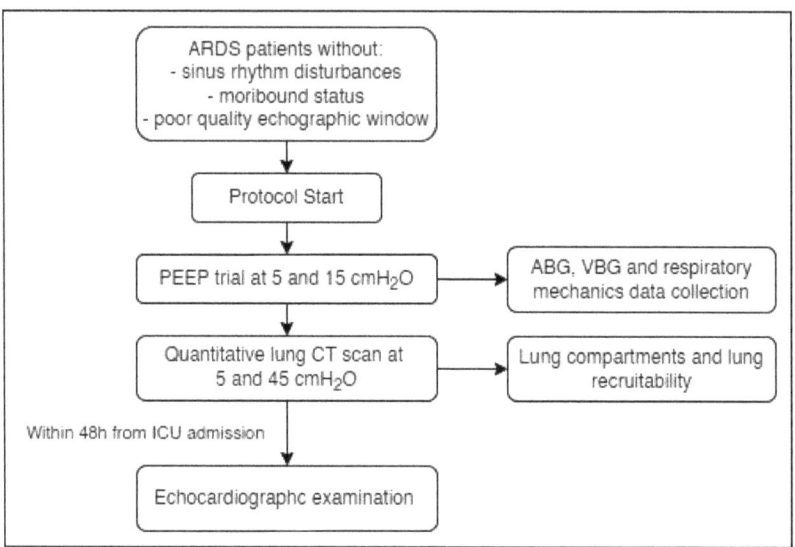

Figure 1. Study protocol flow chart. ARDS: Acute Respiratory Distress Syndrome; ABG: arterial blood gas; VBG: venous blood gas; CT: computed tomography; ICU: intensive care unit.

2.3. Clinical Data

We collected demographic information, vital signs, mechanical ventilation parameters, CT scan quantitative analysis and echocardiographic measurements within 48 h from ICU admission.

2.4. Measurements

Esophageal pressure was measured using a standard balloon catheter (Smart Cath, Viasys, PalmSprings, CA, USA) consisting of a tube 103 cm long with an external diameter of 3 mm and a thin-walled balloon 10 cm long. The esophageal catheter was emptied of air and introduced trans orally into the esophagus to reach the stomach at a depth of 50–55 cm from the mouth. Subsequently the balloon was inflated with 1.5 mL of air. The intragastric position of the catheter was confirmed by a positive pressure deflection of intra-abdominal pressure during an external manual epigastric pressure. Subsequently, the catheter was retracted and positioned in the low esophageal position. The amount of gas in the balloon was periodically checked throughout the experiment. During an end-inspiratory and end-expiratory pause the airway and esophageal pressure were measured. The respiratory system, lung and chest wall elastance were computed according to the standard formulas [24]. To measure the functional residual capacity (FRC), a gas mixture of oxygen and 13.44% helium was manually equilibrated with the patient's lung using a ventilation bag for 10 large insufflations [25]. Thereafter, helium concentration in the bag was analyzed (KG850, Hitech Instruments, Pennsburg, PA, USA). The FRC was computed as:

$$\text{FRC (mL)} = (V_b \times C_i)/C_f - V_b$$

where V_b is the initial volume of the bag, C_i is the initial helium concentration and C_f is the final helium concentration after equilibration.

2.5. Transthoracic Echocardiography

Echocardiography was performed during controlled mechanical ventilation at 5 cmH$_2$O of PEEP within 48 h of ICU admission. All echocardiographic examinations were performed and analyzed by a single trained cardiologist not involved in the patient care and blinded to the treatment and outcome (LM). Transthoracic echocardiography (TTE) was performed using a GE, Vivid E9 (General Electric Horten, Norway) equipped with a 2–5 MHz transducer. All images were obtained with standard techniques using M-mode, two-dimensional, and Doppler measurements in accordance with the ASE/EACVI recommendations [26]. Pulsed Doppler echocardiography was used to evaluate transmitral LV filling velocities at the tips of the mitral valve. The peak early-diastolic flow velocity (E) and the peak late-diastolic velocity (A) shown as the E/A ratio were measured by analyzing trans-mitral flow. The ASE/EACVI recommendations showed the four recommended variables for identifying left ventricular diastolic dysfunction (LVDD), and their abnormal cut-off values were annular e' velocity (septal e' < 7 cm/s or lateral e' < 10 cm/s), average E/e' ratio > 14, LA volume index > 34 mL/m^2, and peak TR velocity > 2.8 m/s. Diastolic function was normal when more than half of the available variables did not meet the cut-off values for identifying abnormal function. LVDD was present when more than half of the available parameters met these cut-off values but was indeterminate when only half met these values. Patients were graded as the DD classification in three groups (I grade–II grade–III grade) according to the algorithm for the diagnosis of LVDD in ASE/EACVI recommendations. In addition to assessing diastolic function, we also measured the following parameters: the LV end-diastolic and end-systolic volumes, diameters and areas, the left ventricular ejection fraction (EF) using biplane modified Simpson's rule, miocardical mass, thickness of septum and posterior wall, the RV end-diastolic diameter, the RV end-diastolic and end-systolic areas, the tricuspidal annular plane systolic excursion (TAPSE), RIMP (right index of myocardial performance) defined as the ratio of isovolumic time divided by Ejection Time (ET), or [(isovolumic relaxation time (IVRT) + isovolumic contraction time (IVCT))/ET].

2.6. Statistical Analysis

Continuous data are expressed as mean ± SD or median [IQR], as appropriate, while categorical data are expressed as %, number. Comparisons between patients with and without diastolic dysfunction for continuous data were performed by Student's T test or the Wilcoxon–Mann–Whitney test. Comparisons between patients with and without diastolic dysfunction for categorical variables were performed by χ^2 test. We investigated the role of diastolic dysfunction and PEEP on respiratory mechanics, gas exchange, hemodynamics and quantitative CT-scan data by two-ways repeated measures analysis of variance (ANOVA) between groups (diastolic dysfunction) and a fixed factor within-subjects PEEP. In case of statistically significant interaction, the comparisons of the two classes of a factor within each class of the other factor were performed with all pairwise multiple comparison procedures (Holm–Šidák method). The statistical analysis was performed using RStudio (R foundation for statistical computing, Vienna, Austria). A *p* value of 0.05 or less was considered statistically significant.

3. Results

A total of 30 patients were enrolled in this study. The baseline characteristics are shown in Table 1. The main sources of ARDS were pulmonary pneumonia (25 patients, 83%). The mean PaO$_2$/FiO$_2$ was 137 ± 52 with a median PEEP level of 10 [9–10] cmH$_2$O; the applied median tidal volume of predicted body weight was 6.9 [6.6–7.3] mL/Kg PBW. The echocardiography study was performed within 48 h after the start of mechanical ventilation. 9 patients (30%) had a diastolic dysfunction with a grade 1, 2 and 3 in 33%, 45% and 22%, respectively. There was no difference in terms of PaO$_2$/FiO$_2$, applied tidal volume predicted body weight and minute ventilation between the two groups at the baseline; the FRC was not different (630 ± 230 vs. 600 ± 410 mL). The 28-day mortality was significantly worse in patients with diastolic dysfunction.

Table 1. Characteristics of the study population within the first 48 h since ICU admission according to the presence or absence of diastolic dysfunction. BMI: body mass index; ICU: intensive care unit; ARDS: acute respiratory distress syndrome; PaO_2: arterial oxygen partial pressure; FiO_2: inspired oxygen fraction; $PaCO_2$: arterial carbon dioxide partial pressure; PEEP: positive end-expiratory pressure; IBW: ideal body weight. Comparisons for continuous variables were performed by Student's T test or Wilcoxon–Mann–Whitney test, as appropriate, while comparisons for categorical variables were performed by χ^2 test.

	Study Population N = 30	Diastolic Dysfunction N = 9	No Diastolic Dysfunction N = 21	p
Age, years	63 ± 16	73 ± 11	60 ± 16	0.018
Male sex, % (number)	80 (24)	78 (7)	81 (17)	0.999
Weight, kg	72 ± 17	72 ± 12	72 ± 19	0.939
BMI, kg/m^2	25 ± 5	26 ± 4	25 ± 6	0.077
History of, % (n)				
Hypertension	57 (17)	55 (5)	57 (12)	0.999
Myocardial infarction	23 (7)	33 (3)	19 (4)	0.706
Chronic kidney failure	17 (5)	11 (1)	19 (4)	0.952
Chronic obstructive pulmonary disease	17 (5)	22 (2)	14 (3)	0.968
Diabetes mellitus	37 (11)	44 (4)	33 (7)	0.869
SAPS II	43 ± 6	43 ± 5	44 ± 6	0.687
SOFA score	4 [2–5]	3 [2–5]	4 [2–5]	0.341
ICU stay, days	16 [12–22]	16 [9–16]	19 [12–27]	0.173
28 days mortality, % (n)	50 [15]	8 (89)	7 (33)	0.017
Diastolic dysfunction grade, % (n)				
Grade I	33 (3)	33 (3)		-
Grade II	45 (4)	45 (4)		
Grade III	22 (2)	22 (2)		
Cause of ARDS, % (number)				
Pulmonary	83 (25)	78 (7)	83 (18)	0.883
Extrapulmonary	17 (5)	22 /2)	17 (3)	0.579
PaO_2/FiO_2, mmHg	137 ± 52	115 ± 47	147 ± 52	0.119
$PaCO_2$, mmHg	50 [41–59]	51 [45–70]	50 [41–56]	0.469
Arterial pH	7.39 ± 0.05	7.39 ± 0.04	7.39 ± 0.06	0.958
PEEP, cmH$_2$O	10 [9–10]	10 [10–10]	10 [8–10]	0.818
Respiratory rate, breaths per minute	16 [15–18]	18 [17–20]	16 [15–17]	0.080
Respiratory system elastance, cmH$_2$O/L	26 ± 7	22.5 ± 6.2	28.2 ± 7.6	0.118
Minute ventilation, L/min	7.6 ± 1.2	8.0 ± 1.4	7.4 ± 1.1	0.225
Tidal volume per IBW, mL/kg IBW	6.9 [6.6–7.3]	6.8 [6.6–7.3]	7.0 [6.5–7.3]	0.803
Functional residual capacity, mL	600 ± 360	630 ± 230	600 ± 410	0.770
Amine requirement, % (n)	66 (20)	78 (7)	62 (13)	0.564
Serum creatinine, mg/dL	1.1 [0.7–1.6]	1.0 [0.7–1.5]	1.2 [0.9–1.7]	0.482
Daily fluid balance, mL	200 [−300–800]	250 [−400–550]	250 [−250–350]	0.437

3.1. Echocardiographic Data

According to the echocardiographic criteria, patients with diastolic dysfunction had a significant higher E/e' ratio and left atrial volume compared to patients without diastolic dysfunction 10.0 [8.9–14.7] versus 7.2 [6.1–9.2] and 65.0 [39.0–98.0] versus 37.0 [26–48] L/m^2. The median ejection fraction 60 [56–61] %, none had an ejection fraction lower than

30% and was not different between two groups and similarly the end diastolic volume was not different between the two groups (Table 2). The TAPSE and the ratio between the RV end diastolic and the LV end diastolic areas were not different among the two groups (20.0 [17.0–24.0] versus 24.0 [20.0–27.0] mL; 0.66 [0.57–0.70] versus 0.66 [0.57–0.88] respectively) (Table 3).

Table 2. Left ventricular and atrial echocardiographic characteristics according to the presence or absence of diastolic dysfunction. E: peak early-diastolic flow velocity; A: peak late-diastolic velocity; e': annular velocity. Comparisons for continuous variables were performed by Student's T test or Wilcoxon–Mann–Whitney, as appropriate, while comparisons for categorical variables were performed by χ^2 test.

	Study Population N = 30	Diastolic Dysfunction N = 9	No Diastolic Dysfunction N = 21	p
Left Ventricle				
End-diastolic diameter (mm)	44.5 [40.2–49-5]	50.0 [47.0–52.0]	42.0 [40.0–47.0]	0.027
End-systolic diameter (mm)	30.0 [25.2–36.0]	40.0 [36.0–42.0]	30.0 [25.0–32.0]	0.044
End-diastolic area (cm^2)	17.0 [13.2–22.8]	20.0 [17.0–23.4]	15.0 [12.0–20.0]	0.442
End-diastolic volume (mL)	81.5 [68.5–108.0]	103.0 [72.0–130.0]	78.0 [66.0–103.0]	0.291
End-systolic volume (mL)	34.0 [25.0–51.5]	53.0 [35.0–67.0]	30.0 [23.0–44.0]	0.114
Ejection fraction (%)	60 [56–61]	57 [39–62]	60 [57–60]	0.396
Septum thickness (mm)	10.0 [8.0–11.0]	10.0 [10.0–13.0]	10.0 [8.0–10.0]	0.040
Posterior wall thickness (mm)	9.0 [8.0–10.0]	10.0 [8.0–10.0]	9.0 [8.0–10.0]	0.482
Myocardical mass (g/m^2)	74.5 [58.5–97.2]	103.0 [91.0–111.0]	60.0 [45.0–87.0]	0.001
Left Atrium				
Left atrial volume index (mL/m^2)	39.5 [32–60]	65.0 [39.0–98.0]	37.0 [26.0–48.0]	0.017
Diastolic function				
E (cm/s)	80.5 [64.0–93.8]	83.0 [67.0–92.0]	80.0 [64.0–95.0]	0.888
A (cm/s)	78.5 [56.0–92.5]	85.0 [54.0–93.0]	78.0 [59.0–91.0]	0.853
E/A ratio	1.1 [0.9–1.4]	0.9 [0.8–1.5]	1.2 [0.9–1.3]	0.910
e' septal (cm/s)	8.0 [6.0–11.0]	6.1 [5.6–7.2]	9.3 [7.0–12.0]	0.085
e' lateral (cm/s)	10.5 [7.8–13.4]	7.6 [6.4–8.6]	12.0 [10.0–14.2]	0.001
E/e' ratio	8.6 [6.3–10.0]	10.0 [8.9–14.7]	7.2 [6.1–9.2]	0.013
Deceleration time (ms)	184 [162–253]	183 [170–253]	185 [160–253]	0.928

Table 3. Right ventricular and pulmonary artery echocardiographic characteristics according to the presence or absence of diastolic dysfunction. RV ED-area: right ventricular end-diastolic area; LV ED-area: left ventricular end-diastolic area; TAPSE: tricuspid annular plane systolic excursion; RIMP: right ventricular index of myocardial performance; PAPs: pulmonary arterial systolic pressure. Comparisons for continuous variables were performed by Student's T test or Wilcoxon–Mann–Whitney, as appropriate, while comparisons for categorical variables were performed by χ^2 test.

	Study Population N = 30	Diastolic Dysfunction N = 9	No Diastolic Dysfunction N = 21	p
Right Ventricle				
End-diastolic diameter (mm)	38.0 [33.5–39.8]	39.5 [29.5–42.0]	37.0 [34.5–38.3]	0.600
End-diastolic area (cm^2)	17.0 [14.0–20.0]	17.0 [15.0–19.0]	17.0 [10.8–20.8]	0.906
RV ED-area/LV ED-area	0.67 [0.56–0.76]	0.66 [0.57–0.70]	0.66 [0.57–0.88]	0.647

Table 3. Cont.

	Study Population N = 30	Diastolic Dysfunction N = 9	No Diastolic Dysfunction N = 21	p
End-systolic area (cm^2)	9.0 [6.0–13.7]	6.5 [6.0–10.0]	10.0 [6.7–15.0]	0.465
Lateral wall (mm)	4.0 [3.0–4.0]	4.0 [4.0–4.0]	4.0 [3.0–4.5]	0.852
TAPSE (mm)	23.5 [19.0–26.5]	20.0 [17.0–24.0]	24.0 [20.0–27.0]	0.253
RIMP	0.30 [0.24–0.37]	0.31 [0.25–0.37]	0.30 [0.22–0.38]	0.662
Fractional shortening (%)	50 [43–57]	58 [47–60]	50 [41–50]	0.153
Pulmonary Artery				
Peak tricuspidal velocity (m/s)	2.5 [2.3–2.9]	2.8 [2.3–3.0]	2.4 [2.1–2.8]	0.404
PAPs (mmHg)	41 [31–46]	43 [31–49]	38 [31–44]	0.748

3.2. Gas Exchange and Respiratory Mechanics Response to PEEP

The oxygenation was similar at 5 cmH$_2$O of PEEP and similarly was the changes at 15 cmH$_2$O of PEEP (Tables 4 and S2). The carbon dioxide and the ratio between the ETCO$_2$ and PaCO$_2$ were not different. Concerning the total, lung and chest wall elastance were not different among the two groups both at 5 and 15 cmH$_2$O of PEEP (Table 4).

Table 4. Respiratory mechanics and gas exchange data according to the presence or absence of diastolic dysfunction. ERS: respiratory system elastance; EL: lung elastance; ECW: chest wall elastance; PaO$_2$: arterial oxygen partial pressure; FiO$_2$: inspired oxygen fraction; PaCO$_2$: arterial carbon dioxide partial pressure; EtCO$_2$: end-tidal carbon dioxide partial pressure. The role of the of PEEP between groups was assessed by two-way repeated-measures analysis of variance (ANOVA) followed by all-pairwise comparisons (Holm–Sidak method).

	Study Population N = 30	Diastolic Dysfunction N = 9	No Diastolic Dysfunction N = 21	p disf	p PEEP	p inter
End Inspiratory Airway Pressure (cmH$_2$O)						
5 cmH$_2$O	16.4 [13.7–18.5]	15.9 [13.4–17.6]	16.4 [13.8–18.5]	0.420	<0.001	0.725
15 cmH$_2$O	24.7 [22.1–26.7]	24.0 [22.0–25.4]	25.2 [23.8–26.8]			
Driving Pressure (cmH$_2$O)						
5 cmH$_2$O	10.1 [7.7–12.9]	8.3 [6.9–9.7]	11.4 [7.8–13.5]	0.226	0.435	0.152
15 cmH$_2$O	9.5 [8.0–11.9]	9.0 [7.6–11.4]	10.1 [8.6–12.0]			
E$_{RS}$ (cmH$_2$O/L)						
5 cmH$_2$O	20.9 [16.7–28.1]	18.7 [16.9–20.5]	26.8 [16.7–29.4]	0.658	0.187	0.211
15 cmH$_2$O	21.4 [18.2–28.5]	20.2 [20.0–28.1]	21.4 [17.0–28.7]			
E$_L$ (cmH$_2$O/L)						
5 cmH$_2$O	16.2 [12.0–25.0]	14.7 [12.8–24.0]	19.0 [11.2–25.2]	0.555	0.140	0.588
15 cmH$_2$O	15.2 [12.0–21.0]	15.8 [14.9–21.4]	14.0 [11.2–19.9]			
E$_{CW}$ (cmH$_2$O/L)						
5 cmH$_2$O	4.8 [3.0–6.3]	4.0 [3.1–5.8]	5.5 [2.9–6.3]	0.585	0.288	0.544
15 cmH$_2$O	5.9 [3.9–10.3]	4.6 [3.8–8.1]	6.3 [5.0–10.5]			

Table 4. Cont.

	Study Population N = 30	Diastolic Dysfunction N = 9	No Diastolic Dysfunction N = 21	p disf	p PEEP	p inter
PaO_2 (mmHg)						
5 cmH$_2$O	70 [63–76]	71 [70–74]	68 [62–79]	0.842	<0.001	0.821
15 cmH$_2$O	88 [75–128]	107 [97–134]	87 [68–100]			
PaO_2/FiO_2						
5 cmH$_2$O	128 [107–146]	117 [84–146]	131 [110–145]	0.274	<0.001	0.745
15 cmH$_2$O	187 [113–237]	195 [94–242]	182 [131–232]			
$PaCO_2$ (mmHg)						
5 cmH$_2$O	47.4 [40.4–56.4]	45.9 [39.4–51.0]	50.2 [41.5–58.0]	0.836	0.808	0.023
15 cmH$_2$O	48.7 [43.2–52.4]	48.9 [45.3–52.0]	47.2 [43.0–52.5]			
$EtCO_2/PaCO_2$						
5 cmH$_2$O	0.74 [0.69–0.82]	0.70 [0.68–0.74]	0.76 [0.70–0.83]	0.073	0.905	0.229
15 cmH$_2$O	0.75 [0.68–0.84]	0.69 [0.66–0.76]	0.77 [0.73–0.89]			
Ventilatory Ratio						
5 cmH$_2$O	1.4 [1.3–1.7]	1.3 [1.2–1.9]	1.5 [1.2–1.8]	0.111	0.089	0.231
15 cmH$_2$O	1.6 [1.5–1.9]	1.7 [1.2–1.8]	1.6 [1.3–1.8]			

3.3. Lung CT Scan Quantitative Data and Recruitability

Patients with diastolic dysfunction had a significantly higher total tissue weight compared to patients without diastolic dysfunction. The percentages of non aerated, poorly aerated, well aerated and overinflated tissue were similar between the two groups. The lung recruitability was similar in patients with diastolic dysfunction (33.3 [27.3–41.4] %) and in patients without diastolic dysfunction (30.6 [20.0–38.8] %) (See Table S1).

4. Discussion

The major findings of this this observational study, which applied a simplified echocardiographic examination in ARDS patients, were: (1) the LV diastolic dysfunction was present in 30% of the patients, and (2) the gas exchange and respiratory mechanics were not different between patients with and without LV diastolic dysfunction, while (3) the 28-day mortality and lung weight were significantly higher in patients with LV diastolic dysfunction. The most severe form of acute respiratory failure is ARDS, which is characterized by a severe deterioration in gas exchange due to an inflammatory pulmonary edema [1]. Pneumonia and sepsis were the most frequent causes of ARDS [27]. In the early phase, ARDS due to infection/inflammation is characterized by hypovolemia due to an increased capillary permeability, higher venous capacitance, vasoplegia and the requirement of mechanical ventilation. These factors associated with the patient's history and comorbidities (age, hypertension, diabetes, renal failure) may promote hemodynamic failure, which has been reported in up to 60% of ARDS patients [3]. Thus, an early evaluation of heart failure of both LV ventricular and diastolic component is of paramount importance to improve the outcome. The diastole is a complex phase of the cardiac cycle that leads to ventricular filling before the ejection, and a normal diastolic phase is essential for ensuring an adequate preload and, consequently, cardiac output. The main determinants of the LV preload are the LV relaxation and compliance of the LV. The best assessment of LV relaxation (i.e., diastolic dysfunction) component is through an invasive measurement of the LV pressure by the pulmonary artery catheter [3,4]. However, based on some negative trials the pulmonary artery catheter, it is rarely used in critically ill patients. Thus, the assessment of possible presence of LV diastolic dysfunction remains challenging [4]. However, in critically ill patients, evidence has suggested performing an echocardiographic examination as soon as signs of hemodynamic failure are suspected [3,4], specifically evaluating the presence of possible diastolic dysfunction by a simplified echocardiographic examination based on the ratio of the early diastolic velocity of transmitral flow to the early myocardial relaxation wave (E/e') [26]. The e' is measured by tissue doppler imaging as the early diastolic mitral anulus velocity and the E reflects the early diastolic transmitral flow velocity, both dependent on LV relaxation. This ratio has been validated as an accurate predictor of pulmonary capillary wedge pressure in patients with cardiogenic shock and in the perioperative patients during cardiac surgery [28,29]. In this vein, Mousavi et al. showed in patients with septic shock a good correlation between the mean E/e' ratio and pulmonary capillary wedge pressure [30]. Previous studies also showed that in septic shock the E/e' ratio had an independent and better prognostic prediction of hospital outcome in septic shock compared to traditional cardiac biomarkers (BNP, NT, proBNP and TnT) [14]. According to previous data, in non-ARDS patients, diastolic dysfunction can be defined accordingly to echocardiographic examinations by an E/e' ratio higher than 14 with a normal left ventricular ejection fraction [26].

In the present study, diastolic dysfunction was found in up to 30% patients, although only 22% of these presented a diastolic dysfunction of high grade. All patients had ARDS of different severity, and echocardiographic examinations were performed within 48 h from the start of mechanical ventilation. Patients with diastolic dysfunction were characterized by a worse 28-day outcome. Applying similar echocardiographic criteria, in severe sepsis/septic shock, LV diastolic dysfunction was found in 9% of the patients and was associated to a worse outcome [22,31]. This study also evaluated the possible associations between the diastolic dysfunction and gas exchange, partitioned respiratory mechanics (lung and chest wall elastance) and quantitative lung CT scan. The response to the change in PEEP in terms of oxygenation and respiratory mechanics from 5 to 15 cm H2O was not affected by the presence of diastolic dysfunction. On the contrary, the lung weight was significantly higher in patients with diastolic dysfunction. This suggested that the presence of diastolic dysfunction, (i.e., a higher filling pressure) could have increased the amount of lung fluid [16]. Similarly, the presence of diastolic dysfunction during the weaning phase associated with a reduction in the intrathoracic pressure and higher venous return promotes an increase in filling pressure. Previous studies and meta-analysis showed that diastolic dysfunction was associated with weaning failure due to the development of pulmonary edema promoted by an increase in filling pressure when the mechanical support was reduced [16,17,19]. However, it is not clear if the left ventricular diastolic dysfunction is mainly promoted by ARDS, pneumonia, sepsis, mechanical ventilation or fluid infusion or is rather only a preexisting condition in critically ill patients worsened by the underlying disease [32].

5. Conclusions

In conclusion, this study showed that LV diastolic dysfunction should be considered in ARDS patients because ARDS patents with left ventricular diastolic dysfunction presented a higher amount of lung edema and worse outcomes. Similar to patients with severe sepsis and septic shock, in whom diastolic dysfunction is one of the strongest independent predictors of mortality, ARDS could be associated with worse outcomes. In addition, the presence of diastolic dysfunction and fluid overload could be particularly harmful, promoting interstitial edema, tissue hypoxia and organ dysfunction [11–13,31]. However, further studies are needed to evaluate the diastolic function in the early phase of ARDS.

Supplementary Materials: The following supporting information can be downloaded at: https://www.mdpi.com/article/10.3390/jcm11205998/s1, Table S1. Quantitative computed-tomography scan data according to the presence or absence of diastolic dysfunction, Table S2. Hemodynamic characteristics according to the presence or absence of diastolic dysfunction.

Author Contributions: Conceptualization, D.C., P.F., S.C. and L.M.; methodology, D.C., P.F., S.C. and L.M.; software, T.P.; validation, P.F., S.C. and L.M.; formal analysis, T.P..; investigation, L.M., P.F., S.C., G.A., L.G. and F.M.; data curation, P.F., L.M.; writing—original draft preparation, D.C., P.F., S.C. and T.P.; supervision, D.C. All authors have read and agreed to the published version of the manuscript.

Funding: This research received no external funding.

Institutional Review Board Statement: The study was conducted in accordance with the Declaration of Helsinki and approved by the Ethics (n. 7185/2019).

Informed Consent Statement: Informed consent was obtained from all subjects involved in the study.

Data Availability Statement: Not applicable.

Conflicts of Interest: The authors declare no conflict of interest.

References

1. Ranieri, V.M.; Rubenfeld, G.D.; Thompson, B.T.; Ferguson, N.D.; Caldwell, E.; Fan, E.; Camporota, L.; Slutsky, A.S. Acute respiratory distress syndrome: The Berlin definition. *JAMA J. Am. Med. Assoc.* **2012**, *307*, 2526–2533. [CrossRef]
2. Cressoni, M.; Chiumello, D.; Chiurazzi, C.; Brioni, M.; Algieri, I.; Gotti, M.; Nikolla, K.; Massari, D.; Cammaroto, A.; Colombo, A.; et al. Lung inhomogeneities, inflation and [18F]2-fluoro-2-deoxy-D-glucose uptake rate in acute respiratory distress syndrome. *Eur. Respir. J.* **2016**, *47*, 233–242. [CrossRef] [PubMed]
3. Vignon, P.; Evrard, B.; Asfar, P.; Busana, M.; Calfee, C.S.; Coppola, S.; Demiselle, J.; Geri, G.; Jozwiak, M.; Martin, G.S.; et al. Fluid administration and monitoring in ARDS: Which management? *Intensive Care Med.* **2020**, *46*, 2252–2264. [CrossRef] [PubMed]
4. Vignon, P. Ventricular diastolic abnormalities in the critically ill. *Curr. Opin. Crit. Care* **2013**, *19*, 242–249. [CrossRef] [PubMed]
5. Brutsaert, D.L.; Sys, S.U.; Gillebert, T.C. Diastolic failure: Pathophysiology and therapeutic implications. *J. Am. Coll. Cardiol.* **1993**, *22*, 318–325. [CrossRef]
6. Moschietto, S.; Doyen, D.; Grech, L.; Dellamonica, J.; Hyvernat, H.; Bernardin, G.; Caille, V.; Amiel, J.-B.; Charron, C.; Belliard, G.; et al. Troponin elevation in severe sepsis and septic shock: The role of left ventricular diastolic dysfunction and right ventricular dilatation. *Crit. Care* **2016**, *14*, 709–714. [CrossRef]
7. Kass, D.A.; Bronzwaer, J.G.F.; Paulus, W.J. What mechanisms underlie diastolic dysfunction in heart failure? *Circ. Res.* **2004**, *94*, 1533–1542. [CrossRef]
8. Mahjoub, Y.; Benoit-Fallet, H.; Airapetian, N.; Lorne, E.; Levrard, M.; Seydi, A.-A.; Amennouche, N.; Slama, M.; Dupont, H. Improvement of left ventricular relaxation as assessed by tissue Doppler imaging in fluid-responsive critically ill septic patients. *Intensive Care Med.* **2012**, *38*, 1461–1470. [CrossRef]
9. Borlaug, B.A.; Paulus, W.J. Heart failure with preserved ejection fraction: Pathophysiology, diagnosis, and treatment. *Eur. Heart J.* **2011**, *32*, 670–679. [CrossRef]
10. Nicoara, A.; Jones-Haywood, M. Diastolic heart failure: Diagnosis and therapy. *Curr. Opin. Anaesthesiol.* **2016**, *29*, 61–67. [CrossRef]
11. Landesberg, G.; Jaffe, A.S.; Gilon, D.; Levin, P.D.; Goodman, S.; Abu-Baih, A.; Beeri, R.; Weissman, C.; Sprung, C.L.; Landesberg, A. Troponin elevation in severe sepsis and septic shock: The role of left ventricular diastolic dysfunction and right ventricular dilatation. *Crit. Care Med.* **2014**, *42*, 790–800. [CrossRef] [PubMed]
12. Jafri, S.M.; Lavine, S.; Field, B.E.; Bahorozian, M.T.; Carlson, R.W. Left ventricular diastolic function in sepsis. *Crit. Care Med.* **1990**, *18*, 709–714. [CrossRef] [PubMed]
13. Brown, S.M.; Pittman, J.E.; Hirshberg, E.L.; Jones, J.P.; Lanspa, M.J.; Kuttler, K.G.; Litwin, S.E.; Grissom, C.K. Diastolic dysfunction and mortality in early severe sepsis and septic shock: A prospective, observational echocardiography study. *Crit. Ultrasound J.* **2012**, *4*, 8. [CrossRef] [PubMed]
14. Sturgess, D.J.; Marwick, T.H.; Joyce, C.; Jenkins, C.; Jones, M.; Masci, P.; Stewart, D.; Venkatesh, B. Prediction of hospital outcome in septic shock: A prospective comparison of tissue Doppler and cardiac biomarkers. *Crit. Care* **2010**, *14*, R44. [CrossRef] [PubMed]
15. Moschietto, S.; Doyen, D.; Grech, L.; Dellamonica, J.; Hyvernat, H.; Bernardin, G. Transthoracic Echocardiography with Doppler Tissue Imaging predicts weaning failure from mechanical ventilation: Evolution of the left ventricle relaxation rate during a spontaneous breathing trial is the key factor in weaning outcome. *Crit. Care* **2012**, *16*, R81. [CrossRef]
16. de Meirelles Almeida, C.A.; Nedel, W.L.; Morais, V.D.; Boniatti, M.M.; de Almeida-Filho, O.C. Diastolic dysfunction as a predictor of weaning failure: A systematic review and meta-analysis. *J. Crit. Care* **2016**, *34*, 135–141. [CrossRef]
17. Papanikolaou, J.; Makris, D.; Saranteas, T.; Karakitsos, D.; Zintzaras, E.; Karabinis, A.; Kostopanagiotou, G.; Zakynthinos, E. New insights into weaning from mechanical ventilation: Left ventricular diastolic dysfunction is a key player. *Intensive Care Med.* **2011**, *37*, 1976–1985. [CrossRef]
18. Caille, V.; Amiel, J.-B.; Charron, C.; Belliard, G.; Vieillard-Baron, A.; Vignon, P. Echocardiography: A help in the weaning process. *Crit. Care* **2010**, *14*, R120. [CrossRef]

19. Roche-Campo, F.; Bedet, A.; Vivier, E.; Brochard, L.; Mekontso Dessap, A. Cardiac function during weaning failure: The role of diastolic dysfunction. *Ann. Intensive Care* **2018**, *8*, 2. [CrossRef]
20. Slama, M.; Maizel, J. Echocardiographic measurement of ventricular function. *Curr. Opin. Crit. Care* **2006**, *12*, 241–248. [CrossRef]
21. Abbate, A.; Arena, R.; Abouzaki, N.; Van Tassell, B.W.; Canada, J.; Shah, K.; Biondi-Zoccai, G.; Voelkel, N.F. Heart failure with preserved ejection fraction: Refocusing on diastole. *Int. J. Cardiol.* **2015**, *179*, 430–440. [CrossRef] [PubMed]
22. Lanspa, M.J.; Gutsche, A.R.; Wilson, E.L.; Olsen, T.D.; Hirshberg, E.L.; Knox, D.B.; Brown, S.M.; Grissom, C.K. Application of a simplified definition of diastolic function in severe sepsis and septic shock. *Crit. Care* **2016**, *20*, 243. [CrossRef] [PubMed]
23. Gattinoni, L.; Caironi, P.; Cressoni, M.; Chiumello, D.; Ranieri, V.M.; Quintel, M.; Russo, S.; Patroniti, N.; Cornejo, R.; Bugedo, G. Lung Recruitment in Patients with the Acute Respiratory Distress Syndrome. *N. Engl. J. Med.* **2006**, *354*, 1775–1786. [CrossRef]
24. Coppola, S.; Froio, S.; Marino, A.; Brioni, M.; Cesana, B.M.; Cressoni, M.; Gattinoni, L.; Chiumello, D. Respiratory Mechanics, Lung Recruitability, and Gas Exchange in Pulmonary and Extrapulmonary Acute Respiratory Distress Syndrome. *Crit. Care Med.* **2019**, *47*, 792–799. [CrossRef] [PubMed]
25. Caironi, P.; Carlesso, E.; Cressoni, M.; Chiumello, D.; Moerer, O.; Chiurazzi, C.; Brioni, M.; Bottino, N.; Lazzerini, M.; Bugedo, G.; et al. Lung recruitability is better estimated according to the Berlin definition of acute respiratory distress syndrome at standard 5 cm H_2O rather than higher positive end-expiratory pressure: A retrospective cohort study. *Crit. Care Med.* **2015**, *43*, 781–790. [CrossRef] [PubMed]
26. Nagueh, S.F.; Smiseth, O.A.; Appleton, C.P.; Byrd, B.F., 3rd; Dokainish, H.; Edvardsen, T.; Flachskampf, F.A.; Gillebert, T.C.; Klein, A.L.; Lancellotti, P.; et al. Recommendations for the Evaluation of Left Ventricular Diastolic Function by Echocardiography: An Update from the American Society of Echocardiography and the European Association of Cardiovascular Imaging. *J. Am. Soc. Echocardiogr. Off. Publ. Am. Soc. Echocardiogr.* **2016**, *29*, 277–314. [CrossRef]
27. Fan, E.; Brodie, D.; Slutsky, A.S. Acute respiratory distress syndrome advances in diagnosis and treatment. *JAMA J. Am. Med. Assoc.* **2018**, *319*, 698–710. [CrossRef]
28. Nagueh, S.F.; Middleton, K.J.; Kopelen, H.A.; Zoghbi, W.A.; Quiñones, M.A. Doppler tissue imaging: A noninvasive technique for evaluation of left ventricular relaxation and estimation of filling pressures. *J. Am. Coll. Cardiol.* **1997**, *30*, 1527–1533. [CrossRef]
29. Firstenberg, M.S.; Levine, B.D.; Garcia, M.J.; Greenberg, N.L.; Cardon, L.; Morehead, A.J.; Zuckerman, J.; Thomas, J.D. Relationship of echocardiographic indices to pulmonary capillary wedge pressures in healthy volunteers. *J. Am. Coll. Cardiol.* **2000**, *36*, 1664–1669. [CrossRef]
30. Mousavi, N.; Czarnecki, A.; Ahmadie, R.; Fang, T.; Kumar, K.; Lytwyn, M.; Kumar, A.; Jassal, D.S. The utility of tissue Doppler imaging for the noninvasive determination of left ventricular filling pressures in patients with septic shock. *J. Intensive Care Med.* **2010**, *25*, 163–167. [CrossRef]
31. Sanfilippo, F.; Corredor, C.; Fletcher, N.; Landesberg, G.; Benedetto, U.; Foex, P.; Cecconi, M. Diastolic dysfunction and mortality in septic patients: A systematic review and meta-analysis. *Intensive Care Med.* **2015**, *41*, 1004–1013. [CrossRef] [PubMed]
32. Eisen, L.A.; Davlouros, P.; Karakitsos, D. Left ventricular diastolic dysfunction in the intensive care unit: Trends and perspectives. *Crit. Care Res. Pract.* **2012**, *2012*, 964158. [CrossRef] [PubMed]

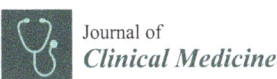

Article

Increased Respiratory Drive after Prolonged Isoflurane Sedation: A Retrospective Cohort Study

Lukas Martin Müller-Wirtz [1,2,*], Dustin Grimm [1], Frederic Walter Albrecht [1], Tobias Fink [1,2], Thomas Volk [1,2] and Andreas Meiser [1,*]

[1] Department of Anaesthesiology, Intensive Care and Pain Therapy, Saarland University Medical Center and Saarland University Faculty of Medicine, 66424 Homburg, Germany
[2] Outcomes Research Consortium, Cleveland, OH 44195, USA
* Correspondence: lukas.mueller-wirtz@uks.eu (L.M.M.-W.); andreas.meiser@uks.eu (A.M.)

Abstract: Low-dose isoflurane stimulates spontaneous breathing. We, therefore, tested the hypothesis that isoflurane compared to propofol sedation for at least 48 h is associated with increased respiratory drive in intensive care patients after sedation stop. All patients in our intensive care unit receiving at least 48 h of isoflurane or propofol sedation in 2019 were included. The primary outcome was increased respiratory drive over 72 h after sedation stop, defined as an arterial carbon dioxide pressure below 35 mmHg and a base excess more than −2 mmol/L. Secondary outcomes were acid–base balance and ventilatory parameters. We analyzed 64 patients, 23 patients sedated with isoflurane and 41 patients sedated with propofol. Patients sedated with isoflurane were about three times as likely to show increased respiratory drive after sedation stop than those sedated with propofol: adjusted risk ratio [95% confidence interval]: 2.9 [1.3, 6.5], $p = 0.010$. After sedation stop, tidal volumes were significantly greater and arterial carbon dioxide partial pressures were significantly lower, while respiratory rates did not differ in isoflurane versus propofol-sedated patients. In conclusion, prolonged isoflurane use in intensive care patients is associated with increased respiratory drive after sedation stop. Beneficial effects of isoflurane sedation on respiratory drive may, thus, extend beyond the actual period of sedation.

Keywords: intensive care; anesthesia; inhaled sedation; respiratory drive; isoflurane; propofol

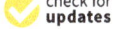

Citation: Müller-Wirtz, L.M.; Grimm, D.; Albrecht, F.W.; Fink, T.; Volk, T.; Meiser, A. Increased Respiratory Drive after Prolonged Isoflurane Sedation: A Retrospective Cohort Study. *J. Clin. Med.* **2022**, *11*, 5422. https://doi.org/10.3390/jcm11185422

Academic Editor: Spyros D. Mentzelopoulos

Received: 29 July 2022
Accepted: 12 September 2022
Published: 15 September 2022

Publisher's Note: MDPI stays neutral with regard to jurisdictional claims in published maps and institutional affiliations.

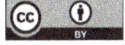

Copyright: © 2022 by the authors. Licensee MDPI, Basel, Switzerland. This article is an open access article distributed under the terms and conditions of the Creative Commons Attribution (CC BY) license (https://creativecommons.org/licenses/by/4.0/).

1. Introduction

Sedation is a central treatment of intensive care, enabling life-saving invasive procedures such as mechanical ventilation. Inhaled isoflurane was recently approved for intensive care sedation in Europe based on a multicentric randomized trial [1]. Use of isoflurane is especially interesting for prolonged periods of sedation [2,3], as intravenous sedatives may accumulate or cause substantial harm after prolonged use [4–6].

Preclinical studies indicate that isoflurane increases respiratory drive [7–9]. Specifically, tidal volume and, thus, minute ventilation are better maintained with isoflurane than with propofol [9]. Consistently, patients sedated with isoflurane are more likely to breathe spontaneously than patients sedated with propofol despite moderate to deep sedation [10]. Own non-published clinical observations suggest that this effect may well extend beyond the actual period of sedation with patients showing increased respiratory drive after discontinuation of prolonged sedation with isoflurane. As an adequate respiratory drive after sedation stop is essential for a successful weaning of the patient from the ventilator, it is of considerable interest to investigate the post sedative effects of prolonged isoflurane use on ventilation.

This study, therefore, aims to investigate the post sedative effects of prolonged isoflurane use on ventilation in intensive care patients. Specifically, we hypothesized that isoflurane compared to propofol sedation for at least 48 h is associated with increased respiratory drive in intensive care patients over 72 h after sedation stop.

2. Materials and Methods

This study was approved by our Institutional Review Board with waived consent (approval date: 4 April 2022, reference number: 67/22, Ethikkommission der Ärztekammer des Saarlandes, Saarbrücken, Germany).

2.1. Study Design

This is a retrospective cohort study performed at a single academic center for surgical intensive care of the Saarland University Medical Center. We screened all patients ventilated for at least 96 h in 2019 for eligibility. All data were digitally extracted from the patient data management system (Copra, Version 5, Copra System, Berlin, Germany). Data were obtained from 48 h before sedation stop until 72 h after sedation stop.

2.2. Inclusion and Exclusion Criteria

Inclusion criteria were mechanical ventilation for at least 96 h with more than 48 h of continuous sedation with isoflurane or propofol as the primary sedative before sedation stop, at least three available blood gas analyses during spontaneous ventilation under sedation, at least 24 h of spontaneous ventilation and no re-sedation after sedation stop, and at least three available blood gas analyzes during spontaneous ventilation after sedation stop. Exclusion criteria were age < 18 years, switch of the sedative within 48 h before sedation stop, severe pulmonary diseases, death within the observation period, and patients under palliative care.

2.3. Drug Administration

Isoflurane (Isoflurane 100%, Piramal Critical Care, West Drayton, UK) was administered via the Sedaconda Anesthetic Conserving Device (ACD, Sedana Medical AB, Danderyd, Sweden) as recommended by the manufacturer. Briefly, the ACD was inserted between the endotracheal tube of the patient and the Y-piece of the breathing circuit of a common intensive care ventilator. The ACD was connected to a syringe pump (Perfusor compact, B. Braun, Melsungen, Germany) that delivered liquid isoflurane. A gas monitor (Vamos, Dräger Medical Deutschland GmbH, Lübeck, Germany) was connected to the ACD to monitor the end-tidal isoflurane concentration. Finally, a charcoal filter (FlurAbsorb, Sedana medical AB, Stockholm, Sweden) was connected to the expiratory port of the ventilator for gas scavenging.

Propofol 20 mg·mL^{-1} (Propofol Hexal, Hexal AG/Sandoz, Holzkirchen, Germany) was infused by a syringe pump (Perfusor Space, B. Braun, Melsungen, Germany) according to common clinical practice.

As natural for retrospective studies, there was no explicit protocol for sedation. However, a written standard operating procedure of our center (provided as Supplementary Materials) stipulates to administer sedative drugs as low as possible according to the patient's needs and to perform daily spontaneous awakening trials for avoidance of overdosing and assessment of neurological function.

2.4. Ventilation

Patients were ventilated with Evita 4 ventilators (Dräger Medical Deutschland GmbH) in pressure-controlled mode (biphasic positive airway pressure) or pressure-support mode. Ventilation parameters were automatically captured by our patient data management system. In the patients that were extubated after sedation stop, ventilation parameters were captured from periods of non-invasive ventilation via a face mask.

2.5. Measurements

All available blood gas analyzes (BGA) within the observation period while patients were breathing spontaneously were included to evaluate respiratory drive. Circulatory and ventilatory measures were extracted from the patient data management system at 12-h intervals. Implausible values, as commonly obtained during periods of nursing or airway leaks, were excluded. Intravenously and orally applied opioids were converted to morphine equivalent doses (μg/kg) as previously published [11] to enable comparison (sufentanil 1:1000; hydromorphone 1:7; remifentanil 1:200). For remifentanil, the equivalent dose was divided by 60 to account for the considerably shorter half-life than morphine. The sum of all morphine equivalent doses over 12-h intervals was divided by 12 to obtain morphine equivalent dose rates (μg/kg/h). Patients that received additional opioid boluses from nurse-controlled analgesia pumps not being electronically recorded after sedation stop were excluded from the analysis of opioid consumption. The Simplified Acute Physiology Score II (SAPS II) was calculated according to Le Gall et al. [12]. The Sequential Organ Failure Assessment (SOFA) score was calculated according to Vincent et al. [13]. Ideal body weight was calculated according to the sex-specific ARDSnet formulas [14].

2.6. Outcomes

The primary outcome was increased respiratory drive after sedation stop, defined as arterial carbon dioxide pressure < 35 mmHg and base excess > −2 mmol/L to exclude potential respiratory compensations of metabolic acidosis. Secondary outcomes were measures of acid-base balance and ventilation including pH, arterial carbon dioxide partial pressure, base excess, tidal volume, respiratory rate, and inspiratory pressure support.

2.7. Statistical Analysis

Data were collected with Excel Version 16.58 (Microsoft, Redmond, WA, USA). Statistical analyses were carried out with R (*v4.0.2*, R Core Team, 2020) using the packages *readxl* (*v1.3.1*, Wickham and Bryan, 2019), *dplyr* (*v1.0.5*, Wickham, François, Henry, and Müller, 2021), *tableone* (*v0.12.0*, Yoshida and Bartel, 2020), *rcompanion* (*v2.4.1*, Mangiafico, 2016), *geepack* (*v1.3-2*; Højsgaard, Halekoh, and Yan, 2006), *parameters* (*v0.14.0*; Lüdecke, Ben-Shachar, Patil and Makowski, 2020), and *ggplot2* (*v3.3.3*; Wickham, 2016).

Normality was assessed by visual assessment of histograms/quantile-quantile plots and Shapiro–Wilk testing. According to data distribution, we present continuous measures as means with standard deviations or medians with interquartile ranges (IQR) for descriptive data and with the corresponding 95% confidence intervals (95% CI) for outcome data. Categorical variables are presented as frequencies (percentages).

Baseline balance is presented as absolute standardized differences, defined as the absolute difference in means divided by the pooled standard deviation. Repeated-measures data were summarized with a mean for each patient for the periods of 48 h before and 72 h after sedation stop and compared between groups by independent samples t-tests or Wilcoxon rank-sum tests. A two-sided $p < 0.05$ was considered statistically significant.

The risk ratio for increased respiratory drive in isoflurane versus propofol-sedated patients was calculated by Poisson generalized estimating equation regression to account for repeated measures. Two separate univariable models were calculated to estimate the crude risk ratio before and after sedation stop. Multivariable models were calculated to adjust for age, total ventilation and sedation time, tracheostomy, hemodialysis, simplified acute physiology score II, and mean morphine equivalent dose rate.

To our knowledge, there are no previous data on the prevalence of increased respiratory drive after sedation stop in intensive care patients. We, therefore, did not estimate sample size in advance and planned to include all qualifying patient records from a one-year cohort.

3. Results

3.1. Study Population Characteristics

A total of 158 patients were ventilated for at least 96 h throughout 2019. After application of inclusion and exclusion criteria, 23 patients sedated with isoflurane and 41 with propofol were included (Figure 1).

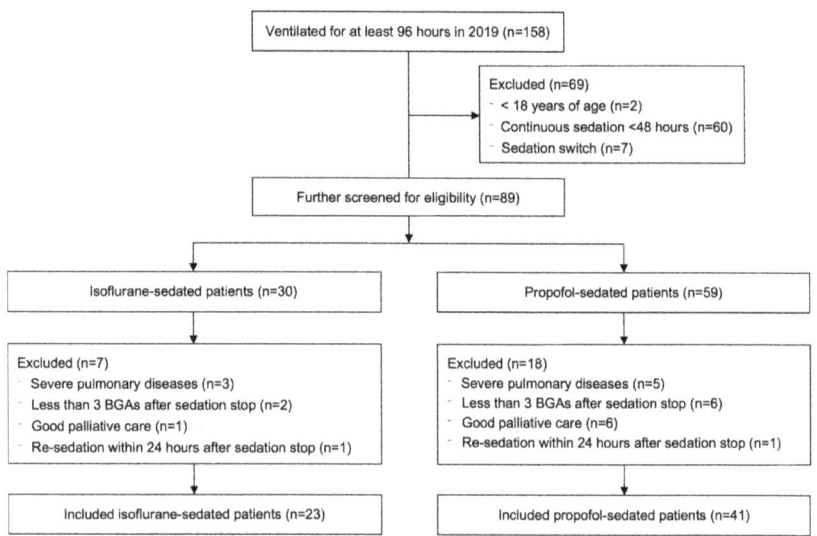

Figure 1. Patient flow chart.

Potential covariates/confounders for respiratory drive including age, total ventilation and sedation times, tracheostomy, hemodialysis, and simplified acute physiology score II were not well balanced between the sedation groups (Table 1), and the analysis of increased respiratory drive was, therefore, adjusted for these variables.

Table 1. Study population characteristics.

Parameter	Isoflurane	Propofol	SMD
n	23	41	-
Sex [male]	20 (87)	24 (58)	0.673
Age [years]	55 [52, 65]	69 [60, 80]	0.833
Height [cm]	175 [171, 180]	170 [165, 178]	0.218
Weight [kg]	85 ± 28	81 ± 23	0.158
BMI	26 [23, 32]	27 [23, 30]	0.028
SAPS II	37 ± 13	41 ± 13	0.313
SOFA	10 ± 4	10 ± 3	0.121
CVVHD [n]	11 (48)	11 (27)	0.445
Death [n]	5 (22)	13 (32)	0.227
Tracheostomy [n]	16 (70)	11 (27)	0.946
Total ventilation time [h]	114 [86, 171]	108 [79, 167]	0.402
Total sedation time [h]	179 [141, 234]	108 [79, 167]	0.845
Surgical patients [n]	20 (87)	38 (93)	-
Visceral [n]	11 (48)	19 (46)	-
Trauma [n]	2 (9)	10 (24)	-
Other [n]	7 (30)	9 (22)	-
Medical patients [n]	3 (13)	3 (7)	-

Data are reported as means ± standard deviations, medians [interquartile ranges], or numbers (percentages). The standardized mean difference (SMD) is presented as a measure of balance. BMI, body mass index. SAPS II, Simplified Acute Physiology Score II (scored at intensive care unit admission). SOFA, sepsis-related organ failure assessment score (scored 24 h before sedation stop). CVVHD, continuous veno-venous hemodialysis.

Circulatory measures were similar in both groups; only heart rate was significantly higher in isoflurane patients during sedation (mean [95% CI]: isoflurane: 95 [87, 101], propofol: 84 [79, 89], $p = 0.012$; Table 2).

Table 2. Circulatory and ventilatory measures within 48 h before and 72 h after sedation stop.

Parameter	Before Sedation Stop			After Sedation Stop		
	Isoflurane	Propofol	P	Isoflurane	Propofol	P
n	23	41	-	23	41	-
Circulation						
Heart rate [bpm] *	95 [87, 101]	84 [79, 89]	0.012	93 [86, 100]	87 [83, 92]	0.157
Mean arterial blood pressure [mmHg]	69 [61, 69]	71 [68, 73]	0.195	80 [71, 88]	78 [72, 80]	0.585
Sedation and analgesia						
End-tidal isoflurane [Vol%]	0.64 [0.55, 0.70]	-	-	-	-	-
Propofol dose [mg/kg/h]	-	1.4 [1.1, 1.7]	-	-	-	-
Morphine equivalent dose [µg/kg/h]	39 [29, 60]	31 [22, 38]	0.087	34 [18, 46] [†]	25 [15, 26] [†]	0.073
Primary outcome—Increased respiratory drive						
Total observations [n]	318	520		515	924	
Observations with increased respiratory drive [n]	9 (3%)	27 (5%)		159 (31%)	110 (12%)	
Risk ratio	0.5 [0.1, 2.1]		0.319	2.6 [1.3, 5.2]		0.005
Adjusted risk ratio [#]	0.9 [0.2, 5.5]		0.926	2.9 [1.3, 6.5]		0.010
Adjusted risk ratio [#,§]	0.9 [0.2, 5.4]		0.925	3.3 [1.3, 8.3] [†]		0.012
Secondary outcomes—Acid–base balance and ventilation						
pH	7.41 [7.38, 7.43]	7.40 [7.37, 7.41]	0.374	7.45 [7.41, 7.46]	7.43 [7.42, 7.44]	0.221
P_aCO_2 [mmHg]	47 [44, 52]	44 [42, 45]	0.096	37 [35, 42]	41 [39, 45]	0.007
Base excess [mmol/L]	4.3 [3.1, 5.0]	1.9 [0.7, 2.7]	0.005	1.7 [0.9, 3.0]	2.5 [1.5, 3.5]	0.297
Tidal volume [ml] *	613 [559, 660]	526 [503, 550]	0.001	609 [556, 668]	503 [471, 540]	0.002
Tidal volume normalized to IBW [ml/kg] *	9.0 [8.4, 9.6]	8.2 [7.8, 8.5]	0.014	9.0 [8.3, 9.7]	7.8 [7.3, 8.2]	0.006
Respiratory rate [bpm]	17 [15, 19]	17 [15, 17]	0.238	19 [15, 19]	19 [16, 20]	0.445
Inspiratory pressure support [cmH$_2$O] *	8 [7, 10]	8 [7, 9]	0.377	6 [5, 7]	7 [6, 8]	0.362

Repeated measures were summarized with a mean for each patient and are reported as means (*) or medians with the corresponding 95% confidence intervals (95% CI) for each sedation group within 48 h before and 72 h after sedation. Groups were compared using independent samples t-tests or Wilcoxon rank-sum tests. Statistical significances ($p < 0.05$) are written in bold. The presented risk ratios [95% CI] were calculated by Poisson generalized estimating equation regression and describe the effect of isoflurane versus propofol sedation on increased respiratory drive within 48 h before or 72 h after sedation stop. Increased respiratory drive was defined as arterial carbon dioxide partial pressure < 35 mmHg and base excess > −2 mmol/L. [#] Adjusted for age, total ventilation and sedation time, tracheostomy, hemodialysis, and simplified acute physiology score II. [§] Additional adjustment for mean morphine equivalent dose rate. [†] 30% (7/23) of patients after isoflurane and 39% (16/41) after propofol sedation were excluded due to opioid intake via a nurse-controlled analgesia system, which was not electronically recorded. P_aCO_2, arterial carbon dioxide partial pressure. SpO$_2$, oxygen saturation by pulse oximetry. IBW, ideal body weight.

Sedatives were applied within a low dosing range with isoflurane applied at around 0.5 minimum alveolar concentration (MAC) and propofol applied below 2 mg/kg/h (Table 2). Opioid consumption was similar with both sedatives before and after sedation stop (Table 2). During sedation, patients received continuous intravenous opioids, either remifentanil, sufentanil, or hydromorphone. After sedation stop, in most patients, the continuous opioid infusion was stopped, and oral opioids or intravenous opioid boluses were applied. Thirty percent (7/23) of patients after isoflurane and 39% (16/41) after propofol sedation received occasional boluses of intravenous opioids via a nurse-controlled analgesia system not being electronically recorded and were, therefore, excluded from the analysis of opioid consumption after sedation stop.

3.2. Primary Outcome—Increased Respiratory Drive after Sedation Stop

We detected increased respiratory drive at 31% (159/515) of the observations in isoflurane-sedated patients compared to only 12% (110/924) in propofol-sedated patients within 72 h after sedation stop. Patients sedated with isoflurane were three times as likely to show increased respiratory drive within 72 h after sedation stop than those sedated with propofol: risk ratio [95% CI]: 2.6 [1.3, 5.2], $p = 0.005$, which remained similar after adjustments for age, total ventilation and sedation times, tracheostomy, hemodialysis, and simplified acute physiology score II: adjusted risk ratio [95% CI]: 2.9 [1.3, 6.5], $p = 0.010$ (Table 2, Figure 2). Additional adjustment for the mean morphine equivalent dose rate for those patients with complete data on opioid intake did not substantially change the association: adjusted risk ratio [95% CI]: 3.3 [1.3, 8.3], $p = 0.012$ (isoflurane: $n = 16$, propofol $n = 25$).

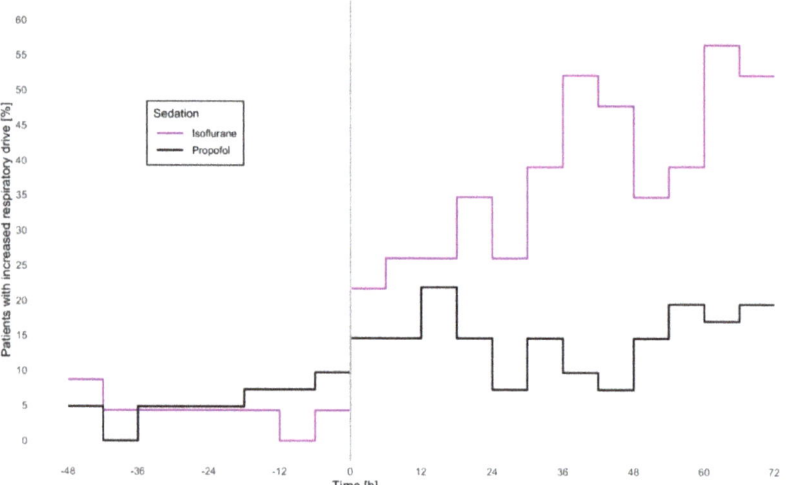

Figure 2. Percentage of patients with increased respiratory drive. Sedation was stopped at time point 0. Data are presented in 6-hour intervals as percentage of patients within each sedation group. The risk for increased respiratory drive after sedation stop was three times higher in patients sedated with isoflurane than in those receiving propofol: adjusted risk ratio [95%CI]: 2.9 [1.3, 6.5], $p = 0.010$. Increased respiratory drive was defined as arterial carbon dioxide partial pressure (P_aCO_2) < 35 mmHg and base excess > −2 mmol/L.

In contrast, increased respiratory drive was equally frequent with both sedatives before sedation was discontinued: adjusted risk ratio [95% CI]: 0.9 [0.2, 5.4], $p = 0.925$ (Table 2, Figure 2).

3.3. Secondary Outcomes—Acid-Base Balance, Ventilation and Opioid Consumption

There was no difference in blood pH between isoflurane-sedated and propofol-sedated patients (Table 2). However, base excess was significantly higher in isoflurane-sedated patients before sedation stop (median [95% CI]: isoflurane: 4.3 [3.1, 5.0], propofol: 1.9 [0.7, 2.7], $p = 0.005$; Table 2), suggesting metabolic compensation of slightly increased arterial carbon dioxide partial pressures before sedation stop (median [95% CI]: isoflurane: 47 [44, 52], propofol: 44 [42, 45], $p = 0.096$; Table 2, Figure 3). Although tidal volumes and respiratory rate did not substantially change after sedation stop, arterial carbon dioxide partial pressure was significantly lower in patients sedated with isoflurane compared to those sedated with propofol after sedation stop (median [95% CI]: isoflurane: 37 [35, 42] mmHg, propofol: 41 [39, 45] mmHg, $p = 0.007$; Table 2, Figure 3).

Tidal volumes were about 100 mL greater in patients sedated with isoflurane than in those sedated with propofol, with nearly identical differences before and after sedation stop (mean [95% CI]: before sedation stop: isoflurane: 613 [559, 660], propofol: 526 [503, 550], $p = 0.001$; after sedation stop: isoflurane: 609 [556, 668], propofol: 503 [471, 540], $p = 0.002$; Table 2, Figure 2). Respiratory rate and inspiratory pressure support did not differ significantly between the sedation groups (Table 2, Figure 3).

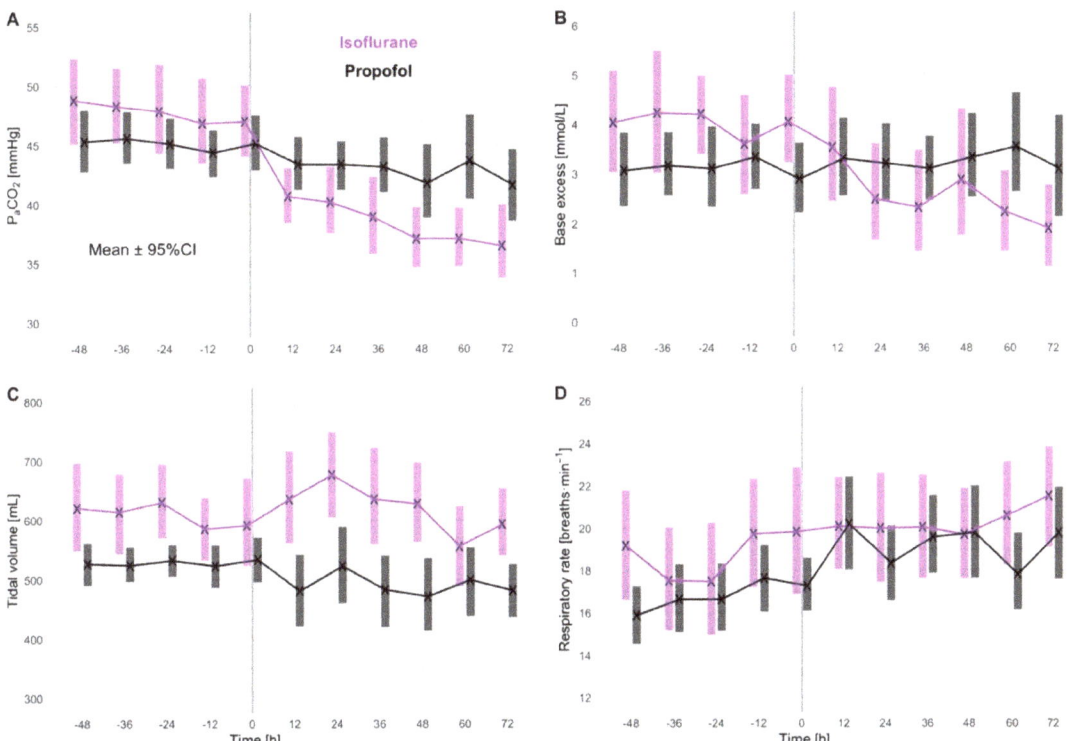

Figure 3. Acid-base balance and ventilation. Sedation was stopped at time point 0. Data are presented in 12-hour intervals as means ± 95% confidence intervals (95%CI). PaCO$_2$, arterial carbon dioxide pressure. (**A**) Arterial carbon dioxide partial pressure; (**B**) Base excess; (**C**) Tidal volume; (**D**) Respiratory rate.

4. Discussion

Isoflurane-sedated patients were about three times as likely to have an arterial carbon dioxide pressure below 35 mmHg during periods of spontaneous breathing after sedation stop than those sedated with propofol. A comparatively better-maintained respiratory drive with isoflurane as opposed to propofol sedation, thus, seems to extend to the post-sedation period. To our knowledge, this is the first report on differential post-sedative effects of prolonged inhaled versus intravenous sedation on ventilation in intensive care patients.

In line with our primary finding, studies in rats showed that minute ventilation is better maintained with isoflurane than with propofol [9]. Most interestingly, isoflurane even increases respiratory drive at subanesthetic doses of 0.5 MAC but decreases respiratory drive at doses exceeding 1 MAC in rats [9]. Consistently, subanesthetic doses of volatile anesthetics promote the transition from controlled to spontaneous ventilation in intensive care patients [10,15,16]. Our study, thus, adds to current evidence that better maintenance of respiratory drive in isoflurane-sedated patients may continue well beyond the actual period of sedation.

Brainstem neurons of the retrotrapezoid nucleus are responsible for the maintenance of spontaneous breathing under general anesthesia [17]. The increased respiratory drive under isoflurane compared to propofol sedation can be explained by diverging effects on the central regulation of breathing; whereby propofol inhibits, isoflurane stimulates neurons of the retrotrapezoid nucleus, and, thus, increases respiratory drive [7,8].

The largest amount of isoflurane is exhaled during the first hours after anesthesia [18,19]. However, modern highly sensitive analytical methods show that volatile anesthetics are exhaled up to two weeks after general anesthesia [20,21]. Isoflurane trace concentrations were even detected in breath up to 130 days after anesthesia [21]. Whereas general anesthesia may last a few hours, we included patients exposed to isoflurane over at least 48 h. Therefore, additional saturation of body tissues with isoflurane leading to even longer final elimination times can be assumed. Residual pharmacologically active isoflurane concentrations could, thus, explain the observed increased respiratory drive after sedation stop in patients exposed to prolonged isoflurane sedation.

Arterial carbon dioxide pressure was slightly higher in isoflurane-sedated patients within the last 48 h before sedation stop, as opposed to being significantly lower within 72 h after sedation stop when compared to propofol-sedated patients. Slightly higher arterial carbon dioxide pressures under isoflurane sedation are explainable by the fact that volatile anesthetic reflection devices increase respiratory dead space resulting in carbon dioxide retention [22–25]. Interestingly, arterial carbon dioxide pressures dropped considerably after sedation stop in patients sedated with isoflurane, while tidal volume and respiratory rate remained almost unchanged, which is consistent with reduced dead space ventilation after removal of the volatile anesthetic reflection device.

Compared to patients sedated with propofol, tidal volumes were higher in patients sedated with isoflurane before and after sedation. While a compensatory increase in tidal volume may be a consequence of increased ventilatory dead space under isoflurane sedation [22–25], tidal volumes remained higher after sedation stop, even though volatile anesthetic reflection devices were removed. Animal data suggest that an isoflurane-induced increase in minute ventilation is largely caused by increased tidal volumes [9]. It, thus, seems likely that the observed phenomenon results from residual isoflurane concentrations increasing respiratory drive. However, this could also reflect a physiological consequence of prolonged exposure of the lung to higher tidal volumes causing adaptations in the neural control of breathing. Consistent with this theory, a lung volume-related habituation and desensitization of the Hering–Breuer inflation reflex was shown in rats [26]. In general, both causes are interesting with potential clinical consequences and should be subject to future studies.

Our study has distinct limitations. At first, age, total ventilation and sedation time, tracheostomy, hemodialysis, and simplified acute physiology score II differed markedly between the sedation groups. However, all of them only marginally influenced the primary outcome—increased respiratory drive after sedation stop. Furthermore, uncaptured adjunct drugs, such as benzodiazepines, may have influenced respiratory drive and ventilatory measures, although unlikely since our center largely dispenses with the administration of benzodiazepines. Of note, our study represents an initial observation of increased respiratory drive after discontinuation of prolonged isoflurane sedation. Future studies with larger sample sizes and distinct treatment protocols for sedation, opioid use, and adjunct drugs may provide more accurate estimates of differences in respiration between isoflurane and propofol sedation.

5. Conclusions

Prolonged isoflurane use in intensive care patients was associated with increased respiratory drive throughout 72 h after sedation stop. Beneficial effects of isoflurane sedation on respiratory drive may, thus, extend beyond the actual period of sedation. However, these results still need confirmation by studies with larger sample sizes and at best by prospective investigations.

Supplementary Materials: The following supporting information can be downloaded at: https://www.mdpi.com/article/10.3390/jcm11185422/s1, The departmental standard operating procedure on analgesia, sedation, and delirium therapy.

Author Contributions: All authors contributed to the conceptualization of the study, whereby A.M. was the driving force in developing the research question. D.G. performed data collection. L.M.M.-W. performed the statistical analysis and wrote the first draft of the manuscript. F.W.A., T.F., T.V. and A.M. helped with interpretation of the results. All authors have read and agreed to the published version of the manuscript.

Funding: Conduction of this study was financed solely from institutional and/or departmental funds. The APC was funded by the Deutsche Forschungsgemeinschaft (DFG, German Research Foundation) and Saarland University.

Institutional Review Board Statement: The study was conducted in accordance with the Declaration of Helsinki and approved by the Ethics Committee of Saarland Physician Board, Saarbrücken, Germany (approval date: 4 April 2022, reference number: 67/22) with waived consent.

Informed Consent Statement: Patient consent was waived due to the retrospective study design.

Data Availability Statement: The datasets analyzed during the current study are available from the corresponding author on reasonable request.

Acknowledgments: This study contains data taken from the thesis presented by Dustin Grimm as part of the requirements for the obtention of the degree "Doctor of Medicine" at Saarland University Medical Center and Saarland University Faculty of Medicine. We acknowledge Nadine Weber and Hanan Kasouha for their help with data collection. We acknowledge support by the Deutsche Forschungsgemeinschaft (DFG, German Research Foundation) and Saarland University within the funding programme Open Access Publishing.

Conflicts of Interest: Thomas Volk and Andreas Meiser received consulting fees from Sedana Medical AB, Danderyd, Sweden.

References

1. Meiser, A.; Volk, T.; Wallenborn, J.; Guenther, U.; Becher, T.; Bracht, H.; Schwarzkopf, K.; Knafelj, R.; Faltlhauser, A.; Thal, S.C.; et al. Inhaled isoflurane via the anaesthetic conserving device versus propofol for sedation of invasively ventilated patients in intensive care units in Germany and Slovenia: An open-label, phase 3, randomised controlled, non-inferiority trial. *Lancet Respir. Med.* **2021**, *9*, 1231–1240. [CrossRef]
2. Jerath, A.; Wong, K.; Wasowicz, M.; Fowler, T.; Steel, A.; Grewal, D.; Huszti, E.; Parotto, M.; Zhang, H.; Wilcox, M.E.; et al. Use of Inhaled Volatile Anesthetics for Longer Term Critical Care Sedation: A Pilot Randomized Controlled Trial. *Crit. Care Explor.* **2020**, *2*, e0281. [CrossRef]
3. Bellgardt, M.; Bomberg, H.; Herzog-Niescery, J.; Dasch, B.; Vogelsang, H.; Weber, T.P.; Steinfort, C.; Uhl, W.; Wagenpfeil, S.; Volk, T.; et al. Survival after long-term isoflurane sedation as opposed to intravenous sedation in critically ill surgical patients. *Eur. J. Anaesthesiol.* **2016**, *33*, 6–13. [CrossRef]
4. Hemphill, S.; McMenamin, L.; Bellamy, M.C.; Hopkins, P.M. Propofol infusion syndrome: A structured literature review and analysis of published case reports. *Br. J. Anaesth.* **2019**, *122*, 448–459. [CrossRef]
5. Naritoku, D.K.; Sinha, S. Prolongation of midazolam half-life after sustained infusion for status epilepticus. *Neurology* **2000**, *54*, 1366–1368. [CrossRef] [PubMed]
6. Wills, R.; Khoo, K.; Soni, P.; Patel, I. Increased volume of distribution prolongs midazolam half-life. *Br. J. Clin. Pharmacol.* **1990**, *29*, 269–272. [CrossRef]
7. Yang, Y.; Ou, M.; Liu, J.; Zhao, W.; Zhuoma, L.; Liang, Y.; Zhu, T.; Mulkey, D.K.; Zhou, C. Volatile anesthetics activate a leak sodium conductance in retrotrapezoid nucleus neurons to maintain breathing during anesthesia in mice. *Anesthesiology* **2020**, *133*, 824–838. [CrossRef]
8. Lazarenko, R.M.; Fortuna, M.G.; Shi, Y.; Mulkey, D.K.; Takakura, A.C.; Moreira, T.S.; Guyenet, P.G.; Bayliss, D.A. Anesthetic activation of central respiratory chemoreceptor neurons involves inhibition of a THIK-1-like background K+ current. *J. Neurosci.* **2010**, *30*, 9324–9334. [CrossRef]
9. Hao, X.; Ou, M.; Li, Y.; Zhou, C. Volatile anesthetics maintain tidal volume and minute ventilation to a greater degree than propofol under spontaneous respiration. *BMC Anesthesiol.* **2021**, *21*, 238. [CrossRef]
10. Müller-Wirtz, L.M.; Behne, F.; Kermad, A.; Wagenpfeil, G.; Schroeder, M.; Sessler, D.I.; Volk, T.; Meiser, A. Isoflurane promotes early spontaneous breathing in ventilated intensive care patients: A post hoc subgroup analysis of a randomized trial. *Acta Anaesthesiol. Scand.* **2022**, *66*, 354–364. [CrossRef]
11. Kermad, A.; Speltz, J.; Danziger, G.; Mertke, T.; Bals, R.; Volk, T.; Lepper, P.M.; Meiser, A. Comparison of isoflurane and propofol sedation in critically ill COVID-19 patients—A retrospective chart review. *J. Anesth.* **2021**, *35*, 625–632. [CrossRef] [PubMed]
12. Le Gall, J.-R. A New Simplified Acute Physiology Score (SAPS II) Based on a European/North American Multicenter Study. *JAMA J. Am. Med. Assoc.* **1993**, *270*, 2957. [CrossRef]

13. Vincent, J.L.; Moreno, R.; Takala, J.; Willatts, S.; De Mendonça, A.; Bruining, H.; Reinhart, C.K.; Suter, P.M.; Thijs, L.G. The SOFA (Sepsis-related Organ Failure Assessment) score to describe organ dysfunction/failure. *Intensive Care Med.* **1996**, *22*, 707–710. [CrossRef] [PubMed]
14. Acute Respiratory Distress Syndrome Network; Brower, R.G.; Matthay, M.A.; Morris, A.; Schoenfeld, D.; Thompson, B.T.; Wheeler, A. Ventilation with lower tidal volumes as compared with traditional tidal volumes for acute lung injury and the acute respiratory distress syndrome. *N. Engl. J. Med.* **2000**, *342*, 1301–1308. [CrossRef]
15. Heider, J.; Bansbach, J.; Kaufmann, K.; Heinrich, S.; Loop, T.; Kalbhenn, J. Does volatile sedation with sevoflurane allow spontaneous breathing during prolonged prone positioning in intubated ARDS patients? A retrospective observational feasibility trial. *Ann. Intensive Care* **2019**, *9*, 41. [CrossRef]
16. Meiser, A.; Groesdonk, H.V.; Bonnekessel, S.; Volk, T.; Bomberg, H. Inhalation Sedation in Subjects With ARDS Undergoing Continuous Lateral Rotational Therapy. *Respir. Care* **2018**, *63*, 441–447. [CrossRef]
17. Bourgeois, T.; Ringot, M.; Ramanantsoa, N.; Matrot, B.; Dauger, S.; Delclaux, C.; Gallego, J. Breathing under Anesthesia. *Anesthesiology* **2019**, *130*, 995–1006. [CrossRef]
18. Yasuda, N.; Lockhart, S.H.; Eger, E.I.; Weiskopf, R.B.; Johnson, B.H.; Frelre, B.A.; Fassoulakl, A. Kinetics of Desflurane, Isoflurane, and Halothane in Humans. *Anesthesiology* **1991**, *74*, 489–498. [CrossRef]
19. Lu, C.C.; Tsai, C.S.; Hu, O.Y.P.; Chen, R.M.; Chen, T.L.; Ho, S.T. Pharmacokinetics of isoflurane in human blood. *Pharmacology* **2008**, *81*, 344–349. [CrossRef]
20. Hüppe, T.; Dreyer, D.B.; Genoux, L.H.; Meiers, K.; Volk, T.; Kreuer, S. Desflurane and Sevoflurane are Detectable in Expired Air Up to 14 Days after General Anesthesia (Conference Abstract, A3161). American Society of Anesthesiologists Annual Meeting. 15 October 2018. Available online: https://www.abstractsonline.com/pp8/#!/4593/presentation/5903 (accessed on 28 July 2022).
21. Fernández Del Río, F.; O'Hara, M.E.; Pemberton, P.; Whitehouse, T.; Mayhew, C.A. Elimination characteristics of post-operative isoflurane levels in alveolar exhaled breath via PTR-MS analysis. *J. Breath Res.* **2016**, *10*, 046006. [CrossRef]
22. Bomberg, H.; Meiser, F.; Zimmer, S.; Bellgardt, M.; Volk, T.; Sessler, D.I.; Groesdonk, H.V.; Meiser, A. Halving the volume of AnaConDa: Initial clinical experience with a new small-volume anaesthetic reflector in critically ill patients-a quality improvement project. *J. Clin. Monit. Comput.* **2018**, *32*, 639–646. [CrossRef] [PubMed]
23. Bomberg, H.; Meiser, F.; Daume, P.; Bellgardt, M.; Volk, T.; Sessler, D.I.; Groesdonk, H.V.; Meiser, A. Halving the Volume of AnaConDa: Evaluation of a New Small-Volume Anesthetic Reflector in a Test Lung Model. *Anesth. Analg.* **2019**, *129*, 371–379. [CrossRef] [PubMed]
24. Bomberg, H.; Veddeler, M.; Volk, T.; Groesdonk, H.V.; Meiser, A. Volumetric and reflective device dead space of anaesthetic reflectors under different conditions. *J. Clin. Monit. Comput.* **2018**, *32*, 1073–1080. [CrossRef] [PubMed]
25. Sturesson, L.W.; Bodelsson, M.; Johansson, A.; Jonson, B.; Malmkvist, G. Apparent dead space with the anesthetic conserving device, AnaConDa®: A clinical and laboratory investigation. *Anesth. Analg.* **2013**, *117*, 1319–1324. [CrossRef]
26. MacDonald, S.M.; Tin, C.; Song, G.; Poon, C.S. Use-dependent learning and memory of the Hering-Breuer inflation reflex in rats. *Exp. Physiol.* **2009**, *94*, 269–278. [CrossRef]

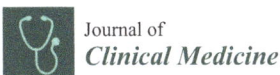

Article

The Potential Impact of Heparanase Activity and Endothelial Damage in COVID-19 Disease

Elisabeth Zechendorf [1,*], Katharina Schröder [1], Lara Stiehler [1], Nadine Frank [1], Christian Beckers [1], Sandra Kraemer [1], Michael Dreher [2], Alexander Kersten [2], Christoph Thiemermann [3], Gernot Marx [1], Tim-Philipp Simon [1,†] and Lukas Martin [1,†]

1 Department of Intensive and Intermediate Care, University Hospital RWTH Aachen, 52074 Aachen, Germany
2 Department of Pneumology and Intensive Care Medicine, University Hospital RWTH Aachen, 52074 Aachen, Germany
3 William Harvey Research Institute, Barts and The London School of Medicine and Dentistry, Queen Mary University of London, London EC1M 6BQ, UK
* Correspondence: ezechendorf@ukaachen.de; Tel.: +49-(0)241-8035484
† These authors contributed equally to this work.

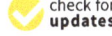

Citation: Zechendorf, E.; Schröder, K.; Stiehler, L.; Frank, N.; Beckers, C.; Kraemer, S.; Dreher, M.; Kersten, A.; Thiemermann, C.; Marx, G.; et al. The Potential Impact of Heparanase Activity and Endothelial Damage in COVID-19 Disease. *J. Clin. Med.* **2022**, *11*, 5261. https://doi.org/10.3390/jcm11185261

Academic Editor: Spyros D. Mentzelopoulos

Received: 30 June 2022
Accepted: 1 September 2022
Published: 6 September 2022

Publisher's Note: MDPI stays neutral with regard to jurisdictional claims in published maps and institutional affiliations.

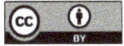

Copyright: © 2022 by the authors. Licensee MDPI, Basel, Switzerland. This article is an open access article distributed under the terms and conditions of the Creative Commons Attribution (CC BY) license (https://creativecommons.org/licenses/by/4.0/).

Abstract: SARS-CoV-2 was first detected in 2019 in Wuhan, China. It has been found to be the most pathogenic virus among coronaviruses and is associated with endothelial damage resulting in respiratory failure. Determine whether heparanase and heparan sulfate fragments, biomarkers of endothelial function, can assist in the risk stratification and clinical management of critically ill COVID-19 patients admitted to the intensive care unit. We investigated 53 critically ill patients with severe COVID-19 admitted between March and April 2020 to the University Hospital RWTH Aachen. Heparanase activity and serum levels of both heparanase and heparan sulfate were measured on day one (day of diagnosis) and day three in patients with COVID-19. The patients were classified into four groups according to the severity of ARDS. When compared to baseline data (day one), heparanase activity increased and the heparan sulfate serum levels decreased with increasing severity of ARDS. The heparanase activity significantly correlated with the lactate concentration on day one ($r = 0.34$, $p = 0.024$) and on day three ($r = 0.43$, $p = 0.006$). Heparanase activity and heparan sulfate levels correlate with COVID-19 disease severity and outcome. Both biomarkers might be helpful in predicting clinical course and outcomes in COVID-19 patients.

Keywords: COVID-19; ARDS; endothelial dysfunction; heparanase; heparan sulfate; biomarker

1. Introduction

Coronaviruses have been known since 1960. A total of seven different coronaviruses have been described, including the coronavirus SARS-CoV-2 [1]. Most coronaviruses are associated with a moderate clinical course with mild respiratory diseases. The coronaviruses SARS-CoV and MERS-CoV are associated with a more severe disease course and higher mortality. SARS-CoV was first identified in 2003. A total of 8422 cases were detected, and 916 fatalities were described [2]. Having a mortality rate of 34.4%, the MERS-CoV virus turned out to be one of the most dangerous viruses of the group of coronaviruses. From 2012 until today, 2500 cases have been confirmed [3]. SARS-CoV-2 was first detected in 2019 in Wuhan, China. It has been found to be the most pathogenic virus among the coronaviruses [4]. SARS-CoV-2 is associated with a variation in respiratory syndromes ranging from mild airway symptoms to life-threatening viral pneumonia. One-third of all lung cells are endothelial cells, which are known to be associated with the severity of lung damage in patients [5]. The endothelial glycocalyx coats the surface layer of endothelial cells. The endothelial glycocalyx interacts with the blood and thereby regulates microcirculatory flow [6]. The endothelium has a key role in the innate immune response in a wide array of critical care conditions [5]. Endothelial cells are also involved in maintaining barrier function and preventing inflammation by limiting their interactions with immune cells and platelets [6]. Endothelial dysfunction is a key driver in the pathogenesis of the organ dysfunction during viral infections [7]. Angiotensin-converting enzyme 2 (ACE2) is expressed by endothelial cells and has been found in a variety of arterial and venous endothelial cells [8]. SARS-CoV-2 enters target cells and initiates infection by binding to ACE2 on the cell membrane of host cells [8,9]. SARS-CoV-2 has been detected in endothelial cells of many organs. For instance, Varga et al. described that patients with COVID-19 exhibit endothelial cell injury in blood vessels of the kidney, liver, heart, and lung [10]. Monteil and colleagues reported that SARS-CoV-2 directly infects engineered human blood vessels in vitro [11]. Most notably, endothelial cell injury has also been confirmed by transmission electron microscopy in blood vessels obtained during autopsy of patients who died from COVID-19 [6].

The endothelial glycocalyx is composed of different glycoproteins, proteoglycans, and glycosaminoglycans. The heparan sulfate proteoglycan is one of these proteoglycans and represents approximately 50–90% of the total amount of proteoglycans present in the glycocalyx [12]. As a consequence of infection, sheddases, such as heparanase, are activated. Heparanase specifically cleaves heparan sulfate fragments from the proteoglycan, resulting in a loss of integrity and, thus, in endothelial dysfunction. Therefore, it is hypothesized that increased heparanase activity may be one of the driving forces in severe COVID-19 manifestations. Indeed, Buijsers and colleagues demonstrated that heparanase activity and heparan sulfate levels are significantly increased in the plasma of COVID-19 patients, which is related to the severity of the disease [13]. Furthermore, another study showed a significantly higher heparanase activity and increased levels of heparan sulfate in plasma of COVID-19 patients [14].

There is strong evidence that endothelial dysfunction plays a critical role in the pathophysiology and clinical course of acute respiratory distress syndrome (ARDS) [15]. However, the role of heparanase activity and heparanase and heparan sulfate serum levels in this context is unclear. Therefore, the aim of this study was to investigate the relationship between heparanase activity and heparan sulfate fragment formation and outcome in COVID-19 patients and to determine the prognostic value of these potential new biomarkers in ARDS.

2. Materials and Methods

2.1. Study Design

After approval by the Ethics Committee of the University Hospital RWTH Aachen (EK 100/20), serum samples were collected between March and April 2020. All patients or their legal representatives provided written informed consent. After excluding patients younger than 18 years of age who were pregnant or under palliative care, 53 patients with positive SARS-CoV-2 PCR results and intensive care admission were included in this study. Identification of infection was carried out using real-time reverse transcription PCR (RT-PCR). Treatment of patients followed the standards of care in our intensive care unit (ICU), including mechanical ventilation, veno-venous extracorporeal membrane oxygenation (ECMO) and renal replacement therapy (RRT) if needed. The decision to use veno-venous ECMO therapy was based on the recently published Extracorporeal Life Support Organization (ELSO) consensus guidelines [16]. All parameters, including demographics, vital signs, laboratory values, blood gas analyses, and organ support, were extracted from the patient data management system (Intellispace Critical Care and Anesthesia (ICCA) system, Philips, The Netherlands).

2.2. Serum Sampling

Serum samples were collected at two different time points after patients were enrolled in the study following a positive SARS-CoV-2 PCR result: on the day of the positive SARS-CoV-2 PCR result (day 1) and two days after COVID-19 diagnosis (day 3). Serum samples were centrifuged at 3000 rpm for 10 min at room temperature after a 10-min clotting period.

Samples were stored at −80 °C until heparanase activity and heparanase as well as heparan sulfate serum levels were measured.

2.3. Heparanase Activity Assay

Heparanase activity was detected using a commercial heparanase assay kit (Cat. #: Ra001-BE-K, Amsbio, Abingdon, UK). The measurements were performed according to the manufacturer's instructions. After rehydration of the microwell plate, 100 µL of the positive control enzyme was added to two wells. For sample analysis, 50 µL of the reaction buffer and 50 µL of the samples were added to each well. All measurements were performed in duplicate. For the negative control, the reaction buffer alone was used. The microwell plate was incubated at 37 °C for one hour on a plate shaker and washed afterwards. Next, 100 µL Strep-HRP was added to each well, and the plate was incubated at 37 °C for 50 min while shaking. The microwell plate was washed again followed by incubation at room temperature with 100 µL peroxidase substrates. The absorbance was measured at intervals of 1 to 2 min at 650 nm using a microplate reader (Infinity 200, Tecan, Männedorf, Switzerland). The reaction was stopped by adding 100 µL of 0.12 M HCl to each well as soon as an optical density of 0.6–0.7 was reached. The optical density was determined at 450 nm.

2.4. Human Enzyme-Linked Immunosorbent Assay

Heparanase and heparan sulfate serum levels were detected using commercial ELISA kits (Cat. #: E01H0100 and Cat. #: E01H1352, amsbio). For analysis, 100 µL of the standard and samples were added to the precoated wells. As negative control, 100 µL of PBS was used. All measurements were performed in duplicate. An additional 50 µL conjugate was added to each well except for the negative control. After mixing, the microplate was incubated for 1 h at 37 °C. The microplate was washed five times with wash solution, and 50 µL substrate was added. The reaction was stopped with 50 µL of the stop solution after 10–15 min of incubation at room temperature. The optical density was determined at 450 nm using a microplate reader (Infinity 200, Tecan, Männedorf, Switzerland). Sample values were interpolated from the 4PL regression standard curve generated by GraphPad Prism 7 (GraphPad by Dotmatics, San Diego, CA, USA).

2.5. Statistics

Values are expressed as medians and interquartile ranges (IQRs) or counts and percentages, as appropriate. Group comparisons of continuous variables were performed using the Kruskal–Wallis test. Post hoc tests were computed according to Siegel and Castellan 1988 [17]. Categorical data were compared using Pearson's chi-squared test for count data. Biomarker data are typically log-normally distributed and were, therefore, log-transformed for statistical analysis. The untransformed data are presented in a boxplot to illustrate the association of continuous variables with categorical variables. The lines inside the boxes represent the median and the box ranges from the lower quartile (Q1) to the upper quartile (Q3). The circles outside the box are values that represent outliers. Any data observation that was more than 1.5 IQR below the first quartile or above the third quartile is considered an outlier. The smallest/largest value that was not an outlier was indicated by a vertical marker or "whisker". The whisker is connected to the box by a horizontal line. Cox proportional hazards regression was used to analyze the effect of the (log-transformed) biomarker on survival in univariable analyses. Survival curves plotted by the Kaplan–Meier method were used for illustrative purposes. Cox models are slightly positively affected by using log-transformed data. All other results (Kruskal–Wallis test, Spearman r, Kaplan–Meier plots) are not affected by the log transformation since they are rank-based. All statistical tests were 2-tailed, and a two-sided p-value of 0.05 was considered significant. Statistical analyses were performed using R version 3.4.3 (http://www.r-project.org (accessed on 27 July 2020), library rms, Hmisc, ROCR, Vienna, Austria) and Statistical Package for the Social Sciences (SPSS) version 22.0 (SPSS Inc., Chicago, IL, USA).

3. Results

In this study, 53 ICU patients with a confirmed SARS-CoV-2 infection were included. The patients were classified into four groups according to the severity of ARDS. Three (5.7%) patients did not develop ARDS, 12 (22.6%) patients developed mild ARDS, 13 (24.5%) developed moderate ARDS, and most patients 25 (47.2%) developed severe ARDS. Patients without ARDS were in the ICU for a mean of 6 days, patients with mild ARDS for 7.5 days, patients with moderate ARDS for 19.5 days and patients with severe ARDS for 17.5 days. Of these, one (7.7%) patient with moderate ARDS and 7 (28.0%) patients with severe ARDS died in the ICU. Thus, the overall mortality of COVID-19 patients admitted to ICU was 15%. Detailed patient characteristics are shown in Table 1.

Table 1. Patient characteristics separated by severity of ARDS.

Variable	None (n = 3)	Mild (n = 12)	Moderate (n = 13)	Severe (n = 25)	p-Value
n(%)	3 (5.7)	12 (22.6)	13 (24.5)	25 (47.2)	
Age (years)	53 [49–65]	61 [59–64]	62 [54–67]	66 [58–72]	0.767
Sex male, n (%)	3 (100.0)	10 (83.3)	6 (46.2)	21 (84.0)	0.039
Body mass index (kg/m^2)	24.9 [24.7–28.2]	29.2 [26.3–34.9]	30.5 [26.7–35.2]	29.3 [24.7–31.3]	0.759
Temperature, max (°C)	38.1 [37.9–38.9]	38.5 [38.2–38.7]	38.15 [37.7–38.8]	38.1 [37.4–38.6]	0.229
Heart rate (bpm)	89.0 [84.5–105.5]	108.0 [99.0–112.0]	108.0 [87.0–123.5]	112.0 [102.0–124.0]	0.519
Respiratory rate (bpm)	24.0 [23.5–25.0]	25.0 [24.0–27.0]	24.0 [23.0–26.0]	24.0 [20.0–27.5]	0.988
SOFA score at day of enrollment (points)	8.5 [7.6–9.3]	8.0 [5.3–9.8]	10.0 [8.0–12.3]	11.0 [9.0–12.0]	0.034
Blood gas analysis (at day of enrollment)					
Arterial pH	7.5 [7.4–7.5]	7.4 [7.4–7.5]	7.4 [7.3–7.4]	7.4 [7.3–7.4]	0.040
pCO$_2$ (mmHg)	48.0 [42.1–52.1]	36.3 [33.0–38.9]	47.5 [42.7–54.0]	49.8 [42.1–61.1]	0.025
pO$_2$ (mmHg)	83.0 [77.0–85.5]	97.0 [80.0–107.0]	71.0 [68.0–74.8]	82.0 [71.0–93.0]	0.188
SpO$_2$ (%)	94.0 [92.5–94.5]	98.0 [95.8–98.3]	96.0 [92.8–99.0]	95.0 [92.0–97.0]	0.053
Horowitz index (mmHg/%)	93.0 [68.5–256.0]	218.0 [179.8–229.3]	120.5 [105.8–135.3]	95.0 [77.0–125.0]	0.001
Biomarker (at day of enrollment, unless stated differently)					
Lactate (mmol/L)	0.7 [0.7–1.0]	0.7 [0.4–0.9]	1.2 [0.8–1.6]	1.4 [1.0–1.6]	0.030
IL-6 (pg/mL)	86.8 [86.8–86.8]	60.3 [37.9–93.3]	496.3 [158.7–623.7]	263.3 [105.6–708.9]	0.018
PCT (ng/mL)	0.1 [0.1–0.1]	0.3 [0.1–0.4]	0.4 [0.2–0.7]	1.5 [0.7–5.7]	<0.001
CRP (mg/L)	103.2 [63.7–142.6]	115.9 [92.7–144,0]	281.6 [200.8–313.4]	277.4 [186.8–337.8]	0.003
Leukocytes (10^3/mm^3) =/nl	10.1 [9.2–11.7]	6.9 [6.3–10.8]	9.2 [7.1–10.6]	8.9 [7.8–14.1]	0.362
Platelets (10/μL)	202.0 [178.5–292.0]	200.0 [168.0–284.0]	276.5 [197.8–338.8]	247.0 [185.0–307.0]	0.551
Creatinine (mg/dL)	0.7 [0.6–0.7]	0.9 [0.7–1.4]	0.9 [0.6–1.2]	1.8 [1.0–2.7]	0.003
Comorbidities					
Arterial hypertension, n (%)	1 (33.3)	5 (41.7)	9 (69.2)	12 (48.0)	0.455
Diabetes mellitus, n (%)	0 (0.0)	1 (8.3)	3 (23.1)	9 (36.0)	0.215
Adipositas, n (%)	0 (0.0)	2 (16.7)	4 (30.8)	6 (24.0)	0.651
Hyper-/Dyslipidemia, n (%)	0 (0.0)	1 (8.3)	3 (23.1)	3 (12.0)	0.606
Ischemic heart disease, n (%)	0 (0.0)	2 (16.7)	4 (30.8)	4 (16.0)	0.557
Embolism/Thrombosis, n (%)	1 (33.3)	1 (8.3)	3 (23.1)	1 (4.0)	0.197
Cardiac arrhythmia, n (%)	0 (0.0)	1 (8.3)	0 (0.0)	5 (20.0)	0.259
Peripheral arterial occlusive disease, n (%)	0 (0.0)	1 (8.3)	1 (7.7)	0 (0.0)	0.506
Cerebral vascular disease, n (%)	0 (0.0)	2 (16.7)	0 (0.0)	3 (12.0)	0.459
COPD, n (%)	1 (33.3)	2 (16.7)	0 (0.0)	2 (8.0)	0.525
bronchial asthma, n (%)	0 (0.0)	0 (0.0)	3 (23.1)	1 (4.0)	0.104
Other lung diseases, n (%)	1 (33.3)	1 (8.3)	0 (0.0)	0 (0.0)	0.025
Chronic kidney disease, n (%)	0 (0.0)	2 (16.7)	3 (23.1)	3 (12.0)	0.708
Tumor disease, n (%)	0 (0.0)	3 (25.0)	1 (7.7)	0 (0.0)	0.057
Smoker, n (%)	0 (0.0)	1 (8.3)	2 (15.4)	0 (0.0)	0.247
Ex-Smoker, n (%)	0 (0.0)	1 (8.3)	2 (15.4)	1 (4.0)	0.604

Table 1. Cont.

Variable	None (n = 3)	Mild (n = 12)	Moderate (n = 13)	Severe (n = 25)	p-Value
Medication at admission					
Anticoagulation, n (%)	1 (33.3)	2 (16.7)	3 (23.1)	9 (36.0)	0.627
Antiplatelet, n (%)	0 (0.0)	4 (33.3)	6 (46.2)	5 (20.0)	0.238
Antihypertensives, n (%)	1 (33.3)	8 (66.7)	10 (76.9)	13 (52.0)	0.343
Immunosupressants, n (%)	1 (33.3)	2 (16.7)	4 (30.8)	2 (8.0)	0.289
Analgesics, n (%)	1 (33.3)	4 (33.3)	1 (7.7)	2 (8.0)	0.143
Treatment on ICU (first 14 days, unless stated differently)					
ICU length of stay (days)	6.0 [4.0–9.5]	7.5 [3.0–10.5]	19.5 [16.5–22.8]	17.5 [15.0–20.8]	0.004
Highest dose of norepinephrine during the first 7 days (µg/kg/min)	0.1 [0.0–0.1]	0.0 [0.0–0.0]	0.1 [0.1–0.2]	0.1 [0.1–0.21]	0.002
Duration of ventilation (hours)	103.0 [51.5–147.0]	0.0 [0.0–218.8]	330.0 [271.0–341.0]	331.0 [246.0–349.0]	<0.001
Duration of RRT (days)	0 [0–0]	0 [0–0]	0.0 [0–8]	12 [1–14]	0.001
ECMO					
never, n (%)	3 (100.0)	12 (100.0)	11 (84.6)	18 (72.0)	0.471
at admission, n (%)	0 (0.0)	0 (0.0)	1 (7.7)	5 (20.0)	
later, n (%)	0 (0.0)	0 (0.0)	1 (7.7)	2 (8.0)	
Ventilation					
Intubation, n (%)	1 (33.3)	5 (41.7)	13 (100.0)	25 (100.0)	
Never	2 (66.7)	7 (58.3)	0 (0.0)	0 (0.0)	
at admission	1 (33.3)	3 (25.0)	12 (92.3)	22 (88.0)	
Later	0 (0.0)	2 (16.7)	1 (7.7)	3 (12.0)	
External intubation, n (%)	1 (33.3)	0 (0.0)	4 (30.8)	19 (76.0)	
Mechanical ventilation, n (%)	2 (66.7)	5 (41.7)	13 (100.0)	25 (100.0)	
FiO$_2$ (%)	87.5 [81.3–93.8]	40.0 [37.5–41.3]	60.0 [55.0–71.3]	70.0 [60.0–86.0]	0.004
PEEP (cmH$_2$O)	15 [15.0–15.0]	8 [7.0–9.0]	13 [12.0–15.0]	15 [13.5–16.0]	0.002
Tidal volume (mL)	600.5 [560.8–640.3]	674.0 [564.0–810.0]	620.0 [521.8–737.8]	503.5 [435.0–600.0]	0.045
NIV, n (%)	2 (66.7)	1 (8.3)	3 (23.1)	2 (8.0)	0.041
Outcome					
Death at 28 days, n (%)	1 (33.3)	0 (0.0)	1 (7.7)	11 (44.0)	0.011
Disposition on day 28					
discharged, n (%)	2 (66.7)	12 (100.0)	11 (84.6)	7 (28.0)	0.001
on ICU post day 28, n (%)	0 (0.0)	0 (0.0)	1 (7.7)	7 (28.0)	
Death at 28 days, n (%)	1 (33.3)	0 (0.0)	1 (7.7)	11 (44.0)	

Variables are given as median [interquartile range] or number (%). Kruskal–Wallis analysis with a significance level of $p < 0.05$ was used for statistical analysis. ARDS, acute respiratory distress syndrome; COPD, chronic obstructive pulmonary disease; CRP, C-reactive protein; ECMO, extracorporeal membrane oxygenation; FiO$_2$, fraction of inspired oxygen; ICU, intensive care unit; IL-6, interleukin-6; pCO$_2$, partial pressure of carbon dioxide; PCT, procalcitonin; pO$_2$, partial pressure of oxygen; RRT, renal replacement therapy; SpO$_2$, peripheral capillary oxygen saturation; SOFA, sequential organ failure assessment.

On day one (the day of inclusion into the study), we measured an increased heparanase activity in patients with a severe ARDS, but no significant difference was detected between patients with different severity of ARDS (Figure 1A, $p = 0.144$). There was no difference in heparanase serum levels detected between patients with different severities of ARDS (Figure 1B, $p = 0.640$). When compared to patients that had not developed ARDS, patients with mild ARDS showed a small, but significant increase in the serum levels of heparan sulfate, while the heparan sulfate serum levels were lower in patients with moderate or severe ARDS (compared to patients with either mild or no ARDS; Figure 1C, $p = 0.022$). Three days after ICU admission, mean heparanase serum levels in patients with moderate ARDS showed a tendency toward slightly lower levels compared with patients with severe

ARDS (Figure 1E). Also, no significant differences in serum heparanase levels were observed on the third day between patients with different severity of ARDS (Figure 1E, $p = 0.140$). Heparanase activity and heparan sulfate serum levels showed similar trends as on day 1 (Figure 1D,F, $p = 0.470$ and $p = 0.129$).

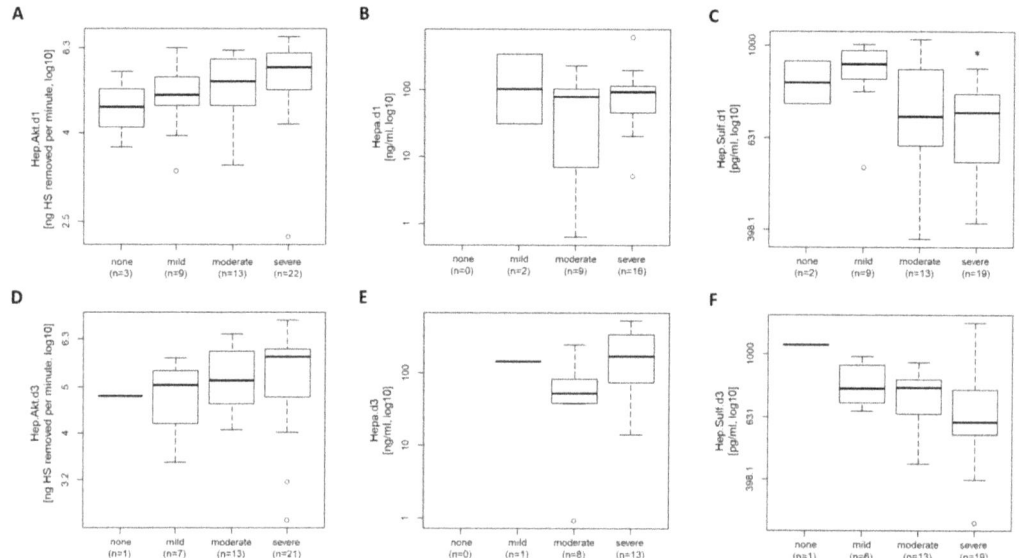

Figure 1. Heparanase activity, heparanase level, and heparan sulfate level in COVID-19 patients in relation to the severity of ARDS. Boxplot of heparanase activity on (**A**) day 1 and (**D**) 3 and heparanase level on (**B**) day 1 and (**E**) 3, as well as the heparanase sulfate level on (**C**) day 1 and (**F**) 3 of COVID-19 patients in relation to the severity of ARDS (none, mild, moderate, or severe ARDS) are shown. The untransformed data are presented as a boxplot. The lines inside the boxes represent the median, and the box is defined by the range of Q1 and Q3. Circles outside the box are values represent outliers. For statistical analysis, Kruskal–Wallis analysis was used with a significance level of $p < 0.05$, with the post hoc test indicating which groups showed a statistical difference by TRUE (significant) or FALSE (not significant). * indicates a significant difference between severe and mild ARDS. ARDS: acute respiratory distress syndrome; Hep.Akt.: heparanase activity; Hepa.: heparanase; Hep.Sulf.: heparan sulfate.

The heparanase activity significantly correlated (positively) with the lactate concentration on day one ($r = 0.34$, $p = 0.024$, CI: 0.07, 0.58) and on day three ($r = 0.43$, $p = 0.006$, CI: 0.01, 0.47). Additionally, a significant positive correlation could be detected with PCT on both days ($r = 0.38$, $p = 0.011$, CI: 0.09, 0.65 and $r = 0.36$, $p = 0.023$, CI: 0.04, 0.60). Furthermore, heparanase activity significantly correlated positively with CRP on day one ($r = 0.34$, $p = 0.020$, CI: −0.03, 0.59) and IL-6 on day three ($r = 0.36$, $p = 0.032$, CI: −0.12, 0.54). Interestingly, a slightly positive non-significant correlation of heparanase serum levels and a negative significant correlation of heparan sulfate serum levels with PCT were measured on day three ($r = 0.40$, $p = 0.065$, CI: −0.04, 0.72; $r = -0.35$, $p = 0.034$, CI: −0.58, −0.02). The heparan sulfate serum level also correlated negatively with the SOFA score on day one ($r = -0.35$, $p = 0.028$, CI: −0.57, −0.06; Table 2).

Table 2. Significant correlations between biomarkers and clinical features.

Variable	Spearman r	p-Value	CI
Heparanase level d1			
Age	−0.34	0.0805	−0.69, 0.06
SpO_2	−0.44	0.0297	−0.77, −0.07
Leucocytes	0.50	0.0103	0.07, 0.79
Heparan sulfate level d1			
BMI	0.31	0.0467	−0.06, 0.57
Respiratory rate	−0.42	0.0201	−0.63, −0.11
SOFA-Score	−0.35	0.0281	−0.57, −0.06
Norepinephrine	−0.31	0.0397	−0.56, 0.02
Heparanase activity d1			
Lactate	0.34	0.0241	0.07, 0.58
PCT	0.38	0.0113	0.09, 0.65
CRP	0.34	0.0200	−0.03, 0.59
Heparanase level d3			
Duration of ventilation	−0.47	0.0273	−0.82, 0.03
Temperature max	−0.51	0.0158	−0.76, −0.13
Heparan sulfate level d3			
PCT	−0.35	0.0341	−0.58, −0.02
Leucocytes	−0.44	0.0055	−0.61, −0.17
Heparanase activity d3			
Lactate	0.43	0.0055	0.01, 0.47
IL-6	0.36	0.0322	−0.12, 0.54
PCT	0.36	0.0226	0.04, 0.60

Shown are significant correlations of heparanase activity, heparanase serum level, and heparan sulfate serum level at days 1 and 3 with various clinical parameters, and Spearman rank correlation coefficient r with 95% confidence interval CI (bootstrap CI, B = 200). BMI, body mass index; CRP, C-reactive protein; IL-6, interleukin-6; PCT, procalcitonin; SpO_2, peripheral capillary oxygen saturation; SOFA, sequential organ failure assessment.

Next, we analyzed the potential of heparan sulfate and heparanase serum levels as well as heparanase activity to predict 28-day mortality. None of the biomarkers showed a linear association with mortality (all $p > 0.20$), nor a consistent non-linear association between day 1 and day 3. For illustration, the biomarker levels were divided into 4 quartiles and analyzed by using a Kaplan–Meier plot with respect to 28-day mortality. Patients with higher heparanase levels [113–600] on day one had a 100% survival rate. In contrast, patients with heparanase levels between 86.3–113.0 ng/mL on day one had a higher probability of dying within 28 days (below 60% survival).

Patients presenting heparan sulfate levels below 583 ng/mL on day one and below 598 ng/mL on day three showed the worst outcome. Patients with heparanase activity in the range of the third quarter on days one [5.39; 5.91] and three [5.28; 5.95] also showed a worse outcome. Patients with heparanase activity in the range of the second quarter [4.63; 5.28] showed an even worse outcome, with only 60% of patients surviving (Figure 2).

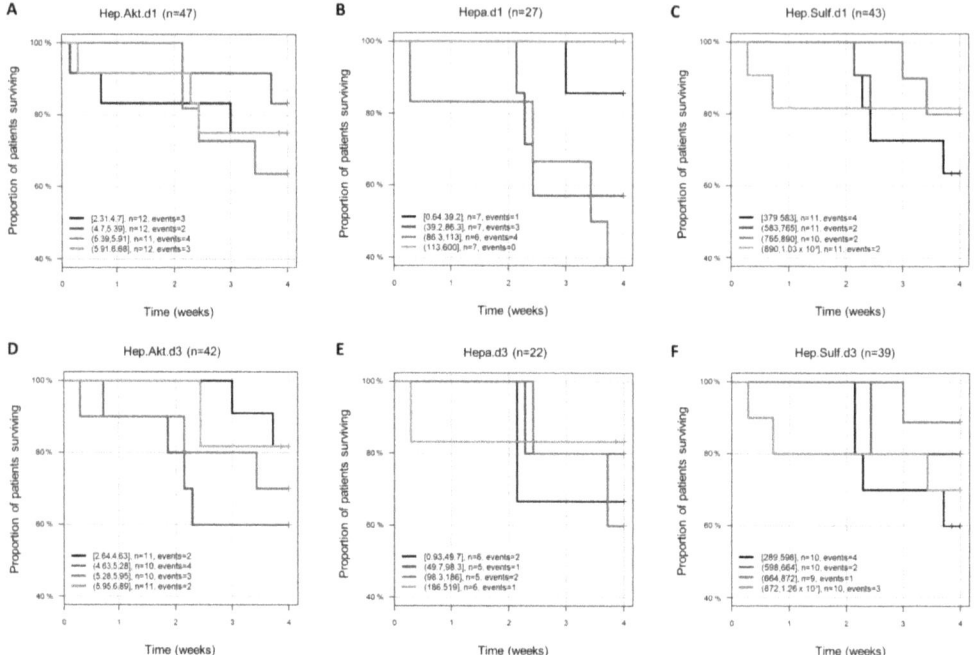

Figure 2. The relationship between heparan sulfate and heparanase serum levels as well as heparanase activity and the 28-day mortality. Presented are Kaplan–Meier plots for 28-day mortality for heparanase activity on (**A**) day 1 and (**D**) day 3 and heparanase level on (**B**) day 1 and (**E**) day 3 as well as the heparanase sulfate level on (**C**) day 1 and (**F**) day 3 of COVID-19 patients. Curves are plotted by quartiles. Hep.Akt.: heparanase activity; Hepa: heparanase; Hep.Sulf.: heparan sulfate.

4. Discussion

The new coronavirus represents a major challenge, especially for intensive care units, because SARS-CoV-2 is one of the most pathogenic coronaviruses, and a high proportion of patients suffer a severe course of disease [18]. Endothelial dysfunction plays a crucial role in ARDS and consequently in the pathophysiology of COVID-19. In a previous study, Buijsers et al. postulated an association between elevated heparanase activity and heparan sulfate plasma levels and the need for intensive care unit admission [13]. In fact, our work confirms and extends this data by showing a clear potential of heparanase activity and heparan sulfate plasma levels as promising biomarkers for the prediction of disease severity and outcome of COVID-19 patients admitted to the ICU.

Consequently, in this work, the role of heparanase and heparan sulfate in COVID-19 patients in relation to the severity of ARDS was investigated. Indeed, in patients with severe ARDS, an increase in the activity of heparanase on day 1 (5.7 [5.1–6.1]) and day 3 (5.8 [4.8–6.0]) was observed when compared to patients with moderate (day 1: 5.3 [4.6–5.9], day 3: 5.2 [4.6–5.9]) and mild ARDS (day 1: 4.9 [4.6–5.4]; day 3: 5.0 [4.3–5.4]) (Figure 1). Unlike with heparanase activity, we did not observe an increase in heparanase levels with an increase in ARDS severity. Along with increasing severity of ARDS, there is an increased expression of proinflammatory cytokines, such as IL-6. Heparanase is activated by proinflammatory cytokines [19]; thus, the increased activity with respect to severe ARDS might be associated with the increased expression of proinflammatory cytokines, rather than with an increase in heparanase levels. On day 3, a correlation of heparanase activity and IL-6 concentration was detected (Table 2). This result confirms the assumption that IL-6 is involved in heparanase activation. However, no elevated heparan sulfate serum levels could be measured in COVID-19 patients with severe ARDS compared to those with moderate or mild ARDS. In line, Buijsers et al. showed that a reduction in heparanase activity due to the prophylactic administration of low molecular weight heparins (LMWH) was not associated with a reduction in heparan sulfate or IL-6 plasma levels [13].

In addition to the fragmentation of heparan sulfate (and its fragments), heparanase is involved in the cleavage of heparan sulfate-bound cytokines and growth factors such as angiopoietin-2 (Ang-2). In various studies, a significantly higher Ang-2 concentration was measured in the serum of septic patients compared to healthy subjects [20,21]. Furthermore, increased heparan sulfate and heparanase levels in the serum of patients and mice with sepsis [22–24] suggests an association between heparanase activity and increased expression of Ang-2. Lukasz and colleagues showed that the Ang-2-mediated breakdown of endothelial glycocalyx thickness depends on heparanase [25]. Furthermore, increased Ang-2 levels were detected in COVID-19 patients [26]. Drost et al. showed that HPSE activity was inversely correlated with HS concentration in healthy volunteers and COVID-19 patients [14]. This would also be in line with our results, as we measured that heparan sulfate levels tended to decrease with increasing severity of ARDS in COVID-19 patients.

5. Limitation/Conclusions

As our investigation was limited to a small patient cohort with a variation in the number of measurements of some variables, further investigations in a larger cohort should be carried out to confirm our data. Moreover, our measurements were limited to heparanase activity and heparanase as well as heparan sulfate serum levels, and the analysis of other biomarkers associated with activation of the heparanase system, such as syndecane-1 concentrations in serum, would strengthen the findings reported here.

Due to the novel SARS-CoV-2 variants, COVID-19 still plays a crucial role today. Therefore, it is still important to identify new biomarkers that indicate the severity of COVID-19 and the severity of COVID-19-associated ARDS. In conclusion, in this study, we showed that heparanase activity increased in patients with severe ARDS on both days in COVID-19 patients. Furthermore, heparanase activity and heparan sulfate levels correlate with COVID-19 disease severity and outcome. Based on these results, there is now good evidence that heparanase activity may play a role in endothelial dysfunction and ARDS associated with COVID-19 and may be a potential biomarker to predict outcome in COVID-19 patients in the ICU. This may also be relevant to newer variants of SARS-CoV-2.

Author Contributions: Conceptualization, E.Z., T.-P.S. and L.M.; methodology, E.Z., K.S., N.F., C.B., T.-P.S. and L.M.; validation, E.Z., T.-P.S. and L.M.; formal analysis E.Z., S.K., T.-P.S., M.D., A.K. and L.M.; resources, E.Z., T.-P.S., L.M. and G.M.; data curation, K.S., N.F., T.-P.S., L.S., E.Z., L.M. and M.D.; writing—review and editing, E.Z., T.-P.S., C.T. and L.M.; supervision, G.M. and C.T.; project administration, E.Z., T.-P.S. and L.M.; funding acquisition, E.Z. and L.M. All authors have read and agreed to the published version of the manuscript.

Funding: This research was funded by a grant from the German Research Foundation to LM (DFG, MA 7082/3-1) and by an intramural grant to EZ (START 113/17).

Institutional Review Board Statement: The study was conducted according to the guidelines of the Declaration of Helsinki, and approved by the local Ethical Committee of RWTH University (EK 100/20).

Informed Consent Statement: Informed consent was obtained from all subjects involved in the study or their legal representatives.

Data Availability Statement: Not applicable.

Acknowledgments: The authors would like to thank Oliver Hartmann for the support with data analysis and Jessica Pezechk as well as Bianca Meier for their excellent technical support.

Conflicts of Interest: The authors declare no conflict of interest. The funders had no role in the design of the study; in the collection, analyses, or interpretation of data; in the writing of the manuscript; or in the decision to publish the results.

References

1. Hasöksüz, M.; Kiliç, S.; Saraç, F. Coronaviruses and SARS-CoV-2. *Turk. J. Med. Sci.* **2020**, *50*, 549–556. [CrossRef]
2. Park, M.; Thwaites, R.S.; Openshaw, P.J.M. COVID-19: Lessons from SARS and MERS. *Eur. J. Immunol.* **2020**, *50*, 308–311. [CrossRef]
3. World Health Organisation. Middle East Respiratory Syndrome Coronavirus (MERS-CoV). 2020. Available online: https://www.who.int/emergencies/mers-cov/en/ (accessed on 1 February 2022).
4. World Health Organisation. WHO Coronavirus Disease (COVID-19) Dashboard. 2020. Available online: https://covid19.who.int (accessed on 1 February 2022).
5. Pons, S.; Fodil, S.; Azoulay, E.; Zafrani, L. The vascular endothelium: The cornerstone of organ dysfunction in severe SARS-CoV-2 infection. *Crit. Care* **2020**, *24*, 353. [CrossRef] [PubMed]
6. Gu, S.X.; Tyagi, T.; Jain, K.; Gu, V.W.; Lee, S.H.; Hwa, J.M.; Kwan, J.M.; Krause, D.S.; Lee, A.I.; Halene, S.; et al. Thrombocytopathy and endotheliopathy: Crucial contributors to COVID-19 thromboinflammation. *Nat. Rev. Cardiol.* **2020**, *18*, 194–209. [CrossRef] [PubMed]
7. Lin, G.-L.; McGinley, J.P.; Drysdale, S.B.; Pollard, A.J. Epidemiology and immune pathogenesis of viral sepsis. *Front. Immunol.* **2018**, *9*, 2147. [CrossRef]
8. Hamming, I.; Timens, W.; Bulthuis, M.L.C.; Lely, A.T.; Navis, G.J.; van Goor, H. Tissue distribution of ACE2 protein, the functional receptor for SARS coronavirus. A first step in understanding SARS pathogenesis. *J. Pathol.* **2004**, *203*, 631–637. [CrossRef]
9. Stein, R.A.; Young, L.M. From ACE2 to COVID-19: A multiorgan endothelial disease. *Int. J. Infect. Dis.* **2020**, *100*, 425–430. [CrossRef]
10. Varga, Z.; Flammer, A.J.; Steiger, P.; Haberecker, M.; Andermatt, R.; Zinkernagel, A.S.; Mehra, M.R.; Schuepbach, R.A.; Ruschitzka, F.; Moch, H. Endothelial cell infection and endotheliitis in COVID-19. *Lancet* **2020**, *395*, 1417–1418. [CrossRef]
11. Monteil, V.; Kwon, H.; Prado, P.; Hagelkrüys, A.; Wimmer, R.A.; Stahl, M.; Leopoldi, A.; Garreta, E.; Del Pozo, C.H.; Prosper, F.; et al. Inhibition of SARS-CoV-2 infections in engineered human tissues using clinical-grade soluble human ACE2. *Cell* **2020**, *181*, 905–913.e7. [CrossRef]
12. Reitsma, S.; Slaaf, D.W.; Vink, H.; van Zandvoort, M.A.M.J.; Oude Egbrink, M.G. The endothelial glycocalyx: Composition, functions, and visualization. *Pflug. Arch.* **2007**, *454*, 345–359. [CrossRef]
13. Buijsers, B.; Yanginlar, C.; de Nooijer, A.; Grondman, I.; Maciej-Hulme, M.L.; Jonkman, I.; Janssen, N.A.F.; Rother, N.; de Graaf, M.; Pickkers, P.; et al. Increased plasma heparanase activity in COVID-19 patients. *Front. Immunol.* **2020**, *11*, 575047. [CrossRef] [PubMed]
14. Drost, C.C.; Rovas, A.; Osiaevi, I.; Rauen, M.; van der Vlag, J.; Buijsers, B.; Salmenov, R.; Lukasz, A.; Pavenstädt, H.; Linke, W.A.; et al. Heparanase Is a putative mediator of endothelial glycocalyx damage in COVID-19—A proof-of-concept study. *Front. Immunol.* **2022**, *13*, 916512. [CrossRef] [PubMed]
15. Spadaro, S.; Park, M.; Turrini, C.; Tunstall, T.; Thwaites, R.; Mauri, T.; Ragazzi, R.; Ruggeri, P.; Hansel, T.T.; Caramori, G.; et al. Biomarkers for acute respiratory distress syndrome and prospects for personalised medicine. *J. Inflamm.* **2019**, *16*, 1. [CrossRef] [PubMed]
16. Bartlett, R.H.; Ogino, M.T.; Brodie, D.; McMullan, D.M.; Lorusso, R.; MacLaren, G.; Stead, C.M.; Rycus, P.; Fraser, J.F.; Belohlavek, J.; et al. Initial ELSO guidance document: ECMO for COVID-19 patients with severe cardiopulmonary failure. *ASAIO J.* **2020**, *66*, 472–474. [CrossRef]
17. Siegel, S.; Castellan, N.J., Jr. *Nonparametric Statistics for the Behavioral Sciences*, 2nd ed.; Mcgraw-Hill Book Company: New York, NY, USA, 1988; 399p.
18. Lai, C.C.; Shih, T.P.; Ko, W.C.; Tang, H.J.; Hsueh, P.R. Severe acute respiratory syndrome coronavirus 2 (SARS-CoV-2) and coronavirus disease-2019 (COVID-19): The epidemic and the challenges. *Int. J. Antimicrob. Agents* **2020**, *55*, 105924. [CrossRef]
19. Chen, G.; Wang, D.; Vikramadithyan, R.; Yagyu, H.; Saxena, U.; Pillarisetti, S.; Goldberg, I.J. Inflammatory cytokines and fatty acids regulate endothelial cell heparanase expression. *Biochemistry* **2004**, *43*, 4971–4977. [CrossRef]
20. Statz, S.; Sabal, G.; Walborn, A.; Williams, M.; Hoppensteadt, D.; Mosier, M.; Rondina, M.; Fareed, J. Angiopoietin 2 levels in the risk stratification and mortality outcome prediction of sepsis-associated coagulopathy. *Clin. Appl. Thromb.* **2018**, *24*, 1223–1233. [CrossRef]
21. Ricciuto, D.R.; dos Santos, C.C.; Hawkes, M.; Toltl, L.J.; Conroy, A.L.; Rajwans, N.; Lafferty, E.I.; Cook, D.J.; Fox-Robichaud, A.; Kahnamoui, K.; et al. Angiopoietin-1 and angiopoietin-2 as clinically informative prognostic biomarkers of morbidity and mortality in severe sepsis. *Crit. Care Med.* **2011**, *39*, 702–710. [CrossRef]
22. Martin, L.B.; De Santis, R.; Koczera, P.; Simons, N.; Haase, H.; Heinbockel, L.; Brandenburg, K.; Marx, G.; Schuerholz, T. The synthetic antimicrobial peptide 19-2.5 interacts with heparanase and heparan sulfate in murine and human sepsis. *PLoS ONE* **2015**, *10*, e0143583. [CrossRef]
23. Martin, L.; Schmitz, S.; De Santis, R.; Doemming, S.; Haase, H.; Hoeger, J.; Heinbockel, L.; Brandenburg, K.; Marx, G.; Schuerholz, T. Peptide 19-2.5 Inhibits heparan sulfate-triggered inflammation in murine cardiomyocytes stimulated with human sepsis serum. *PLoS ONE* **2015**, *10*, e0127584. [CrossRef]
24. Martin, L.; Peters, C.; Schmitz, S.; Moellmann, J.; Martincuks, A.; Heussen, N.; Lehrke, M.; Müller-Newen, G.; Marx, G.; Schuerholz, T. Soluble heparan sulfate in serum of septic shock patients induces mitochondrial dysfunction in murine cardiomyocytes. *Shock* **2015**, *44*, 569–577. [CrossRef] [PubMed]

25. Lukasz, A.; Hillgruber, C.; Oberleithner, H.; Kusche-Vihrog, K.; Pavenstädt, H.; Rovas, A.; Hesse, B.; Goerge, T.; Kümpers, P. Endothelial glycocalyx breakdown is mediated by angiopoietin-2. *Cardiovasc. Res.* **2017**, *113*, 671–680. [CrossRef] [PubMed]
26. Smadja, D.M.; Guerin, C.L.; Chocron, R.; Yatim, N.; Boussier, J.; Gendron, N.; Khider, L.; Hadjadj, J.; Goudot, G.; Debuc, B.; et al. Angiopoietin-2 as a marker of endothelial activation is a good predictor factor for intensive care unit admission of COVID-19 patients. *Angiogenesis* **2020**, *23*, 611–620. [CrossRef] [PubMed]

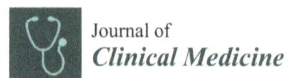 Journal of
Clinical Medicine

Article

Evolution of European Resuscitation and End-of-Life Practices from 2015 to 2019: A Survey-Based Comparative Evaluation

Spyros D. Mentzelopoulos [1,*], Keith Couper [2,3], Violetta Raffay [4,5], Jana Djakow [6,7] and Leo Bossaert [8]

1. First Department of Intensive Care Medicine, National and Kapodistrian University of Athens Medical School, Evaggelismos General Hospital, 45-47 Ipsilandou Street, 10675 Athens, Greece
2. UK Critical Care Unit, University Hospitals Birmingham, NHS Foundation Trust, Birmingham B15 2TH, UK; k.couper@warwick.ac.uk
3. Warwick Medical School, University of Warwick, Coventry CV4 7AL, UK
4. School of Medicine, European University Cyprus, Nicosia 2404, Cyprus; violetta.raffay@gmail.com
5. Serbian Resuscitation Council, 21102 Novi Sad, Serbia
6. Paediatric Intensive Care Unit, NH Hospital, 26801 Hořovice, Czech Republic; jana.djakow@gmail.com
7. Department of Paediatric Anaesthesiology and Intensive Care Medicine, University Hospital Brno and Faculty of Medicine, Masaryk University, 62500 Brno, Czech Republic
8. University of Antwerp, 2000 Antwerp, Belgium; leo.bossaert@erc.edu
* Correspondence: sdmentzelopoulos@yahoo.com or sdmentzelopoulos@gmail.com; Tel.: +30-697-530-4909; Fax: +30-213-204-3307

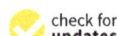

Citation: Mentzelopoulos, S.D.; Couper, K.; Raffay, V.; Djakow, J.; Bossaert, L. Evolution of European Resuscitation and End-of-Life Practices from 2015 to 2019: A Survey-Based Comparative Evaluation. *J. Clin. Med.* **2022**, *11*, 4005. https://doi.org/10.3390/jcm11144005

Academic Editors: Karim Bendjelid and Peter Markus Spieth

Received: 23 May 2022
Accepted: 6 July 2022
Published: 11 July 2022

Publisher's Note: MDPI stays neutral with regard to jurisdictional claims in published maps and institutional affiliations.

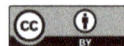

Copyright: © 2022 by the authors. Licensee MDPI, Basel, Switzerland. This article is an open access article distributed under the terms and conditions of the Creative Commons Attribution (CC BY) license (https://creativecommons.org/licenses/by/4.0/).

Abstract: Background: In concordance with the results of large, observational studies, a 2015 European survey suggested variation in resuscitation/end-of-life practices and emergency care organization across 31 countries. The current survey-based study aimed to comparatively assess the evolution of practices from 2015 to 2019, especially in countries with "low" (i.e., average or lower) 2015 questionnaire domain scores. Methods: The 2015 questionnaire with additional consensus-based questions was used. The 2019 questionnaire covered practices/decisions related to end-of-life care (domain A); determinants of access to resuscitation/post-resuscitation care (domain B); diagnosis of death/organ donation (domain C); and emergency care organization (domain D). Responses from 25 countries were analyzed. Positive or negative responses were graded by 1 or 0, respectively. Domain scores were calculated by summation of practice-specific response grades. Results: Domain A and B scores for 2015 and 2019 were similar. Domain C score decreased by 1 point [95% confidence interval (CI): 1–3; $p = 0.02$]. Domain D score increased by 2.6 points (95% CI: 0.2–5.0; $p = 0.035$); this improvement was driven by countries with "low" 2015 domain D scores. In countries with "low" 2015 domain A scores, domain A score increased by 5.5 points (95% CI: 0.4–10.6; $p = 0.047$). Conclusions: In 2019, improvements in emergency care organization and an increasing frequency of end-of-life practices were observed primarily in countries with previously "low" scores in the corresponding domains of the 2015 questionnaire.

Keywords: ethics; resuscitation; terminal care; surveys and questionnaires; emergency care

1. Introduction

Data from multinational, observational studies suggest a substantial variation in end-of-life practices across European countries, and an increasing frequency of decisions to limit life-sustaining treatments, especially in southern Europe [1,2]. End-of-life practices are evolving continuously as a result of new evidence-based guidelines, publication of randomized controlled trials supporting complex advance care planning (ACP), new laws/policies, and educational activities [3–23].

In 2015, we conducted a survey of experts from 31 European countries. We administered a comprehensive questionnaire spanning the following four domains: A: practices/decisions related to end-of-life care; B: access to best available care; C: death diagnosis and organ donation; and D: emergency care organization. Practices and organization of care were scored by numerical summation of positive responses. Results showed substantial variability in country-specific approaches to resuscitation/end-of-life care, indicating the presence of space for evidence-supported progress in all the aforementioned domains [3].

In 2019, we undertook a methodologically improved version of the 2015 survey to address the following questions: (1) How did resuscitation/end-of-life care and emergency care organization evolve over the 2015–2019 period? and (2) Could such evolution, be more marked in countries with "low" (i.e., at or below average) practice/organization scores for 2015?

2. Materials and Methods

The current survey conforms with the Checklist for Reporting Results of Internet E-Surveys (https://www.jmir.org/2004/3/e34/; accessed on 20 July 2019 see Supplementary Materials).

Potential study participants from 33 European countries were contacted via e-mail. Participant inclusion criteria comprised nationally and/or internationally recognized, specific, clinical, and/or research expertise in resuscitation and end-of-life care; pertinent evidence should be classifiable in 1 or more of the following categories: (1) European Resuscitation Council (ERC) National Resuscitation Council representative; and/or member of the European Registry of Cardiac Arrest investigators network or other ERC related clinical research networks (e.g., ERC Dispatch Center Survey, Reappropriate Trial, Euro-call); (2) Established researcher in the field: first, second or last author of published, scholarly articles in this field; and (3) At least 3 years of prior service as lead clinician in emergency and/or intensive care.

To reduce the risk of recall/social desirability bias, we aimed for at least three participants from each country. However, this did not constitute an inclusion criterion for country-specific responses. Consequently, responses from countries with just one or two participants were to be anyway included in the data analyses. Following the obtainment of informed consent (see Supplementary Materials), participants were able to electronically access the study questionnaire (Table 1).

Table 1. The 2019 Ethical Practices Questionnaire.

DOMAIN A. PRACTICES/DECISIONS RELATED TO END-OF-LIFE CARE *
A1. End-of-life practices
1. Do-not-attempt cardiopulmonary resuscitation (DNACPR) orders (legally allowed, supported, and applied in your country (3 questions)? applied in single tier, or first and second tier ambulance [†] (3 questions)? applied in-hospital? written in medical record? reviewed?) No. of discrete questions (N) = 9; Maximum score if all responses positive (Max. Score) = 9.
2. Advance directives (respect for advance directives legally allowed, and supported in your country (2 questions)? applied in the out-of-hospital, and in-hospital setting (2 questions)?) applied to start/stop cardiopulmonary resuscitation (CPR) in single tier, or first and second tier ambulance (3-questions)? applied to start/stop CPR in-hospital? N = 8, 4-choice; Max. Score = 8.
3. Advance Care Planning (same questions as for advance directives). N = 8, 4-choice; Max. Score = 8.
4. Terminal analgesia/sedation (legally allowed in your country? applied?). N = 2; Max. Score = 2.
5. Termination of Resuscitation protocols (TOR) (legally allowed? applied in single tier, or first and second tier ambulance (3-questions)? applied in-hospital? N = 5, 4-choice; Max. Score = 5.
6. Limitation of in-hospital treatment level (If applied, does it pertain to withholding, and withdrawing CPR (2 questions)? does it include TOR, withholding of invasive treatments, and withdrawing of feeding and hydration?). N = 5; Max. Score = 5.
7. Euthanasia in adults (legally allowed in your country? applied?); euthanasia in children (legally allowed in your country? applied? Physician-assisted suicide (legally allowed in your country?). N = 5; Max. Score = 5.
8. During patient transportation: Is CPR continued in the prospect of organ donation? Is CPR continued in the prospect of access to higher-level treatment (e.g., extracorporeal CPR)? N = 2; Max. Score = 2.

Table 1. *Cont.*

Max. Subscore for end-of-life practices (A1) = sum of Max. Scores of 1 to 8 = 44.

A2. End-of-life Decisions

1. Adults/children: Family participating in Decisions? N = 2; Max. Score = 2.
2. Adults/children: Are end-of-life decisions reached through a shared decision-making process? N = 2; Max. Score = 2.

Max. Subscore end-of-life decisions (A2) = sum of Max. Scores of 1 and 2 = 4.

A3. Family presence during CPR

1. Adults: Family present during CPR? Children: Parents present during CPR? Children:

Other family members present during CPR? N = 3; Max. Score = 3.
Max. Subscore for family presence during CPR (A3) = 3.
Max. Score for Domain A = sum of max. Subscores of A1, A2 and A3 = 51.
Questions pertaining to law and those included in A1.6 and A1.7 had 2-choice responses (i.e., *yes* or *no*); Questions pertaining to what is applied had 4-choice responses (i.e., *never*, *sometimes*, *usually*, and *always*).

B. ACCESS TO BEST RESUSCITATION AND POSTRESUSCITATION CARE ‡
B1–B3. Out-of-hospital (B1) and in-hospital (B2) resuscitation care, and postresuscitation care (B3)

1. Is access to best available care (including extracorporeal CPR wherever available) affected by age? race? religion? comorbidity? socioeconomic status? urban-rural (area of occurrence)? type of receiving hospital (out-of-hospital setting) or type of treating hospital (in-hospital setting)? minority? language? high-risk presentation (e.g., acute physiology and chronic health evaluation II score > 25 corresponding to >50% mortality probability)? suicide attempt? knowledge of patient's wish against undergoing CPR? other? The same group of questions was asked about B1, B2, and B3. For each of B1, B2, and B3: N = 13; Max. Score = 13.

Max. Score for Domain B = sum of max. Subscores of B1, B2, and B3 = 39. All questions had 2-choice responses (i.e., *yes* or *no*).

C. DIAGNOSIS OF DEATH AND ORGAN DONATION
C1. Death diagnosis

1. Legally allowed to diagnose death: physician, out-of-hospital or in-hospital (2 questions)? nurse, out-of-hospital or in-hospital (2 questions)? ambulance person [advanced life support (ALS) provider]? ambulance person [basic life support (BLS) provider]? N = 6; Max. Score = 6.
2. Legally allowed to diagnose death in the absence of obvious signs of death such as rigor mortis or decapitation, and after 20 minutes of asystole without reversible cause: same questions as above; N = 6; Max. Score = 6.
3. Diagnostic criteria for death: Brain death criteria used in out-of-hospital cardiac arrest (after hospital admission) or in-hospital cardiac arrest, and written on death certificate (3 questions)? Cardiorespiratory death criteria used in out-of-hospital or in-hospital cardiac arrest, and written on death certificate (3 questions)? N=6; Max. Score=6.

Max. Subscore for death diagnosis (C1) = sum of max. Scores of 1 to 3 = 18.

C2. Organ donation

1. Heart beating organ donation allowed? Non-heart beating organ donation allowed? Organ donation applied by opting in? Organ donation applied by opting out. N = 4; Max. Score = 4.

Max. Subscore for organ donation (C2) = 4.
Max. Score for Domain C = sum of Max. Subscores of C1 and C2 = 22. All questions had 2-choice responses (i.e., *yes* or *no*).

D. EMERGENCY CARE ORGANIZATION †
D1. Access to emergency care

1. Out-of-hospital: rural areas: emergency number 112 or another (2 questions)? ambulance arrival within 10 min? N = 3; Max. Score = 3.
2. Out-of-hospital: urban areas emergency number 112 or another (2 questions)? ambulance arrival within 10 min? N = 3; Max. Score = 3.
3. In-hospital: emergency number 112 or another (2 questions)? cardiac arrest team arrival within 10 min? N = 2; Max. Score = 2.

Max. Subscore for access to emergency care (D1) = sum of Max. Scores of 1 to 3 = 8.

D2. Defibrillation

1. Legally allowed to defibrillate using an automated external defibrillator (AED): physician? nurse? ambulance personnel? police? On-site responder? Citizen? Other (specify)? N = 7; Max. Score = 7.
2. AEDs available in: single tier ambulance? first tier ambulance? fire cars? police cars? public places? mass gatherings? first responder dispatch projects? other? N = 8; Max. Score=8.
3. Are AED data (electrocardiographic sequence, waveform, time) available in the patient record? N = 1; Max. Score = 1.
4. Ongoing public access defibrillation programs in place? home AED? school AED? in-hospital AED?-Is there a registry of all AEDs, at national or regional level (2 questions)? N = 6; Max. Score = 6.

Table 1. *Cont.*

Max. Subscore for defibrillation (D2) = sum of Max. Scores of 1 to 4 = 22.
D3. Organization of out-of-hospital emergency care
1. Is there a system in place to alert trained lay rescuers (and/or first responders) by text message or app? N = 1; Max. Score = 1.
2. [A] Is dispatcher assisted bystander CPR practiced in rural areas? Does guidance include compressions or ventilations (2 questions)? N = 3; Max. Score = 3.
3. [B] Is dispatcher assisted bystander CPR practiced in urban areas? Does guidance include compressions or ventilations (2 questions)? N = 3; Max. Score = 3. Single tier ambulance: ALS? First tier ambulance: BLS plus defibrillation or ALS (2 questions)? Second tier ambulance: ALS? N = 4; Max. Score = 4.
4. In traumatic cardiac arrest: in single tier ambulance, or first and second tier ambulance:

    A. Is the intervention unit qualified for prompt confirmation and management of life-threatening injuries (3 questions, one for each type of ambulance)?
    B. Are specific criteria applied for withholding or terminating resuscitation (3 questions, one for each type of ambulance)? yes-no, specify.

N = 6; Max. Score = 6.
Max. Subscore for level of out-of-hospital care (D3) = sum of Max. Scores of 1 to 4 = 17.
D4. Organization of in-hospital emergency services
1. Are in-hospital Rapid Response Teams Programs in place? N = 1; Max. Score = 1
2. Is CPR feedback, debriefing, and audit applied (3 questions)? N = 3; Max. Score = 3.
3. Is CPR training on the recently dead legally allowed?-is CPR training practiced? N = 2; Max. Score = 2.

Max. Subscore for organization of in-hospital emergency services (D4) = sum of Max. Scores of 1 to 3 = 6.

D. EMERGENCY CARE ORGANIZATION
D5. Registry reporting of cardiac arrest
1. Out-of-hospital or in-hospital cardiac arrest data reported to a Registry? N = 2; Max. Score = 2.

Max. Subscore for registry reporting of cardiac arrest (D5) = 2
D6. Education
1. Are there ongoing programs of (a) theoretical education and (b) practice training (e.g., clinical scenario-based) in the field of ethics at pregraduate level (2 questions)? postgraduate level (2 questions)? medical specialty/subspecialty registrar level (2 questions)? specialist level (2 questions)? N = 8; Max. Score = 8.
2. Certified CPR training mandatory for in-hospital healthcare providers: physicians? nurses? other staff? N = 3; Max. Score = 3.

Max. Subscore education (D6) = sum of Max. Scores of 1 and 2 = 11.
D7. Research
1. Enrollment of adults legally allowed without consent in: observational research? interventional research involving drugs? interventional research involving non-drug interventions? N = 3; Max. Score=3.

Max. Subscore for research (D7) = 3
Max. Score for Domain D = sum of Max. Subscores of D1, D2, D3, D4, D5, D6, and D7 = 67. Questions D1.1-3, D2.3, D3.4A, D4.1-3., and D5.1 had 4-choice responses (i.e., *never, sometimes, usually,* and *always*); all other questions had 2-choice responses (i.e. *yes* or *no*)

*, Related to the application of the following Ethical Principles: Autonomy, Beneficence, Non-maleficence, Dignity, and Honesty. †, the first tier ambulance corresponds to the capability of BLS plus defibrillation, whereas the second tier ambulance corresponds to the capability of ALS and monitored mechanical ventilatory and hemodynamic support offered by specifically trained and certified personnel. ‡, Related to the application of the Principles of Justice and Beneficence. Scores of Domain A subsections A1.3 and A2.2; and scores of Domain subsections D1.3 (question about 112 as emergency number); D2.3; D3.1; D3.2; D3.4, D6, and D7 were not included in the 2019 vs. 2015 comparative analysis, because the corresponding questions were not included in the 2015 Survey [3]. Therefore, for the purpose of this comparative analysis, the Max. Scores for the 2019 domain A and D were 41 and 40, respectively.

Respondents chose either among four options, that is, *never, sometimes, usually* and *always* or between *no* and *yes* [3]. Subsequently, responses of *never/sometimes* and *usually/always* were categorized as *no* and *yes*, respectively. All data were entered in an original, "anonymized" Excel Masterfile. Original responses were received from 1 September 2019, to 25 October 2019. Participants from each country were asked to reconfirm their answers and provide any missing answers, approximately 3 months after the initial email invitation. Participants were also asked whether they agreed or disagreed with answers provided by other participants from the same country. In cases of disagreement, we encouraged resolution through consensus. The process of data finalization lasted from 1 December 2019 to 31 January 2020. Only consensus-based, country-specific responses were ultimately analyzed, besides the case(s) of having to include responses from just one country-specific respondent. This resulted in a final Excel Masterfile that included a single, country-specific response to each one of the survey questions [3]. For data analysis, we used a dichotomous quantizing approach by grading a positive response with 1 and a negative response with 0 [24].

2.1. Questionnaire Structure and Grading

The 2019 questionnaire was organized into four domains (Table 1), precisely like the 2015 questionnaire [3]. Domain A (practices/decisions related to end-of-life care) included subdivisions that included sets of questions pertaining to (1) eight end-of-life practices (e.g., do-not-attempt cardiopulmonary resuscitation (DNACPR), advance directives, advance care planning); (2) end-of life decisions and (3) family presence during resuscitation. Each domain A subdivision could reach a maximum subscore if the responses to all of its subcomponent questions were positive. Domain A score was calculated as the sum of the aforementioned subscores (Table 1).

Domain B, C, and D scores were also calculated by summation of the respective subscores (Table 1). Domain B included subdivisions with sets of questions pertaining to access to (1) best out-of-hospital resuscitation care; (2) best in-hospital resuscitation care; and (3) best postresuscitation care. Domain C subdivisions concerned (1) death diagnosis; and (2) organ donation. Domain D subdivisions included sets of questions related to (1) access to emergency care; (2) defibrillation; (3) organization of out-of-hospital emergency care; 4) organization of in-hospital emergency services; (5) registry reporting of cardiac arrest and (6) education (Table 1).

As further detailed in the footnote of Table 1, Domains A and D of the 2019 questionnaire had a total of 10 sets of questions (concerning specific variables, for example, advance care planning (ACP)) that were not included in the 2015 questionnaire. These "new—2019-only" questions were not taken into account in the calculation of the 2019 Domain A and D scores for the purpose of the below-presented 2019 vs. 2015 comparisons.

2.2. Study Outcomes

The primary outcome was the presence/absence of statistically significant differences between 2015 and 2019 in domain A to D scores of all participating countries.

The secondary outcome was the presence/absence of significant differences between 2015 and 2019 domain A to D scores of countries with "low" domain scores in 2015. "Low" 2015 scores were defined as domain scores equal to or lower than the corresponding, overall mean score values of 2015 [3]; more specifically, "low" 2015 scores for domains A, B, C and D were those not exceeding 18, 7, 12 and 23, respectively [3]. Accordingly, "high" (or above average) 2015 scores for domains A, B, C, and D were those exceeding 18, 7, 12 and 23, respectively [3].

The tertiary outcome was the presence/absence of significant differences between changes in "low" 2015 domain scores from 2015 to 2019, and changes in "high" 2015 domain scores from 2015 to 2019.

2.3. Additional Data Collection in the Context of Un-Prespecified, Exploratory Analyses

In an effort to determine any potential effect of the coronavirus disease-19 (COVID-19), we asked respondents to determine whether the pandemic could have resulted in changes in any of their original responses to the questionnaire (Table 1). Pertinent data collection started on 15 May 2020 and ended on 29 June 2020.

2.4. Protocol Approval and Registration

The study protocol was approved by the Ethics and Scientific Committee of Evaggelismos General Hospital Athens, Greece. The approval was used for study conduct in 32/44 European countries (73%) and Turkey. Countries are listed in the online supplement, along with details for informed consent and personal data protection. The protocol was registered with Clinicaltrials.gov (Identifier: NCT04078815).

2.5. Statistical Analyses

The internal consistency of the 2019 and the 2015 questionnaires was assessed by the determination of domain-specific Cronbach's alpha. The distribution normality of domain scores and subscores was assessed by the Kolmogorov–Smirnov test with Lilliefors significance correction. Data are reported as number, number (percentage) and median (IQR) or mean ± SD unless otherwise specified. Comparisons pertaining to (1) study outcomes; and (2) domain subscores were conducted using an independent samples *t*-test or the Mann–Whitney *U* test.

Bivariate linear regression was used to explore possible associations between (1) the 2019 domain A and D scores with and without the "new—2019-only" questions [3]; and (2) the 2019 variable-specific scores for DNACPR or advance directives and ACP. All analyses were performed using SPSS version 28 (IBM Corporation, Armonk, NY, USA). All reported P values are two-sided. Statistical significance was set at $p < 0.05$.

3. Results

3.1. Respondents and Countries Participating in the Analysis

A study flow diagram is presented in Figure 1. Initial responses were received from 1 September 2019, to 28 October 2019 from 85 respondents originating from 31/33 European countries (93.9%). The median number (IQR) of respondents per country was 2 (1–4) and ranged from 1 (9 countries) to 9 (1 country). Details on conflicting and/or initially missing responses are presented in Supplemental Table S1. Consensus on conflicting responses and provision of initially missing responses was accomplished for 25/33 countries (75.8%), which were ultimately included in the analyses.

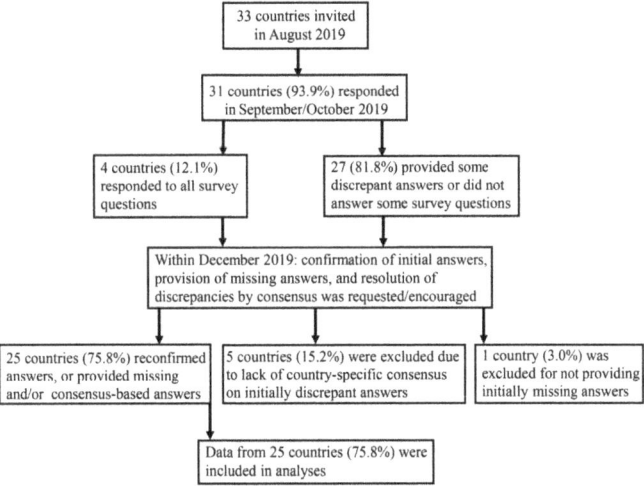

Figure 1. Flow diagram of responses to the 2019 questionnaire.

3.2. Internal Consistency of the 2019 and 2015 Questionnaires

Domains A (end-of-life care practices/decisions), B (access to best resuscitation/postresuscitation care), C (death diagnosis/organ donation) and D (emergency care organization) of the 2019 questionnaire had Cronbach's alpha values of 0.94, 0.94, 0.63 and 0.74, respectively. Domains A, B, C and D of the 2015 questionnaire, had Cronbach's alpha values of 0.94, 0.88, 0.61 and 0.78, respectively. Regarding domain C, deletion of a question regarding "organ donation by opting in" in the 2019 questionnaire (Table 1), and deletion of a question about "use of brain death criteria in "out-of-hospital cardiac arrest" in the 2015 questionnaire [3] (Table 1) would result in respective alpha values of 0.70 and 0.68.

3.3. Results on Study Outcomes

Results on the primary and secondary outcomes are summarized in Figures 2 and 3, respectively; further details, including scores of variable-specific sets of questions, and additional, subgroup-specific data are presented in Supplemental Tables S2–S5.

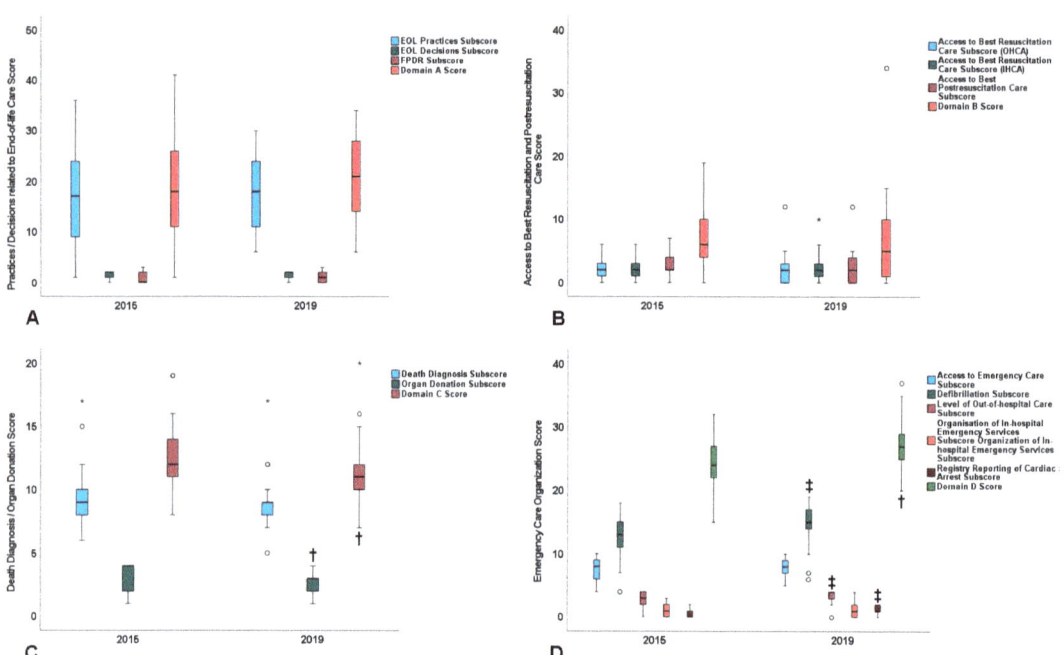

Figure 2. Summary results on the primary study outcome. Boxplot presentation of subscores and scores of domains (**A–D**) of the study questionnaire. Data originate from the 25 participating countries. Bars reflect median value; box height reflects interquartile range; bars on top or bottom of the boxes reflect actual range of values; symbols (circles and asterisk) reflect countries with outlier score values, that is, score values outside the range that corresponds to box height plus the bars. †, $p < 0.05$ vs. 2015; ‡, $p \leq 0.01$ vs. 2015.

Regarding the primary outcome, domain A and B scores did not differ significantly between 2015 and 2019 (Figure 2). However, domain C score was lower by 1 point in 2019 vs. 2015 (95% confidence interval (CI): 1 to 3; $p = 0.02$); this change was driven by a reduction in the organ donation subscore (Figure 2, Table S3). In contrast, from 2015 to 2019, domain D score exhibited a significant increase of 2.6 points (95% CI: 0.2 to 5.0; $p = 0.035$) (Figure 2, Table S3). Regarding domains A and D, the comparable ranges of score values (Figure 2) and coefficients of variation in 2019 (Table S3) suggest the persistence of the considerable variation in end-of-life practices and emergency care organization observed in 2015 [3].

Regarding the secondary outcome, in countries with "low" 2015 domain scores, domain B and C scores did not differ significantly between 2015 and 2019 (Figure 3). However, from 2015 to 2019, the domain A score increased by 5.5 points (95% CI: 0.4 to 10.6; $p = 0.047$) (Figure 3, Table S4). The domain D score also increased by 4.7 points (95% CI: 2.1 to 7.3;

$p = 0.009$) (Figure 3, Table S4), thereby driving the "overall increase" reported above and in Figure 2 and Table S3.

In the context of a "pragmatic", practice-level presentation, Table 2 presents the main, observed, proportional changes in positive responses to variable-specific questions from 2015 to 2019.

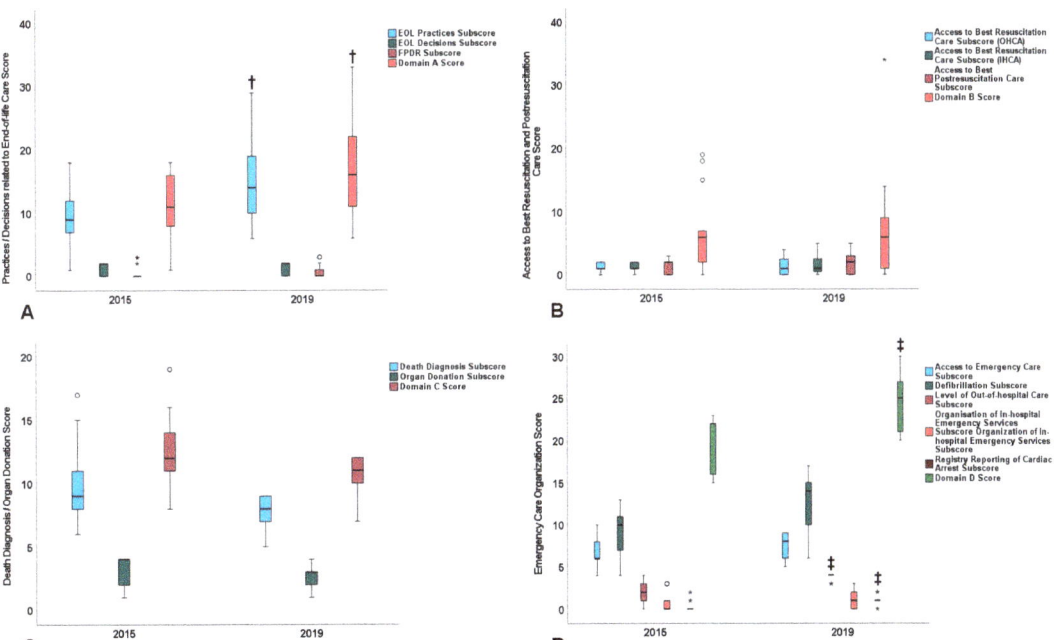

Figure 3. Summary results on the secondary study outcome. Boxplot presentation of subscores and scores of domains (**A–D**) of the study questionnaire. Data originate from countries with "low" 2015 domain scores (n = 13 for domains (**A,C**); n = 15 for domain (**B**); and n = 9 for domain (**D**)). Bars reflect median value; box height reflects interquartile range; bars on top or bottom of the boxes reflect actual range of values; symbols (circles and asterisk) reflect countries with outlier score values, that is, score values outside the range that corresponds to box height plus the bars. †, $p < 0.05$ vs. 2015; ‡, $p \leq 0.01$ vs. 2015.

Table 2. Main proportional (%) changes in positive responses to variable-specific questions from 2015 to 2019.

Domain A—End-of-Life Care Practices/ Decisions	Legally Allowed	Legally Supported	Application out-of-/in-Hospital	Application Related to Start/Stop CPR STIER AMB 1st TIER AMB 2nd TIER AMB Hospital				Written in Medical Records	Reviewed
DNACPR—all countries (n = 25)	16%	0%	+28%/+28%	8%	4%	24%	12%	24%	0%
DNACPR—low 2015 score (n = 13)	31%	23%	+46%/+46%	15%	15%	31%	23%	31%	15%
Ads—all countries (n = 25)	20%	12%	+20%/+24%	0%	−8%	8%	8%		
Ads—low 2015 score (n = 13)	46%	46%	0.794872	8%	15%	23%	31%		
Term. Analg/Sed - all countries (n = 25)	−12%		−12%						

Domain A	Legally allowed	STIER AMB	1st TIER AMB	2nd TIER AMB	Hospital
TOR Protocols—all countries (n = 25)	−4%	−12%	−4%	0%	−28%

Domain C -Death diagnosis/organ donation	Heart beating	Non-heart beating	Opt in	Opt out	Opt in and/or Opt out			
Organ donation—all countries (n = 25)	0%	0%	−48%	−8%	−8%			

Domain D -Emergency care organization	STIER AMB	1st TIER AMB	Fire Cars	Police Cars	Public Places	Mass gatherings	FRDP	Other
Defibrillation Av/ty—all countries (n = 25)	32%	12%	12%	20%	0%	12%	−4%	−8%
Defibrillation Av/ty—low 2015 score (n = 9)	78%	33%	33%	56%	0%	22%	11%	0%

Domain D	PAD programs	Home AED	School AED	In-hospital AED	AED Registry—Nat.	AED Registry—Reg.
PAD—all countries (n = 25)	8%	4%	28%	12%	12%	36%

Domain D	Physician	Nurse	AMB Personnel	Police	On-site Responder	Citizen
Legally allowed to defibrillate—low 2015 score (n = 9)	0%	0%	−11%	0%	−11%	22%

Domain D	STIER—ALS	1st TIER—ALS	1st TIER—Defibrillation	2nd TIER—ALS
AMB level of care—all countries (n = 25)	36%	36%	12%	0%
AMB level of care—low 2015 score (n = 9)	67%	78%	33%	11%

	OHCA	IHCA
Registry reporting—all countries (n = 25)	36%	40%
Registry reporting—low 2015 score (n = 9)	33%	44%

STIER, single tier; AMB, ambulance; DNACPR, do-not-attempt cardiopulmonary resuscitation; ADs, advance directives; Term. Analg/Sed, terminal analgesia/sedation; TOR, termination of resuscitation; Av/ty, availability; FRDP, first responder dispatch project; PAD, public access defibrillation; AED, automated external defibrillator; Nat., national; Reg., regional, ALS, advanced life support; OHCA, out-of-hospital cardiac arrest; IHCA, in-hospital cardiac arrest. Regarding "all participating countries (n = 25)", proportional changes of ≥12% in ≥3 countries are highlighted in bold script. Domain A: regarding "countries with low 2015 scores (n = 13)" proportional changes of ≥15% in ≥2 countries are highlighted in bold script. Domain D: regarding "countries with low 2015 scores (n = 9)" proportional changes of ≥22% in ≥2 countries are highlighted in bold script.

Regarding the tertiary outcome, in countries with "low" 2015 domain A to D scores, all changes in the scores of domains A, C and D from 2015 to 2019 were arithmetically positive and differed significantly from the respective changes determined for countries with "high" 2015 domain A to D scores ($p \leq 0.02$) (Table 3).

Table 3. Summary results on the tertiary outcome.

	Domain A ΔScore 2015 to 2019	Domain B ΔScore 2015 to 2019	Domain C ΔScore 2015 to 2019	Domain D ΔScore 2015 to 2019
Low 2015 score countries, n, median (IQR) or mean ± SD	n = 13 4.0 (−0.5–10.0) *	n = 15 0.8 ± 5.4	n = 13 0.5 ± 1.9 †	n = 9 4.8 ± 4.4 ‡
High 2015 score countries, n median (IQR) or mean ± SD	n = 12 −2.0 (−6.0–−0.3)	n = 10 −2.8 ± 9.0	n = 12 −3.2 ± 4.3	n = 16 1.4 ± 4.6

Domain A, Practices/decisions related to end-of-life care; Domain B, Access to Best Resuscitation and Postresuscitation Care; Domain C, Death Diagnosis and Organ Donation; Domain D, Emergency Care Organization; ΔScore, Change in Score (from 2015 to 2019). The tertiary outcome comprises the comparison of ΔScores from 2015 to 2019 between countries with low 2015 scores and countries with high 2015 scores; low and high 2015 scores are defined in Methods. *, $p = 0.01$ vs. high-score countries †, $p = 0.01$ vs. high-score countries ‡, $p = 0.02$ vs. high score countries.

3.4. Responses Pertaining Only to the 2019 Survey

Responses to questions included only in the 2019 survey are detailed in the supplement. Country-specific, positive response rates of >50% pertained primarily to ACP, shared decision making, dispatcher-assisted CPR and guidance about compressions/ventilation, quality features of prehospital (ambulance) care and educational programs for ethics.

3.5. Exploratory Analyses

Linear regression revealed significant associations between 2019 domain A (end-of-life care practices/decisions) and domain D (emergency care organization) scores (adjusted $r^2 = 0.35$ to 0.43; $p \leq 0.001$; Supplemental Figure S1A,B). There were also strong linear relationships between the 2019 variable-specific score for DNACPR and ACP ($r^2 = 0.68$, $p < 0.001$; supplemental Figure S1C) and the 2019 variable-specific score for advance directives and ACP ($r^2 = 0.79$, $p < 0.001$; Supplemental Figure S1D). Additional details are reported in the supplement.

Results on the effect of COVID-19 were remarkable mainly for changes in access to resuscitation care; for further details see the supplement's text and Table S6.

4. Discussion

The current comparison of responses to the 2015 and 2019 questionnaires from 25 countries revealed no overall significant changes in end-of-life practices and access to best resuscitation/postresuscitation care. There was an apparent decline in organ donation practices in just two countries. There was a significant improvement in the 2019 emergency care organization, driven by countries with "low" 2015 domain D scores. Furthermore, from 2015 to 2019, the frequency of application of end-of-life practices increased significantly in countries with "low" 2015 domain A scores, as opposed to countries with "high" 2015 domain A scores. The considerable variation in practices and emergency care organization noted in 2015 persisted in 2019. As in 2015, a higher 2019 end-of-life practice score was predictive of an improved 2019 emergency care organization [3].

Regarding end-of-life practices, our results are consistent with recent papers on new legislation [25,26] by suggesting a country-level expansion of legal support [3] and application/implementation of DNACPR and advance directives. Integration of DNACPR/advance directives with ACP has been recently advocated in the context of a holistic approach to honoring patient preferences [4,18]. Accordingly, exploratory analyses revealed that the 2019 variable-specific scores for DNACPR and advance directives were predictive of the variable-specific score for ACP.

Current European guidelines support using terminal analgesia and sedation, without hastening death [7,27]. Accordingly, the new Italian law entitled "Rules about informed consent and advance directives" supports prescribing clinically indicated, deep sedation for terminally ill patients, in the presence of valid informed consent [26]. The right to deep continuous sedation is also established by the recent, French Claeys–Leonetti law [28]. The use of sedation and analgesia does not seem to shorten the dying process of terminally ill patients [4,27,29]. Furthermore, terminal sedation and analgesia are recommended by recent Canadian guidelines for the alleviation of any pain/distress after LST withdrawal [30]. This clearly differs from the practice of euthanasia, that is, the intentional and painless termination of the patient's life upon their request [31]. Despite the fundamental difference as regards the main objective of the intervention (i.e., alleviation of distress vs. termination of life), several authors have expressed concerns about a potential "practice overlap" between deep sedation until death and euthanasia [26,28,32–42]. This could partly explain our results of declining legal support/application of terminal analgesia and sedation, despite the recently reported increase of treatment limitation decisions over time in Europe [1]. Indeed, if certain respondents (subjectively/erratically) viewed "terminal analgesia and sedation" as a form of "euthanasia" [40], they might have provided negative responses for legal support/application [2,31].

In Western countries, out-of-hospital termination-of-resuscitation rules perform well, with proportions of cardiac arrest survivors recommended for termination (i.e., miss rates) of <1% [43,44]. However, miss rates may exceed 6% in countries with lower proportions of in-field defibrillation attempts and shorter in-field resuscitation before patient transportation [44]. Furthermore, the application of termination-of-resuscitation protocols may vary widely at the country level (according to legal support) [6,44], regional healthcare system level (depending on the local frequency of witnessed arrest and bystander CPR) [45], emergency medical service (EMS) or hospital level (according to service-specific or institution-specific resuscitation policies) [44,46] and healthcare professional level (according to pertinent knowledge/expertise, confidence and right/responsibility to decide, possible fear of litigation and personal views) [6,47–49]. Such multiple sources of variation and the concurrent inability to issue a "universal/clear-cut" recommendation for a rule [4] may explain our results of the declining application of termination-of-resuscitation protocols.

Organ transplantation prolongs the life of recipients and improves its quality [50]. An ongoing shortage of organs for transplantation has led to the consideration of uncontrolled donation after circulatory death (DCD) [51]. Over the past 16 years, there has been a steady increase in DCD in the United Kingdom, the Netherlands, Belgium and Spain [50,52]. Such country-specific increases in organ donation could not be detected by our survey questions (Table 1).

Automated external defibrillator (AED) availability and use improve survival and neurological outcome after shockable out-of-hospital cardiac arrest [53–58]. Barriers and facilitators of bystander defibrillation are related to knowledge/awareness, training, willingness, AED availability/accessibility, medicolegal issues, AED registration and dispatcher assistance [59]. Major problems contributing to AED underutilization comprise AED retrieval distance and time-dependent availability (e.g., functional AED not available at night) [60,61]. Recently proposed improvements included mathematical optimization of AED placement and AED drone delivery to lay rescuers [62,63]. Our results are consistent with an ongoing and expanding effort to increase AED availability in various locations and emergency vehicles and improve AED data collection by creating new AED registries.

Our results of increased defibrillation availability are consistent with the reported improvements in ambulance/pre-hospital level of care. However, the pertinent key determinant was the reported increase in ambulance advanced life support (ALS) (Table 1). Prehospital ALS is cost-effective [64] and efficient paramedic training in ALS interventions may lead to better patient outcomes [65–68]. Physician-staffed ambulances have been associated with improved neurological outcomes in bystander-witnessed cardiac arrest [69]. EMS physician attendance has been associated with improved survival after cardiac arrest in Norwegian rural areas [70].

As elsewhere detailed [6], registry-based analyses offer valuable insights into regional variation, temporal trends and determinants of cardiac arrest outcomes, the potential efficacy of therapeutic interventions, and the extent of evidence-based clinical practice [70–73]. The EuReCa projects combined data from the national cardiac arrest registries of 28 European countries and have already reported on key modifiable variables (e.g., bystander CPR and defibrillation rates) affecting patient outcomes [73]. Accordingly, our results suggest an improvement in registry reporting of cardiac arrest from 2015 to 2019.

Responses to domain A and D "2019-only" questions suggested variation in end-of-life practices and emergency care organization, respectively. Variable-specific scores for DNACPR and advance directives were predictive of the variable-specific score for ACP, possibly implying increasing integration of advance directives with ACP [6,18]. Overall and "2019-only" results on emergency care organization indicate a need for multilevel improvement in many countries and are consistent with the observed large variation in cardiac arrest outcomes [71,73].

The current questionnaire was not specifically designed to detect pandemic-induced changes in resuscitation practices and patient outcomes [74–76]. Our results are consistent with the recently reported less CPR initiation by bystanders/first aid providers and mobile medical teams, and less AED use [74,75].

Strengths and Limitations

The current survey's strengths include coverage of multiple aspects of resuscitation and end-of-life practices/care and comparative determination of their time-dependent changes [3,31].

Limitations (including subjectivity-related bias) exhibit similarities to those acknowledged in our 2015 survey [3]. In 2019, we attempted to increase the number of 1–2 respondents per country in 2015; this was not feasible for 9/25 countries (36%; Supplemental Table S1). Consequently, the current work is still primarily based on the opinion of just a few experts from each participating country. We also requested confirmation of original answers and provision of missing answers within 3 months (as opposed to 6 months in 2015). Furthermore, in contrast to 2015, we analyzed only consensus-based data from most (i.e., 16/25; 64%) of the participating countries. Arguably, these methodological differences between the current and the 2015 survey may have limited their comparability. Nevertheless, in 2015, we employed similar criteria for respondent selection and also analyzed consensus-based data from 4/25 (16%) participating countries.

As in 2015, we assumed that respondents had a thorough knowledge of multiple aspects of practice/care or access to information concerning survey items [3]. Furthermore, we employed a dichotomous quantizing approach, which may risk the loss of critical information but also limit respondent subjectivity [3,24]. Arguably, our approach could be regarded as more suitable for questions answerable with a "clear yes or no" (e.g., are DNACPR orders legally allowed?) and less suitable for differentiated questions (e.g., are DNACPR orders applied in the out-of-hospital or in-hospital setting?). However, the determined Cronbach's alpha values indicated similarly good-to-strong internal consistency of the 2015 and 2019 survey domains [77–79]; this further suggests homogenous and replicable patterns of participant responses in both surveys [79], thereby also supporting domain scores' comparability.

Our results were derived by simple summation of positive responses and should therefore be interpreted with caution as a higher domain A score may not always indicate better practice. Controversial end-of-life practices such as euthanasia and physician-assisted suicide (PHAD) [80,81] should not be considered equivalent to practices aimed at safeguarding patient autonomy, such as advance directives and ACP [4–6]. However, euthanasia/PHAD are rarely requested/practiced [2], and pertinent positive responses (increasing domain A scores by $\leq 15\%$) were provided by just 4/25 (16%) and 5/25 (20%) countries in 2015 and 2019, respectively.

Finally, in 5/25 countries (20%; respondents, n = 1 and ≥ 3, in three and two countries, respectively), we noted domain A score changes of >10 points from 2015 to 2019 (supplemental Tables S1 and S2); pertinent contributing factors could include improved adherence to ethics/end-of-life guidelines published in 2014 and 2015 [5,7], changes in local legislation [25], and recall/social desirability bias [1].

5. Conclusions

There was a persisting, substantial variation in resuscitation/end-of-life practices across Europe in 2019, indicating a need for progress, preferably through harmonized legislations, governmental policies, and education/training. There was an overall improvement in emergency care organization from 2015 to 2019, driven by countries with "low" 2015 emergency care organization scores. Significant end-of-life practice changes were also noted in countries with "low" 2015 end-of-life practice scores. As in 2015, higher end-of-life practice scores were associated with better emergency care organization in 2019.

Supplementary Materials: The following supporting information can be downloaded at: https://www.mdpi.com/article/10.3390/jcm11144005/s1. Summary of results reported in supplemental Tables S1 to S3; Table S1: Country-specific, initial number of discrepancies in responses and/or missing responses, and outcome of efforts to resolve these issues; Table S2: Country-level domain A to D scores in 2015 and 2019, and corresponding summary results; Table S3: Results on domain scores, subscores and their components in all 25 countries; Table S4: Results on domain total scores and subscores and their components in countries with "low" 2015 domain total scores (as defined in main paper's Methods) Table S5: Results on domain total scores and subscores and their components in countries with "high" 2015 domain total scores (as defined in main paper's Methods); Summary of responses to questions included only in the 2019 survey; Exploratory analyses: summary of results reported in supplemental Figure S1; Figure S1: Graphs of linear relationships between 2019 domain A and domain D scores with (A) and without (B) the questions included only in the 2019 survey; Graphs of linear relationships between 2019 do-not-attempt cardiopulmonary resuscitation (DNACPR) and advance care planning (ACP) variable-specific scores (C), and between 2019 advance directives and ACP variable-specific scores (D); summary of results reported in Table S6; Table S6: Changes in responses to the 2019 questionnaire due to the coronavirus disease-19 (COVID-19) pandemic). Ethics Committee Approval; Study participant eligibility criteria; Compliance with the Checklist for Reporting Results of Internet E-surveys (CHERRIES); Statistical Analysis—additional details on linear regression.

Author Contributions: Study concept: L.B. and S.D.M. Study Design: S.D.M., K.C., V.R., J.D. and L.B. Acquisition of Data: L.B. and S.D.M. Drafting of the manuscript: S.D.M. Critical revision of the manuscript for important intellectual content: all authors. Statistical analyses: S.D.M., Study supervision: L.B. and S.D.M. All authors have read and agreed to the published version of the manuscript.

Funding: This research received no external funding.

Institutional Review Board Statement: The study protocol was approved by the Regional Ethics and Scientific Committee of Evaggelismos General Hospital of Athens, the Athens Eye Clinic, and the Athens Polyclinic (Approval No. 447/29/7/2019). The approval was used to support the conduct of the survey study in 32 European countries and Turkey.

Informed Consent Statement: Informed consent was obtained from all subjects involved in the study.

Data Availability Statement: "De-identified" datasets used and/or analyzed during the current study are available (in the form of Microsoft Excel Worksheets) from the corresponding author on reasonable request.

Acknowledgments: Support from Epidemiology team: Ingvild Tjelmeland, Jan Wnent.

Conflicts of Interest: The authors declare no conflict of interest.

Abbreviations

AED	automated external defibrillator
ACP	advance care planning
COVID-19	coronavirus disease 19
DCD	donation after circulatory death
DNACPR	do-not-attempt cardiopulmonary resuscitation
EMS	emergency medical services

References

1. Sprung, C.L.; Ricou, B.; Hartog, C.S.; Maia, P.; Mentzelopoulos, S.D.; Weiss, M.; Levin, P.D.; Galarza, L.; De La Guardia, V.; Schefold, J.C.; et al. Changes in End-of-Life Practices in European Intensive Care Units From 1999 to 2016. *JAMA* **2019**, *322*, 1692–1704. [CrossRef] [PubMed]
2. Avidan, A.; Sprung, C.L.; Schefold, J.C.; Ricou, B.; Hartog, C.S.; Nates, J.L.; Jaschinski, U.; Lobo, S.M.; Joynt, G.M.; Lesieur, O.; et al. Variations in end-of-life practices in intensive care units worldwide (Ethicus-2): A prospective observational study. *Lancet Respir. Med.* **2021**, *9*, 1101–1110. [CrossRef]
3. Mentzelopoulos, S.D.; Bossaert, L.; Raffay, V.; Askitopoulou, H.; Perkins, G.; Greif, R.; Haywood, K.; Van de Voorde, P.; Xanthos, T. A survey of key opinion leaders on ethical resuscitation practices in 31 European Countries. *Resuscitation* **2016**, *100*, 11–17. [CrossRef] [PubMed]
4. Mentzelopoulos, S.D.; Slowther, A.-M.; Fritz, Z.; Sandroni, C.; Xanthos, T.; Callaway, C.; Perkins, G.D.; Newgard, C.; Ischaki, E.; Greif, R.; et al. Ethical challenges in resuscitation. *Intensiv. Care Med.* **2018**, *44*, 703–716. [CrossRef]
5. Bossaert, L.L.; Perkins, G.D.; Askitopoulou, H.; Raffay, V.I.; Greif, R.; Haywood, K.L.; Mentzelopoulos, S.D.; Nolan, J.P.; Van de Voorde, P.; Xanthos, T.T.; et al. Ethics of resuscitation and end-of-life decisions section Collaborators. European Resuscitation Council Guidelines for Resuscitation 2015: Section 11. The ethics of resuscitation and end-of-life decisions. *Resuscitation* **2015**, *95*, 302–311. [CrossRef]
6. Mentzelopoulos, S.D.; Couper, K.; Van de Voorde, P.; Druwé, P.; Blom, M.; Perkins, G.D.; Lulic, I.; Djakow, J.; Raffay, V.; Lilja, G.; et al. European Resuscitation Council Guidelines for Resuscitation 2021: Section 11. The ethics of resuscitation and end-of-life decisions. *Resuscitation* **2021**, *161*, 408–432. [CrossRef] [PubMed]
7. Council of Europe. Guide on the Decision-Making Process Regarding Medical Treatment in End-of-Life Situations. *Bioethics.net website*. Available online: http://www.bioethics.net/2014/05/council-of-europe-launches-guide-on-decision-making-process-regarding-medical-treatment-in-end-oflife-situations/ (accessed on 21 March 2019).
8. Davidson, J.E.; Aslakson, R.A.; Long, A.C.; Puntillo, K.A.; Kross, E.K.; Hart, J.; Cox, C.E.; Wunsch, H.; Wickline, M.A.; Nunnally, M.E.; et al. Guidelines for Family-Centered Care in the Neonatal, Pediatric, and Adult ICU. *Crit. Care Med.* **2017**, *45*, 103–128. [CrossRef]
9. Kon, A.A.; Davidson, J.E.; Morrison, W.; Danis, M.; White, D.B. American College of Critical Care Medicine; American Thoracic Society. Shared Decision Making in ICUs: An American College of Critical Care Medicine and American Thoracic Society Policy Statement. *Crit. Care Med.* **2016**, *44*, 188–201. [CrossRef]
10. Houben, C.H.; Spruit, M.A.; Groenen, M.T.; Wouters, E.F.; Janssen, D.J. Efficacy of Advance Care Planning: A Systematic Review and Meta-Analysis. *J. Am. Med Dir. Assoc.* **2014**, *15*, 477–489. [CrossRef]
11. Brinkman-Stoppelenburg, A.; Judith, A.C.; Rietjens, J.A.C.; van der Heide, A. The effects of advance care planning on end-of-life care: A systematic review. *Palliat. Med.* **2014**, *28*, 1000–1025. [CrossRef]
12. Kernick, L.A.; Hogg, K.J.; Millerick, Y.; Murtagh, F.E.M.; Djahit, A.; Johnson, M. Does advance care planning in addition to usual care reduce hospitalisation for patients with advanced heart failure: A systematic review and narrative synthesis. *Palliat. Med.* **2018**, *32*, 1539–1551. [CrossRef] [PubMed]
13. El-Jawahri, A.; Paasche-Orlow, M.K.; Matlock, D.; Stevenson, L.W.; Lewis, E.F.; Stewart, G.; Semigran, M.; Chang, Y.; Parks, K.; Walker-Corkery, E.S.; et al. Randomized, Controlled Trial of an Advance Care Planning Video Decision Support Tool for Patients With Advanced Heart Failure. *Circulation* **2016**, *134*, 52–60. [CrossRef] [PubMed]
14. Chan, H.Y.-L.; Ng, J.S.-C.; Chan, K.-S.; Ko, P.-S.; Leung, D.Y.-P.; Chan, C.W.-H.; Chan, L.-N.; Lee, I.F.-K.; Lee, D.T.-F. Effects of a nurse-led post-discharge advance care planning programme for community-dwelling patients nearing the end of life and their family members: A randomised controlled trial. *Int. J. Nurs. Stud.* **2018**, *87*, 26–33. [CrossRef] [PubMed]
15. Cohen, S.M.; Volandes, A.E.; Shaffer, M.L.; Hanson, L.C.; Habtemariam, D.; Mitchell, S.L. Concordance Between Proxy Level of Care Preference and Advance Directives Among Nursing Home Residents With Advanced Dementia: A Cluster Randomized Clinical Trial. *J. Pain Symptom Manag.* **2019**, *57*, 37–46.e1. [CrossRef] [PubMed]
16. Green, M.J.; Van Scoy, L.J.; Foy, A.J.; Dimmock, A.E.; Lehman, E.; Levi, B.H. Patients With Advanced Cancer Choose Less Aggressive Medical Treatment on Vignettes After Using a Computer-Based Decision Aid. *Am. J. Hosp. Palliat. Care* **2020**, *37*, 537–541. [CrossRef]
17. Tolle, S.W.; Teno, J.M. Lessons from Oregon in Embracing Complexity in End-of-Life Care. *N. Engl. J. Med.* **2017**, *376*, 1078–1082. [CrossRef]
18. Fritz, Z.; Slowther, A.-M.; Perkins, G.D. Resuscitation policy should focus on the patient, not the decision. *BMJ* **2017**, *356*, j813. [CrossRef]
19. Hawkes, C.A.; Fritz, Z.; Deas, G.; Ahmedzai, S.H.; Richardson, A.; Pitcher, D.; Spiller, J.; Perkins, G.D.; ReSPECT Working Group Collaborators. Development of the Recommended Summary Plan for eEmergency Care and Treatment (ReSPECT). *Resuscitation* **2020**, *148*, 98–107. [CrossRef]
20. Sulmasy, D.P. Italy's New Advance Directive Law: When in Rome. *JAMA Intern. Med.* **2018**, *178*, 607–608. [CrossRef]
21. Danish Patient Safety Authority. A Guide on Withholding Life Support, Resuscitation and Withdrawing of Treatment. 2012. Available online: https://stps.dk/da/udgivelser/2012/vejledning-om-forudgaaende-fravalg-af-livsforlaengende-behandling,-herunder-genoplivningsforsoeg,-og-om-afbrydelse-af-behandling (accessed on 21 June 2018).

22. The Norwegian Directorate of Health. Decision-Making Process when Limiting Life-Sustaining Treatment. 2013. Available online: https://helsedirektoratet.no/retningslinjer/beslutningsprosesser-ved-begrensning-av-livsforlengende-behandling (accessed on 21 June 2018).
23. Schulz-Quach, C.; Wenzel-Meyburg, U.; Fetz, K. Can elearning be used to teach palliative care?—Medical students' acceptance, knowledge, and self-estimation of competence in palliative care after elearning. *BMC Med. Educ.* **2018**, *18*, 82. [CrossRef]
24. Sandelowski, M.; Voils, C.L.; Knafl, G. On Quantitizing. *J. Mix Methods Res.* **2009**, *3*, 208–222. [CrossRef] [PubMed]
25. Ciliberti, R.; Gorini, I.; Gazzaniga, V.; De Stefano, F.; Gulino, M. The Italian law on informed consent and advance directives: New rules of conduct for the autonomy of doctors and patients in end-of-life care. *J. Crit. Care* **2018**, *48*, 178–182. [CrossRef] [PubMed]
26. Orsi, L.; Gristina, G.R. Palliative sedation: The position statement of the Italian National Committee for Bioethics. *Minerva Anestesiol.* **2017**, *83*, 524–528. [CrossRef] [PubMed]
27. Cherny, N.I.; Radbruch, L. The Board of the European Association for Palliative Care European Association for Palliative Care (EAPC) recommended framework for the use of sedation in palliative care. *Palliat. Med.* **2009**, *23*, 581–593. [CrossRef]
28. Le Dorze, M.; Kandelman, S.; Veber, B.; SFAR's Ethics Committee. End-of-life care in the French ICU: Impact of Claeys-Leonetti law on decision to withhold or withdraw life-supportive therapy. *Anaesth. Crit. Care Pain Med.* **2019**, *38*, 569–570. [CrossRef] [PubMed]
29. Beller, E.M.; van Driel, M.L.; McGregor, L.; Truong, S.; Mitchell, G. Palliative pharmacological sedation for terminally ill adults. *Cochrane Database Syst. Rev.* **2015**, *1*, CD010206. [CrossRef]
30. Downar, J.; Delaney, J.W.; Hawryluck, L.; Kenny, L. Guidelines for the withdrawal of life-sustaining measures. *Intensiv. Care Med.* **2016**, *42*, 1003–1017. [CrossRef]
31. Mentzelopoulos, S.D.; Haywood, K.; Cariou, A.; Mantzanas, M.; Bossaert, L. Evolution of medical ethics in resuscitation and end of life. *Trends Anaesth. Crit. Care* **2016**, *10*, 7–14. [CrossRef]
32. Badarau, D.O.; De Clercq, E.; Elger, B.S. Continuous Deep Sedation and Euthanasia in Pediatrics: Does One Really Exclude the Other for Terminally Ill Patients? *J. Med. Philos.* **2019**, *44*, 50–70. [CrossRef]
33. Bhyan, P.; Pesce, M.B.; Shrestha, U.; Goyal, A. Palliative Sedation. 2 December 2020. In *StatPearls [Internet]*; StatPearls Publishing: Treasure Island, FL, USA, 2020; PMID: 29262025.
34. Benítez-Rosario, M.A.; Ascanio-León, B. Palliative sedation: Beliefs and decision-making among Spanish palliative care physicians. *Support. Care Cancer* **2020**, *28*, 2651–2658. [CrossRef]
35. Riisfeldt, T.D. Weakening the ethical distinction between euthanasia, palliative opioid use and palliative sedation. *J. Med. Ethic* **2019**, *45*, 125–130. [CrossRef] [PubMed]
36. Sulmasy, D.P. Sedation and care at the end of life. *Theor. Med. Bioeth.* **2018**, *39*, 171–180. [CrossRef]
37. Cohen-Almagor, R.; Ely, E.W. Euthanasia and palliative sedation in Belgium. *BMJ Support. Palliat. Care* **2018**, *8*, 307–313. [CrossRef] [PubMed]
38. Horn, R. The 'French exception': The right to continuous deep sedation at the end of life. *J. Med. Ethic-* **2018**, *44*, 204–205. [CrossRef] [PubMed]
39. Kirby, J. Morally-Relevant Similarities and Differences Between Assisted Dying Practices in Paradigm and Non-Paradigm Circumstances: Could They Inform Regulatory Decisions? *J. Bioethical Inq.* **2017**, *14*, 475–483. [CrossRef]
40. den Hartogh, G. Continuous deep sedation and homicide: An unsolved problem in law and professional morality. *Med. Health Care Philos.* **2016**, *19*, 285–297. [CrossRef]
41. Raho, J.A.; Miccinesi, G. Contesting the Equivalency of Continuous Sedation until Death and Physician-assisted Suicide/Euthanasia: A Commentary on LiPuma. *J. Med. Philos.* **2015**, *40*, 529–553. [CrossRef]
42. Seale, C.; Raus, K.; Bruinsma, S.; van der Heide, A.; Sterckx, S.; Mortier, F.; Payne, S.; Mathers, N.; Rietjens, J.; Addington-Hall, J.; et al. The language of sedation in end-of-life care: The ethical reasoning of care providers in three countries. *Health* **2014**, *19*, 339–354. [CrossRef]
43. Ebell, M.H.; Vellinga, A.; Masterson, S.; Yun, P. Meta-analysis of the accuracy of termination of resuscitation rules for out-of-hospital cardiac arrest. *Emerg. Med. J.* **2019**, *36*, 479–484. [CrossRef]
44. Nas, J.; Kleinnibbelink, G.; Hannink, G.; Navarese, E.P.; van Royen, N.; de Boer, M.-J.; Wik, L.; Bonnes, J.L.; Brouwer, M.A. Diagnostic performance of the basic and advanced life support termination of resuscitation rules: A systematic review and diagnostic meta-analysis. *Resuscitation* **2020**, *148*, 3–13. [CrossRef]
45. Verhaert, D.; Bonnes, J.L.; Nas, J.; Keuper, W.; van Grunsven, P.M.; Smeets, J.L.; de Boer, M.J.; Brouwer, M.A. Termination of resuscitation in the prehospital setting: A comparison of decisions in clinical practice vs. recommendations of a termination rule. *Resuscitation* **2016**, *100*, 60–65. [CrossRef] [PubMed]
46. Eckstein, M.; Stratton, S.J.; Chan, L.S. Termination of Resuscitative Efforts for Out-of-hospital Cardiac Arrests. *Acad. Emerg. Med.* **2005**, *12*, 65–70. [CrossRef] [PubMed]
47. Hansen, C.; Lauridsen, K.G.; Schmidt, A.S.; Løfgren, B. Decision-making in cardiac arrest: Physicians' and nurses' knowledge and views on terminating resuscitation. *Open Access Emerg. Med.* **2018**, *11*, 1–8. [CrossRef]
48. Campwala, R.T.; Schmidt, A.R.; Chang, T.P.; Nager, A.L. Factors influencing termination of resuscitation in children: A qualitative analysis. *Int. J. Emerg. Med.* **2020**, *13*, 12–14. [CrossRef] [PubMed]

49. Long, A.C.; Brumback, L.C.; Curtis, J.R.; Avidan, A.; Baras, M.; De Robertis, E.; Efferen, L.; Engelberg, R.A.; Kross, E.K.; Michalsen, A.; et al. Agreement With Consensus Statements on End-of-Life Care: A Description of Variability at the Level of the Provider, Hospital, and Country. *Crit. Care Med.* **2019**, *47*, 1396–1401. [CrossRef] [PubMed]
50. Gardiner, D.; Charlesworth, M.; Rubino, A.; Madden, S. The rise of organ donation after circulatory death: A narrative review. *Anaesthesia* **2020**, *75*, 1215–1222. [CrossRef] [PubMed]
51. Ortega-Deballon, I.; Hornby, L.; Shemie, S.D. Protocols for uncontrolled donation after circulatory death: A systematic review of international guidelines, practices and transplant outcomes. *Crit. Care* **2015**, *19*, 1–15. [CrossRef]
52. Smith, M.; Dominguez-Gil, B.; Greer, D.M.; Manara, A.R.; Souter, M.J. Organ donation after circulatory death: Current status and future potential. *Intensiv. Care Med.* **2019**, *45*, 310–321. [CrossRef]
53. Hallstrom, A.P.; Ornato, J.P.; Weisfeldt, M.; Travers, A.; Christenson, J.; A McBurnie, M.; Zalenski, R.; Becker, L.B.; Schron, E.B.; Proschan, M.; et al. Public-Access Defibrillation and Survival after Out-of-Hospital Cardiac Arrest. *N. Engl. J. Med.* **2004**, *351*, 637–646. [CrossRef]
54. Kitamura, T.; Kiyohara, K.; Sakai, T.; Matsuyama, T.; Hatakeyama, T.; Shimamoto, T.; Izawa, J.; Fujii, T.; Nishiyama, C.; Kawamura, T.; et al. Public-Access Defibrillation and Out-of-Hospital Cardiac Arrest in Japan. *N. Engl. J. Med.* **2016**, *375*, 1649–1659. [CrossRef]
55. Baekgaard, J.S.; Viereck, S.; Møller, T.P.; Ersbøll, A.K.; Lippert, F.; Folke, F. Response by Baekgaard et al to Letters Regarding Article, "The Effects of Public Access Defibrillation on Survival After Out-of-Hospital Cardiac Arrest: A Systematic Review of Observational Studies". *Circulation* **2017**, *137*, 954–965. [CrossRef] [PubMed]
56. Holmberg, M.J.; Vognsen, M.; Andersen, M.S.; Donnino, M.W.; Andersen, L.W. Bystander automated external defibrillator use and clinical outcomes after out-of-hospital cardiac arrest: A systematic review and meta-analysis. *Resuscitation* **2017**, *120*, 77–87. [CrossRef] [PubMed]
57. Pollack, R.A.; Brown, S.P.; Rea, T.; Aufderheide, T.; Barbic, D.; Buick, J.E.; Christenson, J.; Idris, A.H.; Jasti, J.; Kampp, M.; et al. Impact of Bystander Automated External Defibrillator Use on Survival and Functional Outcomes in Shockable Observed Public Cardiac Arrests. *Circulation* **2018**, *137*, 2104–2113. [CrossRef] [PubMed]
58. Kobayashi, D.; Sado, J.; Kiyohara, K.; Kitamura, T.; Kiguchi, T.; Nishiyama, C.; Okabayashi, S.; Shimamoto, T.; Matsuyama, T.; Kawamura, T.; et al. Public location and survival from out-of-hospital cardiac arrest in the public-access defibrillation era in Japan. *J. Cardiol.* **2020**, *75*, 97–104. [CrossRef]
59. Smith, C.M.; Keung, S.N.L.C.; Khan, M.O.; Arvanitis, T.N.; Fothergill, R.; Hartley-Sharpe, C.; Wilson, M.H.; Perkins, G. Barriers and facilitators to public access defibrillation in out-of-hospital cardiac arrest: A systematic review. *Eur. Heart J. Qual. Care Clin. Outcomes* **2017**, *3*, 264–273. [CrossRef]
60. Deakin, C.D.; Shewry, E.; Gray, H.H. Public access defibrillation remains out of reach for most victims of out-of-hospital sudden cardiac arrest. *Heart* **2014**, *100*, 619–623. [CrossRef]
61. Deakin, C.D.; Anfield, S.; Hodgetts, G.A. Underutilisation of public access defibrillation is related to retrieval distance and time-dependent availability. *Heart* **2018**, *104*, 1339–1343. [CrossRef]
62. Sun, C.L.F.; Karlsson, L.; Morrison, L.J.; Brooks, S.C.; Folke, F.; Chan, T.C.Y. Effect of Optimized Versus Guidelines-Based Automated External Defibrillator Placement on Out-of-Hospital Cardiac Arrest Coverage: An In Silico Trial. *J. Am. Heart Assoc.* **2020**, *9*, e016701. [CrossRef]
63. Zègre-Hemsey, J.K.; Grewe, M.E.; Johnson, A.M.; Arnold, E.; Cunningham, C.J.; Bogle, B.M.; Rosamond, W.D. Delivery of Automated External Defibrillators via Drones in Simulated Cardiac Arrest: Users' Experiences and the Human-Drone Interaction. *Resuscitation* **2020**, *157*, 83–88. [CrossRef]
64. Von Vopelius-Feldt, J.; Powell, J.; Benger, J.R. Cost-effectiveness of advanced life support and prehospital critical care for out-of-hospital cardiac arrest in England: A decision analysis model. *BMJ Open* **2019**, *9*, e028574. [CrossRef]
65. Baker, T.W.; King, W.; Soto, W.; Asher, C.; Stolfi, A.; Rowin, M.E. The Efficacy of Pediatric Advanced Life Support Training in Emergency Medical Service Providers. *Pediatr. Emerg. Care* **2009**, *25*, 508–512. [CrossRef] [PubMed]
66. Pilbery, R.; Teare, M.D.; Lawton, D. Do RATs save lives? A service evaluation of an out-of-hospital cardiac arrest team in an English ambulance service. *Br. Paramedic J.* **2019**, *3*, 32–39. [CrossRef] [PubMed]
67. Park, J.-H.; Moon, S.; Cho, H.; Ahn, E.; Kim, T.-K.; Bobrow, B.J. Effect of team-based cardiopulmonary resuscitation training for emergency medical service providers on pre-hospital return of spontaneous circulation in out-of-hospital cardiac arrest patients. *Resuscitation* **2019**, *144*, 60–66. [CrossRef] [PubMed]
68. Naito, H.; Yumoto, T.; Yorifuji, T.; Tahara, Y.; Yonemoto, N.; Nonogi, H.; Nagao, K.; Ikeda, T.; Sato, N.; Tsutsui, H. Improved outcomes for out-of-hospital cardiac arrest patients treated by emergency life-saving technicians compared with basic emergency medical technicians: A JCS-ReSS study report. *Resuscitation* **2020**, *153*, 251–257. [CrossRef]
69. Sato, N.; Matsuyama, T.; Akazawa, K.; Nakazawa, K.; Hirose, Y. Benefits of adding a physician-staffed ambulance to bystander-witnessed out-of-hospital cardiac arrest: A community-based, observational study in Niigata, Japan. *BMJ Open* **2019**, *9*, e032967. [CrossRef]
70. Gräsner, J.-T.; Lefering, R.; Koster, R.W.; Masterson, S.; Böttiger, B.W.; Herlitz, J.; Wnent, J.; Tjelmeland, I.B.; Ortiz, F.R.; Maurer, H.; et al. EuReCa ONE-27 Nations, ONE Europe, ONE Registry: A prospective one month analysis of out-of-hospital cardiac arrest outcomes in 27 countries in Europe. *Resuscitation* **2016**, *105*, 188–195. [CrossRef]
71. Gräsner, J.-T.; Masterson, S. EuReCa and international resuscitation registries. *Curr. Opin. Crit. Care* **2015**, *21*, 215–219. [CrossRef]

72. Donnino, M.W.; Salciccioli, J.D.; Howell, M.D.; Cocchi, M.N.; Giberson, B.; Berg, K.; Gautam, S.; Callaway, C. For the American Heart Association's Get With The Guidelines-Resuscitation Investigators Time to administration of epinephrine and outcome after in-hospital cardiac arrest with non-shockable rhythms: Retrospective analysis of large in-hospital data registry. *BMJ* **2014**, *348*, g3028. [CrossRef]
73. Gräsner, J.-T.; Wnent, J.; Herlitz, J.; Perkins, G.D.; Lefering, R.; Tjelmeland, I.; Koster, R.W.; Masterson, S.; Rossell-Ortiz, F.; Maurer, H.; et al. Survival after out-of-hospital cardiac arrest in Europe—Results of the EuReCa TWO study. *Resuscitation* **2020**, *148*, 218–226. [CrossRef]
74. Lim, Z.J.; Reddy, M.P.; Afroz, A.; Billah, B.; Shekar, K.; Subramaniam, A. Incidence and outcome of out-of-hospital cardiac arrests in the COVID-19 era: A systematic review and meta-analysis. *Resuscitation* **2020**, *157*, 248–258. [CrossRef]
75. Baert, V.; Jaeger, D.; Hubert, H.; Lascarrou, J.-B.; Debaty, G.; Chouihed, T.; Javaudin, F.; on behalf of the GR-RéAC. Assessment of changes in cardiopulmonary resuscitation practices and outcomes on 1005 victims of out-of-hospital cardiac arrest during the COVID-19 outbreak: Registry-based study. *Scand. J. Trauma Resusc. Emerg. Med.* **2020**, *28*, 119. [CrossRef] [PubMed]
76. Coleman, J.J.; Botkai, A.; Marson, E.J.; Evison, F.; Atia, J.; Wang, J.; Gallier, S.; Speakman, J.; Pankhurst, T. Bringing into focus treatment limitation and DNACPR decisions: How COVID-19 has changed practice. *Resuscitation* **2020**, *155*, 172–179. [CrossRef] [PubMed]
77. Heale, R.; Twycross, A. Validity and reliability in quantitative studies. *Évid. Based Nurs.* **2015**, *18*, 66–67. [CrossRef]
78. Taber, K.S. The Use of Cronbach's Alpha When Developing and Reporting Research Instruments in Science Education. *Res. Sci. Educ.* **2018**, *48*, 1273–1296. [CrossRef]
79. Bolarinwa, O.A. Principles and methods of validity and reliability testing of questionnaires used in social and health science researches. *Niger. Postgrad. Med. J.* **2015**, *22*, 195–201. [CrossRef] [PubMed]
80. WMA Declaration on Euthanasia and Physician-Assisted Suicide. Adopted by the 70 WMA General Assembly, Tbilisi, Georgia. October 2019. Available online: https://www.wma.net/policies-post/declaration-on-euthanasia-and-physician-assisted-suicide/ (accessed on 23 May 2022).
81. American Medical Association. Ethics. *Euthanasia*. Available online: https://www.ama-assn.org/delivering-care/euthanasia (accessed on 23 May 2022).

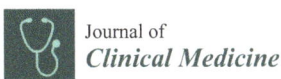

Article

Impaired Antibody Response Is Associated with Histone-Release, Organ Dysfunction and Mortality in Critically Ill COVID-19 Patients

Rickard Lagedal [1,*], Oskar Eriksson [2,3], Anna Sörman [2], Joram B. Huckriede [4], Bjarne Kristensen [5], Stephanie Franzén [1], Anders Larsson [6], Anders Bergqvist [7,8], Kjell Alving [9], Anders Forslund [9], Barbro Persson [2], Kristina N. Ekdahl [2,10], Pablo Garcia de Frutos [11], Bo Nilsson [2], Gerry A. F. Nicolaes [4], Miklos Lipcsey [1,12], Michael Hultström [1,13] and Robert Frithiof [1]

1. Department of Surgical Sciences, Anaesthesia and Intensive Care, Uppsala University, 752 36 Uppsala, Sweden; stephanie.franzen@surgsci.uu.se (S.F.); miklos.lipcsey@surgsci.uu.se (M.L.); michael.hultstrom@mcb.uu.se (M.H.); robert.frithiof@surgsci.uu.se (R.F.)
2. Department of Immunology, Genetics and Pathology, Uppsala University, 752 36 Uppsala, Sweden; oskar.eriksson@igp.uu.se (O.E.); anna.sorman@igp.uu.se (A.S.); barbro.persson@igp.uu.se (B.P.); kristina.nilsson_ekdahl@igp.uu.se (K.N.E.); bo.nilsson@igp.uu.se (B.N.)
3. Department of Medical Biochemistry and Microbiology, Uppsala University, 752 36 Uppsala, Sweden
4. Department of Biochemistry, Cardiovascular Research Institute Maastricht (CARIM), Maastricht University, 6211 LK Maastricht, The Netherlands; j.huckriede@maastrichtuniversity.nl (J.B.H.); g.nicolaes@maastrichtuniversity.nl (G.A.F.N.)
5. Thermo Fisher Scientific, 3450 Allerod, Denmark; bjarne.kristensen@thermofisher.com
6. Department of Medical Sciences, Uppsala University, 752 36 Uppsala, Sweden; anders.larsson@akademiska.se
7. Department of Medical Sciences, Section of Clinical Microbiology, Uppsala University, 752 36 Uppsala, Sweden; anders.bergqvist@akademiska.se
8. Clinical Microbiology and Hospital Infection Control, Uppsala University Hospital, 752 36 Uppsala, Sweden
9. Department of Women's and Children's Health, Uppsala University, 752 36 Uppsala, Sweden; kjell.alving@kbh.uu.se (K.A.); anders.forslund@kbh.uu.se (A.F.)
10. Linneus Centre for Biomaterials Chemistry, Linneus University, 392 31 Kalmar, Sweden
11. Department of Cell Death and Proliferation, IIBB-CSIC, IDIBAPS and CIBERCV, 08036 Barcelona, Spain; pablo.garcia@iibb.csic.es
12. Hedenstierna Laboratory, Anesthesiology and Intensive Care, Department of Surgical Sciences, Uppsala University, 752 36 Uppsala, Sweden
13. Unit for Integrative Physiology, Department of Medical Cell Biology, Uppsala University, 752 36 Uppsala, Sweden
* Correspondence: rickard.lagedal@surgsci.uu.se

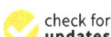

Citation: Lagedal, R.; Eriksson, O.; Sörman, A.; Huckriede, J.B.; Kristensen, B.; Franzén, S.; Larsson, A.; Bergqvist, A.; Alving, K.; Forslund, A.; et al. Impaired Antibody Response Is Associated with Histone-Release, Organ Dysfunction and Mortality in Critically Ill COVID-19 Patients. *J. Clin. Med.* 2022, 11, 3419. https://doi.org/10.3390/jcm11123419

Academic Editors: Spyros D. Mentzelopoulos and Richard Mario Pino

Received: 6 April 2022
Accepted: 10 June 2022
Published: 14 June 2022

Publisher's Note: MDPI stays neutral with regard to jurisdictional claims in published maps and institutional affiliations.

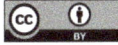

Copyright: © 2022 by the authors. Licensee MDPI, Basel, Switzerland. This article is an open access article distributed under the terms and conditions of the Creative Commons Attribution (CC BY) license (https://creativecommons.org/licenses/by/4.0/).

Abstract: Purpose: the pathophysiologic mechanisms explaining differences in clinical outcomes following COVID-19 are not completely described. This study aims to investigate antibody responses in critically ill patients with COVID-19 in relation to inflammation, organ failure and 30-day survival. Methods: All patients with PCR-verified COVID-19 and gave consent, and who were admitted to a tertiary Intensive care unit (ICU) in Sweden during March–September 2020 were included. Demography, repeated blood samples and measures of organ function were collected. Analyses of anti-SARS-CoV-2 antibodies (IgM, IgA and IgG) in plasma were performed and correlated to patient outcome and biomarkers of inflammation and organ failure. Results: A total of 115 patients (median age 62 years, 77% male) were included prospectively. All patients developed severe respiratory dysfunction, and 59% were treated with invasive ventilation. Thirty-day mortality was 22.6% for all included patients. Patients negative for any anti-SARS-CoV-2 antibody in plasma during ICU admission had higher 30-day mortality compared to patients positive for antibodies. Patients positive for IgM had more ICU-, ventilator-, renal replacement therapy- and vasoactive medication-free days. IgA antibody concentrations correlated negatively with both SAPS3 and maximal SOFA-score and IgM-levels correlated negatively with SAPS3. Patients with antibody levels below the detection limit had higher plasma levels of extracellular histones on day 1 and elevated levels of kidney and cardiac biomarkers, but showed no signs of increased inflammation, complement activation or cytokine release. After adjusting for age, positive IgM and IgG antibodies were still associated with increased

30-day survival, with odds ratio (OR) 7.1 (1.5–34.4) and 4.2 (1.1–15.7), respectively. Conclusion: In patients with severe COVID-19 requiring intensive care, a poor antibody response is associated with organ failure, systemic histone release and increased 30-day mortality.

Keywords: COVID-19; SARS-CoV-2; critical care; antibody response; NET; histones

1. Background

The ongoing COVID-19 pandemic, caused by the novel SARS-CoV-2 virus, has caused millions of deaths worldwide and left the healthcare system in many countries in the worst crisis for decades. Since the virus phenotype is novel for humans, no patients have previous antibodies specific for the virus, creating a situation where, in theory, all humans are susceptible for infection and severe disease. Despite this, the clinical course of SARS-CoV-2 infection varies substantially, from asymptomatic carriers to severe multiple organ dysfunction syndrome (MODS) and death, probably explained by individual variations in the immune response.

Several risk factors, both for the development of severe disease but also for death, have been identified [1]. Age is the strongest risk factor, but several others such as male sex, cardiovascular disease, obesity, chronic obstructive pulmonary disease (COPD), Alzheimer's disease and genetic predisposition are now known to increase the risk of poor outcomes following COVID-19 disease [2–6]. Even if part of the increased risk is due to physiologic fragility, for example, very old patients have lower cardiopulmonary reserve to cope with a pneumonia regardless of the causative agent, the immune response to the infection is likely of great importance [7,8]. Several studies have described the immune response during COVID-19 and defined differences between patients developing severe disease and patients with asymptomatic or mild disease [9,10]. However, somewhat conflicting results concerning antibody responses have been presented, perhaps reflecting sampling site, varying cohorts or the timing of blood sampling [11–16]. It appears that an adequate, early response from the innate immune system, including expression of type I interferons (IFN), is important for reducing viral replication, allowing the slower adaptive immune system to become fully activated [17]. SARS-CoV-2 has the ability to suppress the expression of type I IFN, and hence inhibit the innate immune response to the virus [18]. A delayed innate immune response might also lead to a longer activation time for the adaptive immune response, since the two systems are dependent on each other for optimal function. We hypothesised that a delayed or absent adaptive immune response in critically ill patients with COVID-19 would cause higher mortality and organ failure. Several groups have also reported that SARS-CoV-2 can induce neutrophil extracellular trap (NET) formation in neutrophiles and that NET-formation could be part of the immunopathology in severe COVID-19 [19–25].

Our group previously reported that a weak anti-SARS-CoV-2 antibody response was associated with increased mortality in a small cohort of intensive care patients with COVID-19 disease [26]. The aim of this study is to describe the effects of an impaired antibody response, with regard to 30-day survival, organ failure and activation of other parts of the immune system, identifying key pathophysiological mechanisms in a large group of intensive care patients.

2. Materials and Methods

2.1. Study Design

This single centre, prospective observational investigation is a sub-study of the PronMed-study, approved by the Swedish National Ethical Review Agency (EPM; No. 2020-01623). Informed consent was obtained either by the patient or by a next-of-kin if the patient was unable to receive information due to their clinical status. The Declaration of Helsinki and its subsequent revisions were followed. The protocol of the study was registered a priori (ClinicalTrials ID: NCT04316884). STROBE guidelines were followed for reporting.

2.2. Data Collection

All patients admitted to the central intensive care unit at Uppsala University Hospital during the first wave of the pandemic in 2020, with suspected COVID-19 infection, were screened for inclusion.

Background characteristics of the patients were obtained through patients' electronic medical records. Clinical data were collected prospectively daily. Blood samples were taken at ICU admission and three times per week during the time patients were treated in the ICU. Simplified Acute Physiology Score 3 (SAPS3) on admission and daily Sequential Organ Failure Assessment (SOFA) score were calculated prospectively [27,28]. Acute kidney injury (AKI) was diagnosed according to the Kidney Disease: Improving Global Outcome (KDIGO) creatinine criteria [29].

2.3. Plasma Analyses

Peripheral blood from patients with COVID-19 was collected into EDTA- and citrate-containing tubes and plasma was separated using centrifugation at $3000\times g$ for 10 min. After separation, all plasma samples were stored at $-80\ ^\circ C$.

Complete blood cell counts (CBC), plasma C-reactive protein (CRP), procalcitonin, IL-6, fibrin D-dimer, troponin I and N-terminal pro-brain natriuretic peptide (NT-pro-BNP), kidney function tests (plasma creatinine and cystatin C), liver function tests (plasma bilirubin, alanine aminotransferase (ALT), aspartate aminotransferase (AST), alkaline phosphatase (ALP)) were performed in the hospital central laboratory. CBC was analysed on a Sysmex XN instrument (Sysmex, Kobe, Japan) while plasma CRP, ferritin, troponin I, kidney and liver markers were analysed on an Architect ci16200 (Abbott Laboratories, Abbott Park, IL, USA). IL-6 was measured by a commercial sandwich ELISA kit (D6050, R&D Systems, Minneapolis, MN, USA). IgA, IgG and IgM antibodies against SARS-CoV-2 Spike-1 protein were quantified by FluoroEnzymeImmunoassay (FEIA), Phadia AB, Uppsala, Sweden. The analyses were performed on the last sample obtained during the stay at the ICU but within 30 days from symptoms onset to maximise the probability to discover plasma-antibodies. The lower limit of detection was 5 and 20 ug/L for IgA and IgM, respectively, and 10 U/L for IgG.

Cytokine and complement analyses are described in detail in the Supplementary Material.

SARS-CoV-2 RNA in plasma was determined by reverse transcription qPCR as previously described [30]. For qualitative and quantitative detection of viral RNA, we used the 2019-nCoV N1 reagent set from the published protocol from the Center for Disease Control (CDC) of the United States [31]. For quantitative analysis, the ISO 13485 certified molecular standard Quantitative Synthetic SARS-CoV-2 RNA: ORF, E, N (VR-3276SD, American Tissue Type Collection) was used as external calibrator. The reaction showed linearity over 6 orders of magnitude with 10^9 copies/mL and 300 copies/mL as the upper and lower limits of quantitative detection, respectively. The viral RNA analyses were performed at samples taken between day 1 and day 7 in the ICU.

2.4. Histone Analyses

The presence of histones was determined via a semi-quantitative Western blotting method as previously described [32,33]. In short, plasma was diluted 10 times and separated via SDS-PAGE gel electrophoresis (4–15% gradient gel), and transferred to a PVDF membrane (Bio-Rad Laboratories, Hemel Hempstead, UK) using semi-dry blotting. After blocking, the membranes were incubated overnight with a primary rabbit anti-histone H3 antibody (1:10,000, sc-8654-R, Santa Cruz Biotechnology, Heidelberg, Germany), followed by 1 h incubation with a secondary biotin-conjugated donkey anti-rabbit IgG antibody (1:10,000, ab97083, Abcam, Cambridge, UK), and 30 min with a streptavidin-biotin complex (1:500, Vectastain, Vector Laboratories, Burlingame, CA, USA). Histone H3 bands were visualised by the WesternBright ECL substrate (Advansta, San Jose, CA, USA) on the iBright CL1500 Imaging System (ThermoFisher Scientific, Waltham, MA, USA). The band densities were quantified by iBright Analysis Software, compared to known standard concentrations of purified calf thymus H3 (Roche, Basel, Switzerland).

2.5. Statistics

Categorical variables are presented as number of observations (percentage of total number of observations) and continuous variables as medians and interquartile range (IQR). Comparison between dichotomous variables were made with Pearson's Chi2-test or Fischer's exact test as appropriate. Continuous variables were compared with the Mann–Whitney U test. Correlation between antibody levels and SAPS3/SOFA were assessed with Spearman correlation. Analyses of survival in relation to whether patients were positive or negative for antibodies were further assessed with multiple logistic regression while controlling for age. For calculations and figures, SPSS Statistics software, version 23 (IBM) was used. $p < 0.05$ was considered significant.

3. Results

Between 13 March and 28 September 2020, 125 patients were included. After the exclusion of patients without verified COVID-19 infection, patients where no blood samples were obtained and patients where the diagnoses of COVID-19 were considered a secondary finding, 115 patients were included in the final analyses. The vast majority (88%) of the patients in the study were admitted during March–May.

3.1. Patient Characteristics

The median age for all patients was 62 years and 77% were male (Table 1). Median time from onset of symptoms until ICU admission was 10 days. Ninety percent of the total cohort developed anti-SARS-CoV-2 antibodies during their time in the ICU. Eighty-nine patients (77%) were alive after 30 days. Five (4%) of the included patients had a known immune deficiency prior to admission, either due to immune suppressive treatment or disease (previous organ transplant, lymphoma or B-cell suppressive treatment). Two of these patients did not develop antibodies and two only expressed IgM and IgM + IgG, respectively. Four of these patients were alive at 30 days from ICU admission. Thus, 110 out of 115 patients had no known reason for impaired antibody responses. For the groups with negative vs. positive SARS-CoV-2 antibodies, there was no difference in median time from ICU admission to blood sampling for antibody analyses.

Table 1. Patient characteristics.

		All Patients $n = 115$	Alive at 30 Days	
			Yes $n = 89$	No $n = 26$
Age		62 (52–71)	57 (51–67)	73 (68–79)
Male sex		88 (77%)	67 (75%)	21 (81%)
SAPS3 on ICU arrival		53 (47–57)	50.5 (46–56)	60 (55–65)
Days with symptoms on ICU arrival		10 (8–12)	10 (9–12)	10 (8–12)
BMI		28.6 (25.6–33.2)	28.8 (26.6–33.8)	27.4 (23.9–30.8)
Pulmonary disease		29 (25%)	21 (24%)	8 (31%)
Hypertension		62 (54%)	41 (46%)	21 (81%)
Diabetes		32 (28%)	24 (46%)	8 (31%)
Smoker	Ongoing	7 (6%)	5 (6%)	2 (9%)

Table 1. Cont.

		All Patients $n = 115$	Alive at 30 Days Yes $n = 89$	Alive at 30 Days No $n = 26$
	Previous	20 (18%)	15 (17%)	5 (23%)
Alive at 30 days		89 (77%)	89 (100%)	0 (0%)
IgG positive		98 (85%)	80 (90%)	18 (69%)
IgA positive		96 (83%)	80 (90%)	16 (62%)
IgM positive		103 (90%)	85 (96%)	18 (69%)

Results are expressed as n (%) or median (interquartile range, IQR). Abbreviations: BMI: Body mass index (kg/m^2), Alive at 30 days: 30 days from ICU admission. Age counted in years. Antibody-positive: Before ICU discharge.

3.2. Survival and Organ Dysfunction

Fifty-nine percent of the included patients were treated with mechanical ventilation and 15% received renal replacement therapy. Patients positive for anti-SARS-CoV2 antibodies had higher 30-day survival (which was the main outcome in the present analysis) compared to patients negative for antibodies (30-day survival for IgM 83% vs. 33%, IgG 82% vs. 53% and IgA 83% vs. 47%). As a complementary analyses, 90-day survival was analysed. This confirmed the findings with higher survival rates in the patient groups positive for anti-SARS-CoV2 antibodies. (Figure 1 and Table 2).

Table 2. Comparison between patients with or without anti-SARS-CoV-2 antibodies.

	All Patients	Iga Positive Yes $n = 96$	Iga Positive No $n = 19$	p	Igm Positive Yes $n = 103$	Igm Positive No $n = 12$	p	Igg Positive Yes $n = 98$	Igg Positive No $n = 17$	p
Alive at 30 days	89 (77%)	80 (83%)	9 (47%)	0.002	85 (83%)	4 (33%)	0.001	80 (82%)	9 (53%)	0.02
Alive at 90 days	84 (73%)	78 (79%)	6 (38%)	0.001	82 (79%)	2 (18%)	<0.001	79 (79%)	5 (33%)	0.01
Male sex	88 (77%)	79 (82%)	9 (47%)	0.002	83 (81%)	5 (42%)	0.007	79 (81%)	9 (53%)	0.03
Thrombotic events	15 (13%)	15 (16%)	0 (0%)	n.s.	15 (15%)	0 (0%)	n.s	15 (15%)	0 (0%)	n.s.
Critical illness	15 (13%)	14 (15%)	1 (5%)	n.s.	13 (13%)	2 (17%)	n.s	14 (14%)	1 (6%)	n.s.
Secondary infection	58 (51%)	51 (54%)	7 (37%)	n.s.	52 (51%)	6 (50%)	n.s	50 (52%)	8 (47%)	n.s.
Vasoactive medication	75 (65%)	65 (68%)	10 (53%)	n.s.	67 (65%)	8 (67%)	n.s	65 (66%)	10 (59%)	n.s.
Invasive ventilation	68 (59%)	62 (65%)	6 (32%)	0.007	61 (59%)	7 (58%)	n.s	60 (61%)	8 (47%)	n.s.
Renal replacement therapy	17 (15%)	16 (17%)	1 (5%)	n.s.	15 (15%)	2 (17%)	n.s	16 (16%)	1 (6%)	n.s.
AKI	68 (62%)	57 (62%)	11 (65%)	n.s.	61 (62%)	7 (64%)	n.s	60 (63%)	8 (62%)	n.s.
Severe AKI	19 (17%)	17 (18%)	2 (12%)	n.s.	18 (18%)	1 (9%)	n.s	19 (20%)	0 (0%)	n.s.
SARS-CoV-2 Plasma	57 (64%)	53 (64%)	4 (67%)	n.s.	52 (63%)	5 (83%)	n.s	50 (62%)	7 (88%)	n.s.
Days with symptoms on ICU arrival	10 (8–12)	10 (8–12)	10 (8–13)	n.s.	10 (9–12)	9 (7–11)	n.s.	10 (9–12)	9 (7–11)	n.s.
BMI	28.6 (25.6–33.2)	29.0 (26.6–33.4)	26.4 (22.9–29.2)	n.s.	28.6 (25.6–32.8)	28.7 (26.4–38.3)	n.s.	28.7 (26.2–33.4)	26.9 (22.9–32.3)	n.s.

Data are expressed as n (%) or median (interquartile range, IQR). Statistically significant differences between groups marked in red. Antibody-positive: Before ICU discharge. Abbreviations: Alive at 30 days: 30 days from ICU admission. AKI: Acute kidney injury. Severe AKI: AKI $\geq$ stage III. SARS-CoV-2 plasma: Patients with SARS-CoV-2 virus detected in plasma. BMI: Body mass index (kg/m^2). n.s.: Not significant. Groups compared with Z-test or Mann-Whiney U test.

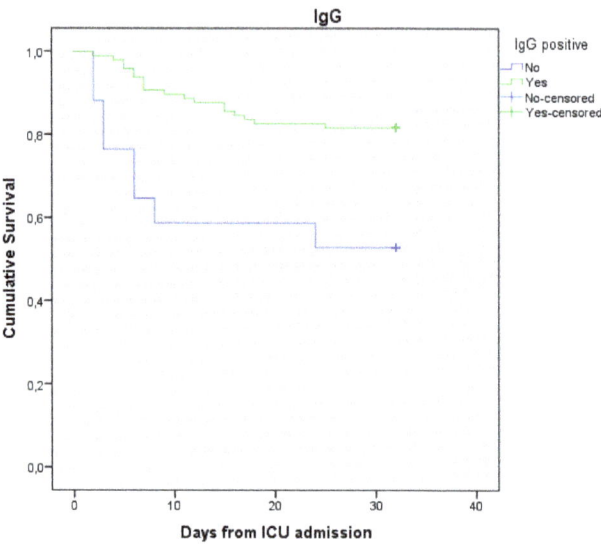

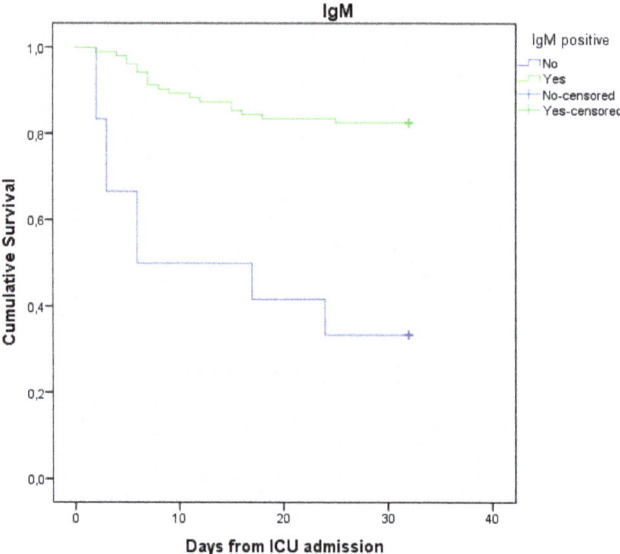

Figure 1. *Cont.*

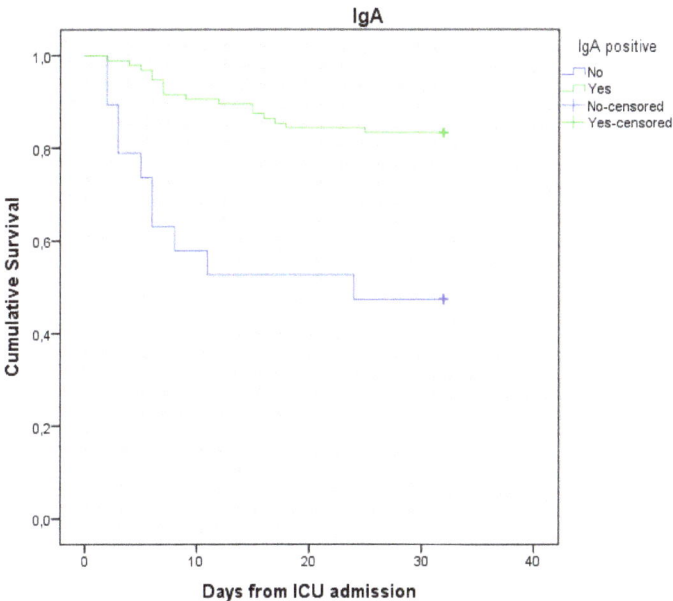

Figure 1. Kaplan–Meier curves describing survival after hospital admission for patients positive vs. negative for SARS-CoV-2 antibodies in plasma.

Patients positive for IgM also had more ICU-free days, ventilator-free days, renal replacement-free days and vasoactive medication-free days. For IgG and IgA, antibody-positive patients had more renal replacement-free days. (Table 3)

Table 3. Organ support in relation to positivity for anti-SARS-CoV-2 antibodies.

	Total	IgM Positive		p
		Yes $n = 103$	No $n = 12$	
ICU-free days	17 (0–24)	18 (0–24)	0 (0–0)	0.002
RRT-free days	30 (15–30)	30 (28–30)	0 (0–15)	<0.001
Ventilator-free days	24 (6–30)	25 (15–30)	0 (0–11)	0.002
Vasoactive-free days	25 (15–30)	26 (19–30)	0 (0–19)	0.002
Lowest p/f-ratio	78.8 (69.8–95.3)	78.8 (69.8–95.3)	76.5 (66.0–105.5)	n.s.
SARS-CoV-2 plasma (copies/mL)	0 (0–800)	0 (0–800)	600 (0–1100)	n.s.
		IgG positive		
	Total	Yes $n = 98$	No $n = 17$	p
ICU-free days	17 (0–24)	18 (0–23)	0 (0–26)	n.s.
RRT-free days	30 (15–30)	30 (28–30)	0 (0–30)	0.012
Ventilator-free days	24 (6–30)	25 (12–30)	11 (0–30)	n.s.
Vasoactive-free days	25 (15–30)	26 (19–30)	19 (0–30)	n.s.
Lowest p/f-ratio	78.8 (69.8–95.3)	78.0 (69.8–94.5)	89.3 (68.3–105.8)	n.s.
SARS-CoV-2 plasma (copies/mL)	0 (0–800)	0 (0–800)	450 (0–2000)	n.s.

Table 3. *Cont.*

		IgM Positive		
	Total	Yes $n = 103$	No $n = 12$	*p*
		IgA positive		
	Total	Yes $n = 96$	No $n = 19$	*p*
ICU-free days	17 (0–24)	18 (0–23)	0 (0–27)	n.s.
RRT-free days	30 (15–30)	30 (26–30)	30 (0–30)	0.039
Ventilator-free days	24 (6–30)	24 (12–30)	21 (0–30)	n.s.
Vasoactive-free days	25 (15–30)	26 (19–30)	22 (0–30)	n.s.
Lowest p/f-ratio	78.8 (69.8–95.3)	78.0 (69.0)–93.0)	89.3 (70.5–113.3)	n.s.
SARS-CoV-2 plasma (copies/mL)	0 (0–800)	0 (0–800)	150 (0–2600)	n.s.

Data are expressed as median (interquartile range, IQR). Statistically significant differences between groups marked in red. Antibody-positive: Before ICU discharge. Abbreviations: RRT: Renal replacement therapy. Vasoactive-free days: Days without vasoactive treatment. p/f-ratio: mmHg/FiO$_2$ SARS-CoV-2 plasma: Viral copies in plasma.

In a simple logistic regression model, odds ratios (confidence interval, CI) for 30-day survival were 9.4 (2.6–34.8), 4.0 (1.3–11.6) and 5.6 (1.9–15.9) for patients positive for IgM, IgG and IgA, respectively. When adjusting for age in a multiple logistic regression model, positive tests for IgM and IgG antibodies were still correlated with higher OR for 30-day survival, whereas no difference between the groups were seen for IgA. (Figure 2)

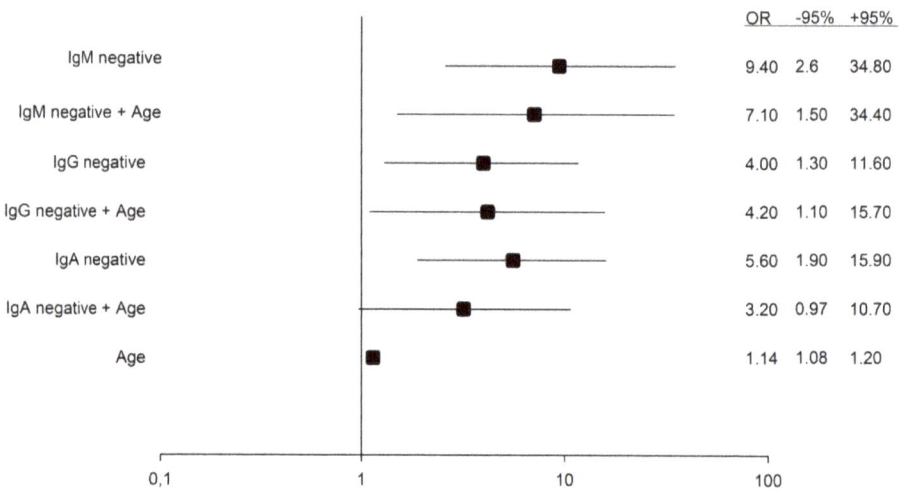

Figure 2. Odds ratios for death in single and multiple logistic regression models with antibody negativity and patient age as independent variables. Increasing age (counted in years) is associated with higher mortality rates.

In the correlation analyses, IgA antibody concentrations correlated negatively with both SAPS3 (r = −0.233, *p* = 0.013) and maximal SOFA score (r = −0.231, *p* = 0.014). No correlation was seen between IgG and SAPS3 or SOFA whereas the levels of IgM antibodies correlated negatively with SAPS3 (r = −0.231, *p* = 0.014).

3.3. Plasma Biomarkers in Relation to Antibody Response

Next, we analysed plasma biomarkers and their relation to antibody response. Clinical chemistry tests and blood cell counts analysed during ICU care were extracted from the patients' medical records, and ICU entry and peak values were calculated.

To corroborate the association between antibody response and organ support, biomarkers of organ failure were compared among antibody-negative and -positive patients. Significant associations were observed for kidney (Creatinine, Cystatin C) and cardiac biomarkers (NT-proBNP). A prominent activation of the coagulation system with elevated D-dimer and platelet counts is an important feature of severe COVID-19 [34]. However, antibody-negative subjects had significantly lower platelet counts, and a non-significant trend towards lower D-dimer levels was observed. Furthermore, antibody-negative patients had lower CRP levels, indicating an attenuation of systemic inflammation in patients with an impaired antibody response.

To further characterise the immune response in relation to antibody positivity, biomarkers of the innate immune system, including cytokines, systemic histone release and complement activation, and white blood cell differential counts were analysed.

Antibody-negative patients had significantly higher plasma levels of extracellular histones on day 1 compared to antibody-positive patients, and elevated extracellular histone levels were observed irrespective of the antibody class (Figure 3). We could not find strong associations between antibody levels in plasma and any of the analysed cytokines (Supplementary Material).

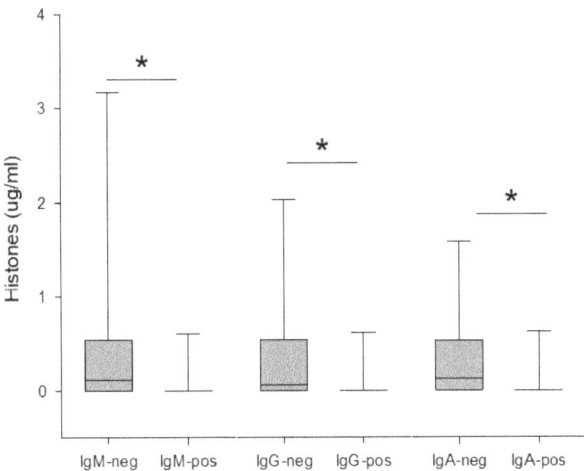

Figure 3. Concentration of Histones H3 in plasma in relation to positivity/negativity for SARS-CoV-2 antibodies in plasma. Antibody-positive: Before ICU discharge. Statistically significant differences between groups are marked by *.

Complement factors and activation markers were analysed in plasma samples taken upon ICU admission (Supplementary Material). There was no difference in the degree of complement activation between antibody-positive and -negative patients, as measured by C3a, C3d and sC5b9 levels in plasma. In contrast, IgG and IgA antibody-negative patients had significantly lower circulating levels of intact complement factor C3 and factor B.

4. Discussion

The main finding of this study is that a poor antibody response is associated with increased mortality in patients with severe SARS-CoV-2-infection. Furthermore, patients with poor antibody response have higher rates of organ failure based on SAPS3 and SOFA score, even if the correlations are weak and should be interpreted with caution, and also based on the duration of organ support such as renal replacement therapy and vasoactive medication.

These clinical associations were corroborated by biomarker analyses, where the strongest associations were seen for kidney function and cardiac biomarkers. In particular, antibody-negative patients had strongly elevated NT-proBNP levels during ICU care, which could indicate an increased rate of circulatory failure in agreement with a trend towards longer duration of vasoactive support in these patients.

The strongest signal in our cohort for the associations with outcome is seen for IgM antibodies and it is reasonable to believe that this is due to the natural course of the B-cell development in the germinal centre (GC) reaction. Additionally, IgM, in its pentameric form, has the highest complement-activating capacity among all immunoglobulin subclasses, thus it has a very high neutralising capacity [35].

There was no significant difference in the concentration of viral copies in blood between the analysed groups, although patients negative for antibodies in this study did have numerically higher levels of viral copies in blood. The non-significance might reflect a lack of power in the study, and it would be interesting to analyse this in a larger group of ICU patients. However, we have previously described a lack of strong association between viremia and organ failure in COVID-19 [30,36].

As the production of antibodies is a result of a close and simultaneous collaboration between the innate and adaptive immune systems, alterations in the innate immune system due to age, gender and/or genetic variations will skew the adaptive responses in different directions [37]. It has been previously described that COVID-19 patients who develop a mild disease responds with a fast antibody response of short duration. Patients with severe disease instead have a slower antibody response with a longer duration [9]. Measurable antigen-specific antibodies in plasma from patients are a result of a successful GC-reaction. When it comes to viral infections, the GC-reaction is dependent on antigen-specific T-cells [38]. T-cell studies on patients with mild versus severe COVID-19 have in both cases shown a robust specific T-cell response (both CD4+ and CD8+ T-cells) but the T-cell phenotypes (e.g., cytokine production and dominant T-cell subset) differ between the two disease severity groups [39,40]. It is thus plausible that differences in T-cell responses would mirror any difference in priming of the GC-reaction and hence the antibody response. From the results in our study, it seems that among patients developing severe the disease who require intensive care, patients with a higher antibody response have a better chance of survival, suggesting that an adequate response from both T- and B-cells is of great importance in the defence against SARS-CoV-2 infections. The individual differences in the total immune response to the virus causing COVID-19 might be due to several, not mutually exclusive, mechanisms, e.g., it is described that the SARS-CoV-2 virus can inhibit the initial innate immune response through suppression of type I IFN [41]. This can lead to a slower activation of the adaptive immune system. In patients with an inherent poor type I IFN-response this effect can give rise to a greater initial viral replication causing more severe disease [42]. Thus, the slow activation of the adaptive immune system may reflect an initial suboptimal innate immune response.

This hypothesis is supported by our biomarker analysis, which by several measures indicated a lower degree of inflammation in antibody-negative subjects, possibly due to an unknown inborn or acquired immune defect.

Our complement analyses revealed no differences in complement activation between antibody-negative and -positive subjects, but they demonstrated significantly lower circulating levels of intact complement protein C3 and Factor B in antibody-negative patients. These factors are well-known to display an acute phase response pattern and are elevated during systemic inflammation, hence lower plasma levels are agreement with an attenuated inflammatory response in antibody-negative subjects. Furthermore, a recent study on bronkoalveolar lavage in patients with severe COVID-19 describes a more aggravated local immune response in the lung, suggesting plasma analyses might be misleading in compement analyses [43].

Another hypothesis is that patients with a suboptimal adaptive immune response, instead, develop a more powerful non-specific innate immune response, partly supported by previous research [44], with increased neutrophil activation and a powerful activation of the complement system [45]. We could not find any sign of increased complement activation or cytokine release in patients with poor antibody response, but those patients had more circulating cell-free histones. SARS-CoV-2 is able to induce neutrophil extracellular trap (NET) formation in healthy neutrophils, suggesting a role for NETs in driving cytokine release, respiratory failure, and microvascular injury in COVID-19 [19,20]. In this study, patients that did not express anti-SARS-CoV-2 antibodies in the ICU had increased extracellular histones in their blood at ICU admission, which may signal systemic neutrophil activation and NET formation [21]. Although we only measured histone H3, this could be seen as a proxy for all other histones. However, it is possible that the increased levels of histones are a marker of unspecific cell damage and are not linked to NET formation. Previous research shows that the number of neutrophils and markers of NETosis are elevated in severe COVID-19 patients [22], and a link has been suggested between NETosis and poor outcome [23], indicating a crucial contribution of NETs to the severity of the COVID-19 disease [24,25]. An association has also been described between anti-SARS-CoV-2 IgA2, NET formation and poor outcome [46]. As lymphopenia and inadequate T-cell responses are found to be predictors of COVID-19 severity, [47] our findings of an association between poor antibody response and amount of histones in blood in ICU patients suggests a link between poor adaptive immune activation and NET formation. Furthermore, patients with impaired antibody responses and increased number of free histones also have lower thrombocyte values. This could be an indirect sign of platelet consumption in NET-containing microthrombi as neutrophil-platelet infiltration has been observed in pulmonary autopsies from COVID-19 patients [48].

Our findings that a poor antibody response is associated with a poor outcome in ICU patients with COVID-19 could have clinical implications. If we could identify patients that are likely to have a slow antibody response early in the disease process, these might be the patients benefiting the most from immune-modulating treatment, as studies, in which patients treated as early as 72 h after COVID-19 diagnosis with convalescent plasma or monoclonal anti-SARS-CoV-2 antibodies, have shown [49,50]. In addition, specific organ failure, such as AKI, is common in severe COVID-19 and may cause long-term effects in surviving patients [51,52]. Together with common clinical variables, these data may prove useful in improving recognition of patients at risk of extra pulmonary organ failure.

The strength of this study is the large number of intensive care patients included and the high quality of clinical data prospectively collected in combination with analyses of both antibodies, cytokines, and components of the complement system. The major weakness is that samples for antibody analyses were not taken on the same day as for the other analyses; instead, we chose to analyse the last available blood sample taken in the ICU. The reason for this was to maximise the chance to have samples taken after the patients had developed an antibody response and hopefully also switched antibody class. This might have impacted the results, but there was no difference between the compared groups in median time from admission to sample day.

5. Conclusions

This study confirms that a weak anti-SARS-CoV-2 antibody response in intensive care patients with COVID-19 is associated with increased 30-day mortality and our results suggest that this may be due to multiple organ dysfunction and NETosis.

Supplementary Materials: The following supporting information can be downloaded at: https://www.mdpi.com/article/10.3390/jcm11123419/s1, Methods describing analyses of cytokines end complement factors. Tables over complement factors and complement activation factors, clinical chemistry tests including inflammation and organ damage markers. Figure describing correlation of cytokine concentration and antibody concentration. Reference [53] is cited in the supplementary materials.

Author Contributions: R.L, B.K., K.A., A.F., M.H., M.L., G.A.F.N. and R.F. conceived the study. B.K., A.L., O.E., B.P., J.B.H., A.B. and S.F. analysed the blood samples. R.L., M.H., O.E. and R.F. performed data analysis. R.L. drafted the manuscript. All authors commented on previous versions of the manuscript. All authors have read and agreed to the published version of the manuscript.

Funding: SciLifeLab/KAW national COVID-19 research program project grant (KAW 2020.0182 and KAW 2020.0241) and from the Swedish Heart-Lung Foundation (20210089) to MH. The Swedish Research Council (2014-02569 and 2014-07606) and The Swedish Kidney Foundation (F2020-0054) to RF. The study was supported by the Netherlands Thrombosis Foundation (2016_01) and Thrombosestichting (2016-1) to GN. OE was supported by grants from the Göran Gustafsson Foundation, the Swedish Society of Medicine (SLS-943007) and the Swedish Research Council (2015-06429).

Informed Consent Statement: Informed consent was obtained either by the patient or by a next-of-kin if the patient was unable to receive information due to their clinical status.

Data Availability Statement: Individual level data is available from the authors on reasonable request as detailed at https://doi.org/10.17044/scilifelab.14229410.v1.

Acknowledgments: We thank the study nurses Joanna Wessbergh and Elin Söderman for their expertise in compiling the study. We are also indebted to the biobank research assistants Erik Danielsson, Labolina Spång, Amanda Svensson and Philip Karlsson for organising the sample analysis and the Uppsala Intensive Care COVID-19 research group: Sara Bülow Anderberg, Tomas Luther, Katja Hanslin, Anna Gradin, Sarah Galien and Jacob Rosén for patient inclusion.

Conflicts of Interest: The authors declare no conflict of interest.

References

1. Niemi, M.E.; Karjalainen, J.; Liao, R.G.; Neale, B.M.; Daly, M.; Ganna, A.; Pathak, G.A.; Andrews, S.J.; Kanai, M.; Veerapen, K.; et al. Mapping the human genetic architecture of COVID-19. *Nature* **2021**, *600*, 472–477.
2. Grasselli, G.; Zangrillo, A.; Zanella, A.; Antonelli, M.; Cabrini, L.; Castelli, A.; Cereda, D.; Coluccello, A.; Foti, G.; Fumagalli, R.; et al. Baseline Characteristics and Outcomes of 1591 Patients Infected With SARS-CoV-2 Admitted to ICUs of the Lombardy Region, Italy. *JAMA* **2020**, *323*, 1574–1581. [CrossRef] [PubMed]
3. Ahlström, B.; Frithiof, R.; Hultström, M.; Larsson, I.M.; Strandberg, G.; Lipcsey, M. The swedish COVID-19 intensive care cohort: Risk factors of ICU admission and ICU mortality. *Acta Anaesthesiol. Scand.* **2021**, *65*, 525–533. [CrossRef] [PubMed]
4. Nakanishi, T.; Pigazzini, S.; Degenhardt, F.; Cordioli, M.; Butler-Laporte, G.; Maya-Miles, D.; Bujanda, L.; Bouysran, Y.; Niemi, M.E.; Palom, A.; et al. Age-dependent impact of the major common genetic risk factor for COVID-19 on severity and mortality. medRxiv: The preprint server for health sciences. *J. Clin. Investig.* **2021**, *131*. [CrossRef]
5. Anderberg, S.B.; Luther, T.; Berglund, M.; Larsson, R.; Rubertsson, S.; Lipcsey, M.; Larsson, A.; Frithiof, R.; Hultström, M. Increased levels of plasma cytokines and correlations to organ failure and 30-day mortality in critically ill COVID-19 patients. *Cytokine* **2021**, *138*, 155389. [CrossRef] [PubMed]
6. Eriksson, O.; Hultström, M.; Persson, B.; Lipcsey, M.; Ekdahl, K.N.; Nilsson, B.; Frithiof, R. Mannose-Binding Lectin is Associated with Thrombosis and Coagulopathy in Critically Ill COVID-19 Patients. *Thrombosis and haemostasis* **2020**, *120*, 1720–1724. [PubMed]
7. Brodin, P. Immune determinants of COVID-19 disease presentation and severity. *Nat. Med.* **2021**, *27*, 28–33. [CrossRef]
8. Gradin, A.; Andersson, H.; Luther, T.; Anderberg, S.B.; Rubertsson, S.; Lipcsey, M.; Åberg, M.; Larsson, A.; Frithiof, R.; Hultström, M. Urinary cytokines correlate with acute kidney injury in critically ill COVID-19 patients. *Cytokine* **2021**, *146*, 155589. [CrossRef]
9. Carsetti, R.; Zaffina, S.; Piano Mortari, E.; Terreri, S.; Corrente, F.; Capponi, C.; Palomba, P.; Mirabella, M.; Cascioli, S.; Palange, P.; et al. Different innate and adaptive immune response to SARS-CoV-2 infection of asymptomatic, mild and severe cases. *Front. Immunol.* **2020**, *11*, 610300. [CrossRef]
10. Kuri-Cervantes, L.; Pampena, M.B.; Meng, W.; Rosenfeld, A.M.; Ittner, C.A.G.; Weisman, A.R.; Agyekum, R.S.; Mathew, D.; Baxter, A.E.; Vella, L.A.; et al. Comprehensive mapping of immune perturbations associated with severe COVID-19. *Sci. Immunol.* **2020**, *5*, eabd7114. [CrossRef]
11. Kowitdamrong, E.; Puthanakit, T.; Jantarabenjakul, W.; Prompetchara, E.; Suchartlikitwong, P.; Putcharoen, O.; Hirankarn, N. Antibody responses to SARS-CoV-2 in patients with differing severities of coronavirus disease 2019. *PLoS ONE* **2020**, *15*, e0240502. [CrossRef] [PubMed]
12. Schlesinger, T.; Weißbrich, B.; Wedekink, F.; Notz, Q.; Herrmann, J.; Krone, M.; Sitter, M.; Schmid, B.; Kredel, M.; Stumpner, J.; et al. Biodistribution and serologic response in SARS-CoV-2 induced ARDS: A cohort study. *PLoS ONE* **2020**, *15*, e0242917. [CrossRef] [PubMed]
13. Li, K.; Huang, B.; Wu, M.; Zhong, A.; Li, L.; Cai, Y.; Wang, Z.; Wu, L.; Zhu, M.; Li, J.; et al. Dynamic changes in anti-SARS-CoV-2 antibodies during SARS-CoV-2 infection and recovery from COVID-19. *Nat. Commun.* **2020**, *11*, 6044. [CrossRef]

14. Cunningham, J.L.; Virhammar, J.; Rönnberg, B.; Castro Dopico, X.; Kolstad, L.; Albinsson, B.; Kumlien, E.; Nääs, A.; Klang, A.; Westman, G.; et al. Anti-SARS-CoV2 antibody responses in serum and cerebrospinal fluid of COVID-19 patients with neurological symptoms. *J. Infect. Dis.* **2022**, *225*, 965–970. [CrossRef] [PubMed]
15. Wang, Y.; Zhang, L.; Sang, L.; Ye, F.; Ruan, S.; Zhong, B.; Song, T.; Alshukairi, A.N.; Chen, R.; Zhang, Z.; et al. Kinetics of viral load and antibody response in relation to COVID-19 severity. *J. Clin. Investig.* **2020**, *130*, 5235–5244. [CrossRef] [PubMed]
16. Dispinseri, S.; Secchi, M.; Pirillo, M.F.; Tolazzi, M.; Borghi, M.; Brigatti, C.; De Angelis, M.L.; Baratella, M.; Bazzigaluppi, E.; Venturi, G.; et al. Neutralizing antibody responses to SARS-CoV-2 in symptomatic COVID-19 is persistent and critical for survival. *Nat. Commun.* **2021**, *12*, 2670. [CrossRef]
17. Zhou, S.; Butler-Laporte, G.; Nakanishi, T.; Morrison, D.R.; Afilalo, J.; Afilalo, M.; Laurent, L.; Pietzner, M.; Kerrison, N.; Zhao, K.; et al. A Neanderthal OAS1 isoform protects individuals of European ancestry against COVID-19 susceptibility and severity. *Nat. Med.* **2021**, *27*, 659–667. [CrossRef]
18. Sette, A.; Crotty, S. Adaptive immunity to SARS-CoV-2 and COVID-19. *Cell* **2021**, *184*, 861–880. [CrossRef]
19. Schönrich, G.; Raftery, M.J.; Samstag, Y. Devilishly radical NETwork in COVID-19: Oxidative stress, neutrophil extracellular traps (NETs), and T cell suppression. *Adv. Biol. Regul.* **2020**, *77*, 100741. [CrossRef]
20. Veras, F.P.; Pontelli, M.C.; Silva, C.M.; Toller-Kawahisa, J.E.; de Lima, M.; Nascimento, D.C.; Schneider, A.H.; Caetité, D.; Tavares, L.A.; Paiva, I.M.; et al. SARS-CoV-2–triggered neutrophil extracellular traps mediate COVID-19 pathologySARS-CoV-2 directly triggers ACE-dependent NETs. *J. Exp. Med.* **2020**, *217*, e20201129. [CrossRef]
21. Brinkmann, V.; Reichard, U.; Goosmann, C.; Fauler, B.; Uhlemann, Y.; Weiss, D.S.; Weinrauch, Y.; Zychlinsky, A. Neutrophil extracellular traps kill bacteria. *Science* **2004**, *303*, 1532–1535. [CrossRef] [PubMed]
22. Bülow Anderberg, S.; Lipcsey, M.; Hultström, M.; Eriksson, A.K.; Venge, P.; Frithiof, R. Systemic Human Neutrophil Lipocalin Associates with Severe Acute Kidney Injury in SARS-CoV-2 Pneumonia. *J. Clin. Med.* **2021**, *10*, 4144. [CrossRef] [PubMed]
23. Cani, E.; Dwivedi, D.J.; Liaw, K.-L.; Fraser, D.D.; Yeh, C.H.; Martin, C.; Slessarev, M.; Cerroni, S.E.; Fox-Robichaud, A.A.; Weitz, J.I.; et al. Immunothrombosis Biomarkers for Distinguishing Coronavirus Disease 2019 Patients From Noncoronavirus Disease Septic Patients with Pneumonia and for Predicting ICU Mortality. *Crit. Care Explor.* **2021**, *3*, e0588. [CrossRef] [PubMed]
24. Wang, D.; Hu, B.; Hu, C.; Zhu, F.; Liu, X.; Zhang, J.; Wang, B.; Xiang, H.; Cheng, Z.; Xiong, Y.; et al. Clinical Characteristics of 138 Hospitalized Patients With 2019 Novel Coronavirus—Infected Pneumonia in Wuhan, China. *JAMA* **2020**, *323*, 1061–1069. [CrossRef] [PubMed]
25. Zuo, Y.; Yalavarthi, S.; Shi, H.; Gockman, K.; Zuo, M.; Madison, J.A.; Blair, C.; Weber, A.; Barnes, B.J.; Egeblad, M.; et al. Neutrophil extracellular traps in COVID-19. *JCI Insight.* **2020**, *5*, e138999. [CrossRef] [PubMed]
26. Asif, S.; Frithiof, R.; Lipcsey, M.; Kristensen, B.; Alving, K.; Hultström, M. Weak anti-SARS-CoV-2 antibody response is associated with mortality in a Swedish cohort of COVID-19 patients in critical care. *Crit. Care* **2020**, *24*, 639. [CrossRef]
27. Moreno, R.P.; Metnitz, P.G.H.; Almeida, E.; Jordan, B.; Bauer, P.; Campos, R.A.; Iapichino, G.; Edbrooke, D.; Capuzzo, M.; Le Gall, J.-R. SAPS 3—From evaluation of the patient to evaluation of the intensive care unit. Part 2: Development of a prognostic model for hospital mortality at ICU admission. *Intensiv. Care Med.* **2005**, *31*, 1345–1355. [CrossRef]
28. Vincent, J.L.; Moreno, R.; Takala, J.; Willatts, S.; De Mendonça, A.; Bruining, H.; Reinhart, C.K.; Suter, P.; Thijs, L.G. The SOFA (Sepsis-related Organ Failure Assessment) score to describe organ dysfunction/failure. On behalf of the Working Group on Sepsis-Related Problems of the European Society of Intensive Care Medicine. *Intensive Care Med.* **1996**, *22*, 707–710. [CrossRef]
29. Kellum, J.A.; Lameire, N.; Aspelin, P.; Barsoum, R.S.; Burdmann, E.A.; Goldstein, S.L. Section 2: AKI Definition. *Kidney Int. Suppl.* **2012**, *2*, 19–36.
30. Järhult, J.D.; Hultström, M.; Bergqvist, A.; Frithiof, R.; Lipcsey, M. The impact of viremia on organ failure, biomarkers and mortality in a Swedish cohort of critically ill COVID-19 patients. *Sci. Rep.* **2021**, *11*, 7163. [CrossRef]
31. CDC. Research Use Only 2019-Novel Coronavirus (2019-nCoV) Real-Time RT-PCR Primers and Probes. 2020. Available online: https://www.cdc.gov/coronavirus/2019-ncov/lab/rt-pcr-panel-primer-probes.html (accessed on 1 March 2020).
32. Wildhagen, K.C.; Wiewel, M.A.; Schultz, M.J.; Horn, J.; Schrijver, R.; Reutelingsperger, C.P.; van der Poll, T.; Nicolaes, G.A. Extracellular histone H3 levels are inversely correlated with antithrombin levels and platelet counts and are associated with mortality in sepsis patients. *Thromb. Res.* **2015**, *136*, 542–547. [CrossRef] [PubMed]
33. Huckriede, J.; Vries, F.D.; Hultström, M.; Wichapong, K.; Reutelingsperger, C.; Lipcsey, M.; Garcia de Frutos, P.; Frithiof, R.; Nicolaes, G.A. Histone H3 Cleavage in Severe COVID-19 ICU Patients. *Front. Cell. Infect. Microbiol.* **2021**, *11*, 694186. [CrossRef] [PubMed]
34. Pawlowski, C.; Wagner, T.; Puranik, A.; Murugadoss, K.; Loscalzo, L.; Venkatakrishnan, A.; Pruthi, R.K.; Houghton, D.; O'Horo, J.C.; Morice, W.G.; et al. Inference from longitudinal laboratory tests characterizes temporal evolution of COVID-19-associated coagulopathy (CAC). *eLife* **2020**, *9*, e59209. [CrossRef] [PubMed]
35. Czajkowsky, D.M.; Shao, Z. The human IgM pentamer is a mushroom-shaped molecule with a flexural bias. *Proc. Natl. Acad. Sci. USA* **2009**, *106*, 14960–14965. [CrossRef]
36. Frithiof, R.; Bergqvist, A.; Järhult, J.D.; Lipcsey, M.; Hultström, M. Presence of SARS-CoV-2 in urine is rare and not associated with acute kidney injury in critically ill COVID-19 patients. *Crit. Care* **2020**, *24*, 587. [CrossRef]
37. Gubbels Bupp, M.R.; Potluri, T.; Fink, A.L.; Klein, S.L. The Confluence of Sex Hormones and Aging on Immunity. *Front. Immunol.* **2018**, *9*, 1269. [CrossRef]
38. Victora, G.D. SnapShot: The germinal center reaction. *Cell* **2014**, *159*, 700–700.e1. [CrossRef]

39. Peng, Y.; Mentzer, A.J.; Liu, G.; Yao, X.; Yin, Z.; Dong, D.; Dejnirattisai, W.; Rostron, T.; Supasa, P.; Liu, C.; et al. Broad and strong memory CD4(+) and CD8(+) T cells induced by SARS-CoV-2 in UK convalescent individuals following COVID-19. *Nat. Immunol.* **2020**, *21*, 1336–1345. [CrossRef]
40. Sekine, T.; Perez-Potti, A.; Rivera-Ballesteros, O.; Strålin, K.; Gorin, J.-B.; Olsson, A.; Llewellyn-Lacey, S.; Kamal, H.; Bogdanovic, G.; Muschiol, S.; et al. Robust T cell immunity in convalescent individuals with asymptomatic or mild COVID-19. *Cell* **2020**, *183*, 158–168.e14. [CrossRef]
41. Arunachalam, P.S.; Wimmers, F.; Mok, C.K.P.; Perera, R.A.P.M.; Scott, M.; Hagan, T.; Sigal, N.; Feng, Y.; Bristow, L.; Tsang, O.T.-Y.; et al. Systems biological assessment of immunity to mild versus severe COVID-19 infection in humans. *Science* **2020**, *369*, 1210–1220. [CrossRef]
42. Bermejo-Martin, J.F.; González-Rivera, M.; Almansa, R.; Micheloud, D.; Tedim, A.P.; Domínguez-Gil, M.; Resino, S.; Martín-Fernández, M.; Murua, P.R.; Pérez-García, F.; et al. Viral RNA load in plasma is associated with critical illness and a dysregulated host response in COVID-19. *Crit. Care* **2020**, *24*, 691. [CrossRef] [PubMed]
43. Nossent, E.J.; Schuurman, A.R.; Reijnders, T.D.; Saris, A.; Jongerius, I.; Blok, S.G.; de Vries, H.; Duitman, J.; Noordegraaf, A.V.; Meijboom, L.J.; et al. Pulmonary Procoagulant and Innate Immune Responses in Critically Ill COVID-19 Patients. *Front. Immunol.* **2021**, *12*, 664209. [CrossRef] [PubMed]
44. Janssen, N.A.F.; Grondman, I.; de Nooijer, A.H.; Boahen, C.K.; Koeken, V.A.C.M.; Matzaraki, V.; Kumar, V.; He, X.; Kox, M.; Koenen, H.J.P.M.; et al. Dysregulated Innate and Adaptive Immune Responses Discriminate Disease Severity in COVID-19. *J. Infect. Dis.* **2021**, *223*, 1322–1333. [CrossRef] [PubMed]
45. Karawajczyk, M.; Douhan Håkansson, L.; Lipcsey, M.; Hultström, M.; Pauksens, K.; Frithiof, R.; Larsson, A. High expression of neutrophil and monocyte CD64 with simultaneous lack of upregulation of adhesion receptors CD11b, CD162, CD15, CD65 on neutrophils in severe COVID-19. *Ther. Adv. Infect. Dis.* **2021**, *8*, 20499361211034065. [CrossRef]
46. Staats, L.A.; Pfeiffer, H.; Knopf, J.; Lindemann, A.; Fürst, J.; Kremer, A.E.; Hackstein, H.; Neurath, M.F.; Muñoz, L.E.; Achenbach, S.; et al. IgA2 Antibodies against SARS-CoV-2 Correlate with NET Formation and Fatal Outcome in Severely Diseased COVID-19 Patients. *Cells* **2020**, *9*, 2676. [CrossRef]
47. Wang, F.; Nie, J.; Wang, H.; Zhao, Q.; Xiong, Y.; Deng, L.; Song, S.; Ma, Z.; Mo, P.; Zhang, Y. Characteristics of Peripheral Lymphocyte Subset Alteration in COVID-19 Pneumonia. *J. Infect. Dis.* **2020**, *221*, 1762–1769. [CrossRef]
48. Middleton, E.A.; He, X.-Y.; Denorme, F.; Campbell, R.A.; Ng, D.; Salvatore, S.P.; Mostyka, M.; Baxter-Stoltzfus, A.; Borczuk, A.C.; Loda, M.; et al. Neutrophil extracellular traps contribute to immunothrombosis in COVID-19 acute respiratory distress syndrome. *Blood* **2020**, *136*, 1169–1179. [CrossRef]
49. Libster, R.; Marc, G.P.; Wappner, D.; Coviello, S.; Bianchi, A.; Braem, V.; Esteban, I.; Caballero, M.T.; Wood, C.; Berrueta, M.; et al. Early High-Titer Plasma Therapy to Prevent Severe COVID-19 in Older Adults. *New Engl. J. Med.* **2021**, *384*, 610–618. [CrossRef]
50. Gottlieb, R.L.; Nirula, A.; Chen, P.; Boscia, J.; Heller, B.; Morris, J.; Huhn, G.; Cardona, J.; Mocherla, B.; Stosor, V.; et al. Effect of Bamlanivimab as Monotherapy or in Combination With Etesevimab on Viral Load in Patients With Mild to Moderate COVID-19: A Randomized Clinical Trial. *JAMA* **2021**, *325*, 632–644. [CrossRef]
51. Luther, T.; Bülow-Anderberg, S.; Larsson, A.; Rubertsson, S.; Lipcsey, M.; Frithiof, R.; Hultström, M. COVID-19 patients in intensive care develop predominantly oliguric acute kidney injury. *Acta Anaesthesiol. Scand.* **2020**, *65*, 364–372. [CrossRef]
52. Hultström, M.; Lipcsey, M.; Wallin, E.; Larsson, I.-M.; Larsson, A.; Frithiof, R. Severe acute kidney injury associated with progression of chronic kidney disease after critical COVID-19. *Crit. Care* **2021**, *25*, 37. [CrossRef] [PubMed]
53. Lipcsey, M.; Persson, B.; Eriksson, O.; Blom, A.M.; Fromell, K.; Hultström, M.; Huber-Lang, M.; Ekdahl, K.N.; Frithiof, R.; Nilsson, B. The Outcome of Critically Ill COVID-19 Patients Is Linked to Thromboinflammation Dominated by the Kallikrein/Kinin System. *Front. Immunol.* **2021**, *12*, 627579. [CrossRef] [PubMed]

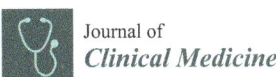

Article

Impact of Renal Replacement Therapy on Mortality and Renal Outcomes in Critically Ill Patients with Acute Kidney Injury: A Population-Based Cohort Study in Korea between 2008 and 2015

Subin Hwang [1,†], Danbee Kang [2,3,†], Hyejeong Park [2,3], Youngha Kim [2,3], Eliseo Guallar [2,4], Junseok Jeon [5], Jung-Eun Lee [5], Wooseong Huh [5], Gee-Young Suh [6], Juhee Cho [2,3,*] and Hye-Ryoun Jang [5,*]

1. Department of Internal Medicine, Seoul Paik Hospital, Inje University School of Medicine, Seoul 04551, Korea; subin.151719@gmail.com
2. Center for Clinical Epidemiology, Samsung Medical Center, Sungkyunkwan University School of Medicine, Seoul 06531, Korea; dbee.kang@skku.edu (D.K.); hj.park219@sbri.co.kr (H.P.); youngha1223@gmail.com (Y.K.); eguallar@jhu.edu (E.G.)
3. Department of Clinical Research Design and Evaluation, Samsung Advanced Institute for Health Science and Technology, Sungkyunkwan University School of Medicine, Seoul 06531, Korea
4. Department of Epidemiology and Medicine and Welch Center for Prevention, Epidemiology and Clinical Research, Johns Hopkins Medical Institutions, Baltimore, MD 21287, USA
5. Division of Nephrology, Department of Medicine, Samsung Medical Center, Sungkyunkwan University School of Medicine, Seoul 06531, Korea; uncleimdr@gmail.com (J.J.); jungeun34.lee@samsung.com (J.-E.L.); wooseong.huh@samsung.com (W.H.)
6. Department of Critical Care Medicine, Samsung Medical Center, Sungkyunkwan University School of Medicine, Seoul 06351, Korea; smccritcare@gmail.com
* Correspondence: jcho@skku.edu (J.C.); shinehr@skku.edu (H.-R.J.); Tel.: +82-2-3410-1448 (J.C.); +82-2-3410-0782 (H.-R.J.)
† These authors contributed equally to this work.

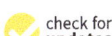

Citation: Hwang, S.; Kang, D.; Park, H.; Kim, Y.; Guallar, E.; Jeon, J.; Lee, J.-E.; Huh, W.; Suh, G.-Y.; Cho, J.; et al. Impact of Renal Replacement Therapy on Mortality and Renal Outcomes in Critically Ill Patients with Acute Kidney Injury: A Population-Based Cohort Study in Korea between 2008 and 2015. *J. Clin. Med.* **2022**, *11*, 2392. https://doi.org/10.3390/jcm11092392

Academic Editors: Spyros D. Mentzelopoulos and Jesús Villar

Received: 29 March 2022
Accepted: 19 April 2022
Published: 24 April 2022

Publisher's Note: MDPI stays neutral with regard to jurisdictional claims in published maps and institutional affiliations.

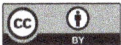

Copyright: © 2022 by the authors. Licensee MDPI, Basel, Switzerland. This article is an open access article distributed under the terms and conditions of the Creative Commons Attribution (CC BY) license (https://creativecommons.org/licenses/by/4.0/).

Abstract: The outcomes depending on the type of renal replacement therapy (RRT) or pre-existing kidney disease in critically ill patients with acute kidney injury (AKI) have not been fully elucidated. All adult intensive care unit patients with AKI in Korea from 2008 to 2015 were screened. A total of 124,182 patients, including 21,165 patients with pre-existing kidney disease, were divided into three groups: control (no RRT), dialysis, and continuous RRT (CRRT). In-hospital mortality and progression to end-stage kidney disease (ESKD) were analyzed according to the presence of pre-existing kidney disease. The CRRT group had a higher risk of in-hospital mortality. Among the patients with pre-existing kidney disease, the dialysis group had a lower risk of in-hospital mortality compared to other groups. The risk of ESKD was higher in the dialysis and CRRT groups compared to the control group. In the CRRT group, the risk of ESKD was even higher in patients without pre-existing kidney disease. Although both dialysis and CRRT groups showed a higher incidence of ESKD, in-hospital mortality was lower in the dialysis group, especially in patients with pre-existing kidney disease. Our study supports that RRT and pre-existing kidney disease may be important prognostic factors for overall and renal outcomes in patients with AKI.

Keywords: acute kidney injury; chronic kidney disease; continuous renal replacement therapy; end-stage of kidney disease; intermittent hemodialysis; mortality; renal replacement therapy

1. Introduction

Acute kidney injury (AKI) is a common complication of critically ill patients suffering from various diseases such as heart failure or septic shock and is associated with high mortality and progression to chronic kidney disease (CKD) [1,2]. Renal replacement therapy (RRT) is frequently required in patients with severe AKI [3]. Given the evident advances in critical care medicine, the application of RRT has significantly increased [4]. Although a number of studies have reported renal prognosis and mortality according to the modality of RRT, current clinical data do not support the superiority of specific RRT modalities [5]. The RRT modality is usually determined according to patients' conditions and institutional availability of dialysis or continuous RRT (CRRT) equipment.

Moreover, although AKI is usually regarded as a consequence of serious conditions or a component of multiorgan failure in critically ill patients, the most important factor affecting renal outcomes may be the presence of an underlying kidney disease, which increases susceptibility to AKI or impairs renal recovery [6]. Several studies have reported that renal function after AKI affects long-term outcomes. An et al. [7] showed that renal functional assessment at 3 months after CRRT initiation can help predict progression to end-stage kidney disease (ESKD) and long-term survival. Further, a retrospective cohort study reported an estimated glomerular filtration rate of <30 mL/min per 1.73 m^2 at hospital discharge after CRRT as a strong risk factor for poor long-term survival and a poor renal prognosis [8]. However, only a few recent studies have analyzed renal and patient outcomes after AKI depending on the modality of RRT and pre-existing kidney diseases in a representative large cohort of critically ill patients.

In this study, we analyzed a large database from a nationwide cohort including virtually all intensive care unit (ICU) admissions in Korea to investigate the impact of application and modality of RRT and pre-existing kidney diseases on in-hospital mortality, progression to ESKD, and length of stay (LOS) in hospitals and ICUs.

2. Materials and Methods

2.1. Data Source

We retrospectively analyzed the cohort of the Korean ICU National Data (KIND) study [9] based on the Health Insurance Review and Assessment (HIRA) database of the Korean Ministry of Health. This database includes all ICU admissions in Korea. The HIRA database contains health insurance claims data generated in the process of reimbursing healthcare services under the National Health Insurance (NHI) system in Korea. The HIRA database contains information on almost 50 million patients as of 2014 in Korea, covering 98% of the total population through the universal health coverage system [10]. The study was reviewed by the Institutional Review Board (IRB) of Samsung Medical Center (IRB protocol 2015-11-17). The informed consent was waived because only previously collected deidentified administrative data were used.

2.2. Study Population

The study population included all adult patients older than 18 years from the KIND study (n = 131,988), who were diagnosed with AKI during the first ICU admission from 1 January 2008 to 31 May 2015. These patients had no history of AKI, dialysis, CRRT treatment, or ICU admission within a year prior to hospitalization.

Patients with the following characteristics were excluded: (1) those who received CRRT due to mental and behavioral disorders, intoxication, or organ donation (n = 1800); (2) those who received CRRT for less than 3 days, which could not be confirmed as AKI because of the possibility of applying CRRT for other diseases such as drug intoxication (n = 5867); and (3) ESKD patients who received dialysis prior to hospitalization, or patients who had been observed for less than 12 months during a one-year washout period (n = 139). Finally, a total of 124,182 patients (73,512 men and 50,670 women) were included (Figure 1).

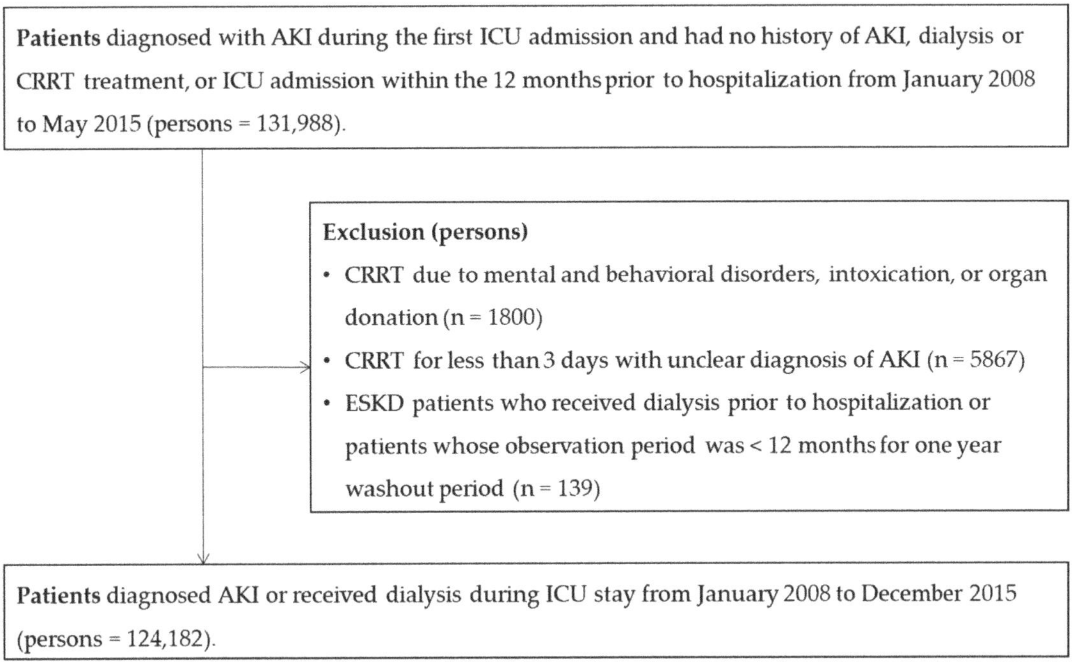

```
┌─────────────────────────────────────────────────────────────────────┐
│ Patients diagnosed with AKI during the first ICU admission and had   │
│ no history of AKI, dialysis or CRRT treatment, or ICU admission     │
│ within the 12 months prior to hospitalization from January 2008     │
│ to May 2015 (persons = 131,988).                                     │
└─────────────────────────────────────────────────────────────────────┘
            │
            │         ┌──────────────────────────────────────────────┐
            │         │ Exclusion (persons)                          │
            │────────▶│ • CRRT due to mental and behavioral          │
            │         │   disorders, intoxication, or organ          │
            │         │   donation (n = 1800)                        │
            │         │ • CRRT for less than 3 days with unclear     │
            │         │   diagnosis of AKI (n = 5867)                │
            │         │ • ESKD patients who received dialysis prior  │
            │         │   to hospitalization or patients whose       │
            │         │   observation period was < 12 months for     │
            │         │   one year washout period (n = 139)          │
            │         └──────────────────────────────────────────────┘
            ▼
┌─────────────────────────────────────────────────────────────────────┐
│ Patients diagnosed AKI or received dialysis during ICU stay from    │
│ January 2008 to December 2015 (persons = 124,182).                  │
└─────────────────────────────────────────────────────────────────────┘
```

Figure 1. Flowchart of study participants (n = 124,182).

2.3. Study Variables

ICU admission was defined by examining the claim codes that all hospitals in Korea are required to use when they submit cost claims of ICU admissions to the HIRA service (codes AJ100-AJ590900). These codes are based on the Korean Classification of Diseases 6th edition, a modified version of the International Classification of Diseases 10th revision (ICD-10), adapted for use in the Korean health system [11]. All ICU stays during the same hospitalization were considered as a single ICU admission. Similarly, hospital stays separated by <2 days were considered the same hospital admission.

AKI was defined as the presence of codes that identified AKI (ICD-10 codes N17), RRT including CRRT (Korean NHI procedure codes O7031-O7035, O7051-O7055), or dialysis. Dialysis was defined as intermittent hemodialysis (O7020-O7021, O2011-O2012, O2081-O2083, or O9991) or peritoneal dialysis (O7061-O7062, O7071-O7075, E6581, E6582, or E6593) using Korean NHI procedure codes.

Initiation timing and the modality of RRT were decided considering patients' overall conditions and RRT equipment status of each center. Indications for RRT were symptomatic uremia, severe electrolyte imbalance including hyperkalemia, severe metabolic acidosis, and volume overload according to guidelines [12,13]. CRRT was preferentially initiated in these patients with hemodynamic instability, multiorgan failure, or risk of increased intracerebral pressure.

We collected claim codes regarding information on comorbidities, management procedures during ICU admission, prescriptions, and demographic characteristics. Comorbidities, including pre-existing kidney disease within the year prior to hospitalization, were summarized using the Charlson index [14,15]. Kidney diseases were additionally defined using codes for chronic or unspecified nephritic syndromes (ICD-10 codes N030, N031, N038, N039, N050, N051, N058, or N059), which are not included in the Charlson Comorbidity Index.

The management procedures included mechanical ventilation (MV; Korean NHI procedure codes M5857, M5858, or M5860) and extracorporeal membrane oxygenation (ECMO, Korean NHI procedure codes O1901-O1904, material codes CAPIOX EBS CIRCUIT G5401008, QUADROX PLS G5501050, or CAPIOX EBS PMP CIRCUIT G5501008). Administration of inotropic or vasopressor drugs such as dobutamine, dopamine, epinephrine, and norepinephrine for more than 2 days was also identified using Korean drug and anatomical therapeutic chemical codes (148201BIJ, 38900BIJ, 148701BIJ, 148702BIJ, 429500BIJ, 152601BIJ, or 203101BIJ) [16].

We obtained information regarding hospital characteristics from the HIRA Medical Care Institution Database, which included the type of institution, location, number of hospital beds, facilities, and physicians. The type of hospital was classified according to the capacity, based on the number of hospital beds and the number of specialties as defined by the Korean Health Law [17]. In general, hospitals are defined as healthcare institutions with more than 30 inpatient beds. General hospitals are hospitals with more than 100 beds and more than seven specialty departments, including internal medicine, surgery, pediatrics, obstetrics and gynecology, anesthesiology, pathology, and laboratory medicine. Tertiary hospitals are general hospitals with more than 20 specialty departments that serve as teaching hospitals to medical students and nurses.

Total cost was the amount of money reimbursed by Korean NHI to hospitals, including ICU stay and for patients' medical services endorsed by HIRA, and then was converted into US dollars using the exchange rate of 1 December 2015 (1158 won/dollar).

2.4. Definition of Outcomes

The primary outcome was in-hospital mortality, defined as the death code of the billing statement. We also compared hospital and ICU LOS (days) and the incidence of ESKD after discharge among survivors ($n = 77,185$). To define post-discharge outcomes, we linked the personal identification number of each study participant to the inpatient claims data in the admission result database. The progression to ESKD as the long-term outcome of AKI was evaluated between hospitalization and 1 year after discharge. ESKD was defined in patients who received dialysis for >3 months (codes O7020, O9991, O7075) with registration for a copayment decreasing policy for ESKD patients (codes V001 and V003) or patients who underwent kidney transplantation (codes R3280).

2.5. Statistical Analysis

All patients were divided into three groups according to the RRT modality: control (no RRT), dialysis, and CRRT groups. Patients who received both dialysis and CRRT were categorized into the CRRT group. Continuous variables are presented as mean and standard deviation (SD) or median and interquartile range (IQR) and compared using one-way analysis of variance (ANOVA). Categorical variables are presented as numbers and proportions and compared using the χ^2 test.

Because patients' outcomes could be clustered by a hospital [18], we used the hospital as a random intercept in mixed-effects logistic regression models to estimate odds ratios (ORs) with 95% confidence intervals (CIs).

Patients who died during hospitalization were excluded from the analyses of progression to ESKD, as well as from the hospital and ICU LOS analysis to avoid the inclusion of censored patients due to death. A total of 77,185 patients were included in the final analysis. For hospital and ICU LOS in survivors, we used multiple linear regression models to compare the three groups. Since hospital LOS and ICU LOS were markedly right-skewed, $\log_e$-transformed outcomes and the estimated ratio with 95% CI comparing the three groups were used.

The long-term outcome of this study was the incidence of ESKD between hospitalization and 1 year after discharge. Person-time was calculated from the date of hospital admission to ESKD or the last follow-up date. Survival curves were generated using the Kaplan–Meier product-limit method and compared using log-rank tests. We used Cox proportional hazards regression models to estimate the hazard ratio (HR) with 95% CI for ESKD. We examined the proportional hazards assumption using plots of the log (−log) survival function and Schoenfeld residuals.

Age, sex, type of hospital, history of comorbidities (myocardial infarction, congestive heart failure, peripheral vascular disease, cerebrovascular disease, rheumatologic disease, liver disease, diabetes mellitus, kidney disease, cancer, and acquired immune deficiency syndrome/human immunodeficiency virus), and the use of MV, vasopressor drugs, and ECMO were adjusted in the final model. In addition, we conducted a subgroup analysis to evaluate the association of RRT with each outcome, depending on pre-existing kidney diseases.

All analyses were two-sided, and p-values < 0.05 were considered statistically significant. Statistical analyses were performed using SAS version 9.2 (SAS Institute, Inc., Cary, NC, USA) and R software (version 3.3.2; Free Software Foundation, Inc., Boston, MA, USA).

3. Results

A total of 124,182 ICU patients who were diagnosed with AKI were analyzed: 56.5%, 12.2%, and 31.3% in the control, dialysis, and CRRT groups, respectively (Table 1). The average proportion of AKI patients who received CRRT was 31.1% during the study period, which increased steadily from 24.1% in 2008 to 36.7% in 2014. During the same period, the in-hospital mortality rate of patients who received CRRT increased by 1% (58.9–59.7%) (Figure 2).

Table 1. Patient characteristics.

	Control	Dialysis	CRRT	p-Value
Number of patients	70,096	15,174	38,912	
Gender				<0.001
Male	40,259 (57.4)	9120 (60.1)	24,133 (62.0)	
Female	29,837 (42.6)	6054 (39.9)	14,779 (38.0)	
Age, years	69.4 (14.9)	64.5 (15.1)	64.0 (15.1)	<0.001
Pre-existing kidney disease	7720 (11.0)	5964 (39.3)	7481 (19.2)	<0.001
Comorbidity				
Myocardial infarction	4131 (5.9)	897 (5.9)	2444 (6.3)	0.03
Congestive heart failure	10,827 (15.4)	3006 (19.8)	5990 (15.4)	<0.001
Peripheral vascular disease	12,776 (18.2)	3108 (20.5)	7001 (18.0)	<0.001
Cerebrovascular disease	18,740 (26.7)	3598 (23.7)	8134 (20.9)	<0.001
Rheumatologic disease	3657 (5.2)	805 (5.3)	2516 (6.5)	<0.001
Liver disease	21,710 (31.0)	5135 (33.8)	15,127 (38.9)	<0.001
Diabetes	28,606 (40.8)	8355 (55.1)	17,908 (46.0)	<0.001
Cancer	10,527 (15.0)	2453 (16.2)	9306 (23.9)	<0.001
AIDS/HIV	51 (0.1)	8 (0.1)	36 (0.1)	0.279
Type of hospital				<0.001
Tertiary	20,157 (28.8)	6162 (40.6)	22,390 (57.5)	
General	46,978 (67.0)	8857 (58.4)	16,297 (41.9)	
Nursing care hospital	96 (0.1)	17 (0.1)	7 (0.0)	
Other	2865 (4.1)	138 (0.9)	218 (0.6)	
Management procedures				
Mechanical ventilation	26,662 (38.0)	5564 (36.7)	31,248 (80.3)	<0.001
ECMO	271 (0.4)	25 (0.2)	2002 (5.1)	<0.001
Vasopressor drugs	15,868 (22.6)	3206 (21.1)	19,278 (49.5)	<0.001
Total cost, USD 10 *	490 (229–971)	807 (433–1459)	1450 (720–2805)	<0.001

Values are numbers and proportions, except for age, Charlson index (mean and standard deviation), and total cost (median and interquartile range). CRRT, continuous renal replacement therapy; ECMO, extracorporeal membrane oxygenation. Dialysis was defined as intermittent hemodialysis and peritoneal dialysis. * USD 1 = KRW 1158 (exchange rate as of 1 December 2015).

The mean patient age (SD) was 67.1 ± 15.2 years, and 59.2% of the patients were men. The dialysis and CRRT groups included younger patients (control vs. dialysis and CRRT: 69.4% vs. 64.5% and 64.0%, $p < 0.001$), were more likely to include males (57.4% vs. 60.1% and 62.0%, $p < 0.001$), had a higher proportion of pre-existing kidney diseases (11.0% vs. 39.3% and 19.2%, $p < 0.001$), and showed more frequent admission in tertiary hospitals (28.8% vs. 40.6% and 57.5%, $p < 0.001$) than the control group. Among the three groups, MV (80.3%), ECMO (5.1%), and vasopressor drugs (49.5%) were most frequently used in the CRRT group.

The in-hospital mortality rate was significantly higher in the CRRT group than in the control and dialysis groups (control vs. dialysis vs. CRRT; 30.8% vs. 24.4% vs. 59.0%; $p < 0.001$) (Table 2). Even after adjustment for several confounders, the CRRT group had a significantly higher in-hospital mortality than the control and dialysis groups (fully adjusted or compared with the control group 2.04 (95% CI, 1.98–2.11, $p < 0.001$)). When the association between RRT and in-hospital mortality was evaluated depending on the pre-existing kidney disease, the CRRT group showed a significantly higher risk of in-hospital mortality in both subgroups (fully adjusted or compared with the control group; 2.10 (95% CI, 2.03–2.17) in the subgroup without pre-existing kidney disease vs. 1.70 (95% CI, 1.56–1.84) in the subgroup with pre-existing kidney disease). In the dialysis group, the in-hospital mortality of the subgroup without pre-existing kidney disease was comparable with that of the control group (fully adjusted or compared with the control group 0.98 (95% CI, 0.93–1.03)). However, the dialysis subgroup with pre-existing kidney disease showed lower in-hospital mortality (fully adjusted OR compared with the control group 0.67 (95% CI, 0.61–0.74)).

The median hospital LOS among survivors ($n = 77,185$) was 17 days (IQR, 9–31), 25 days (IQR, 14–43), and 29 days (IQR, 16–53) in the control, dialysis, and CRRT groups, respectively (Table 3). The dialysis group was more likely to have a longer hospital and ICU LOS than the control group. ICU LOS in the CRRT group was 43% longer than that in the control group. The association between RRT and LOS was consistent regardless of pre-existing kidney diseases.

In all patients who were discharged, the median follow-up of AKI patients was 365 days (IQR 128–365 days). During the 47,141.1 person-years of follow-up period, 3433 (4.45%) patients progressed to ESKD (incidence rate 72.8/1000 person-years). The incidence rate of ESKD was higher in the dialysis and CRRT groups than in the control group (control vs. dialysis vs. CRRT groups; 16.2 vs. 463.8 vs. 126.5 per 1000 person-years). In the Kaplan–Meier survival analyses, the cumulative incidence of ESKD was significantly higher in the dialysis group than in the control and CRRT groups (log-rank test, $p < 0.001$) (Figure 3).

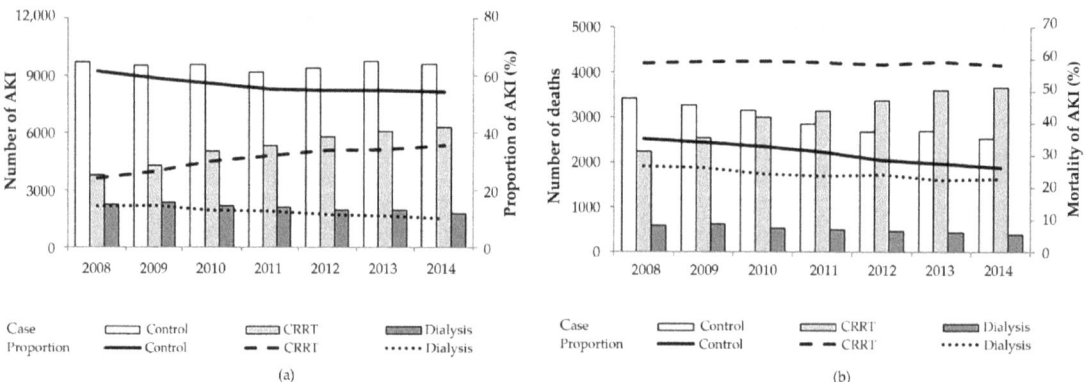

Figure 2. Yearly trends of acute kidney injury and in-hospital mortality according to renal replacement therapy modality: (a) Bars and lines represent the absolute numbers and the proportion of critically ill patients with AKI among all intensive care unit patients, respectively. The proportion of patients who received CRRT increased steadily from 24.1% in 2008 to 36.7% in 2014.; (b) Bars and lines represent the absolute number of deaths and the mortality of critically ill patients with AKI, respectively. In-hospital mortality rate of patients who received CRRT increased by 1% for 7 years (58.9% in 2008 to 59.7% in 2014).

Compared with the control group, the age- and gender-adjusted HRs for ESKD were 25.48 (95% CI, 21.30–30.48) and 7.74 (95% CI, 6.59–9.10) in the dialysis and CRRT groups, respectively. This association remained significant after further adjustment for multiple confounders (fully adjusted HR compared with the control group: 17.67 (95% CI, 15.06–20.72) in the dialysis group and 7.28 (95% CI, 6.29–8.41) in the CRRT group) (Table 4). In patients with pre-existing kidney disease, the risk of ESKD in the dialysis and CRRT groups was higher than that in the control group (fully adjusted HR compared with the control group; dialysis vs. CRRT groups, 15.15 (95% CI, 12.88–17.83) vs. 5.83 (95% CI, 4.89–6.96); $p < 0.001$). In patients without pre-existing kidney disease, the risk of ESKD was even higher in both dialysis and CRRT groups than in the control group (fully adjusted HR; dialysis vs. CRRT groups, 20.06 (95% CI, 16.06–25.05) vs. 8.86 (95% CI, 7.30–10.76); $p < 0.001$).

Table 2. Risk of hospital mortality according to RRT modalities and pre-existing kidney disease.

	Control	Dialysis	CRRT	p-Value
Number of patients	70,096	15,174	38,912	
Gender				<0.001
Male	40,259 (57.4)	9120 (60.1)	24,133 (62.0)	
Female	29,837 (42.6)	6054 (39.9)	14,779 (38.0)	
Age, years	69.4 (14.9)	64.5 (15.1)	64.0 (15.1)	<0.001
Pre-existing kidney disease	7720 (11.0)	5964 (39.3)	7481 (19.2)	<0.001
Comorbidity				
Myocardial infarction	4131 (5.9)	897 (5.9)	2444 (6.3)	0.03
Congestive heart failure	10,827 (15.4)	3006 (19.8)	5990 (15.4)	<0.001
Peripheral vascular disease	12,776 (18.2)	3108 (20.5)	7001 (18.0)	<0.001
Cerebrovascular disease	18,740 (26.7)	3598 (23.7)	8134 (20.9)	<0.001
Rheumatologic disease	3657 (5.2)	805 (5.3)	2516 (6.5)	<0.001
Liver disease	21,710 (31.0)	5135 (33.8)	15,127 (38.9)	<0.001
Diabetes	28,606 (40.8)	8355 (55.1)	17,908 (46.0)	<0.001
Cancer	10,527 (15.0)	2453 (16.2)	9306 (23.9)	<0.001
AIDS/HIV	51 (0.1)	8 (0.1)	36 (0.1)	0.279
Type of hospital				<0.001
Tertiary	20,157 (28.8)	6162 (40.6)	22,390 (57.5)	
General	46,978 (67.0)	8857 (58.4)	16,297 (41.9)	
Nursing care hospital	96 (0.1)	17 (0.1)	7 (0.0)	
Other	2865 (4.1)	138 (0.9)	218 (0.6)	
Management procedures				
Mechanical ventilation	26,662 (38.0)	5564 (36.7)	31,248 (80.3)	<0.001
ECMO	271 (0.4)	25 (0.2)	2002 (5.1)	<0.001
Vasopressor drugs	15,868 (22.6)	3206 (21.1)	19,278 (49.5)	<0.001
Total cost, USD 10 *	490 (229–971)	807 (433–1459)	1450 (720–2805)	<0.001

Values are numbers and proportions, except for age, Charlson index (mean and standard deviation), and total cost (median and interquartile range). CRRT, continuous renal replacement therapy; ECMO, extracorporeal membrane oxygenation. Dialysis was defined as intermittent hemodialysis and peritoneal dialysis. * USD 1= KRW 1158 (exchange rate as of 1 December 2015).

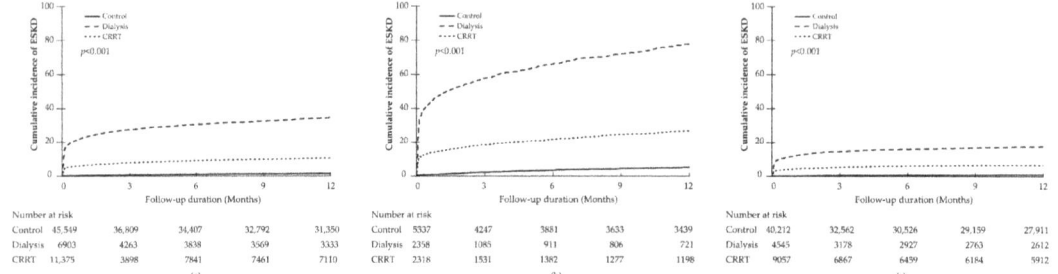

Figure 3. Cumulative incidence of end-stage kidney disease (ESKD) according to the modality of renal replacement therapy: All patients (**a**); patients with pre-existing kidney disease (**b**); and patients without pre-existing kidney disease (**c**); the risk of ESKD was the highest in the dialysis group with pre-existing kidney disease.

Table 3. Hospital and ICU length of stay according to RRT modalities and pre-existing kidney disease.

	Length of Stay, Days	Crude Model		Adjusted Model [a]	
	Median (IQR)	Ratio [b] (95% CI)	p-Value	Ratio [b] (95% CI)	p-Value
Hospital length of stay					
Overall					
Control	17 (9–31)	Reference		Reference	
Dialysis	25 (14–43)	1.40 (1.37–1.43)	<0.001	1.46 (1.43–1.49)	<0.001
CRRT	29 (16–53)	1.45 (1.42–1.48)	<0.001	1.22 (1.2–1.25)	<0.001
Pre-existing kidney disease					
With pre-existing kidney disease					
Control	16 (9–30)	Reference		Reference	
Dialysis	24 (14–41)	1.42 (1.37–1.47)	<0.001	1.48 (1.43–1.53)	<0.001
CRRT	28 (16–48)	1.57 (1.51–1.64)	<0.001	1.35 (1.3–1.41)	<0.001
Without pre-existing kidney disease					
Control	17 (9–32)	Reference		Reference	
Dialysis	25 (15–46)	1.44 (1.40–1.48)	<0.001	1.46 (1.42–1.50)	<0.001
CRRT	30 (16–55)	1.43 (1.40–1.46)	<0.001	1.19 (1.16–1.22)	<0.001
ICU length of stay					
Overall					
Control	6 (2–14)	Reference		Reference	
Dialysis	6 (3–15)	0.95 (0.93–0.97)	<0.001	1.10 (1.08–1.13)	<0.001
CRRT	18 (8–34)	2.06 (2.02–2.11)	<0.001	1.43 (1.40–1.46)	<0.001
Pre-existing kidney disease					
With pre-existing kidney disease					
Control	5 (2–12)	Reference		Reference	
Dialysis	5 (2–10)	0.88 (0.85–0.92)	<0.001	0.98 (0.94–1.01)	0.239
CRRT	14 (6–28)	2.18 (2.08–2.28)	<0.001	1.52 (1.45–1.58)	<0.001
Without pre-existing kidney disease					
Control	6 (2–14)	Reference		Reference	
Dialysis	8 (4–20)	1.13 (1.10–1.17)	<0.001	1.20 (1.17–1.23)	<0.001
CRRT	18 (8–37)	2.10 (2.05–2.15)	<0.001	1.40 (1.37–1.43)	<0.001

ICU, intensive care unit; RRT, renal replacement therapy; CRRT, continuous renal replacement therapy; IQR, interquartile range; CI, confidence interval. [a] Adjusted for differences in type of hospital, history of comorbidity (myocardial infarction, congestive heart failure, peripheral vascular disease, cerebrovascular disease, rheumatologic disease, liver disease, diabetes, kidney disease (adjusted only overall group), cancer, AIDS/HIV), mechanical ventilator, vasopressor drugs, and extracorporeal membrane oxygenation. [b] Ratios and 95% CI were estimated from linear regression with log transformed variable as the outcome.

Table 4. Risk of end-stage kidney disease (ESKD) according to RRT modalities and pre-existing kidney disease.

	Person Years	No. of Cases	Incidence Rate (per 1000 Person-Years)	Model 1 HR (95% CI)	Model 2 HR (95% CI)
Overall					
Control	35,140.5	570	16.2	Reference	Reference
Dialysis	3986.5	1849	463.8	25.48 (21.30–30.48)	17.67 (15.06–20.72)
CRRT	8014.1	1014	126.5	7.74 (6.59–9.10)	7.28 (6.29–8.41)
p-value				<0.001	<0.001
With pre-existing kidney disease					
Control	3984.4	222	55.7	Reference	Reference
Dialysis	974	1168	1199.2	15.76 (13.37–18.58)	15.15 (12.88–17.83)
CRRT	1426.5	480	336.5	5.37 (4.52–6.38)	5.83 (4.89–6.96)
p-value				<0.001	<0.001
Without pre-existing kidney disease					
Control	31,156.1	348	11.2	Reference	Reference
Dialysis	3012.5	681	226.1	19.22 (15.39–24.01)	20.06 (16.06–25.05)
CRRT	6587.6	534	81.1	7.30 (6.03–8.85)	8.86 (7.30–10.76)
p-value				<0.001	<0.001

RRT, renal replacement therapy; CRRT, continuous renal replacement therapy. Model 1 was adjusted for age and gender. Model 2 was further adjusted for type of hospital, history of comorbidity (myocardial infarction, congestive heart failure, peripheral vascular disease, cerebrovascular disease, rheumatologic disease, liver disease, diabetes, kidney disease (adjusted only overall group), cancer, AIDS/HIV), mechanical ventilator, vasopressor drugs, and extracorporeal membrane oxygenation.

4. Discussion

This study investigated the overall outcomes of AKI depending on the type of RRT and pre-existing kidney disease in critically ill adult patients using a nationwide population-based cohort in Korea during a 7-year period. The CRRT group had a significantly higher risk of in-hospital mortality, whereas the dialysis group showed lower in-hospital mortality than the control group. Specifically, among the patients without pre-existing kidney disease, in-hospital mortality was higher in the CRRT group, and the incidence of ESKD was also higher in both dialysis and CRRT groups than in the control group. These results suggest that severe AKI that develops as a consequence of multiorgan failure may exert a critically adverse impact on patient survival and renal outcomes. Further, the lower in-hospital mortality in the dialysis group may indicate the importance of appropriate RRT in the treatment of AKI in critically ill patients.

Previous prospective randomized studies comparing the effects of dialysis and CRRT showed no difference in mortality between the two treatment modalities [19–21]. One meta-analysis of 30 randomized controlled trials and eight prospective cohort studies found no difference in all-cause mortality between patients treated with intermittent hemodialysis and those treated with CRRT [22]. In a recent meta-analysis of 21 studies, the modality of RRT was not associated with in-hospital and ICU mortality [23]. According to a retrospective population-based matched cohort study comparing outcomes according to CRRT and hemodialysis (propensity-matched patients with no difference in mechanical ventilation, number of days between hospitalization and initiation of RRT, and baseline characteristics), there was no difference in mortality between the two groups [24]. In contrast to these reports, our results showed that the CRRT group had significantly higher mortality than both the control and dialysis groups. In clinical practice, CRRT has been preferentially used in AKI patients with unstable vital signs or poor overall medical conditions; thus, these patients are expected to show a higher mortality rate. Further, in an 8-year observational cohort study by De Corte et al., non-survivors had worse profiles of disease severity, and CRRT as the initial RRT modality was associated with long-term mortality [25]. In our study, although it was not possible to obtain severity scores directly from our database, ECMO, mechanical ventilation, and vasopressor were used more frequently in the CRRT group than in the dialysis or the control groups, suggesting that patients with higher severity scores were included in the CRRT group. Unlike other previous studies with no difference in mortality between the dialysis group and the CRRT group, the CRRT group in our study had a higher mortality. We believe that our result was more representative of real-world practice reflecting the overall severity of patients.

Few studies have investigated the impact of pre-existing kidney disease and RRT modality on AKI outcomes among critically ill patients. In our study, the dialysis group with pre-existing kidney disease showed lower in-hospital mortality than the control group. A prospective cohort study of AKI in critically ill patients reported that patients with pre-existing kidney disease had a lower mortality rate but were more likely to be dialysis-dependent at hospital discharge [26]. CKD is known to increase susceptibility to AKI, and AKI on CKD is associated with a worse renal outcome [27]. Patients with pre-existing kidney disease may take a relatively shorter time to reach the indications for RRT during the course of AKI, or early RRT can be considered based on their medical history of kidney disease. Our hypothesis is that multiorgan failure might be more frequent in AKI patients without pre-existing kidney disease, and RRT might be performed relatively earlier in patients with pre-existing kidney disease, resulting in reduced in-hospital mortality in our study population. Moreover, the mortality at day 60 was significantly higher in patients who received late RRT (61.8%) than in those who received early RRT (48.5%) in the Artificial Kidney Initiation in Kidney Injury (AKIKI) trial [28], which supports our hypothesis. The Early versus Late Initiation of Renal Replacement Therapy in Critically Ill Patients with AKI (ELAIN) trial also demonstrated that early initiation of RRT significantly reduced 90-day and 1-year all-cause mortality compared to delayed initiation of RRT [29,30].

Furthermore, intrarenal alterations at a molecular, cellular, and tissue level related to pre-existing kidney diseases seem to affect not only the severity of AKI but also the degree of the renal repair process, including fibrosis [6]. Previous studies reported that AKI contributes to the deterioration of renal function in CKD patients [31,32]. In a retrospective cohort study including patients older than 67 years, those with AKI on CKD showed a significantly higher risk of ESKD than those with AKI or CKD alone [26]. Further, in a cohort study of 9425 patients with postoperative AKI, patients with pre-existing kidney disease had higher risks of long-term mortality and dialysis dependency than those without pre-existing kidney disease [32]. Additionally, in several studies, the CRRT group showed better renal recovery and lower rate of dialysis dependency than the dialysis group [24,33–36]. Similarly, our results showed that the cumulative incidence of ESKD was higher in the dialysis group than in the CRRT group, especially in the subgroup with pre-existing kidney disease. The incidence rate of ESKD was significantly higher in patients with pre-existing kidney disease, regardless of the RRT modality received. However, the dialysis group showed lower in-hospital mortality than the control group. These results support the clinical importance of timely RRT to improve the survival of critically ill patients with AKI, although maintenance dialysis reduces the quality of life and increases the burden of medical costs [37]. Our results also suggest the necessity of further study focusing on overall outcomes of AKI in critically ill patients stratified by the presence of pre-existing kidney disease.

This study has several limitations. First, detailed clinical data, such as etiology of AKI, serum creatinine, and urine volume could not be analyzed because of the inherent limitations of the national registry database used in our study. However, the main purpose of this study was to compare hard outcomes such as in-hospital mortality and the risk of ESKD development depending on the application of RRT or RRT modalities. Although a contemporary consensus-based definition of AKI could not be used, we believe that our large database was sufficient to investigate the primary aim of our study. Second, the overall severity scores of critically ill patients, such as sequential organ failure assessment (SOFA) and acute physiology and chronic health evaluation (APACHE) scores, were not measured. However, considering that MV, ECMO, and vasopressor drugs were used more frequently in the CRRT group than in the dialysis group, the CRRT group seemed to include patients with hemodynamic instability and worse medical conditions. Unlike previous studies showing similar mortality in both CRRT and dialysis groups, our study showed higher mortality in the CRRT group after adjusting for confounding variables. We believe that our study reveals a difference in mortality among critically ill patients with AKI according to the modality of RRT in the real world. Third, the definition of 'kidney disease' was based on diagnostic codes. The NHIS department regularly audits claims in the Korean health insurance system, and the government provides special insurance coverage by evaluating the procedures and treatment under disease codes. Therefore, our HIRA database is considered reliable and has been widely used for research purposes [10].

Despite these limitations, our study has clinically important strengths including the study's design and statistical methods based on the analysis of a large population-based cohort. This enables a meaningful report of mortality and progression to ESKD considering both available RRT modalities and the presence of pre-existing kidney disease. Additionally, medical treatments associated with relevant critically-ill patient conditions such as MV, ECMO, and vasopressor drugs were comprehensively analyzed.

5. Conclusions

Among critically ill patients with AKI in Korea, patients with pre-existing kidney disease in the dialysis group had relatively lower in-hospital mortality and a greater risk of progression to ESKD than those with pre-existing kidney disease in both the control and CRRT groups. In-hospital mortality was the highest in the CRRT group without pre-existing kidney disease, while the risk of ESKD was higher in the subgroup without pre-existing kidney disease. Our findings may support the critical impact of severe AKI requiring RRT on both mortality and long-term renal outcome in critically ill patients, including those without pre-existing kidney disease. Further prospective studies considering pre-existing kidney disease are required to elucidate the clinical impact of RRT modality on overall and renal outcomes in clinically ill patients with AKI.

Author Contributions: Conceptualization, J.C. and H.-R.J.; methodology, J.C. and H.-R.J.; software, D.K., H.P. and Y.K.; validation, S.H. and H.-R.J.; formal analysis, D.K., H.P. and Y.K.; investigation, S.H., D.K., H.P. and Y.K.; resources, J.J., J.-E.L., W.H., G.-Y.S. and H.-R.J.; data curation, S.H. and D.K.; writing—original draft preparation, S.H. and D.K.; writing—review and editing, S.H., D.K., J.C. and H.-R.J.; visualization, S.H. and H.P.; supervision, E.G., J.-E.L. and W.H.; project administration, G.-Y.S. and H.-R.J.; funding acquisition, H.-R.J. All authors have read and agreed to the published version of the manuscript.

Funding: This research was supported by a grant from the Korea Health Technology R&D Project through the Korea Health Industry Development Institute (KHIDI), funded by the Ministry of Health & Welfare, Republic of Korea (grant number: HC20C0085).

Institutional Review Board Statement: The study was reviewed by the IRB of Samsung Medical Center (IRB protocol 2015-11-17).

Informed Consent Statement: Informed consent was waived because only previously collected de-identified administrative data were used.

Data Availability Statement: The datasets used and/or analyzed in this study are available from the corresponding author upon reasonable request.

Acknowledgments: The authors would like to thank the CRRT nursing team of Samsung Medical Center for their dedicated efforts to perform CRRT properly.

Conflicts of Interest: The authors declare no conflict of interest. The results presented in this article have not been published previously in whole or part, except in abstract format.

References

1. Uchino, S.; Kellum, J.A.; Bellomo, R.; Doig, G.S.; Morimatsu, H.; Morgera, S.; Schetz, M.; Tan, I.; Bouman, C.; Macedo, E.; et al. Acute renal failure in critically ill patients: A multinational, multicenter study. *JAMA* **2005**, *294*, 813–818. [CrossRef] [PubMed]
2. Liborio, A.B.; Leite, T.T.; Neves, F.M.; Teles, F.; Bezerra, C.T. AKI complications in critically ill patients: Association with mortality rates and RRT. *Clin. J. Am. Soc. Nephrol.* **2015**, *10*, 21–28. [CrossRef] [PubMed]
3. Elseviers, M.M.; Lins, R.L.; Van der Niepen, P.; Hoste, E.; Malbrain, M.L.; Damas, P.; Devriendt, J.; the SHARF Investigators. Renal replacement therapy is an independent risk factor for mortality in critically ill patients with acute kidney injury. *Crit. Care* **2010**, *14*, R221. [CrossRef]
4. Siew, E.D.; Davenport, A. The growth of acute kidney injury: A rising tide or just closer attention to detail? *Kidney Int.* **2015**, *87*, 46–61. [CrossRef] [PubMed]
5. Chawla, L.S.; Bellomo, R.; Bihorac, A.; Goldstein, S.L.; Siew, E.D.; Bagshaw, S.M.; Bittleman, D.; Cruz, D.; Endre, Z.; Fitzgerald, R.L.; et al. Acute kidney disease and renal recovery: Consensus report of the Acute Disease Quality Initiative (ADQI) 16 Workgroup. *Nat. Rev. Nephrol.* **2017**, *13*, 241–257. [CrossRef] [PubMed]
6. He, L.; Wei, Q.; Liu, J.; Yi, M.; Liu, Y.; Liu, H.; Sun, L.; Peng, Y.; Liu, F.; Venkatachalam, M.A.; et al. AKI on CKD: Heightened injury, suppressed repair, and the underlying mechanisms. *Kidney Int.* **2017**, *92*, 1071–1083. [CrossRef] [PubMed]
7. An, J.N.; Hwang, J.H.; Kim, D.K.; Lee, H.; Ahn, S.Y.; Kim, S.; Park, J.T.; Kang, S.W.; Oh, Y.K.; Kim, Y.S.; et al. Chronic Kidney Disease After Acute Kidney Injury Requiring Continuous Renal Replacement Therapy and Its Impact on Long-Term Outcomes: A Multicenter Retrospective Cohort Study in Korea. *Crit. Care Med.* **2017**, *45*, 47–57. [CrossRef]
8. Stads, S.; Fortrie, G.; van Bommel, J.; Zietse, R.; Betjes, M.G. Impaired kidney function at hospital discharge and long-term renal and overall survival in patients who received CRRT. *Clin. J. Am. Soc. Nephrol.* **2013**, *8*, 1284–1291. [CrossRef]
9. Park, J.; Jeon, K.; Chung, C.R.; Yang, J.H.; Cho, Y.H.; Cho, J.; Park, C.M.; Park, H.; Cho, J.; Guallar, E.; et al. A nationwide analysis of intensive care unit admissions, 2009–2014—The Korean ICU National Data (KIND) study. *J. Crit. Care* **2018**, *44*, 24–30. [CrossRef]
10. Kim, J.A.; Yoon, S.; Kim, L.Y.; Kim, D.S. Towards Actualizing the Value Potential of Korea Health Insurance Review and Assessment (HIRA) Data as a Resource for Health Research: Strengths, Limitations, Applications, and Strategies for Optimal Use of HIRA Data. *J. Korean Med. Sci.* **2017**, *32*, 718–728. [CrossRef]
11. Lee, Y.S.; Lee, Y.R.; Chae, Y.; Park, S.Y.; Oh, I.H.; Jang, B.H. Translation of Korean Medicine Use to ICD-Codes Using National Health Insurance Service-National Sample Cohort. *Evid. Based Complement. Alternat. Med.* **2016**, *2016*, 8160838. [CrossRef] [PubMed]
12. Bagshaw, S.M.; Wald, R. Strategies for the optimal timing to start renal replacement therapy in critically ill patients with acute kidney injury. *Kidney Int.* **2017**, *91*, 1022–1032. [CrossRef] [PubMed]
13. Kdigo, A. Work Group. KDIGO clinical practice guideline for acute kidney injury. *Kidney Int. Suppl.* **2012**, *2*, 1–138.
14. Charlson, M.E.; Pompei, P.; Ales, K.L.; MacKenzie, C.R. A new method of classifying prognostic comorbidity in longitudinal studies: Development and validation. *J. Chronic Dis.* **1987**, *40*, 373–383. [CrossRef]
15. Kim, K.H. Comparative study on three algorithms of the ICD-10 Charlson comorbidity index with myocardial infarction patients. *J. Prev. Med. Public Health* **2010**, *43*, 42–49. [CrossRef]
16. Morgan, J.H.; Kallen, M.A.; Okike, K.; Lee, O.C.; Vrahas, M.S. PROMIS Physical Function Computer Adaptive Test Compared With Other Upper Extremity Outcome Measures in the Evaluation of Proximal Humerus Fractures in Patients Older Than 60 Years. *J. Orthop. Trauma* **2015**, *29*, 257–263. [CrossRef]
17. Overbeek, C.L.; Nota, S.P.; Jayakumar, P.; Hageman, M.G.; Ring, D. The PROMIS physical function correlates with the QuickDASH in patients with upper extremity illness. *Clin. Orthop. Relat. Res.* **2015**, *473*, 311–317. [CrossRef]
18. Shulman, L.N.; Palis, B.E.; McCabe, R.M.; Gay, E.G.; Mallin, K.; Loomis, A.; Winchester, D.P.; McKellar, D.P. Survival as a measure of quality of cancer care and advances in therapy: Lessons learned from analyses of the National Cancer Data Base (NCDB). *J. Clin. Oncol.* **2016**, *34*, 173. [CrossRef]
19. Vinsonneau, C.; Camus, C.; Combes, A.; Costa de Beauregard, M.A.; Klouche, K.; Boulain, T.; Pallot, J.L.; Chiche, J.D.; Taupin, P.; Landais, P.; et al. Continuous venovenous haemodiafiltration versus intermittent haemodialysis for acute renal failure in patients with multiple-organ dysfunction syndrome: A multicentre randomised trial. *Lancet* **2006**, *368*, 379–385. [CrossRef]
20. Lins, R.L.; Elseviers, M.M.; Van der Niepen, P.; Hoste, E.; Malbrain, M.L.; Damas, P.; Devriendt, J.; the SHARF Investigators. Intermittent versus continuous renal replacement therapy for acute kidney injury patients admitted to the intensive care unit: Results of a randomized clinical trial. *Nephrol. Dial. Transpl.* **2009**, *24*, 512–518. [CrossRef]
21. Gaudry, S.; Grolleau, F.; Barbar, S.; Martin-Lefevre, L.; Pons, B.; Boulet, E.; Boyer, A.; Chevrel, G.; Montini, F.; Bohe, J.; et al. Continuous renal replacement therapy versus intermittent hemodialysis as first modality for renal replacement therapy in severe acute kidney injury: A secondary analysis of AKIKI and IDEAL-ICU studies. *Crit Care* **2022**, *26*, 93. [CrossRef] [PubMed]
22. Pannu, N.; Klarenbach, S.; Wiebe, N.; Manns, B.; Tonelli, M.; Alberta Kidney Disease, N. Renal replacement therapy in patients with acute renal failure: A systematic review. *JAMA* **2008**, *299*, 793–805. [CrossRef] [PubMed]
23. Nash, D.M.; Przech, S.; Wald, R.; O'Reilly, D. Systematic review and meta-analysis of renal replacement therapy modalities for acute kidney injury in the intensive care unit. *J. Crit. Care* **2017**, *41*, 138–144. [CrossRef] [PubMed]

24. Wald, R.; Shariff, S.Z.; Adhikari, N.K.; Bagshaw, S.M.; Burns, K.E.; Friedrich, J.O.; Garg, A.X.; Harel, Z.; Kitchlu, A.; Ray, J.G. The association between renal replacement therapy modality and long-term outcomes among critically ill adults with acute kidney injury: A retrospective cohort study*. *Crit. Care Med.* **2014**, *42*, 868–877. [CrossRef]
25. De Corte, W.; Dhondt, A.; Vanholder, R.; De Waele, J.; Decruyenaere, J.; Sergoyne, V.; Vanhalst, J.; Claus, S.; Hoste, E.A. Long-term outcome in ICU patients with acute kidney injury treated with renal replacement therapy: A prospective cohort study. *Crit. Care* **2016**, *20*, 256. [CrossRef]
26. Khosla, N.; Soroko, S.B.; Chertow, G.M.; Himmelfarb, J.; Ikizler, T.A.; Paganini, E.; Mehta, R.L.; Program to Improve Care in Acute Renal Disease. Preexisting chronic kidney disease: A potential for improved outcomes from acute kidney injury. *Clin. J. Am. Soc. Nephrol.* **2009**, *4*, 1914–1919. [CrossRef]
27. Chawla, L.S.; Eggers, P.W.; Star, R.A.; Kimmel, P.L. Acute kidney injury and chronic kidney disease as interconnected syndromes. *N. Engl. J. Med.* **2014**, *371*, 58–66. [CrossRef]
28. Gaudry, S.; Hajage, D.; Schortgen, F.; Martin-Lefevre, L.; Pons, B.; Boulet, E.; Boyer, A.; Chevrel, G.; Lerolle, N.; Carpentier, D.; et al. Initiation Strategies for Renal-Replacement Therapy in the Intensive Care Unit. *N. Engl. J. Med.* **2016**, *375*, 122–133. [CrossRef]
29. Zarbock, A.; Kellum, J.A.; Schmidt, C.; Van Aken, H.; Wempe, C.; Pavenstadt, H.; Boanta, A.; Gerss, J.; Meersch, M. Effect of Early vs Delayed Initiation of Renal Replacement Therapy on Mortality in Critically Ill Patients With Acute Kidney Injury: The ELAIN Randomized Clinical Trial. *JAMA* **2016**, *315*, 2190–2199. [CrossRef]
30. Meersch, M.; Kullmar, M.; Schmidt, C.; Gerss, J.; Weinhage, T.; Margraf, A.; Ermert, T.; Kellum, J.A.; Zarbock, A. Long-Term Clinical Outcomes after Early Initiation of RRT in Critically Ill Patients with AKI. *J. Am. Soc. Nephrol.* **2018**, *29*, 1011–1019. [CrossRef]
31. Ishani, A.; Xue, J.L.; Himmelfarb, J.; Eggers, P.W.; Kimmel, P.L.; Molitoris, B.A.; Collins, A.J. Acute kidney injury increases risk of ESRD among elderly. *J. Am. Soc. Nephrol.* **2009**, *20*, 223–228. [CrossRef] [PubMed]
32. Wu, V.C.; Huang, T.M.; Lai, C.F.; Shiao, C.C.; Lin, Y.F.; Chu, T.S.; Wu, P.C.; Chao, C.T.; Wang, J.Y.; Kao, T.W.; et al. Acute-on-chronic kidney injury at hospital discharge is associated with long-term dialysis and mortality. *Kidney Int.* **2011**, *80*, 1222–1230. [CrossRef] [PubMed]
33. Bell, M.; Granath, F.; Schön, S.; Ekbom, A.; Martling, C.R. Continuous renal replacement therapy is associated with less chronic renal failure than intermittent haemodialysis after acute renal failure. *Intensive Care Med.* **2007**, *33*, 773–780. [CrossRef] [PubMed]
34. Schneider, A.G.; Bellomo, R.; Bagshaw, S.M.; Glassford, N.J.; Lo, S.; Jun, M.; Cass, A.; Gallagher, M. Choice of renal replacement therapy modality and dialysis dependence after acute kidney injury: A systematic review and meta-analysis. *Intensive Care Med.* **2013**, *39*, 987–997. [CrossRef] [PubMed]
35. Bonnassieux, M.; Duclos, A.; Schneider, A.G.; Schmidt, A.; Bénard, S.; Cancalon, C.; Joannes-Boyau, O.; Ichai, C.; Constantin, J.M.; Lefrant, J.Y.; et al. Renal Replacement Therapy Modality in the ICU and Renal Recovery at Hospital Discharge. *Crit. Care Med.* **2018**, *46*, e102–e110. [CrossRef]
36. Wang, Y.; Gallagher, M.; Li, Q.; Lo, S.; Cass, A.; Finfer, S.; Myburgh, J.; Bouman, C.; Faulhaber-Walter, R.; Kellum, J.A.; et al. Renal replacement therapy intensity for acute kidney injury and recovery to dialysis independence: A systematic review and individual patient data meta-analysis. *Nephrol. Dial. Transpl.* **2018**, *33*, 1017–1024. [CrossRef]
37. Ethgen, O.; Schneider, A.G.; Bagshaw, S.M.; Bellomo, R.; Kellum, J.A. Economics of dialysis dependence following renal replacement therapy for critically ill acute kidney injury patients. *Nephrol. Dial. Transpl.* **2015**, *30*, 54–61. [CrossRef]

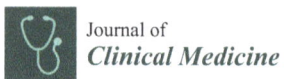

Review

The Role of the Intravenous IgA and IgM-Enriched Immunoglobulin Preparation in the Treatment of Sepsis and Septic Shock

Giorgio Berlot [1,2,*], Silvia Zanchi [1], Edoardo Moro [1], Ariella Tomasini [1] and Mattia Bixio [3]

1. Azienda Sanitaria Universitaria Giuliano Isontina, Department of Anesthesia and Intensive Care, 34148 Trieste, Italy; zanchi.sil1@gmail.com (S.Z.); edoardo.moro@gmail.com (E.M.); ariella.tpmasini9@gmail.com (A.T.)
2. UCO Anestesia Rianimazione e Terapia Antalgica, Azienda Sanitaria Universitaria Giuliano Isontina, Strada di Fiume 447, 34149 Trieste, Italy
3. Ospedale Policlinico San Martino, Department of Anesthesia and Intensive Care, 16132 Genova, Italy; mattia.bixio@gmail.com
* Correspondence: berlotg@virgilio.it; Tel.: +39-04039904540; Fax: +39-040912278

Abstract: Polyclonal Intravenous Immunoglobulins (IvIg) are often administered to critically ill patients more as an act of faith than on the basis of relevant clinical studies. This particularly applies to the treatment of sepsis and septic shock because the current guidelines recommend against their use despite many investigations that have demonstrated their beneficial effects in different subsets of patients. The biology, mechanisms of action, and clinical experience related to the administration of IvIg are reviewed, which aim to give a more in-depth understanding of their properties in order to clarify their possible indications in sepsis and septic shock patients.

Keywords: sepsis; septic shock; immunotherapy

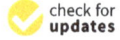

Citation: Berlot, G.; Zanchi, S.; Moro, E.; Tomasini, A.; Bixio, M. The Role of the Intravenous IgA and IgM-Enriched Immunoglobulin Preparation in the Treatment of Sepsis and Septic Shock. *J. Clin. Med.* 2023, 12, 4645. https://doi.org/10.3390/jcm12144645

Academic Editors: Spyros D. Mentzelopoulos and Bernard Allaouchiche

Received: 15 April 2023
Revised: 4 July 2023
Accepted: 11 July 2023
Published: 12 July 2023

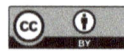

Copyright: © 2023 by the authors. Licensee MDPI, Basel, Switzerland. This article is an open access article distributed under the terms and conditions of the Creative Commons Attribution (CC BY) license (https://creativecommons.org/licenses/by/4.0/).

1. Introduction

Although not all their indications are based on studies fulfilling the evidence-based medicine (EBM) criteria, intravenous immunoglobulins (IvIgs) are currently used in a number of diseases in Intensive Care Unit (ICU) patients. These clinical conditions include (a) autoimmune reactions directed against some tissue target(s), such as Myasthenia Gravis, Guillain-Barre Syndrome, etc.; or (b) a systemic response to an infection, including sepsis and septic shock [1].

The rationale for their administration derives from their biological properties, consisting of both the down-regulation of an exaggerated immune response and the enhancement of the immunological capabilities. As far as the use of IvIg in septic and septic shock patients is concerned, ICU physicians can be subdivided into non-believers, who do not use these preparations due to the lack of robust studies fulfilling the strict EBM rules and believers, who instead use them on the basis of a number of investigations and meta-analyses (MAs) demonstrating a positive effect on the outcome.

The aim of this review is to provide a detailed overview of the possible role of IvIg in critically ill septic patients.

2. Structures and Function of Immunoglobulins

The immune system works via two different but cooperating arms [2] whose activation is triggered by the adhesion of foreign substances on the receptors located on the surface of the cells involved in the response. The innate system is based on the cells of the reticuloendothelial complex, the wide number of mediators produced by these cells during the interaction between the host and the invading organisms and the complement cascade. Yet, as the number of the receptors is genetically determined and not implementable, the innate arm cannot cope with the almost infinite variety of microbial epitopes and acts as a first responder, aiming to circumscribe the infection and impede its spread. The second arm, known as adaptative immunity, is more flexible and is based on the production of the Ig, which is encoded by genes that are able to undergo somatic recombination and hypermutations in order to face the myriad of substances coming in contact with the host. The Ig are secreted by plasma cells, which are derived from B lymphocytes that are activated by trapping antigens on a cell-surface receptor and stimulation with CD4$^+$ T lymphocytes. Antibodies belong to five different classes of Ig (G, A, M, E, and D, respectively) (Figure 1) [3].

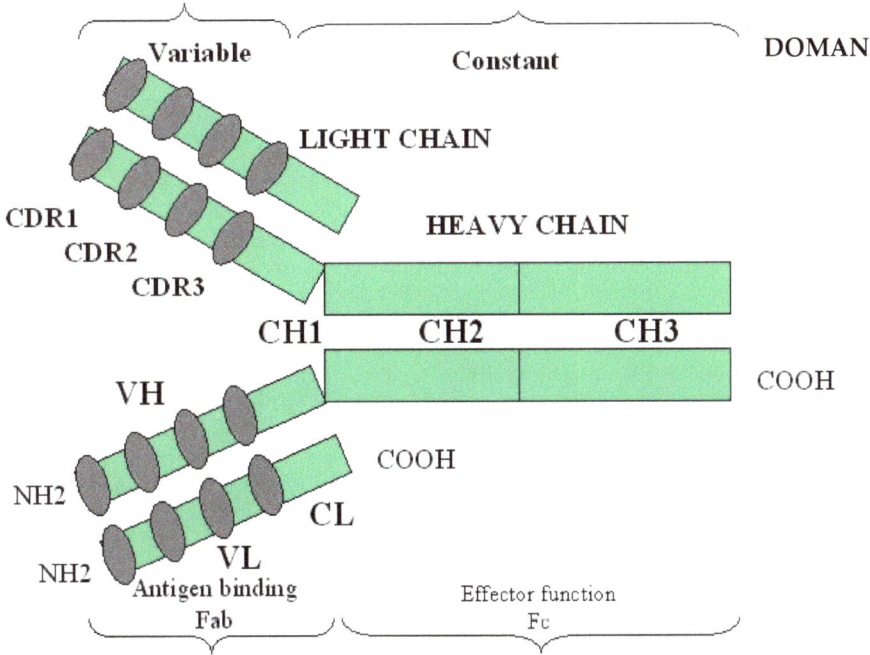

Figure 1. Two-dimensional structure of an IgG molecule. VH and VL indicate the variable regions of the heavy and light chains, respectively. The variable regions located on both the light and heavy chains recognize the epitopes (Fab region). The hypervariable segments located in the Fab regions, which are separated from each other by relatively constant polypeptide chains, are denominated CDR (Complementary Determining Region) domains. The Fc region binds to complement and to the receptors located on the surface of the reticulo-endothelial cells triggering their activation. The region connecting the two functional parts can undergo conformational changes in order to re-shape the molecule according to antigen variability [1].

The molecules belonging to the IgG class are considered the prototypical structure and consist of a Y-shaped molecule formed by two identical heavy (H) and light (L) peptide chains. Both chains are divided into a variable (V) domain that reacts with the antigen, and a constant (C) region that activates the various components of the innate immune system, triggering its response (for example, phagocytosis, antibody-mediated and cell-mediated cytotoxicity, and complement-mediated lysis) (Figure 1). The V regions contain three hypervariable regions that are ultimately responsible for the specific shape of each molecule of Ig. Electrostatic forces in association with disulphuric bridges link the H and L regions together.

Therefore, Ig can be considered biochemical transducers able to exert many different actions (Table 1).

Table 1. Mechanisms of action of the immunoglobulins. ↑: increase; ↓: decrease.

Mechanism	Aims
Toxin inactivation	↑ Clearance of endotoxin and exotoxins ↓ Bacterial cell adherence, invasion, and migration
Stimulation of the leukocytes and serum bactericidal action	↑ Endotoxin-induced neutrophil oxidative burst (7S-IvIgG) ↓ Endotoxin-induced neutrophil oxidative burst (5S-IvIgG; F(ab′)2 fragments and IgM) Enhancement of serum opsonic activity
Modulation of cytokine effect	↓ Pro-Inflammatory mediators ↑ Anti-Inflammatory mediators Cytokine neutralization by anti-cytokine antibodies

For the believers, the different effects exerted by the native Ig on both arms of the immune system could justify the use of IvIgs in clinical circumstances characterized either by (a) an immunodepression due to different causes making the patient prone to newly acquired infections or to the reactivation of latent germs and viruses (see later); or (b) an exaggerated inflammatory response and/or the production of autoantibodies directed against the host's own tissues, including Guillain-Barrè syndrome, Myasthenia Gravis, thrombotic thrombocytopenic purpura (TTP), etc. As far as the former point is concerned, it should be remarked that, besides other causes of immunodepression, this clinical profile is increasingly recognized in chronic critically ill patients, which are often elderly with a number of comorbidities and frailties who survive the initial insult (i.e., septic shock due peritonitis caused by a colon perforation, pneumonia, etc.) but fail to recover and succumb many days if not weeks after the admission [4–8]. This latter condition is characterized by persistent low-grade inflammation, causing muscle wasting that prevents the weaning from mechanical ventilation, which is associated with an overall down-regulation of the immune capabilities with the subsequent occurrence of ICU-acquired infections (see later).

3. The Case of IgM and IgA

Then, once the different actions of the native Ig molecules have been stated, it is worthwhile to describe with more detail the biological properties of the IgM and of IgA. The former is the first Ig to be produced during an infection and has been found throughout all classes of vertebrates, and is present in a dimeric form on the surface of B lymphocytes and circulates as a pentamer (occasionally as a hexamer) in the blood. IgM molecules are the first antibodies produced during infection and appear first during ontogenesis; IgM molecules. Due to their unique structure, IgM molecules form strong interactions with different ligands and have a higher affinity for the complement as compared with IgG [9]. Experimentally, IgMs allow the clearance of apoptotic cells of the reticulo-endothelial system and of the peritoneal macrophages [4]. On the basis of these observations, it is likely that the circulating pentameric IgM molecules bind ligands more avidly than those present on the surface of the B-cells surface but it is not known if, in the presence of reduced blood IgM concentrations, their role could be replaced by the latter [9]. Some investigators demonstrated that IgM concentrations are decreased in septic shock patients and particularly in those with a poor prognosis [10,11]; actually, it appears that reduced levels of this molecule when combined with diminished numbers of natural killer cells (<58 mg/dL and 140 cell/mL, respectively) are associated with an increased risk of death also in non-septic critically ill patients. Should these findings be confirmed in other studies, the supplementation of IgM could be indicated in life-threatening conditions other than sepsis [12].

The IgA molecules are present both in the serum, where they represent the second most prevalent circulating Ig after the IgG, and in the secretions covering the mucosal surface lining the respiratory and the digestive tract, with an overall surface of ~400 m^2 in the adult. These antibodies are present in two different subclasses, named IgA1 and

IgA2 [13]. The IgA molecules exist in multiple forms: in human serum, the prevalent form is monomeric with a subclass distribution of 90% IgA1 and the remaining 10% of IgA2; conversely, in mucosal surfaces, the dimeric form prevails with a more balanced distribution of the two subclasses (40% IgA1 and 60 IgA2). The IgA molecules block or neutralized a number of toxins, bacteria, and viruses and prevent their attachment to the hosts' cells. In contrast to IgG, IgA does not activate the classical complement pathway and likely activates the alternate one via the lectin pathway.

Overall, it appears that the combined administration of IgA and IgM is valuable as it takes advantage of their dual effect in the bloodstream and in the mucosae.

4. Discussion

The history of intensive care medicine is characterized by several hotly debated issues, including the colloid-crystalloids controversy (actually recently replaced by discussions about the best crystalloid solution available), the use of steroids, the appropriate levels of oxygen delivery in critically ill patients, the selective decontamination of the digestive tract, etc. The very same considerations apply to the use of IvIg in septic shock patients and especially for those preparations enriched with supra-normal concentrations of IgM and IgA (eIg). Actually, despite a number of MAs and systematic reviews (SRs) that have demonstrated their efficacy, the current guidelines of the Surviving Sepsis Campaign (SSC) [14] strongly discourage their use primarily due to the absence of large studies robust enough to fulfill the EBM criteria. This notwithstanding, these preparations are widely used in septic shock patients as an add-on treatment aiming not to replace antibiotics or surgery but to enhance the immune capabilities.

To better define the possible role of IvIg and eIg and their possible rules of engagement (ROE) in the treatment of septic shock, it is worthwhile to split the description in different sections.

4.1. Why to Give eIg?

According to the current definition, sepsis and septic shock are life-threatening conditions caused by a dysregulated host's response to an infection leading to multiple organ dysfunctions [15]. Patients with sepsis often present multiple features of immunological alterations, including an initial hyperinflammatory condition that can be followed later on by immunosuppressive events, complement consumption, defects in neutrophil-mediated immunity, and decreased serum levels of immunoglobulins [12]. Sepsis is initiated by the activation of multiple signaling pathways following the recognition and specific cell-surface receptors on cells (toll-like receptors) of pathogen-associated molecular patterns or damage-associated molecular patterns (PAMPs and DAMPs, respectively); the subsequent step consists of the activation of genes involved in inflammation, adaptive immunity, and cellular metabolism, that ultimately determine to the production and release of a huge array of mediators with either pro- and anti-inflammatory capabilities whose respective concentrations vary according to the different phases of the clinical course [5,8].

A number of investigations demonstrated that in septic shock patients, the levels of IgG, IgA, and IgM were decreased, albeit with different effects on the outcome [16–21], and that their contemporaneal reduction was associated with reduced survival [22–24]. Different mechanisms acting alone or in combination can account for these findings, including (a) the reduced secretion of Ig; (b) their leakage into the interstitial space due to the endothelial dysfunction; (c) their redistribution into the inflamed tissues; and (d) their consumption by the complement system [16,21,22,25,26]. However, in a more advanced phase of sepsis, independently from the initial trigger(s), the hyperinflammatory response subsides and in several cases is replaced by a down-regulation of the immune capabilities. Different factors account for these findings, including (a) the increase in the circulating levels of myeloid-derived suppressor cells (MDSCs) that secrete multiple anti-inflammatory cytokines, such as IL-10 and transforming growth factor-β (TGF-β), which blunts the immune function [27,28]; (b) the reduction in committed antigen-presenting dendritic cells and monocytes with the subsequent loss or severe reduction in the associated production of proinflammatory cytokine [29–33]; (c) the depletion of human leukocyte-antigen D related (HLA-DR) in monocytes and dendritic cells also decreases, with the subsequent reduction in responsiveness [34]; (d) the depletion of circulating lymphocytes along with an increase in the apoptosis of dendritic, l cells, T- and B-cells [8]; (e) the upregulation of the immunosuppressant molecules programmed death protein 1 (PD-1), the programmed death ligand 1 (PD-L1) in monocytes and T lymphocytes that eventually determine (a) the expansion of the regulatory T (T-reg) and unresponsive T-cells [28,35,36]; and (b) a down regulation of both the adaptive and innate immune responses [37–39]. The clinical consequence induced by these mechanisms is a persisting low-grade inflammatory state accompanied by an unrelenting hypercatabolism with subsequent muscle wasting and difficult weaning from the mechanical ventilation, the occurrence of re-infections with low-virulence germs, such as Acinetobacter baumanii and the reactivation of viral strains, including Cytomegalovirus and different Herpesviridae.

4.2. Which Are the Available Preparation?

As stated above, the available IvIg preparations can be subdivided into those containing the different classes of immunoglobulins roughly at or slightly above their plasmatic levels and eIg and those containing increased concentrations of IgM and IgA (Table 2).

Table 2. Ig concentration in different preparations. * Not yet available.

Variable		Standard Preparations		IgM and IgA-Enriched Preparations	
Ig Class (%)	Normal Plasma Values	Privigen® CLS Behring, Bern, Switzerland	Polyglobin® Bayer Biol. Prod., Leverkusen, Germany	Pentaglobin® Biotest, Dreiech, Germany	Triglobin® * Biotest, Dreiech, Germany
Ig G	80	>98	>97	56	76
Ig M	7	Traces	Traces	12	23
Ig A	13	Traces	Traces	12	21
Clinical experiences in ICU patients		Septic shock Autoimmune disorders	Septic shock Autoimmune disorders	Septic shock	Severe Community-Acquired Pneumonia

Presently, standard IvIgs and Pentaglobin® have been used in the treatment of septic shock from multiple causes, whereas Triglobin® has been used in an RCT involving septic patients with severe community-acquired pneumonia [40].

Although all polyclonal IvIgs share similar effects on the inflammatory and immune mechanisms and represent a valuable approach to modulate both the pro- and anti-inflammatory processes, differences exist among the various available preparations. Actually, while different studies demonstrated that the administration of IvIg preparations containing only IgG was not associated with improved mortality rates in patients with sepsis [41–43], some MAs and SRs have concluded that patients given eIg presented a reduction in mortality of up to 18% [44–47].

4.3. Who Are the Best Candidates for eIg (and Who Are Not)?

As stated above, it appears that possible candidates for eIg can be basically subdivided into two groups according to their clinical features (Table 3).

The former includes patients at the onset of septic shock who can take advantage both from the antibacterial properties of eIg and of their modulation of the early hyperinflammatory response, whereas the latter includes those with an immunocompromised phenotype, often with a prolonged length-of-stay in the ICU who develop a chronic critical illness whose features have been described in the preceding paragraphs. Due to the unrelenting aging of the population in Western countries, it is likely that in the next few years, the number of these patients will increase [48]. As far as the responsible germs are concerned, septic shock patients due to Gram-negative infections are most likely to take advantage of eIg; among Gram-positive strains, a positive effect on the outcome has been reported in patients with severe invasive group A streptococci infections, especially in streptococcal toxic shock syndrome associated with myositis or fasciitis [49]. As far as either the site of infection or non-responding patients are concerned, it appears that (a) the eIg have been successfully used independently from the initial inoculum; but (b) in different studies, patients with hematological diseases did not benefit from their administration [50].

Table 3. Different clinical courses of septic patients. Legend: ↑: Increase; ↓: Decrease; ↑↑: Marked increase.

Variable	Early Response	Late Response
Patient population	Young, middle-aged	Elderly
Comorbidities	Often absent, no or few frailties	Present, often multiples
Microorganisms	Highly virulent, toxin releasing	Low virulence, opportunistic Viral reactivation
Clinical phenotype	Septic shock, high fever, ARDS, fast-evolving MODS, community-acquired infections	Altered mental status
Laboratory findings	↑↑/↓ White blood cell ↑ Lactate levels	↓ Lymphocytes
Possible clinical trajectories	Resolution of sepsis Restoration of the immunitary capabilities Early deaths	Protracted ICU length of stay Hypercatabolism and protein waste Difficult weaning from the mechanical ventilation Late deaths

Legend: ARDS: acute respiratory distress syndrome; MODS: multiple-organ dysfunction syndrome.

4.4. When to Treat?

The SSC guidelines consider sepsis and septic shock as time-dependent clinical entities [14]. This assumption is based on different investigations that demonstrated an association between each hour of delay in the administration of (appropriate) antibiotics and a measurable increase in the mortality rate [51–53]. That said, due to the absence of clinical evidence, the most appropriate window of opportunity for the administration of eIg remains substantially undetermined. Consequently, it appears that different approaches can be used (Table 4).

Table 4. Possible criteria for the initiation of eIg.

Trigger	Pros	Cons
Low circulating Ig levels	Physiological basis	Long turnaround time not available on a H24-basis throughout the week; Unknown appropriate levels of IgA and IgM in septic shock
Prediction of septic shock (TO-PIRO)	Easy to assess	None
Time lag since the onset of septic shock	Easy to assess	Time lag often approximated

The first is based on the measurement of circulating concentrations of the different classes of Ig that are frequently reduced in septic shock patients; actually, as stated above, several if not all investigations demonstrated an association between low blood levels of native Ig and the outcome of septic patients. This issue appears somewhat controversial because, whereas some investigators found that either isolated or combined low levels of IgG, IgM, and IgA were associated with a decreased survival [16–20] and Giomarellos-Bourboulis et al. [11] showed that the transition from severe sepsis to septic shock and death was marked by decreased blood levels of IgM, other authors reported different results; actually, in a recent meta-analysis (MA), Shankar-Hari et al. [21] demonstrated that low levels of IgG and IgM in septic patients were not associated with a poor outcome. Then, whereas it appears reasonable to restore abnormally low levels of Ig, it is not clear (yet) whether "normal" levels can be considered appropriate in septic shock as their consumption is likely increased as compared to non-septic conditions [54].

Another potential method of guiding the administration of IgM-enriched immunoglobulins is the use of a scoring system, such as the Torino (TO)-PIRO score [55]. This has been developed on the basis of multiple investigations and differs from the original PIRO system [56] as it does not describe the clinical course but rather the underlying medical conditions favoring the occurrence of septic shock, such as the underlying chronic disorders (predisposition), the possible precipitating factors (insult), the host's reaction to the infection (response), and the possible systemic complications (organ) (Table 5).

Table 5. The TO-PIRO score.

Items	Criteria	Score
Predisposition	Uncontrolled cancer	1
	Colonization with MDR bacteria and/or candida	1
	Neutropenia or immunosuppression or allogenic stem cell transplant or splenectomy	2
Insult	Necrotizing fasciitis, invasive meningococcal or pneumococcal disease, MRSA	5
	MDR infections or nosocomial infections	2
	Secondary or tertiary peritonitis	2
Response	Leukocytes < 600/mL	2
	IgM < 60 mg/dL	2
	PCT > 10 ng/L or CRP > 20 mg/dL	1
	PCT > 100 ng/L–Il-6 > 1000 pg/mL–endotoxin > 06–presepsin > 1400 ng/L	2
	Disseminated intravascular coagulation	1
Organ	Septic shock	3
	Sepsis with >1 organ failure	2
	Infection without sepsis	1

Legend; MDR: multiple-drug resistant; IgM: M-class immunoglobulin; MRSA: methicillin-resistant S. aureus; PCT: procalcitonin; CRP: C-reactive protein.

Then, on the basis of the score, it could be possible to identify patients who could benefit from the administration of eIg (Table 6).

Table 6. Possible approaches according to the score values.

TO-PIRO Score	Suggestions	Timing
<5	The administration of eIg may be beneficial	Undetermined
5–10	The administration of eIg is suggested	Possibly within 24 h of clinical presentation
>10	The administration of eIg is recommended *	As soon as possible and within 6 h

* Evidence showed reduced mortality in septic shock patients treated with eIg as compared with non-treated patients.

The last approach basically consists of the administration of eIg immediately after the diagnosis of septic shock. Berlot et al. [57] demonstrated that in 355 septic shock patients, there was an increase of ~2% mortality rate for each 24 h delay in the administration of eIg; however, as stated by the authors, this approach is flawed, which is an inherent risk of approximation as the onset of septic shock is not always immediately recognizable especially when it occurs outside the ICU. However, the score has its own inherent limitations and requires validation in clinical practice and using results gathered from large databases.

4.5. Which Dosage?

The summary of product characteristics currently recommends eIg therapy at a dose of 0.25 g/kg body weight/day for 3 consecutive days, but further infusions may be required according to the clinical course. Actually, even if the appropriate levels of immunoglobulins are far from being established, it is reasonable to increase their levels rapidly. To this aim, Rodriguez et al. [55] used a higher dose of eIg (1–2 mg/kg/day for 5 days) in a group of severe sepsis and septic shock surgical patients and observed an improved outcome in the treatment as compared to the control group. Moreover, in order to adapt the treatment to the patients and not vice versa, two different RCTs are currently underway; in the former, the dose of eIg is titrated on the levels of native IgM [58], and in the latter, on the concentrations of some immunologic biomarkers [59]. In order to achieve a patient-tailored treatment, it could be useful to perform repeated measurements during the eIg infusion to measure the circulating levels of the different classes of Ig in order to make sure the dose is adequate according to their and/or variations. Recently, Berlot et al. [54] demonstrated in a group of septic shock patients that the trajectories of IgM and IgA differed between survivors and non-survivors since, whereas the IgG and the IgA increased in both groups, in survivors, the IgM more than doubled at the end of the infusion and almost tripled 7 days later. Different mechanisms can account for these findings, including (a) the ongoing production of endogenous IgG and IgA possibly associated with the reduced production and/or the consumption of IgM in non-survivors; (b) a higher pathogen or PAMP load and the consequent increased opsonization and clearance of the IgM molecule; and (c) the leaking from the bloodstream into the interstitial space of IgM through a more permeable capillary endothelium of non-survivors.

5. Original Sins & Open Issues

The skepticism of the SSC guidelines concerning the use of eIg stems from the original sins of the published studies that prevent definite conclusions from being drawn from these studies. The main limitations of these investigations include:

(a) The uncertainness of the timing of administration in relationship with the onset of septic shock appears to be a relevant issue as the outcome of these patients appears to be a time-dependent variable.
(b) The not always indicated appropriateness of the concomitant treatments, such as antibiotics and surgical drainage of septic foci.
(c) The lack of risk stratification of patients, which is very often lumped together without taking into consideration the underlying chronic diseases and subsequent frailties.
(d) The clinical phase of their administration; actually, as stated above, the immune conditions of septic patients can vary according to the time elapsed from the initial insult.
(e) The absence of information about the blood concentrations of native Ig, as well as of other immunological variables before the administration of the eIg.

6. Frequently Asked Questions

(a) Is it possible to give eIg to patients undergoing renal replacement treatments and/or other forms of blood purification? Yes, because their molecular weight is too high to be removed or absorbed by commonly used devices; however, they can be removed by plasma exchange [60]. In this case. the eIg should be given after the procedure.
(b) What are the possible harmful side effects? The eIg are well tolerated; however, either a hyperviscosity syndrome or acute renal failure have been occasionally reported, which were likely due to the stabilizers rather than the Ig molecules [61]. Both occurrences can be prevented by adequate hydration.

7. Conclusions

Independently from their composition, the use of IvIgs in sepsis is a widespread practice not encouraged by the current SSC as the published studies are flawed by a number of biases, including the heterogeneity of the enrolled patients, the different ROE, the often unspecified timing of initiation, the appropriateness of the antibiotic treatments, etc. [62]. Even taking into account these original sins, they are valuable adjunctive measures if administered as soon as possible after the onset of septic shock. A step toward precision medicine could be constituted by the titration of the dose according to the patient's immunological or biochemical response aiming for a personalized approach rather than a "one-size-fits-all" policy.

Funding: This research received no external funding.

Institutional Review Board Statement: Not applicable.

Informed Consent Statement: Not applicable.

Data Availability Statement: All data are available.

Conflicts of Interest: The authors declare no conflict of interest.

References

1. Berlot, G.; Rossini, P.; Turchet, F. Biology of immunoglobulins. *Transl. Med. UniSa* **2014**, *11*, 24–27.
2. Mantovani, A.; Garlanda, C. Humoral Innate Immunity and Acute-Phase Proteins. *N. Engl. J. Med.* **2023**, *388*, 439–452. [CrossRef] [PubMed]
3. Medzhitov, R.; Janeway, C. Advances in immunology: Innate immunity. *N. Engl. J. Med.* **2000**, *343*, 337–344. [CrossRef] [PubMed]
4. Späth, P.J. Structure and function of immunoglobulins. *Sepsis* **1999**, *3*, 197–218. [CrossRef]
5. Cecconi, M.; Evans, L.; Levy, M.; Rhodes, A. Sepsis and septic shock. *Lancet* **2018**, *392*, 75–87. [CrossRef] [PubMed]
6. Hotchkiss, R.S.; Karl, I.E. The pathophysiology and treatment of sepsis. *N. Engl. J. Med.* **2003**, *348*, 138–150. [CrossRef]
7. Hotchkiss, R.S.; Monneret, G.; Payen, D. Immunosuppression in sepsis: A novel understanding of the disorder and a new therapeutic approach. *Lancet Infect. Dis.* **2013**, *13*, 260–268. [CrossRef]
8. Jarczak, D.; Kluge, S.; Nierhaus, A. Sepsis-Pathophysiology and Therapeutic Concepts. *Front. Med.* **2021**, *8*, 628302. [CrossRef]
9. Ehrenstein, M.R.; Notley, C.A. The importance of natural IgM: Scavenger, protector and regulator. *Nat. Rev. Immunol.* **2010**, *10*, 778–786. [CrossRef]
10. Venet, F.; Gebeile, R.; Bancel, J.; Guignant, C.; Poitevin-Later, F.; Malcus, C.; Lepape, A.; Monneret, G. Assessment of plasmatic immunoglobulin G, A and M levels in septic shock patients. *Int. Immunopharmacol.* **2011**, *11*, 2086–2090. [CrossRef]
11. Giamarellos-Bourboulis, E.J.; Apostolidou, E.; Lada, M. Kinetics of circulating immunoglobulin M in sepsis: Relationship with final outcome. *Crit. Care* **2013**, *17*, R247–R256. [CrossRef] [PubMed]
12. Andaluz-Ojeda, D.; Iglesias, V.; Bobillo, F.; Nocito, M.; Loma, A.M.; Nieto, C.; Ramos, E.; Gandía, F.; Rico, L.; Bermejo-Martin, J.F. Early levels in blood of immunoglobulin M and natural killer cells predict outcome in nonseptic critically ill patients. *J. Crit. Care* **2013**, *28*, 1110.e7–1110.e10. [CrossRef] [PubMed]
13. de Sousa-Pereira, P.; Woof, J.M. IgA: Structure, Function, and Developability. *Antibodies* **2019**, *8*, 57. [CrossRef]
14. Evans, L.; Rhodes, A.; Alhazzani, W.; Antonelli, M.; Coopersmith, C.M.; French, C.; Machado, F.R.; Mcintyre, L.; Ostermann, M.; Prescott, H.C.; et al. Surviving sepsis campaign: International guidelines for management of sepsis and septic shock 2021. *Intensive Care Med.* **2021**, *47*, 1181–1247. [CrossRef]
15. Singer, M.; Deutschman, C.S.; Seymour, C.W.; Shankar-Hari, M.; Annane, D.; Bauer, M.; Bellomo, R.; Bernard, G.R.; Chiche, J.D.; Coopersmith, C.M.; et al. The Third International Consensus Definitions for Sepsis and Septic Shock (Sepsis-3). *JAMA* **2016**, *315*, 801–810. [CrossRef] [PubMed]
16. Bermejo-Martin, J.F.; Andaluz-Ojeda, D.; Almansa, R.; Gandía, F.; Gómez-Herreras, J.I.; Gomez-Sanchez, E.; Heredia-Rodríguez, M.; Eiros, J.M.; Kelvin, D.J.; Tamayo, E. Defining immunological dysfunction in sepsis: A requisite tool for precision medicine. *J. Infect.* **2016**, *72*, 525–536. [CrossRef]
17. Taccone, F.S.; Stordeur, P.; De Backer, D.; Creteur, J.; Vincent, J.L. Gamma-globulin levels in patients with community-acquired septic shock. *Shock* **2009**, *32*, 379–385. [CrossRef] [PubMed]
18. Andaluz-Ojeda, D.; Iglesias, V.; Bobillo, F.; Almansa, R.; Rico, L.; Gandía, F.; Loma, A.M.; Nieto, C.; Diego, R.; Ramos, E.; et al. Early natural killer cell counts in blood predict mortality in severe sepsis. *Crit. Care* **2011**, *15*, R243. [CrossRef]
19. Tamayo, E.; Fernández, A.; Almansa, R.; Carrasco, E.; Goncalves, L.; Heredia, M.; Andaluz-Ojeda, D.; March, G.; Rico, L.; Gómez-Herreras, J.I.; et al. Beneficial role of endogenous immunoglobulin subclasses and isotypes in septic shock. *J. Crit. Care* **2012**, *27*, 616–622. [CrossRef]
20. Průcha, M.; Zazula, R.; Herold, I.; Dostál, M.; Hyánek, T.; Bellingan, G. Presence of hypogammaglobulinemia—A risk factor of mortality in patients with severe sepsis, septic shock, and SIRS. *Prague Med. Rep.* **2013**, *114*, 246–257. [CrossRef]
21. Shankar-Hari, M.; Culshaw, N.; Post, B.; Tamayo, E.; Andaluz-Ojeda, D.; Bermejo-Martín, J.F.; Dietz, S.; Werdan, K.; Beale, R.; Spencer, J.; et al. Endogenous IgG hypogammaglobulinaemia in critically ill adults with sepsis: Systematic review and meta-analysis. *Intensive Care Med.* **2015**, *41*, 1393–1401. [CrossRef] [PubMed]

22. Bermejo-Martín, J.F.; Rodriguez-Fernandez, A.; Herrán-Monge, R.; Andaluz-Ojeda, D.; Muriel-Bombín, A.; Merino, P.; García-García, M.M.; Citores, R.; Gandía, F.; Almansa, R.; et al. Immunoglobulins IgG1, IgM and IgA: A synergistic team influencing survival in sepsis. *J. Intern. Med.* **2014**, *276*, 404–412. [CrossRef] [PubMed]
23. Bermejo-Martin, J.F.; Giamarellos-Bourboulis, E.J. Endogenous immunoglobulins and sepsis: New perspectives for guiding replacement therapies. *Int. J. Antimicrob. Agents* **2015**, *46* (Suppl. S1), S25–S28. [CrossRef] [PubMed]
24. Krautz, C.; Maier, S.L.; Brunner, M.; Langheinrich, M.; Giamarellos-Bourboulis, E.J.; Gogos, C.; Armaganidis, A.; Kunath, F.; Grützmann, R.; Weber, G.F. Reduced circulating B cells and plasma IgM levels are associated with decreased survival in sepsis—A meta-analysis. *J. Crit. Care* **2018**, *45*, 71–75. [CrossRef]
25. Shankar-Hari, M.; Spencer, J.; Sewell, W.A.; Rowan, K.M.; Singer, M. Bench-to-bedside review: Immunoglobulin therapy for sepsis e biological plausibility from a critical care perspective. *Crit. Care* **2012**, *16*, 206. [CrossRef]
26. Almansa, R.; Tamayo, E.; Heredia, M.; Gutierrez, S.; Ruiz, P.; Alvarez, E.; Gomez-Sanchez, E.; Andaluz-Ojeda, D.; Ceña, R.; Rico, L.; et al. Transcriptomic evidence of impaired immunoglobulin G production in fatal septic shock. *J. Crit. Care* **2014**, *29*, 307–309. [CrossRef]
27. Cuenca, A.G.; Delano, M.J.; Kelly-Scumpia, K.M.; Moreno, C.; Scumpia, P.O.; LaFace, D.M.; Heyworth, P.G.; Efron, P.A.; Moldawer, L.L. A paradoxical role for myeloid-derived suppressor cells in sepsis and trauma. A study demonstrating that the expansion of MDSCs in sepsis can be associated with the preservation of innate immunity, even in the presence of adaptive immune suppression. *Mol. Med.* **2011**, *17*, 281–292. [CrossRef]
28. Hotchkiss, R.S.; Moldawer, L.L.; Opal, S.M.; Reinhart, K.; Turnbull, I.R.; Vincent, J.L. Sepsis and septic shock. *Nat. Rev. Dis. Primers* **2016**, *2*, 16045. [CrossRef]
29. Cazalis, M.A.; Friggeri, A.; Cavé, L.; Demaret, J.; Barbalat, V.; Cerrato, E.; Lepape, A.; Pachot, A.; Monneret, G.; Venet, F. Decreased HLA-DR antigen-associated invariant chain (CD74) mRNA expression predicts mortality after septic shock. *Crit. Care* **2013**, *17*, R287. [CrossRef]
30. Bhardwaj, N.; Mathur, P.; Kumar, S.; Gupta, A.; Gupta, D.; John, N.V.; Varghese, P.; Misra, M.C. Depressed monocytic activity may be a predictor for sepsis. *J. Lab. Physicians* **2015**, *7*, 26.e31. [CrossRef]
31. Fan, X.; Liu, Z.; Jin, H.; Yan, J.; Liang, H.P. Alterations of dendritic cells in sepsis: Featured role in immunoparalysis. *Biomed. Res. Int.* **2015**, *2015*, 903720. [CrossRef] [PubMed]
32. Kjaergaard, A.G.; Nielsen, J.S.; Tønnesen, E.; Krog, J. Expression of NK cell and monocyte receptors in critically ill patients-potential biomarkers of sepsis. *Scand. J. Immunol.* **2015**, *81*, 249–258. [CrossRef] [PubMed]
33. Shalova, I.N.; Lim, J.Y.; Chittezhath, M.; Zinkernagel, A.S.; Beasley, F.; Hernández-Jiménez, E.; Toledano, V.; Cubillos-Zapata, C.; Rapisarda, A.; Chen, J.; et al. Human monocytes undergo functional re-programming during sepsis mediated by hypoxia-inducible factor-1a. *Immunity* **2015**, *42*, 484.e98. [CrossRef] [PubMed]
34. Hynninen, M.; Pettilä, V.; Takkunen, O.; Orko, R.; Jansson, S.E.; Kuusela, P.; Renkonen, R.; Valtonen, M. Predictive value of monocyte histocompatibility leukocyte antigen-DR expression and plasma interleukin-4 and -10 levels in critically ill patients with sepsis. *Shock* **2003**, *20*, 1–4. [CrossRef]
35. Guignant, C.; Lepape, A.; Huang, X.; Kherouf, H.; Denis, L.; Poitevin, F.; Malcus, C.; Chéron, A.; Allaouchiche, B.; Gueyffier, F.; et al. Programmed death-1 levels correlate with increased mortality, nosocomial infection and immune dysfunctions in septic shock patients. *Crit. Care* **2011**, *15*, R99. [CrossRef]
36. Zhang, Y.; Li, J.; Lou, J.; Zhou, Y.; Bo, L.; Zhu, J.; Wan, X.; Cai, Z.; Deng, X. Upregulation of programmed death-1 on T cells and programmed death ligand-1 on monocytes in septic shock patients. *Crit. Care* **2011**, *15*, R70. [CrossRef]
37. Monneret, G.; Debard, A.L.; Venet, F.; Bohe, J.; Hequet, O.; Bienvenu, J.; Lepape, A. Marked elevation of human circulating CD4+CD25+ regulatory T cells in sepsis-induced immunoparalysis. *Crit. Care Med.* **2003**, *31*, 2068–2071. [CrossRef]
38. Hein, F.; Massin, F.; Cravoisy-Popovic, A.; Barraud, D.; Levy, B.; Bollaert, P.E.; Gibot, S. The relationship between CD4+CD25+CD127- regulatory T cells and inflammatory response and outcome during shock states. *Crit. Care* **2010**, *14*, R19. [CrossRef]
39. Cao, C.; Ma, T.; Chai, Y.F.; Shou, S.T. The role of regulatory T cells in immune dysfunction during sepsis. *World J. Emerg. Med.* **2015**, *6*, 5–9. [CrossRef]
40. Welte, T.; Dellinger, R.P.; Ebelt, H.; Ferrer, M.; Opal, S.M.; Singer, M.; Vincent, J.L.; Werdan, K.; Martin-Loeches, I.; Almirall, J.; et al. Efficacy and safety of trimodulin, a novel polyclonal antibody preparation, in patients with severe community-acquired pneumonia: A randomized, placebo-controlled, double-blind, multicenter, phase II trial (CIGMA study). *Intensive Care Med.* **2018**, *44*, 438–448. [CrossRef]
41. Busani, S.; Damiani, E.; Cavazzuti, I.; Donati, A.; Girardis, M. Intravenous immunoglobulin in septic shock: Review of the mechanisms of action and meta-analysis of the clinical effectiveness. *Minerva Anestesiol.* **2016**, *82*, 559–572.
42. Werdan, K.; Pilz, G.; Bujdoso, O.; Fraunberger, P.; Neeser, G.; Schmieder, R.E.; Viell, B.; Marget, W.; Seewald, M.; Walger, P.; et al. Score-based immunoglobulin G therapy of patients with sepsis: The SBITS study. *Crit. Care Med.* **2007**, *35*, 2693–2701.
43. Werdan, K.; Pilz, G.; Müller-Werdan, U.; Maas Enriquez, M.; Schmitt, D.V.; Mohr, F.W.; Neeser, G.; Schöndube, F.; Schäfers, H.J.; Haverich, A.; et al. Immunoglobulin G treatment of postcardiac surgery patients with score-identified severe systemic inflammatory response syndrome—The ESSICS study. *Crit. Care Med.* **2008**, *36*, 716–723. [CrossRef]
44. INIS Collaborative Group; Brocklehurst, P.; Farrell, B.; King, A.; Juszczak, E.; Darlow, B.; Haque, K.; Salt, A.; Stenson, B.; Tarnow-Mordi, W. Treatment of neonatal sepsis with intravenous immune globulin. *N. Engl. J. Med.* **2011**, *365*, 1201–1211.

45. Alejandria, M.M.; Lansang, M.A.; Dans, L.F.; Mantaring, J.B., 3rd. Intravenous immunoglobulin for treating sepsis, severe sepsis and septic shock. *Cochrane Database Syst. Rev.* **2013**, *2013*, CD001090. [CrossRef]
46. Kreymann, K.G.; de Heer, G.; Nierhaus, A.; Kluge, S. Use of polyclonal immunoglobulins as adjunctive therapy for sepsis or septic shock. *Crit. Care Med.* **2007**, *35*, 2677–2685. [PubMed]
47. Cui, J.; Wei, X.; Lv, H.; Li, Y.; Li, P.; Chen, Z.; Liu, G. The clinical efficacy of intravenous IgM-enriched immunoglobulin (pentaglobin) in sepsis or septic shock: A meta-analysis with trial sequential analysis. *Ann. Intensive Care* **2019**, *9*, 27. [CrossRef] [PubMed]
48. Yende, S.; Kellum, J.A.; Talisa, V.B.; Peck Palmer, O.M.; Chang, C.H.; Filbin, M.R.; Shapiro, N.I.; Hou, P.C.; Venkat, A.; LoVecchio, F.; et al. Long-term Host Immune Response Trajectories among Hospitalized Patients with Sepsis. *JAMA Netw. Open* **2019**, *2*, e198686. [CrossRef] [PubMed]
49. Nierhaus, A.; Berlot, G.; Kindgen-Milles, D.; Müller, E.; Girardis, M. Best-practice IgM- and IgA-enriched immunoglobulin use in patients with sepsis. *Ann. Intensive Care* **2020**, *10*, 132. [CrossRef]
50. Fernandes, P.A.; Russo, F.T.; da Silva, L.A.M.; Ramos, L.W.F.; de Almeida Simões, A.; Okada, L.Y.; Cavalcante, J.N.; Ferreira Lopes, M.A.V.; de Almeida Macedo, M.C.M.; da Silva, R.L. The Role of IgM-Enriched Immunoglobulin (Pentaglobin) in Septic Patients with Hematological Disease. *Int. J. Hematol. Oncol. Stem Cell Res.* **2021**, *15*, 103–113. [CrossRef]
51. Kumar, A.; Roberts, D.; Wood, K.E.; Light, B.; Parrillo, J.E.; Sharma, S.; Suppes, R.; Feinstein, D.; Zanotti, S.; Taiberg, L.; et al. Duration of hypotension before initiation of effective antimicrobial therapy is the critical determinant of survival in human septic shock. *Crit. Care Med.* **2006**, *34*, 1589–1596. [CrossRef] [PubMed]
52. Seymour, C.W.; Kahn, J.M.; Martin-Gill, C.; Callaway, C.W.; Yealy, D.M.; Scales, D.; Angus, D.C. Delays From First Medical Contact to Antibiotic Administration for Sepsis. *Crit. Care Med.* **2017**, *45*, 759–765. [CrossRef] [PubMed]
53. Gaieski, D.F.; Mikkelsen, M.E.; Band, R.A.; Pines, J.M.; Massone, R.; Furia, F.F.; Shofer, F.S.; Goyal, M. Impact of time to antibiotics on survival in patients with severe sepsis or septic shock in whom early goal-directed therapy was initiated in the emergency department. *Crit. Care Med.* **2010**, *38*, 1045–1053. [CrossRef]
54. Berlot, G.; Scamperle, A.; Istrati, T.; Dattola, R.; Longo, I.; Chillemi, A.; Baronio, S.; Quarantotto, G.; Zanchi, S.; Roman-Pognuz, E.; et al. Kinetics of Immunoglobulins in Septic Shock Patients Treated with an IgM- and IgA-Enriched Intravenous Preparation: An Observational Study. *Front. Med.* **2021**, *8*, 605113. [CrossRef]
55. De Rosa, F.G.; Corcione, S.; Tascini, C.; Pasero, D.; Rocchetti, A.; Massaia, M.; Berlot, G.; Solidoro, P.; Girardis, M. A position paper on IgM-enriched intravenous immunoglobulin adjunctive therapy in severe acute bacterial infections: The TO-PIRO SCORE proposal. *New Microbiol.* **2019**, *41*, 176–180.
56. Rubulotta, F.; Marshall, J.C.; Ramsay, G.; Nelson, D.; Levy, M.; Williams, M. Predisposition, insult/infection, response, and organ dysfunction: A new model for staging severe sepsis. *Crit. Care Med.* **2009**, *37*, 1329–1335. [CrossRef] [PubMed]
57. Berlot, G.; Vassallo, M.C.; Busetto, N.; Nieto Yabar, M.; Istrati, T.; Baronio, S.; Quarantotto, G.; Bixio, M.; Barbati, G.; Dattola, R.; et al. Effects of the timing of administration of IgM- and IgA-enriched intravenous polyclonal immunoglobulins on the outcome of septic shock patients. *Ann. Intensive Care* **2018**, *8*, 122, Erratum in: *Ann Intensive Care* **2019**, *9*, 33. [CrossRef]
58. Busani, S.; Roat, E.; Tosi, M.; Biagioni, E.; Coloretti, I.; Meschiari, M.; Gelmini, R.; Brugioni, L.; De Biasi, S.; Girardis, M. Adjunctive Immunotherapy with Polyclonal Ig-M Enriched Immunoglobulins for Septic Shock: From Bench to Bedside. The Rationale for a Personalized Treatment Protocol. *Front. Med.* **2021**, *8*, 616511. [CrossRef]
59. Kalvelage, C.; Zacharowski, K.; Bauhofer, A.; Gockel, U.; Adamzik, M.; Nierhaus, A.; Kujath, P.; Eckmann, C.; Pletz, M.W.; Bracht, H.; et al. Personalized medicine with IgGAM compared with standard of care for treatment of peritonitis after infectious source control (the PEPPER trial): Study protocol for a randomized controlled trial. *Trials* **2019**, *20*, 156. [CrossRef]
60. Berlot, G.; Di Bella, S.; Tomasini, A.; Roman-Pognuz, E. The Effects of Hemoadsorption on the Kinetics of Antibacterial and Antifungal Agents. *Antibiotics* **2022**, *11*, 180. [CrossRef]
61. Dantal, J. Intravenous immunoglobulins: In-depth review of excipients and acute kidney injury risk. *Am. J. Nephrol.* **2013**, *38*, 275–284. [CrossRef] [PubMed]
62. Di Rosa, R.; Pietrosanti, M.; Luzi, G.; Salemi, S.; D'Amelio, R. Polyclonal intravenous immunoglobulin: An important additional strategy in sepsis? *Eur. J. Intern. Med.* **2014**, *25*, 511–516. [CrossRef] [PubMed]

Disclaimer/Publisher's Note: The statements, opinions and data contained in all publications are solely those of the individual author(s) and contributor(s) and not of MDPI and/or the editor(s). MDPI and/or the editor(s) disclaim responsibility for any injury to people or property resulting from any ideas, methods, instructions or products referred to in the content.

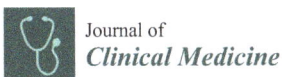

Review

General Critical Care, Temperature Control, and End-of-Life Decision Making in Patients Resuscitated from Cardiac Arrest

Athanasios Chalkias [1,2,*], Georgios Adamos [3] and Spyros D. Mentzelopoulos [3]

1. Department of Anesthesiology, Faculty of Medicine, University of Thessaly, 41500 Larisa, Greece
2. Outcomes Research Consortium, Cleveland, OH 44195, USA
3. First Department of Intensive Care Medicine, National and Kapodistrian University of Athens Medical School, 10675 Athens, Greece; george.adamos1983@gmail.com (G.A.); sdmentzelopoulos@yahoo.com (S.D.M.)
* Correspondence: thanoschalkias@yahoo.gr

Abstract: Cardiac arrest affects millions of people per year worldwide. Although advances in cardiopulmonary resuscitation and intensive care have improved outcomes over time, neurologic impairment and multiple organ dysfunction continue to be associated with a high mortality rate. The pathophysiologic mechanisms underlying the post-resuscitation disease are complex, and a coordinated, evidence-based approach to post-resuscitation care has significant potential to improve survival. Critical care management of patients resuscitated from cardiac arrest focuses on the identification and treatment of the underlying cause(s), hemodynamic and respiratory support, organ protection, and active temperature control. This review provides a state-of-the-art appraisal of critical care management of the post-cardiac arrest patient.

Keywords: cardiac arrest; post-resuscitation care; intensive care medicine; critical care; outcome

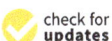

Citation: Chalkias, A.; Adamos, G.; Mentzelopoulos, S.D. General Critical Care, Temperature Control, and End-of-Life Decision Making in Patients Resuscitated from Cardiac Arrest. *J. Clin. Med.* 2023, 12, 4118. https://doi.org/10.3390/jcm12124118

Academic Editors: Federico Franchi and Andrea Fabbri

Received: 5 May 2023
Revised: 2 June 2023
Accepted: 14 June 2023
Published: 18 June 2023

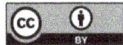

Copyright: © 2023 by the authors. Licensee MDPI, Basel, Switzerland. This article is an open access article distributed under the terms and conditions of the Creative Commons Attribution (CC BY) license (https://creativecommons.org/licenses/by/4.0/).

1. Introduction

For decades, the main focus of resuscitation research was the quality and effectiveness of cardiopulmonary resuscitation (CPR), which led to an increased probability of a return of spontaneous circulation (ROSC). In recent years, optimizing neurologically intact survival from cardiac arrest has been established as the primary aim of resuscitation scientists. Nevertheless, survival rates with good neurological outcomes vary substantially and depend on the location and circumstances of the arrest, the medical team's ability to restore perfusion to the heart, and the quality of post-resuscitation care [1–3].

The unique and complex pathophysiologic mechanisms underlying post-resuscitation disease increase the complexity of management. Patient-related factors, etiology of cardiac arrest, and initial rhythm can further complicate medical care and have a critical impact on outcomes. Unfortunately, the variation in post-cardiac arrest management and the lack of well-organized regional cardiac arrest centers remain important concerns and hamper international efforts toward the standardization of care.

Despite advances in resuscitation science, neurologic impairment, and multiple organ dysfunction cause considerable mortality and morbidity. High-quality post-resuscitation care has significant potential to reduce early mortality but requires major diagnostic and therapeutic resources and specific training. This review provides a state-of-the-art appraisal of critical care management of the post-cardiac arrest patient.

2. Pathophysiology

Post-cardiac arrest syndrome is a complex entity, including myocardial dysfunction, brain injury, the effects of ischemia and reperfusion, and the precipitating pathology or comorbidities as key features. Furthermore, this syndrome can involve injuries caused during the peri-arrest period and several systemic complications that may occur after

ROSC, such as acute respiratory distress syndrome, acute renal failure, refractory shock, and disseminated intravascular coagulation [4].

Post-resuscitation myocardial dysfunction is observed in up to two-thirds of patients resuscitated from cardiac arrest, even in the absence of prior cardiac disease, and is characterized by the absence of irreversible damage, as well as normal or near-normal coronary flow [5]. Systolic dysfunction of variable severity is commonly identified, but diastolic dysfunction is less frequently reported [6–8]. However, in almost all patients, the syndrome is characterized by reduced global contractility, decreased myocardial compliance, and increased microvascular permeability with myocardial edema, all affecting cardiac output. The latter is further impaired due to myocardial injury, metabolic deviation, energy depletion, electrolyte disorders, and the increased formation of reactive oxygen species, which destabilize membrane depolarization and electrical activity [5,6,9].

Post-cardiac arrest brain injury involves a complex cascade of molecular mechanisms, most of which remain unknown. After ROSC, several cytokines are upregulated and promote neutrophil infiltration, while the endothelium becomes more dysfunctional and nitric oxide formation decreases. These result in impaired vasodilation and platelet/neutrophil accumulation, increasing the cerebral microvessel vascular tone and extending tissue injury [5]. The enhancement of blood coagulation, which has already begun during CPR, enhances microthrombosis, while the opening of mitochondrial permeability transition pore results in mitochondrial dysfunction, cytochrome c leakage into the cytoplasm, and activation of delayed neuronal death pathways [10–12]. Post-cardiac arrest brain injury may be further exacerbated by microcirculatory failure, impaired autoregulation, hypercarbia, hypo- or hyperoxia, pyrexia, hyperglycemia, anemia, and seizures [5,13–15]. In most patients, cerebral blood flow is low within 20 min to 12 h after ROSC (hypoperfusion phase), while the disturbed post-ROSC autoregulation may contribute to the development of secondary brain damage [16].

Peri-arrest ischemia and reperfusion injury can also aggravate outcomes. Shortly after reperfusion, cellular edema, altered gene expression, activation of inflammation, and increased production of reactive oxygen species result in tissue trauma and endothelial dysfunction [17–20]. The latter enhances vascular permeability, vasoconstriction, and local inflammation, creating a vicious cycle that ultimately leads to cell death [21–23].

Among organ systems, gastrointestinal tract dysfunction is common and characterized by loss of barrier integrity and bacterial translocation. The passage of viable bacteria or endotoxins from the gastrointestinal lumen, through the mucosal epithelium, to extra-luminal tissues, such as the mesenteric lymph nodes and other distant organs, can aggravate inflammation and cause secondary infections [24–26]. This phenomenon is usually observed after intestinal ischemia-reperfusion injury [27], but the timing and the associated pathophysiological mechanisms have not been elucidated.

Cardiac arrest and CPR induce a marked increase in pro-inflammatory cytokines, which activate pattern recognition receptors (e.g., Toll-like receptors) and inflammasomes, thereby amplifying the inflammatory response in ischemia-reperfusion injury [28]. The enhanced inflammatory response subsequently activates the hypothalamic–pituitary–adrenal axis [5,29,30]. Furthermore, sudden exposure to large quantities of endotoxin entering the bloodstream can contribute to the potentially devastating cascade of the sepsis-like syndrome, with possible concurrent immune suppression or paralysis [31–35]. Whether induced hypothermia after cardiac arrest attenuates the inflammatory response and increases the risk of subsequent infection remains unknown. However, data from mixed surgical–medical intensive care unit (ICU) patients suggest that induced hypothermia does not affect the immune response in patients with cardiac arrest [36]. Additional research is critically needed to elucidate whether all or only a subset of post-arrest patients will benefit from immune modulation and develop strategies to enhance only the beneficial aspects of the immune response following cardiac arrest.

3. Immediate Management following Restoration of Cardiac Activity

Conscious patients with stable hemodynamics and good neurological function usually have an uneventful course while undergoing further diagnostic testing. Unconscious or unstable patients must be repeatedly evaluated using the airway, breathing, circulation, disability, and exposure (ABCDE) approach, and their physiology should be optimized on an individual basis. Further diagnostic evaluation, e.g., transfer to the catheterization laboratory, should follow physiological and vital function stabilization. Another key first step is the re-evaluation of the etiology of cardiac arrest. After ROSC, there is usually more time to re-evaluate the patient and the conditions of cardiac arrest and collect more information from emergency medical services, witnesses, and family. Reversible causes should be rapidly investigated to prevent deterioration and relapse of the arrest.

Electrolyte derangements may be among the most common clinical problems encountered during the post-resuscitation period. Hyper- or hyponatremia may be associated with cellular dehydration and central nervous system damage, while dyskalemias may induce severe arrhythmias. Other abnormalities, such as hypocalcemia, hypomagnesemia, and hypophosphatemia may also be associated with increased adverse events. All physiological derangements should be identified and corrected since they can lead to fatal consequences in the resuscitated cardiac arrest patient (Table 1).

Table 1. Common causes of cardiac arrest and their management after admission to the intensive care unit.

Cause	Management
Electrolyte derangements	Urgent correction; medical treatment; continuous renal replacement therapy
Acidosis	Urgent correction; mechanical ventilation; maintain plasma pH > 7.20 and avoid pH normalization (mild acidosis facilitates tissue oxygenation); avoid normal saline (hyperchloremia); use of the anion gap corrected for albumin; initiation of renal replacement therapy when pH < 7.15 in the absence of severe respiratory acidosis and despite other medical treatment interventions
Acute coronary syndrome	Percutaneous coronary intervention; coronary artery bypass graft; optimization of myocardial perfusion; anticoagulation; thrombolysis
Heart failure	Advanced hemodynamic monitoring; deresuscitation/fluid removal; early point-of-care (POCUS) and venous excess ultrasound (VexUS); optimization of intravascular volume, preload, afterload, and heart-lung interactions; medical treatment; mechanical circulatory support; cardiac transplantation
Arrhythmia	Early rate control; correction of electrolyte disorders, acidosis, and other metabolic processes; diagnosis and treatment of abnormal conduction syndromes; medical treatment; cardioversion; pacing
Myocardial trauma	Resuscitative thoracotomy; surgical intervention
Pericardial tamponade	Emergency pericardiocentesis; resuscitative thoracotomy; surgical pericardiectomy or pericardial window
Tension pneumothorax	Emergency decompression; surgical intervention
Pulmonary embolus	Thrombolysis; embolus aspiration; mechanical circulatory support; prevention and treatment of pulmonary hypertension and acute right ventricular failure; surgical intervention
Airway obstruction	Removal of obstacle (e.g., mucus plug); endotracheal intubation; endotracheal/tracheostomy tube exchange; cricothyroidotomy
Asthma/COPD exacerbation	Medical therapies; non-invasive ventilation; high flow oxygen therapy; mechanical ventilation (aiming at improving gas exchange abnormality and avoiding auto-positive end-expiratory pressure); bronchial thermoplasty (within the context of a clinical trial or registry)

Table 1. Cont.

Cause	Management
Hemorrhage/hypovolemia	Advanced hemodynamic monitoring; fluid resuscitation (patients with maximal vasoconstriction and increased endogenous vasopressin levels may need less fluid); massive transfusion; avoid overload, hemostatic resuscitation, vasopressor use targeted at maintaining perfusion of vital organs *; surgical intervention
Poisoning	Antidote administration; medical treatment; extracorporeal blood purification interventions (e.g., continuous veno-venous hemodiafiltration or hemoadsorption); volume expansion; vasopressor therapy; correction of electrolyte and acid-base disturbances; mechanical circulatory support
Sepsis	30 mL kg^{-1} of crystalloid within 3 h; assess for fluid responsiveness/tolerance; early norepinephrine use; vasopressin when norepinephrine > 0.15 µg^{-1} kg^{-1} min^{-1}; use of point-of-care (POCUS) and venous excess ultrasound (VexUS); medical management; source control; early antibiotics; lung-protective ventilation #

* There are more α-1 adrenergic receptors in the veins than in the arteries, and they are abundant in the hepatic veins. In patients with severe hypovolemia, exogenous administration of pure α1-adrenergic receptor agonists will further constrict the already constricted hepatic veins, increasing the impedance of the outflow of blood from the splanchnic system into systemic circulation and leading to sequestration of blood within the liver (preventing auto-transfusion) [37]. In maximally vasoconstricted individuals, large doses of α1-adrenergic receptor agonists would not further increase venoconstriction and will constrict only arteries [37], aggravating the Fåhræus effect (decaying of the relative hematocrit in small vessels as the vessel diameter decreases) and organ perfusion [38,39]. # Tidal volume should be set between 6 and 8 mL kg^{-1} predicted body weight (volume or pressure controlled); respiratory rate should be initially based on the underlying physiology and thereafter aimed at maintaining normocapnia or mild hypercapnia; plateau pressure should be maintained <30 cmH$_2$O and corrected for intra-abdominal pressure when clinically indicated; avoid high positive end-expiratory pressures (set at ≤5 cmH$_2$O in patients with ROSC and hemodynamic failure and then individualize); driving pressure should be maintained <14 cmH$_2$O; mechanical power should be kept <17 J min^{-1}; fraction of inspired oxygen should be titrated to maintain normoxia [40,41].

4. Airway and Anesthesia Management

Post-cardiac arrest patients have an increased risk of cardiovascular collapse and other complications during the peri-intubation period [42]. These physiological derangements may occur due to pre-existing circulatory failure, chronic diseases, effects of anesthetic agents, and transition to positive pressure ventilation. Although the role of skills in airway management and the presence of a second operator remain important [43,44], expertise in peri-intubation physiological optimization is crucial, and endotracheal intubation should be performed by well-trained physicians [45]. Standard periprocedural monitoring includes peripheral oxygen saturation, waveform capnography, blood pressure, electrocardiogram, heart rate, end-tidal oxygen concentration, and, whenever required, invasive monitoring [46].

Peri-intubation desaturation carries a four-fold increase in the adjusted odds of re-arrest, and significant efforts should be made to improve denitrogenation and functional residual capacity and minimize shunting [42,47,48]. High-flow nasal cannula, non-invasive ventilation, and the 'ramped' position can be used to optimize the delivery of apneic oxygenation and first-pass success, provided that they do not impair hemodynamics and are tolerated by the patient [49–51]. In addition, endotracheal intubation is frequently associated with hemodynamic impairment, especially in post-cardiac arrest patients, and peri-procedural individualized hemodynamic optimization can decrease the risk of cardiovascular collapse [42,52,53]. Peri-intubation optimization of venous return and cardiac contractility in these individuals is crucial. Of note, fluid boluses may be ineffective, and early infusion of norepinephrine with or without an inotrope is usually required [54,55]. In patients with right ventricular failure and/or pulmonary hypertension who cannot tolerate further catecholamine-associated increases in pulmonary vascular resistance, vasopressin could be regarded as the vasopressor agent of choice.

The choice of sedative and induction agents should be also individualized based on the underlying hemodynamic status and comorbidities [42,52]. Although the merits of direct laryngoscopy vs. videolaryngoscopy for airway management in critically ill patients have been a matter of debate over the last few years, videolaryngoscopy may be of high value for overcoming anatomical difficulties but may also lead to life-threatening complications, including apnea and systemic hypotension. In clinical practice, there are several uncontrollable factors that may deteriorate a patient's physiology during videolaryngoscopy, such as secretions or blood in the airway, reflux of gastric contents, and failure to recognize profound desaturation/hypotension in the setting of clear laryngeal view [56,57].

Maintenance of anesthesia after intubation is usually achieved by a combination of hypnotics, opioids, and neuromuscular blocking agents. Although no definitive evidence exists regarding the best sedation regimen or optimal duration after cardiac arrest, patients must be adequately sedated using agents with short elimination half-life, the lowest possible doses, multimodal monitoring, and daily sedation breaks [58,59]. Midazolam and propofol are the most widely used sedatives, with the former allowing a faster neurological recovery; however, it is associated with a higher need for vasopressor therapy [60,61]. Of note, neuromuscular blocking agents are very useful and can facilitate mechanical ventilation, prevent shivering, and help achieve the target temperature quickly in comatose patients [62].

Patients treated with targeted temperature management (TTM) must be deeply sedated. However, TTM is associated with significant pharmacokinetic and pharmacodynamic alterations, which may result in sedative accumulation [63–66]. Therefore, the dosing of anesthetics may have to be reduced during TTM. The depth of anesthesia should always be monitored using frequent clinical assessment, continuous processed electroencephalogram monitoring and nerve stimulators, and should be carefully adjusted to tailoring drug administration to the individual patient.

5. Respiratory Management

The aim of positive pressure ventilation after ROSC is to improve oxygenation whilst minimizing circulatory impairment and other adverse events. Large tidal volumes, high respiratory rate and positive end-expiratory pressure (PEEP), and higher airway pressures may increase ventilator-induced lung injury and worsen hypotension and cerebral blood flow; therefore, they should be avoided, especially in the case of intravascular volume depletion or cardiogenic pulmonary edema [46,67]. Immediately after endotracheal intubation, patients should be mechanically ventilated using a lung-protective strategy with a tidal volume of 6–8 mL·kg^{-1}, PEEP of ≤ 5 cmH$_2$O, plateau pressure < 30 cmH$_2$O, and driving pressure < 14 cmH$_2$O. After hemodynamic optimization, PEEP levels can be titrated on an individualized basis, while mechanical power should be kept below 17 J·min^{-1}, taking into account the driving pressure and respiratory rate [40,41,68].

Furthermore, an arterial blood gas sample should be obtained as soon as possible, and the fraction of inspired oxygen should be individualized and titrated upon ROSC to an arterial oxygen saturation of 94% to 96% or even lower in some patients [69]. Specifically, hyperoxia (i.e., arterial partial pressure of oxygen (PaO$_2$) > 100 mmHg) and hypoxemia (i.e., PaO$_2$ < 65 mmHg) should both be avoided. Although extreme hyperoxia is associated with poor neurologic outcomes [70–73], "critical" hypoxia does not equate to a specific oxygen concentration. Of note, many tissues function physiologically at levels equivalent to an atmosphere of 5% oxygen, and some at levels as low as 1% oxygen [74,75], and therefore, optimizing perfusion may be more important than setting a specific oxygenation target in anesthetized patients [76–78].

Whether oxygenation and ventilation targets should be modified in patients treated with TTM remains unknown. However, at a core temperature of 33 °C, the PaO$_2$ (and arterial partial pressure of carbon dioxide (PaCO$_2$)) determined via an analysis of a warmed sample may be higher than the patient's actual PaO$_2$ (and PaCO$_2$); therefore, maintaining an arterial blood gas analysis PaO$_2$ between 70 and 100 mmHg may be reasonable in these patients. Furthermore, ventilation may be adjusted to maintain normocapnia (or even mild hypercapnia), especially in anesthetized patients treated with temperature control to 32–34 °C or in patients with decreased metabolism and carbon dioxide production [79].

Indeed, when the core temperature is 33 °C, the patient's actual $PaCO_2$ may be 6 to 7 mmHg lower than the value reported by the blood gas machine [80], while patients with chronic hypercapnia (e.g., chronic obstructive pulmonary disease) may require ventilator adjustments to achieve prehospitalization $PaCO_2$ values.

Notably, mild hypercapnia may improve cerebral perfusion and have anticonvulsant, anti-inflammatory, and anti-oxidant effects [81,82]. An observational cohort study of 16,542 patients found a greater likelihood of survival to discharge to home in the hypercapnic group and no difference in in-hospital mortality compared to normocapnic and hypocapnic patients [83]. Another study with 5258 cardiac arrest patients reported that unadjusted hospital mortality was the highest in the hypocapnic group (58.4%), compared with the hypercapnic (56.8%) and normocapnic (49.3%) group ($p < 0.001$). Analyses adjusted for age, lowest glucose, and PaO_2 revealed that hypocapnia (but not hypercapnia) was significantly associated with in-hospital mortality ($p < 0.001$) [84]. A post hoc analysis of the Japanese Association for Acute Medicine out-of-hospital cardiac arrest (OHCA) registry reported that severe hypocapnia, mild hypocapnia, severe hypercapnia, and exposure to both hypocapnia and hypercapnia were more likely to have a 1-month poor neurologic status compared with mild hypercapnia (reference: exposure to mild hypercapnia, respective adjusted odds ratios (ORs) [95% CI]: 6.68 [2.16–20.67], 2.56 [1.30–5.04], 2.62 [1.06–6.47], and 5.63 [2.21–14.34]) [85]. The clinical practice recommendations on the management of perioperative cardiac arrest (PERIOPCA) also recommend a lung-protective ventilation strategy (reducing tidal volume, plateau pressure, and driving pressure) and a $PaCO_2$ of 40–50 mmHg after perioperative cardiac arrest, especially in individuals with cerebral vasospasm or generalized atherosclerosis [86].

6. Circulatory Management

Myocardial stunning, vasoplegia, and capillary leaks are the main causes of circulatory failure after cardiac arrest and resuscitation, and advanced monitoring may be required in unstable patients to optimize oxygen delivery. Reversible post-cardiac arrest myocardial dysfunction, with a depressed left ventricular ejection fraction and an increased left ventricular end-diastolic pressure, may occur in the hours following ROSC, especially in patients with a longer duration of no-flow or CPR [5]. This impairment may persist for 48–72 h, and early echocardiography can quantify its extent, which may require the use of inotropes [5,87–89]. Beta-adrenergic blockade may be necessary as well, as sustained catecholamine-induced β-adrenergic induction produces adverse effects relevant to post-resuscitation management. Indeed, there is evidence suggesting that relative tachycardia is associated with poor neurological outcomes in post-cardiac arrest patients, independently of TTM, and with higher serum lactate levels and admission Sequential Organ Failure Assessment (SOFA) scores [90]. In another study, administration of beta-blocking agents (metoprolol i.v./per os or bisoprolol per os) during the first 72 h of post-resuscitation care was associated with survival at 6 months from the event in both the univariate ($p < 0.001$) and multiple logistic regression analyses ($p = 0.002$) [91]. However, classic β-blockers, such as metoprolol, are not easy to dose in such situations since they may lose their selectivity in the upper standard dose range or when given intravenously, while their longer duration of action may also lead to significant adverse events [92,93]. Ultra-short acting β-blockers, such as esmolol and landiolol, provide significant advantages in these circumstances since their effect can be terminated in a very short time [94,95]. Among these two i.v. agents, landiolol seems to be the most effective for decreasing heart rate in patients with acute heart failure and can be used alongside positive inotropic agents [96–104], e.g., in patients with left ventricular dysfunction and increased heart rate. Landiolol is also the only i.v. β-blocker with a specific dose recommendation for these patients [105]. Consequently, landiolol has been used in intensive care patients in conjunction with positive inotropic agents with positive outcomes (Figure 1) [106–112].

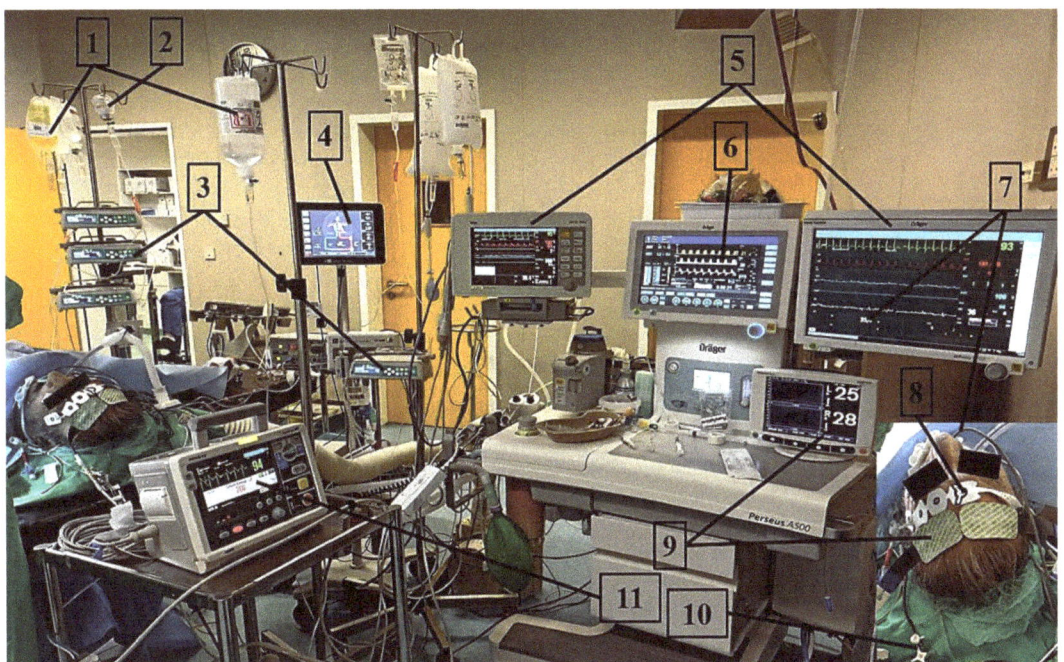

Figure 1. Post-resuscitation care after intraoperative cardiac arrest. A 67-year-old man with a history of end-stage renal disease, heart failure, and pulmonary hypertension underwent emergency surgery (American Society of Anaesthesiologists physical status 5E) due to uncontrolled hemorrhage from an infected axillary-axillary synthetic loop graft. The patient was in hemorrhagic and septic shock upon arrival to the operating room. Two hours after induction of anesthesia, he suffered an intraoperative pulseless electrical activity cardiac arrest. The patient was resuscitated according to the PERSEUS treatment strategy (NCT04428060) [106] and received two i.v. bolus doses of epinephrine 500 µg in order to maintain a diastolic arterial pressure > 40 mmHg during CPR and hydrocortisone 200 mg. A systemic vascular resistance of 1000–1100 dynes s^{-1} cm^{-5}, end-tidal carbon dioxide of 15–18 mmHg, and central venous pressure (CVP) of 6–7 mmHg were recorded during CPR. Spontaneous circulation was restored after 2 min of CPR. Post-resuscitation cardiac ultrasound revealed left ventricular hypertrophy with severe systolic dysfunction (LVEF: ~30%, TR: $3^+/4^+$) and a systolic pulmonary artery pressure of 65–70 mmHg. Inferior vena cava diameter and CVP were 2 cm and 18 mmHg, respectively. The patient was initially supported with noradrenaline 1 µg kg^{-1} min^{-1} and dobutamine 4.17 µg kg^{-1} min^{-1}. Depth of anesthesia was adjusted to maintain bispectral index between 39 and 44 with full neuromuscular blockade. Lung-protective ventilation and targeted temperature management (35.2–35.5 °C) were applied. Esmolol infusion was started due to increased heart rate (sinus rhythm 138 beats min^{-1}; noradrenaline 1 µg kg^{-1} min^{-1}, dobutamine 4.17 µg kg^{-1} min^{-1}, esmolol 14.58 µg kg^{-1} min^{-1}). Subsequently, arginine vasopressin (AVP) was added to facilitate decatecholaminisation and mitigate the effects of noradrenaline on pulmonary vasculature (noradrenaline 0.4 µg kg^{-1} min^{-1}, AVP 0.05 IU min^{-1}, dobutamine 2.92 µg kg^{-1} min^{-1}, esmolol 14 µg kg^{-1} min^{-1}). Thereafter, esmolol was replaced by landiolol in an effort to lower the ventricular rate without markedly deteriorating hemodynamics (noradrenaline 0.37 µg kg^{-1} min^{-1}, AVP 0.05 IU min^{-1}, dobutamine 2.7 µg kg^{-1} min^{-1}, landiolol 6 µg kg^{-1} min^{-1}).

Tranexamic acid was administrated, and the patient was transfused with a packed red blood cell/fresh frozen plasma/platelets ratio of 2:1:1 (total 6:3:3). Intraoperative time (skin-to-skin) was four hours. After another two-hour intensive care in the operating room, the patient was transferred to the intensive care unit, from which he was discharged 7 days later with a cerebral performance category score of 1. 1: fluid resuscitation and transfusion; 2: total intravenous anesthesia; 3: medical infusion pumps; 4: FloTrac/EV1000 clinical platform; 5: patient monitors providing information in numerical and waveform formats; 6: mechanical ventilator parameters and waveforms; 7: temperature control; 8: bispectral index (BIS) monitoring; 9: regional cerebral oxygen saturation (rSO2); 10: internal jugular vein cannulation; 11: manual external defibrillator/pacemaker.

Although dobutamine is the first choice for short-term intravenous inotropic support in patients with decreased contractility, the mechanism of action of levosimendan makes it an attractive alternative [113,114]. Levosimendan increases the sensitivity of myocytes to calcium and improves contractility without increasing intracellular calcium levels; the latter is a key pathophysiological mechanism of post-resuscitation myocardial stunning and ischemic contracture, and attenuating this phenomenon seems important [5,115]. Whether post-resuscitation stable dysrhythmias must be treated immediately after their diagnosis remains unknown. However, they are commonly caused by focal cardiac ischemia, and patients with a new-onset dysrhythmia must be evaluated for percutaneous coronary intervention.

In critically ill patients, mean arterial pressure (MAP) represents the entry pressure for the perfusion of most organs and should be maintained >65–70 mmHg [116–118]. Although higher MAP levels may be required in patients with brain injury or persistent hypoperfusion (e.g., progressing acute kidney injury or altered mental status) [119,120], adequate circulatory volume, absence of left ventricular outflow tract obstruction, and microcirculatory flow and responsiveness (if possible) should be ideally assessed before using a vasopressor challenge, especially in patients treated with TTM [77,121–123]. Considering that organ perfusion pressure is influenced by MAP and venous pressure, maintaining an optimal central venous pressure may facilitate adequate oxygen delivery. Additionally, it is important to remember that diastolic arterial pressure is key for coronary perfusion pressure, and its evaluation is also crucial. Patients with significant or unstable coronary artery disease and those with chronic pulmonary hypertension at a risk of low coronary perfusion pressure may require higher diastolic pressures [124].

Vasodilation should be actively treated with vasopressors, initially targeting a MAP of >65–70 mmHg, followed by an individualized approach. Norepinephrine is recommended as a first-choice agent to increase stressed volume and systemic vascular resistance whilst decreasing inflammation-induced capillary permeability [125,126]. Vasopressin can be used as an adjunct to limit the side effects of catecholamines or when agents with a different mechanism of action are needed; however, vasopressin may be the preferred option in patients with pulmonary hypertension, right ventricular failure, and/or vasopressin deficiency [127,128]. Moreover, vasopressin decreases the risk of atrial fibrillation and may improve renal function in patients with vasodilatory shock [129]. Few data are available regarding angiotensin II, limiting its use as a third- or fourth-choice agent in patients with angiotensin II deficiency or altered expression of angiotensin receptors [130,131]. Of note, hypoxic hypercapnia significantly affects the intra- and extrasplanchnic vascular capacitance system, and the dose of exogenous vasopressors should be possibly decreased in these patients to maintain adequate venous return and afterload [132–134]. Whether TTM affects hemodynamics remains a topic of discussion as these patients often have diverse requirements in vasopressor support [87,135].

In the context of the vasopressin–steroids–epinephrine (VSE) protocol, early post-ROSC, stress dose steroids may contribute to hemodynamic stabilization, especially in patients requiring high doses of vasopressors (e.g., norepinephrine equivalent ≥ 0.25 µg kg^{-1} min^{-1}) and who have multiple organ failure [136,137]. In addition, a re-analysis of combined data from the two randomized VSE trials reported that exposure to stress dose steroids was associated with a lower risk of post-resuscitation lethal septic shock [138]. Nevertheless, a more recent, two-center, randomized trial of stress dose steroids (alone) vs. placebo did not confirm any steroid-associated physiological benefit [139].

Optimizing preload during the post-resuscitation period may be difficult, and high doses of balanced crystalloids are often needed. However, avoiding congestion and the injurious effects of fluid over-resuscitation is imperative. An effective fluid resuscitation strategy may necessitate the adoption of a complex, multimodal cardiovascular model capable of primarily integrating both the arterial and venous sides of the circulation, including microcirculatory flow and oxygen extraction [140].

Perhaps the most important to recognize is the patient who is fluid responsive but not fluid tolerant because this patient will be harmed by a fluid responsiveness-based strategy [138]. As multiple factors can impact the ability of different organs and compartments to accommodate fluids and maintain their function, and different patient phenotypes exist, frequent multimodal and comprehensive clinical assessments of fluid responsiveness and tolerance are necessary. This assessment may include medical history and physical examination, radiographic evaluation, advanced hemodynamic monitoring, intraabdominal pressure measurement, point of care ultrasound (POCUS), and assessment of abnormalities in splanchnic venous flow patterns (i.e., venous excess ultrasound score—VexUS) [141,142].

In patients with refractory circulatory failure, treatment with assistive devices, such as Impella, intra-aortic balloon pump, or veno-arterial extracorporeal membrane oxygenator pumps, may be indicated. However, these devices are often associated with compilations and should therefore be used in selected individuals [143–146].

7. Antibiotic Therapy

Over one-third of adults with OHCA may be bacteremic upon presentation to the Emergency Department [147]. In addition, patients undergoing TTM may develop insulin resistance [148,149], which may impair tissue perfusion and increase the risk of infection. More specifically, clinical and experimental studies suggest that hyperglycemia induces excessive vasoconstriction, endothelial dysfunction, oxidative stress, and inflammatory response, which contribute to microcirculatory dysfunction [77,150–153]. However, bacteremia and antibiotic administration during resuscitation has not been associated with key outcomes [154]. Therefore, routine prophylactic antibiotics are not recommended despite the possibly increased risk for the development of pneumonia and other infections after cardiac arrest and should be reserved for those with evidence of infection. If antibiotics are administered, significant efforts must be made to improve tissue perfusion and local flow, and thus antibiotic delivery to the potential source of infection.

8. Active Temperature Control

In most patients, the primary neurologic injury occurs during cardiac arrest and may continue after ROSC [13]. However, the complex pathophysiology, diverse population, and lack of standardized protocols are major limitations in optimizing neuroprotection. Consequently, post-resuscitation neurological management requires a coordinated multidisciplinary approach aiming at attenuating the progression of cerebral injury.

Targeted temperature management has been described as the most effective neuroprotective strategy, and current recommendations suggest that it improves neurologic outcomes [69,155,156]. However, the recently published "Hypothermia versus Normothermia after Out-of-Hospital Cardiac Arrest" trial, the largest trial to date, found no difference in survival at 6 months or in health-related quality of life between TTM at 33 °C followed by controlled rewarming or targeted normothermia at 36 °C with early treatment of fever (body temperature > 37.7 °C) [157]. Similar results were reported in the CAPITAL CHILL trial, in which patients were randomly assigned to TTM of 31 °C or 34 °C for a period of 24 h [158]. Nevertheless, that study was underpowered to detect a clinically important difference of ≤3%.

Although the international guidelines recommend a target core body temperature of 32 to 36 °C and avoiding fever for at least 72 h [69], considerable debate exists on the optimal timing and temperature target, including whether just avoiding fever is enough or whether TTM is also effective for non-shockable rhythms. A target temperature on the higher end of the aforementioned range may be appropriate for patients with mild brain injury, higher bleeding risk, trauma, recent surgery, or septic shock. On the other hand, patients who may benefit from a temperature target of 32–33 °C include those with severe brain injury, subarachnoid hemorrhage, or stroke [159–166]. In addition, the HYPERION trial reported that moderate therapeutic hypothermia at 33 °C for 24 h led to a higher percentage of patients who survived with a favorable neurologic outcome at day 90 compared to targeted normothermia at 37 °C [167]. In a recent randomized trial of nearly 800 patients who received TTM targeting 36 °C for 24 h after resuscitation from cardiac arrest, the composite outcome of death from any cause or hospital discharge at 90 days with either severe neurologic disability or coma was similar for patients who subsequently underwent fever prevention for an additional 12 h (36 h total TTM duration) versus 48 h (72 h total TTM duration) [168] (Table 2).

Table 2. Randomized controlled trials on targeted temperature management in adult patients.

Author, Year	Intervention	Inclusion Criteria	Exclusion Criteria	No of Patients	Primary Outcome	Adverse Events	Net Effect of TTM
Bernard et al., 2002 [155].	33 °C vs. 37 °C	Age > 18 y (>50 y for women), OHCA with the initial cardiac rhythm of VF, persistent coma after ROSC	Cardiogenic shock, drug overdose, trauma, cerebrovascular accident, pregnancy	77	Discharge with good neurologic outcome: 49% (hypothermia), 26% (normothermia) ($p = 0.046$); for each 2-year increase in age, 9% decrease in likelihood of good outcome (OR, 0.91; $p = 0.014$); for each 1.5 min in time from collapse to ROSC, 14% decrease in likelihood of good outcome (OR, 0.86; $p = 0.001$); multivariate log regression analysis for good outcome: OR, 5.25 in hypothermia group ($p = 0.011$)	No clinically significant arrythmias in the hypothermia group, no statistically significant differences in platelet and white cell count	Positive
Hachimi-Idrissi et al., 2005 [169].	33 °C vs. 37 °C	Short study period: asystole or in pulseless electrical activity, >18 y, tympanic temperature > 30 °C, GCS < 7; Long study period: age 18–75 y, witnessed cardiac arrest, VF or non-perfusing VT, estimated interval of 5–15 min from collapse to first attempt at CPR, interval of <60 min from collapse to ROSC	Short study period: history of central nervous system depressant drug prior to cardiac arrest, pregnancy, coagulopathy; Long study period: cardiac arrest resulting from intoxication or trauma, responding to verbal command after ROSC, with tympanic temperature <30 °C at admission, evidence of hypotension (mean arterial pressure < 60 mmHg for more than 30 min on admission), terminal illness, pre-existing coagulopathy, pregnancy, unavailability for follow up	28	TTM 33 °C: survival until six months (57%), favorable neurological outcome (43%); Controls: survival until six months (43%); favorable neurological outcome (21%)	N/A	Positive
Laurent et al., 2005 [170].	32–33 °C vs. 37 °C	OHCA apparently related to heart disease, age between 18 and 75 years, initial ventricular fibrillation or asystole, estimated interval of <10 min from cardiac arrest to initiation of CPR, and interval of <50 min from initiation of CPR to ROSC	Pregnancy, response to verbal commands after ROSC, or a terminal illness present before the cardiac arrest	42	TTM 33 °C: survival until six months (32%), favorable neurological outcome (32%); Controls: survival until six months (45%); favorable neurological outcome (45%)	Hypokalemia (45%) Hypophosphatemia (<0.70 mmol L^{-1}) occurred in 20 patients (9 in the HF group and 12 in the HF + HT group) and was corrected by intravenous infusion of disodium phosphate, 8 mmol h^{-1}, during HF. During the first 24 h in ICU, ventricular tachycardia occurred in 6 patients in the HF + HT group, in 2 patients in HF group, and 3 patients in the control group ($p = 0.31$)	Positive

Table 2. Cont.

Author, Year	Intervention	Inclusion Criteria	Exclusion Criteria	No of Patients	Primary Outcome	Adverse Events	Net Effect of TTM
Hypothermia After Cardiac Arrest Study Group, 2002 [156].	32–34 °C vs. 37–37.5 °C	Age 18–75 y, witnessed cardiac arrest with shockable initial rhythm (VT, VF), arrest of presumed cardiac cause, estimated interval of 5–15 min from collapse to first resuscitation attempt, <60 min from collapse to ROSC	Spontaneous hypothermia < 30 °C, pregnancy, known coagulopathy, terminal disease, comatose state before cardiac arrest, response to verbal commands after ROSC, hypotension for >30 min after ROSC, hypoxemia for >15 min after ROSC	247	Favorable neurologic outcome (CPC 1–2) at 6 mo: 55% (hypothermia), 39% (normothermia) ($p = 0.009$)	Number of patients with any complication: 73% (hypothermia), 70% (normothermia) ($p = 0.7$); sepsis: 13% (hypothermia), 7% (normothermia); lethal or long-lasting arrhythmia: 36% (hypothermia), 32% (normothermia)	Positive
Castrén et al., 2010 [171].	34 °C vs. 35.8 °C	Age > 18 y, OHCA irrespective of initial rhythm, witnessed arrest, CPR initiated within 20 min of collapse	Trauma, drug overdose, cerebrovascular accident, known coagulopathy, asphyxia, or known requirement for supplemental oxygen, electrocution, spontaneous hypothermia, ROSC before randomization, DNR order, transnasal obstruction	194	Median interval from collapse to transnasal cooling: 26 min; median interval from collapse to systemic cooling: 113 min; median time to target core temperature (34 °C): 115 min (transnasal cooling), 284 min (control); mean core temperature on hospital arrival: 35.1 °C (transnasal cooling), 35.8 °C (control) ($p = 0.01$)	Nasal whitening: 14% (resolved in all survivors); epistaxis: 3.2% (serious bleeding in 1 patient with underlying coagulopathy); periorbital emphysema: 1% (resolved within 24 h); total serious adverse events: n = 7 (transnasal cooling), n = 14 (control) ($p = 0.23$)	Neutral
Bernard et al., 2010 [172].	Prehospital TTM 33 °C vs. in-hospital TTM 33 °C	Age > 15 y, OHCA with initial cardiac rhythm of VF, ROSC, systolic blood pressure > 90 mm Hg, cardiac arrest time > 10 min, established IV access	Patient not intubated, dependent on others for activities of daily living before cardiac arrest, spontaneous hypothermia < 34 °C, pregnancy	234	Rate of favorable outcome (discharge home or to rehabilitation facility): 47.5% (early hypothermia), 52.6% (hospital hypothermia) ($p = 0.43$)	No adverse events related to early hypothermia reported	Neutral
Nielsen et al., 2013 [173].	33 °C vs. 36 °C	Age > 18 y, OHCA of presumed cardiac cause irrespective of initial rhythm, >20 min of ROSC	>240 min from ROSC to screening, unwitnessed arrest with asystole as initial rhythm, intracranial hemorrhage or stroke, spontaneous hypothermia < 30 °C	939	All-cause mortality: 50% (33 °C), 48% (36 °C) ($p = 0.51$)	Number of patients with 1 or more complications: 93% (33 °C), 90% (36 °C) ($p = 0.09$); hypokalemia: 19% (33 °C), 13% (36 °C) ($p = 0.02$)	Neutral
Lilja et al., 2014 [174].	33 °C vs. 36 °C	Age > 18 y, OHCA of presumed cardiac cause irrespective of initial rhythm, >20 min of spontaneous circulation after resuscitation	>240 min from ROSC to screening, unwitnessed arrest with asystole as initial rhythm, intracranial hemorrhage or stroke, spontaneous hypothermia < 30 °C	652	Cognitive function assessed by memory, executive function, and attention/mental speed test did not differ between 33 °C and 36 °C group; attention/mental speed was more affected in all patients with cardiac arrest compared with STEMI controls	N/A	Neutral

Table 2. Cont.

Author, Year	Intervention	Inclusion Criteria	Exclusion Criteria	No of Patients	Primary Outcome	Adverse Events	Net Effect of TTM
Kim et al., 2014 [175].	Prehospital TTM <34 °C vs. in-hospital <34 °C	Age > 18 y, ROSC after OHCA irrespective of initial rhythm, endotracheal intubation, established i.v. access, successful placement of esophageal temperature probe, unconsciousness	Trauma, spontaneous hypothermia < 34 °C	1359	Survival to hospital discharge: 62.7% (prehospital hypothermia), 64.3% (control) ($p = 0.69$) (VF); 19.2% (prehospital hypothermia), 16.3% (control) ($p = 0.30$) (non-VF); full recovery or mild neurological impairment at discharge: 57.5% (prehospital hypothermia), 61.9% (control) ($p = 0.69$) (VF); 14.4% (prehospital hypothermia), 13.4% (control) ($p = 0.30$) (non-VF)	Rearrest in the field: 26% (prehospital hypothermia), 21% (control) ($p = 0.008$); use of diuretics within 12 h of hospital admission: 18% (prehospital hypothermia), 13% (control) ($p = 0.009$); PaO$_2$ on first arterial blood gas: 189 mm Hg (prehospital hypothermia), 218 mm Hg (control) ($p < 0.001$); evidence of pulmonary edema on first chest x-ray: 41% (prehospital hypothermia), 30% (control) ($p < 0.001$)	Neutral
Debaty et al., 2014 [176].	Intra-arrest TTM 32–34 °C vs. in-hospital TTM 32–34 °C	Age > 18 y, patients with OHCA eligible for advanced life support irrespective of initial rhythm	Trauma, hemorrhage, asphyxia, spontaneous hypothermia < 34 °C, ROSC before randomization, DNR order, pregnancy	245	Median NSE at 24 h: 96.7 μg L^{-1} (intra-arrest hypothermia), 97.6 μg L^{-1} (hospital hypothermia) ($p = 0.64$)	Pulmonary edema: n = 7 (intra-arrest), n = 8 (hospital) ($p = 0.59$); pneumonia: n = 7 (intra-arrest), n = 3 (hospital) ($p = 0.24$); hyperthermia: n = 9 (intra-arrest), n = 5 (hospital) ($p = 0.36$); bacteriemia: n = 1 (intra-arrest), n = 0 (hospital) ($p = 1$); hemorrhage: n = 3 (intra-arrest), n = 3 (hospital) ($p = 0.88$); arrhythmia: n = 5 (intra-arrest), n = 7 (hospital) ($p = 0.39$); convulsion: n = 8 (intra-arrest), n = 2 (hospital) ($p = 0.06$)	Neutral
Maynard et al., 2015 [177].	Kim et al. 2014 substudy (Prehospital TTM <34 °C vs. in-hospital <34 °C)	Age > 18 y, ROSC after OHCA irrespective of initial rhythm, endotracheal intubation, established i.v. access, successful placement of esophageal temperature probe, unconsciousness	Trauma, spontaneous hypothermia <34 °C	508	No difference between CPC or mRS scores 3 mo after randomization ($p = 0.70$ and $p = 0.49$, respectively)	N/A	Neutral

Table 2. Cont.

Author, Year	Intervention	Inclusion Criteria	Exclusion Criteria	No of Patients	Primary Outcome	Adverse Events	Net Effect of TTM
Deye et al., 2015 [178].	Advanced endovascular cooling system (34 °C) vs. basic external group (34 °C)	Age 18–79 y, OHCA of presumed cardiac cause, estimated interval of <60 min from collapse to ROSC, <4 h from ROSC to cooling initiation, unconscious patient, availability of endovascular cooling device	Terminal disease, DNR order, pregnancy, uncontrolled bleeding, known coagulopathy, spontaneous hypothermia < 30 °C, OHCA of extracardiac cause, in-hospital cardiac arrest, contraindication to endovascular device, immediate need for ECLS or renal replacement therapy	400	Survival without major neurological damage (CPC 1–2) at day 28: 36.0% (endovascular), 28.4% (external) ($p = 0.107$)	Minor bleeding, hematoma, or Arteriovenous fistula: 43.9% (endovascular), 29.4% (external); microbiological colonization of central venous catheters: 38.5% (endovascular), 26.4% (external); patients experiencing at least 1 cooling-related side effect: 24.6% (endovascular), 14.2% (external) ($p = 0.0086$); 3 patients experienced deep accidental hypothermia (all in external group)	Neutral
Cronberg et al., 2015 [179].	33 °C vs. 36 °C	Age > 18 y, OHCA of presumed cardiac cause irrespective of initial rhythm, >20 min of ROSC	>240 min from ROSC to screening, unwitnessed arrest with asystole as initial rhythm, intracranial hemorrhage or stroke, spontaneous hypothermia < 30 °C	939	Median Mini-Mental State Examination score for all patients, including non-survivors: 14 (33 °C), 17 (36 °C) ($p = 0.77$); median IQCODE score for all patients Including non-survivors: 115 (33 °C), 115 (36 °C) ($p = 0.57$)	N/A	Neutral
Pang et al., 2016 [180].	ECLS TTM 34 °C vs. ECLS TTM 37 °C	Age > 21 y, cardiac arrest irrespective of initial rhythm, interval < 45 min from onset of arrest to ACLS initiation, comatose state, and unresponsiveness after ROSC, intubated with mechanical ventilation, total ACLS time < 60 min	CPR duration > 45 min, severe coagulopathy, drug overdose, head trauma, stroke, pregnancy, terminal illness, spontaneous hypothermia < 30 °C	21	Survival to hospital discharge: 33.3% (hypothermia), 18.2% (normothermia) ($p = 0.44$); survival with good neurologic function (CPC 1–2): 22.2% (hypothermia), 8.3% (normothermia) ($p = 0.37$)	N/A	Neutral
Bernard et al., 2016 [181].	33 °C vs. 36 °C	Age > 18 y, OHCA, established i.v. access, cardiac arrest sustained after initial resuscitation treatment	Trauma, suspected intracranial bleeding, pregnancy, spontaneous hypothermia < 34.5 °C, DNR order	1198	Number of patients transported with ROSC: 33.5% (hypothermia), 39.1% (standard) ($p = 0.04$); overall survival to discharge: 10.2% (hypothermia), 11.4% (standard) ($p = 0.51$)	Acute pulmonary edema: 10.0% (hypothermia), 4.5% (standard) ($p < 0.001$)	Neutral—may cause harm
Scales et al., 2017 [182].	Prehospital cooling at 32–34 °C vs. no prehospital cooling	Age > 18 y, OHCA with sustained ROSC > 5 min, unresponsive to verbal stimuli or requiring intubation	Trauma, burn, spontaneous hypothermia, severe bleeding, severe sepsis, known coagulopathy, DNR order, pregnancy, prisoner status	585	Rate of TT 32 °C–34 °C reached: 30% (prehospital cooling), 25% (standard care) ($p = 0.22$); first temperature measured at hospital admission: 35.1 °C (prehospital cooling), 35.2 °C (standard care) ($p = 0.53$)	Pulmonary edema: 12% (prehospital cooling), 18% (standard care) ($p = 0.04$); use of vasopressors during first 24 h: 54% (prehospital cooling), 62% (standard care) ($p = 0.04$)	Neutral—may increase the application of TTM in hospital

Table 2. Cont.

Author, Year	Intervention	Inclusion Criteria	Exclusion Criteria	No of Patients	Primary Outcome	Adverse Events	Net Effect of TTM
Look et al., 2017 [183].	Internal vs. external cooling	Age 18–80 y, OHCA or IHCA irrespective of initial rhythm, ROSC for >30 min, unresponsiveness after ROSC	Trauma, intracranial hemorrhage, women <50 y, pregnancy, terminal illness, hemodynamic instability	45	Survival to hospital discharge: OR, 3.36 (1.13–10.41) (internal cooling vs. control); OR, 1.96 (0.59–6.86) (internal vs. external); OR, 2.44 (0.95–6.30) (intervention vs. control)	Any cardiac arrhythmias: OR, 0.18 (0.04–0.63) (internal cooling vs. control); OR, 0.26 (0.10–0.70) (intervention vs. control)	Internal cooling method of providing TTM resulted in better survival outcomes compared to controls. No significant difference in outcomes for external cooling compared to internal cooling
Kirkegaard et al., 2017 [184].	33 °C for 48 h vs. 33 °C for 24 h	Age 17–80 y, OHCA of presumed cardiac cause irrespective of initial rhythm, sustained ROSC for >20 min, GCS < 8	Unwitnessed cardiac arrest, asystole as initial rhythm	355	Favorable neurologic outcome (CPC 1–2) at 6 mo: 69% (48 h), 64% (24 h) ($p = 0.33$)	Number of patients with 1 or more complications: 97% (48 h), 91% (24 h) ($p = 0.03$); hypotension: 62% (48 h), 49% (24 h) ($p = 0.013$); pneumonia: 49% (48 h), 43% (24 h) ($p = 0.24$); severe bleeding: 4% (48 h), 1% (24 h) ($p = 0.03$)	Neutral
Lopez-de-Sa et al., 2018 [185].	32 °C vs. 33 °C vs. 34 °C	Age 18–80 y, witnessed OHCA of presumed cardiac cause, shockable initial rhythm, interval < 20 min from collapse to CPR initiation, interval < 60 min from collapse to ROSC	Trauma, toxicological cause, pregnancy, DNR order, interval > 240 min from ROSC to randomization, Spontaneous hypothermia < 34 °C, intracranial bleeding, stroke, neurological disability before event, terminal illness	150	Favorable neurologic outcome (mRS ≤ 3) at 90 d: 63.3% (32 °C), 68.2% (33 °C), 65.1% (34 °C) (ns)	Number of patients with 1 or more complications: 84.6% (32 °C), 79.6% (33 °C), 87.8% (34 °C) (ns); respiratory tract infections: 21.2% (32 °C), 49.0% (33 °C), 36.7% (34 °C) ($p = 0.012$)	Neutral

Table 2. Cont.

Author, Year	Intervention	Inclusion Criteria	Exclusion Criteria	No of Patients	Primary Outcome	Adverse Events	Net Effect of TTM
Nordberg et al., 2019 [186].	Prehospital trans-nasal evaporative intra-arrest cooling vs. prehospital standard care Patients admitted to the hospital in both groups received therapeutic hypothermia at 32–34 °C for 24 h	Age 18–80 y, witnessed cardiac arrest irrespective of initial rhythm	Trauma, severe bleeding, drug overdose, cerebrovascular accident, drowning, smoke inhalation, electrocution, hanging, spontaneous hypothermia, anatomical contraindications for nasal catheter, DNR order, terminal illness, pregnancy, known coagulopathy, ROSC before randomization, interval > 15 min from collapse to EMS arrival, need for supplemental oxygen	677	90-day survival with good Neurologic outcome (CPC 1–2): 16.6% (transnasal cooling), 13.5% (control) ($p = 0.25$); 90-d survival with good neurologic outcome (CPC 1–2) in patients with initial shockable rhythm: 34.8% (transnasal cooling), 25.9% (control) ($p = 0.11$); overall 90-day survival rate: 17.8% (transnasal cooling), 15.6% (control) ($p = 0.44$)	Severe cooling-related nose bleeding in 4 patients, pneumocephalus in 1 patient (resolved, patient survived with good neurologic outcome), adverse event rate within 7 d after randomization: 50.4% (transnasal cooling), 48.8% (control)	Neutral
Lascarrou et al., 2019 [167].	32 °C vs. 33 °C Cardiac arrest with non-shockable rhythm	Age >18 y, OHCA or IHCA with non-shockable initial rhythm (asystole or pulseless electrical activity), GCS ≤ 8	Interval > 10 min from collapse to CPR initiation, interval > 60 min from CPR to ROSC, hemodynamic instability, interval of >300 min from cardiac arrest to screening, terminal illness, severe hepatic dysfunction, pregnancy/breast-feeding, lack of insurance	581	Favorable neurologic Outcome (CPC 1–2) at 90 d: 10.2% (hypothermia), 5.7% (normothermia) ($p = 0.04$)	Severe cardiac arrhythmia between 0 and 7 d: 12.3% (hypothermia), 10.4% (normothermia) ($p = 0.48$); seizures between 0 and 7 d: 23.6% (hypothermia), 24.2% (normothermia) ($p = 0.73$); acute pulmonary edema: 6.7% (hypothermia), 8.7% (normothermia) ($p = 0.33$)	Positive
Le May et al., 2021 [158].	31 °C vs. 34 °C	Age ≥ 18 y, OHCA, all cardiac arrest rhythms	Inability to perform activities of daily living, cardiac arrest secondary to intracranial bleeding, severe coagulopathy with clinical evidence of major bleeding, coma not attributable to the cardiac arrest, life expectancy of <1 y due to reasons unrelated to the cardiac arrest	366	All-cause mortality or poor neurologic outcome at 180 d: 89 (48.4%) patients in 31 °C group vs. 83 (45.4%) patients in 34 °C group (risk difference, 3.0% [95% CI, −7.2% to 13.2%]; RR, 1.07 [95% CI, 0.86–1.33]; $p = 0.56$)	Deep vein thrombosis: 21 (11.4%) patients in 31 °C group vs. 20 (10.9%) patients in 34 °C group (risk difference, 0.5% [95% CI, −6.0% to 6.9%]; RR, 1.04 [95% CI, 0.59–1.86]; $p = 0.88$). Thrombus in the inferior vena cava: 7 (3.8%) patients in 31 °C group vs. 14 (7.7%) patients in 34 °C group (risk difference, −3.9% [95% CI, −8.6% to 0.9%]; RR, 0.50 [95% CI, 0.21–1.20]; $p = 0.11$).	Neutral
Dankiewicz et al., 2021 [157].	33 °C vs. 36.5–37.7 °C	Age > 18 y, OHCA of presumed cardiac or unknown cause irrespective of initial rhythm, unconsciousness without response to verbal commands or pain, >20 min of spontaneous circulation after resuscitation	Interval of >180 min from ROSC to screening, unwitnessed cardiac arrest, asystole as initial rhythm, limitations in care, spontaneous hypothermia < 30 °C, ECMO initiation before ROSC, pregnancy, intracranial hemorrhage, severe COPD	1861	6-mo mortality rate: 50% (hypothermia), 48% (normothermia) ($p = 0.37$)	Arrhythmias resulting in Hemodynamic compromise: 24% (hypothermia), 17% (normothermia) ($p < 0.001$); bleeding: 5% (hypothermia), 5% (normothermia) ($p = 0.81$); skin complication: 1% (hypothermia), <1% (normothermia) ($p = 0.21$); pneumonia: 36% (hypothermia), 35% (normothermia) ($p = 0.75$); sepsis: 11% (hypothermia), 9% (normothermia) ($p = 0.23$)	Neutral

Table 2. Cont.

Author, Year	Intervention	Inclusion Criteria	Exclusion Criteria	No of Patients	Primary Outcome	Adverse Events	Net Effect of TTM
Hassager et al., 2023 [168].	Device-based temperature control targeting 36 °C for 24 h followed by targeting of 37 °C for either 12 or 48 h (for total intervention times of 36 and 72 h, respectively) or until the patient regained consciousness	Age ≥ 18 years, OHCA of presumed cardiac cause, Sustained ROSC, unconsciousness (GCS < 8) (patients not able to obey verbal commands) after sustained ROSC	Conscious patients (obeying verbal commands), Females of childbearing potential (unless a negative HCG test can rule out pregnancy within the inclusion window), IHCA, OHCA of presumed non-cardiac cause, e.g., after trauma or dissection/rupture of major artery or cardiac arrest caused by initial hypoxia (i.e., drowning, suffocation, hanging), known bleeding diathesis (medically induced coagulopathy (e.g., warfarin, NOAC, clopidogrel) does not exclude the patient), Suspected or confirmed acute intracranial bleeding, Suspected or confirmed acute stroke, Unwitnessed asystole, known limitations in therapy and Do Not Resuscitate-order, known disease making 180 days survival unlikely, Known pre-arrest CPC 3 or 4, >4 h (240 min) from ROSC to screening, Systolic blood pressure < 80 mm Hg in spite of fluid loading/vasopressor and/or inotropic medication/intra-aortic balloon pump/axial flow device, Temperature on admission < 30 °C	789	Death from any cause or CPC of 3 or 4 at discharge within 90 days (TTM 36 h 32.3%–TTM 72 h 33.6%, $p = 0.70$)	Infection in ICU (TTM 36 h 26.0%–TTM 72 h 27.8%, $p = 0.56$); Arrhythmia in ICU (TTM 36 h 15.8%–TTM 72 h 11.9%, $p = 0.11$); Any bleeding (TTM 36 h 21.4%–TTM 72 h 22.7%, $p = 0.65$); Uncontrolled bleeding (TTM 36 h 4.3%–TTM 72 h 5.3%, $p = 0.52$); Acute kidney injury with renal-replacement therapy (TTM 36 h 9.9%–TTM 72 h 10.6%, $p = 75$; Electrolyte disorder (TTM 36 h 7.6%–TTM 72 h 6.8, $p = 0.66$); Metabolic disorder (TTM 36 h 8.7%–TTM 72 h 7.1%, $p = 0.41$); Seizure (TTM 36 h 21.4%–TTM 72 h 20.2%, $p = 0.69$)	Neutral

OHCA, out-of-hospital cardiac arrest; ROSC, return of spontaneous circulation; GCS, Glasgow coma scale; TTM, targeted temperature management; N/A, not available; VF, ventricular fibrillation; VT, ventricular tachycardia; CPR, cardiopulmonary resuscitation; DNR, do not resuscitate; STEMI, acute ST-elevation myocardial infarction; CPC, cerebral performance category; ECLS, extracorporeal life support; mRS, modified Rankin Scale; ECLS, extracorporeal life support; IQCODE, informant questionnaire of cognitive decline for the elderly; ACLS, advanced cardiac life support; IHCA, in-hospital cardiac arrest; EMS, emergency medical services; ECMO, extracorporeal membrane oxygenation; COPD, chronic obstructive pulmonary disease; HCG, human chorionic gonadotropin; NOAC, novel oral anticoagulants.

Based on current evidence and recommendations, the target temperature should be maintained stable for at least 24 h, avoiding variations and shivering, while fever should be avoided for at least 72 h after cardiac arrest [178,184,187,188]. Additionally, patients should be rewarmed at a slow rate (i.e., <0.5 °C h^{-1}) [189,190].

Interestingly, several recent systematic reviews and meta-analyses of randomized trials do not support the use of TTM. Elbadawi et al. analyzed eight randomized studies with a total of 2927 patients and a weighted follow-up period of 4.9 months and reported that TTM was not associated with improved survival or neurological outcomes compared with normothermia in comatose patients after cardiac arrest [191]. Another systematic review and network meta-analysis of temperature targets found that mild, moderate, or deep hypothermia may not improve survival or functional outcome after OHCA and may be associated with more harm than benefit [192]. Granfeldt et al. assessed all aspects of TTM, including timing, temperature, duration, method of induction and maintenance, and rewarming in 32 trials and reported that the use of TTM at 32–34 °C, when compared to normothermia, did not result in improved outcomes [193]. In another recent systematic review and Bayesian meta-analysis of seven adult cardiac arrest trials, TTM at 32–34 °C for ≥12 h versus normothermia with active control of fever had a chance of ≤53% to ≤78% to reduce the risk of death or unfavorable neurological outcome by 2–4% [194]. Consequently, more high-quality, large, randomized studies are warranted to further clarify the value of targeted hypothermia versus targeted normothermia.

9. Prognostication

The overall prognosis of patients following cardiac arrest remains poor, with only half of them surviving to discharge [173,195]. Early prognostication can be difficult, and clinical examination should be initially performed after ROSC and thereafter on a daily basis to assess the neurological status and guide decision making. However, assessments may be confounded by physiological derangements such as hypoxia, hypothermia, circulatory failure, and metabolic acidosis. Most in-hospital deaths in comatose patients are caused by hypoxic-ischemic brain injury [69]. Therefore, the overall prognosis depends on the no-flow time, the quality and duration of CPR, and the quality of post-resuscitation care. Furthermore, the combination of patient characteristics, e.g., age and frailty, components of medical care, anesthesia, TTM, and organ injury mandate that prognosis be determined in most patients only after the first five to seven days after ICU admission [69,196–198]. Notably, late awakening may be due to ongoing cardiovascular instability or multiple organ failure and does not preclude full neurological recovery [199–201].

As accurate prognostication is essential, a multimodal approach should be used in all comatose patients. Brain-computed tomography, measurements of biomarkers such as protein S100B or neuron-specific enolase, evoked potentials, electroencephalogram, and frequent clinical examination are important tools [202]. However, several factors can limit prognostication; for example, TTM may affect the predictive value of computed tomography, while continuous electroencephalogram may have a limited predictive value for a good outcome [203–206]. Additionally, no clear cut-off has been identified for neuron-specific enolase, and serial sampling at 24, 48, and 72 h after ROSC are necessary to assess trends.

In general, the neurological outcome depends on the prompt restoration of the systemic circulation and adequate oxygen delivery to meet cerebral oxygen demands [207,208]. Until recently, it was assumed that under normal circumstances, autoregulation maintains a constant cerebral blood flow, and changes in mean blood pressure within a range of 50–150 mmHg have a minor influence on cerebral blood flow [209,210]. However, recent evidence suggests that autoregulation maintains cerebral blood flow within a smaller range above baseline MAP [16,211]. After cardiac arrest, the evidence is conflicting, with several studies showing that cerebral autoregulation is preserved after cardiac arrest [212,213], while other studies reported the absence of autoregulation [214].

Monitoring cerebral perfusion with transcranial Doppler sonography (TCD) may enhance clinicians' ability to optimize individual cerebral perfusion, minimize secondary brain damage, and improve prognostication among patients admitted to the ICU after cardiac arrest. This technology allows the measurement of key parameters, e.g., cerebral blood flow velocity and pulsatility index, that allow ongoing, real-time assessments of patients' autoregulatory indices, intracranial pressure, compliance, and cerebral blood flow, and can identify potentially treatable derangements [215,216]. Various studies have provided conflicting results concerning the association between initial TCD values and neurological outcomes [208,212,217–221].

Although the interpretation of an elevated pulsatility index is complex, values > 1.19 are typically associated with increased downstream cerebrovascular resistance [222]. However, the pulsatility index may increase in the context of decreasing cerebrovascular resistance [217,223]. Transcranial Doppler sonography parameters may complement other available neuromonitoring tools, such as intracranial pressure monitors and near-infrared spectroscopy [224,225]. Of note, TCDs are non-invasive, and their validity may be superior to near-infrared spectroscopy [226]. Real-time data interpretation requires substantial bioinformatic infrastructure and clinician expertise. The GOODYEAR trial (NCT04000334) is anticipated to shed more light on the feasibility of an early goal-directed hemodynamic management with TCD during the first 12 h after ROSC.

10. Ethics of Critical Care and End-of-Life Decisions following Cardiac Arrest

Maximizing the benefit of critical care for patients and their families is a key aspect of post-cardiac arrest management. Apart from high-quality organ support, preventing pertinent harm and early end-of-life care decisions are tightly related to the application of patient-centered care. In this context, discussions with the patient or family members following cardiac arrest may affect the quality of care and should rely on a shared decision-making process [227]. The latter can support and optimize the appropriate allocation of resources, decrease ICU/hospital length of stay, aid in the selection of palliative care pathways, and reduce health care costs.

Effective communication is very important for patient relatives, who may be severely impacted by the illness and critical care stay of their loved ones, experiencing various phycological disorders, such as anxiety, acute stress, post-traumatic stress disorder, and depression [228,229]. Communication in the context of shared decision-making is associated with higher patient/family satisfaction and increased decisional confidence [227,230,231]. However, communication with families is not always easy, and structured communication tools may improve shared decision-making and patient/family satisfaction [232,233]. Consequently, family support interventions that can help reduce these psychological impacts and family-centered communication and care should be key objectives of post-resuscitation management [230–232,234–236]. Indeed, post-ICU admission-focused discussions with relatives can increase documentation of patient preferences and facilitate advance care planning and end-of-life care [232,237–239].

Of note, advance care planning is associated with improvements in symptom control and quality of life, decreases in family carers' decisional conflict, improvements in ICU care and post-resuscitation suffering, lower caregiver burden, and higher patient/family satisfaction [240]. However, an important limitation in the implementation and research in advanced care planning is the lack of a standardized approach; this is also a main cause for the inconsistent findings between studies [238,241–245]. In addition, advanced care planning and shared decision-making may increase organ donation pathways and rates after ensuring family members that donation will be considered only when ongoing treatment cannot improve outcome.

On the other hand, specific and adequate training of healthcare professionals is imperative for improving critical care and end-of-life decisions following cardiac arrest [246]. However, this type of training is often inadequate during medical training or time of specialization/subspecialization. Easily accessible relevant training programs or workshops to improve the delivery of end-of-life care must be available amongst all hospital staff. For example, the 'End-of-life Care for All (e-ELCA)' program is an e-learning library that provides resources to enhance the training and education of the health and social care workforce. The e-ELCA has been highlighted as a resource to help with the implementation of the NICE Guidelines on improving care for people who are in their last days of life [247]. Similarly focused programs created for cardiac arrest patients and their families may enhance the quality of post-resuscitation care.

11. Conclusions

A substantial proportion of cardiac arrest deaths can be attributed to the development of post-cardiac arrest syndrome, and post-resuscitation care is the fourth link in the chain of survival. Critical care management requires highly specialized resources and should be based on a multidisciplinary approach ensuring best-practice critical care.

Author Contributions: Conceptualization, A.C., G.A. and S.D.M.; methodology, A.C. and S.D.M.; validation, A.C., G.A. and S.D.M.; resources, A.C., G.A. and S.D.M.; data curation, A.C., G.A. and S.D.M.; writing—original draft preparation, A.C.; writing—review and editing, A.C., G.A. and S.D.M.; visualization, A.C. and S.D.M.; supervision, S.D.M. All authors have read and agreed to the published version of the manuscript.

Funding: This research received no external funding.

Institutional Review Board Statement: Not applicable.

Informed Consent Statement: Not applicable.

Data Availability Statement: Not applicable.

Conflicts of Interest: The authors declare no conflict of interest.

References

1. Wissenberg, M.; Lippert, F.K.; Folke, F.; Weeke, P.; Hansen, C.M.; Christensen, E.F.; Jans, H.; Hansen, P.A.; Lang-Jensen, T.; Olesen, J.B.; et al. Association of national initiatives to improve cardiac arrest management with rates of bystander intervention and patient survival after out-of-hospital cardiac arrest. *JAMA* **2013**, *310*, 1377–1384. [CrossRef] [PubMed]
2. Girotra, S.; Nallamothu, B.K.; Spertus, J.A.; Li, Y.; Krumholz, H.M.; Chan, P.S.; American Heart Association Get with the Guidelines–Resuscitation Investigators. Trends in survival after in-hospital cardiac arrest. *N. Engl. J. Med.* **2012**, *367*, 1912–1920. [CrossRef] [PubMed]
3. Nolan, J.P.; Soar, J.; Smith, G.B.; Gwinnutt, C.; Parrott, F.; Power, S.; Harrison, D.A.; Nixon, E.; Rowan, K.; National Cardiac Arrest Audit. Incidence and outcome of in-hospital cardiac arrest in the United Kingdom National Cardiac Arrest Audit. *Resuscitation* **2014**, *85*, 987–992. [CrossRef] [PubMed]
4. Kim, J.H.; Oh, Y.M.; So, B.H.; Hong, T.Y.; Lee, W.J.; Choi, S.P.; Park, K.N. Systemic complications of comatose survivors following cardiopulmonary resuscitation. *J. Korean Soc. Emerg. Med.* **2008**, *19*, 88–93.
5. Chalkias, A.; Xanthos, T. Pathophysiology and pathogenesis of post-resuscitation myocardial stunning. *Heart Fail. Rev.* **2012**, *17*, 117–128. [CrossRef]
6. Ruiz-Bailén, M.; Aguayo de Hoyos, E.; Ruiz-Navarro, S.; Díaz-Castellanos, M.A.; Rucabado-Aguilar, L.; Gómez-Jiménez, F.J.; Martínez-Escobar, S.; Moreno, R.M.; Fierro-Rosón, J. Reversible myocardial dysfunction after cardiopulmonary resuscitation. *Resuscitation* **2005**, *66*, 175–181. [CrossRef]
7. Kern, K.B.; Hilwig, R.W.; Berg, R.A.; Rhee, K.H.; Sanders, A.B.; Otto, C.W.; Ewy, G.A. Postresuscitation left ventricular systolic and diastolic dysfunction. Treatment with dobutamine. *Circulation* **1997**, *95*, 2610–2613. [CrossRef]
8. Xu, T.; Tang, W.; Ristagno, G.; Wang, H.; Sun, S.; Weil, M.H. Postresuscitation myocardial diastolic dysfunction following prolonged ventricular fibrillation and cardiopulmonary resuscitation. *Crit. Care Med.* **2008**, *36*, 188–192. [CrossRef]
9. Lopaschuk, G.D.; Ussher, J.R.; Folmes, C.D.; Jaswal, J.S.; Stanley, W.C. Myocardial fatty acid metabolism in health and disease. *Physiol. Rev.* **2010**, *90*, 207–258. [CrossRef]
10. Friberg, H.; Wieloch, T. Mitochondrial permeability transition in acute neurodegeneration. *Biochimie* **2002**, *84*, 241–250. [CrossRef]
11. Lefer, A.M.; Lefer, D.J. The role of nitric oxide and cell adhesion molecules on the microcirculation in ischaemia–reperfusion. *Cardiovasc. Res.* **1996**, *32*, 743–751. [CrossRef]
12. Goldhaber, J.I.; Qayyum, M.S. Oxygen free radicals and excitation–contraction coupling. *Antioxid. Redox. Signal.* **2000**, *2*, 55–64. [CrossRef]
13. Sekhon, M.S.; Ainslie, P.N.; Griesdale, D.E. Clinical pathophysiology of hypoxic ischemic brain injury after cardiac arrest: A "two-hit" model. *Crit. Care* **2017**, *21*, 90. [CrossRef] [PubMed]

14. Panchal, A.R.; Bartos, J.A.; Cabañas, J.G.; Donnino, M.W.; Drennan, I.R.; Hirsch, K.G.; Kudenchuk, P.J.; Kurz, M.C.; Lavonas, E.J.; Morley, P.T.; et al. Part 3: Adult Basic and Advanced Life Support: 2020 American Heart Association Guidelines for Cardiopulmonary Resuscitation and Emergency Cardiovascular Care. *Circulation* **2020**, *142*, S366–S468. [CrossRef] [PubMed]
15. Hare, G.M.T.; Mazer, C.D.; Hutchison, J.S.; McLaren, A.T.; Liu, E.; Rassouli, A.; Ai, J.; Shaye, R.E.; Lockwood, J.A.; Hawkins, C.E.; et al. Severe hemodilutional anemia increases cerebral tissue injury following acute neurotrauma. *J. Appl. Physiol.* **2007**, *103*, 1021–1029. [CrossRef]
16. van den Brule, J.M.D.; van der Hoeven, J.G.; Hoedemaekers, C.W.E. Cerebral Perfusion and Cerebral Autoregulation after Cardiac Arrest. *Biomed. Res. Int.* **2018**, *2018*, 4143636. [CrossRef]
17. Traystman, R.J.; Kirsch, J.R.; Koehler, R.C. Oxygen radical mechanisms of brain injury following ischemia and reperfusion. *J. Appl. Physiol.* **1991**, *71*, 1185–1195. [CrossRef] [PubMed]
18. Lipton, P. Ischemic Cell Death in Brain Neurons. *Physiol. Rev.* **1999**, *79*, 1431–1568. [CrossRef]
19. Morley, P.; Hogan, M.J.; Hakim, A.M. Calcium-Mediated Mechanisms of Ischemic Injury and Protection. *Brain Pathol.* **2008**, *4*, 37–47. [CrossRef]
20. Adrie, C.; Laurent, I.; Monchi, M.; Cariou, A.; Dhainaou, J.F.; Spaulding, C. Postresuscitation disease after cardiac arrest: A sepsis-like syndrome? *Curr. Opin. Crit. Care* **2004**, *10*, 208–212. [CrossRef]
21. Adams, J.A. Endothelium and cardiopulmonary resuscitation. *Crit. Care Med.* **2006**, *34*, S458–S465. [CrossRef] [PubMed]
22. Eckle, T.; Faigle, M.; Grenz, A.; Laucher, S.; Thompson, L.F.; Eltzschig, H.K. A2B adenosine receptor dampens hypoxia-induced vascular leak. *Blood* **2008**, *111*, 2024–2035. [CrossRef] [PubMed]
23. Hotchkiss, R.S.; Strasser, A.; McDunn, J.E.; Swanson, P.E. Cell Death. *N. Engl. J. Med.* **2009**, *361*, 1570–1583. [CrossRef] [PubMed]
24. Chalkias, A.; Scheetz, M.H.; Gulati, A.; Xanthos, T. Periarrest intestinal bacterial translocation and resuscitation outcome. *J. Crit. Care* **2016**, *31*, 217–220. [CrossRef]
25. Tassopoulos, A.; Chalkias, A.; Papalois, A.; Iacovidou, N.; Xanthos, T. The effect of antioxidant supplementation on bacterial translocation after intestinal ischemia and reperfusion. *Redox. Rep.* **2017**, *22*, 1–9. [CrossRef]
26. Hsing, C.H.; Lin, M.C.; Choi, P.C.; Huang, W.C.; Kai, J.I.; Tsai, C.C.; Cheng, Y.L.; Hsieh, C.Y.; Wang, C.Y.; Chang, Y.P.; et al. Anesthetic propofol reduces endotoxic inflammation by inhibiting reactive oxygen species-regulated Akt/IKKβ/NF-κB signaling. *PLoS ONE* **2011**, *6*, e17598. [CrossRef]
27. Tassopoulos, A.; Chalkias, A.; Papalois, A.; Karlovasiti, P.; Zanda, J.S.A.; Chatzidakis, S.; Gazouli, M.; Iacovidou, N.; Fanni, D.; Xanthos, T. Assessment of Post-Resuscitation Intestinal Injury and Timing of Bacterial Translocation in Swine Anaesthetized with Propofol-Based Total Intravenous Anaesthesia. *Cureus* **2020**, *12*, e10362. [CrossRef]
28. Asmussen, A.; Fink, K.; Busch, H.J.; Helbing, T.; Bourgeois, N.; Bode, C.; Grundmann, S. Inflammasome and toll-like receptor signaling in human monocytes after successful cardiopulmonary resuscitation. *Crit. Care* **2016**, *20*, 170. [CrossRef]
29. Zhao, Q.; Shen, Y.; Li, R.; Wu, J.; Lyu, J.; Jiang, M.; Lu, L.; Zhu, M.; Wang, W.; Wang, Z.; et al. Cardiac arrest and resuscitation activates the hypothalamic-pituitary-adrenal axis and results in severe immunosuppression. *J. Cereb. Blood Flow Metab.* **2021**, *41*, 1091–1102. [CrossRef]
30. Chalkias, A.; Xanthos, T. Post-cardiac arrest syndrome: Mechanisms and evaluation of adrenal insufficiency. *World J. Crit. Care Med.* **2012**, *1*, 4–9. [CrossRef]
31. del Campo, R.; Martínez, E.; del Fresno, C.; Alenda, R.; Gómez-Piña, V.; Fernández-Ruíz, I.; Siliceo, M.; Jurado, T.; Toledano, V.; Arnalich, F.; et al. Translocated LPS might cause endotoxin tolerance in circulating monocytes of cystic fibrosis patients. *PLoS ONE* **2011**, *6*, e29577. [CrossRef] [PubMed]
32. López-Collazo, E.; del Fresno, C. Pathophysiology of endotoxin tolerance: Mechanisms and clinical consequences. *Crit. Care* **2013**, *17*, 242. [CrossRef] [PubMed]
33. Cunningham, C.A.; Coppler, P.J.; Skolnik, A.B. The immunology of the post-cardiac arrest syndrome. *Resuscitation* **2022**, *179*, 116–123. [CrossRef] [PubMed]
34. Cavaillon, J.M.; Adib-Conquy, M. Bench-to-bedside review: Endotoxin tolerance as a model of leukocyte reprogramming in sepsis. *Crit. Care* **2006**, *10*, 233. [CrossRef]
35. Qi, Z.; Liu, Q.; Zhang, Q.; Liu, B.; Li, C. Overexpression of programmed cell death-1 and human leucocyte antigen-DR on circulatory regulatory T cells in out-of-hospital cardiac arrest patients in the early period after return of spontaneous circulation. *Resuscitation* **2018**, *130*, 13–20. [CrossRef]
36. Beurskens, C.J.; Horn, J.; de Boer, A.M.; Schultz, M.J.; van Leeuwen, E.M.; Vroom, M.B.; Juffermans, N.P. Cardiac arrest patients have an impaired immune response, which is not influenced by induced hypothermia. *Crit. Care* **2014**, *18*, R162. [CrossRef]
37. Gelman, S. Venous Circulation: A Few Challenging Concepts in Goal-Directed Hemodynamic Therapy (GDHT). In *Perioperative Fluid Management*; Farag, E., Kurz, A., Troianos, C., Eds.; Springer Nature: Basel, Switzerland, 2020; pp. 365–385.
38. Yen, R.T.; Fung, Y.C. Inversion of Fahraeus effect and effect of mainstream flow on capillary hematocrit. *J. Appl. Physiol. Respir. Environ. Exerc. Physiol.* **1977**, *42*, 578–586. [CrossRef]
39. Farina, A.; Fasano, A.; Rosso, F. A theoretical model for the Fåhræus effect in medium-large microvessels. *J. Theor. Biol.* **2023**, *558*, 111355. [CrossRef]
40. Battaglini, D.; Pelosi, P.; Robba, C. Ten rules for optimizing ventilatory settings and targets in post-cardiac arrest patients. *Crit. Care* **2022**, *26*, 390. [CrossRef]

41. Robba, C.; Badenes, R.; Battaglini, D.; Ball, L.; Brunetti, I.; Jakobsen, J.C.; Lilja, G.; Friberg, H.; Wendel-Garcia, P.D.; Young, P.J.; et al. Ventilatory settings in the initial 72 h and their association with outcome in out-of-hospital cardiac arrest patients: A preplanned secondary analysis of the targeted hypothermia versus targeted normothermia after out-of-hospital cardiac arrest (TTM2) trial. *Intensive Care Med.* **2022**, *48*, 1024–1038.
42. Russotto, V.; Myatra, S.N.; Laffey, J.G.; Tassistro, E.; Antolini, L.; Bauer, P.; Lascarrou, J.B.; Szuldrzynski, K.; Camporota, L.; Pelosi, P.; et al. Intubation Practices and Adverse Peri-intubation Events in Critically Ill Patients From 29 Countries. *JAMA* **2021**, *325*, 1164–1172. [CrossRef] [PubMed]
43. Cook, T.M.; Woodall, N.; Harper, J.; Benger, J.; Fourth National Audit Project. Major complications of airway management in the UK: Results of the Fourth National Audit Project of the Royal College of Anaesthetists and the Difficult Airway Society. Part 2: Intensive care and emergency departments. *Br. J. Anaesth.* **2011**, *106*, 632–642. [CrossRef] [PubMed]
44. Quintard, H.; l'Her, E.; Pottecher, J.; Adnet, F.; Constantin, J.M.; De Jong, A.; Diemunsch, P.; Fesseau, R.; Freynet, A.; Girault, C.; et al. Experts' guidelines of intubation and extubation of the ICU patient of French Society of Anaesthesia and Intensive Care Medicine (SFAR) and French-speaking Intensive Care Society (SRLF): In collaboration with the pediatric Association of French-speaking Anaesthetists and Intensivists (ADARPEF), French-speaking Group of Intensive Care and Paediatric emergencies (GFRUP) and Intensive Care physiotherapy society (SKR). *Ann. Intensive Care* **2019**, *9*, 13. [PubMed]
45. Myatra, S.N.; Divatia, J.V.; Brewster, D.J. The physiologically difficult airway: An emerging concept. *Curr. Opin. Anaesthesiol.* **2022**, *35*, 115–121. [CrossRef]
46. Higgs, A.; McGrath, B.A.; Goddard, C.; Rangasami, J.; Suntharalingam, G.; Gale, R.; Cook, T.M., on behalf of the Difficult Airway Society, Intensive Care Society, Faculty of Intensive Care Medicine, Royal College of Anaesthetists. Guidelines for the management of tracheal intubation in critically ill adults. *Br. J. Anaesth.* **2018**, *120*, 323–352. [CrossRef]
47. De Jong, A.; Rolle, A.; Molinari, N.; Paugam-Burtz, C.; Constantin, J.M.; Lefrant, J.Y.; Asehnoune, K.; Jung, B.; Futier, E.; Chanques, G.; et al. Cardiac Arrest and Mortality Related to Intubation Procedure in Critically Ill Adult Patients: A Multicenter Cohort Study. *Crit. Care Med.* **2018**, *46*, 532–539. [CrossRef]
48. Mosier, J.M.; Hypes, C.D.; Sakles, J.C. Understanding preoxygenation and apneic oxygenation during intubation in the critically ill. *Intensive Care Med.* **2017**, *43*, 226–228. [CrossRef]
49. Semler, M.W.; Janz, D.R.; Russell, D.W.; Casey, J.D.; Lentz, R.J.; Zouk, A.N.; deBoisblanc, B.P.; Santanilla, J.I.; Khan, Y.A.; Joffe, A.M.; et al. A Multicenter, Randomized Trial of Ramped Position vs Sniffing Position During Endotracheal Intubation of Critically Ill Adults. *Chest* **2017**, *152*, 712–722. [CrossRef]
50. Frat, J.P.; Ricard, J.D.; Quenot, J.P.; Pichon, N.; Demoule, A.; Forel, J.M.; Mira, J.P.; Coudroy, R.; Berquier, G.; Voisin, B.; et al. Non-invasive ventilation versus high-flow nasal cannula oxygen therapy with apnoeic oxygenation for preoxygenation before intubation of patients with acute hypoxaemic respiratory failure: A randomised, multicentre, open-label trial. *Lancet Respir. Med.* **2019**, *7*, 303–312. [CrossRef]
51. Guitton, C.; Ehrmann, S.; Volteau, C.; Colin, G.; Maamar, A.; Jean-Michel, V.; Mahe, P.J.; Landais, M.; Brule, N.; Bretonnière, C.; et al. Nasal high-flow preoxygenation for endotracheal intubation in the critically ill patient: A randomized clinical trial. *Intensive Care Med.* **2019**, *45*, 447–458. [CrossRef]
52. Chalkias, A.; Pavlopoulos, F.; Papageorgiou, E.; Tountas, C.; Anania, A.; Panteli, M.; Beloukas, A.; Xanthos, T. Development and Testing of a Novel Anaesthesia Induction/Ventilation Protocol for Patients with Cardiogenic Shock Complicating Acute Myocardial Infarction. *Can. J. Cardiol.* **2018**, *34*, 1048–1058. [CrossRef] [PubMed]
53. Natt, B.; Mosier, J. Airway Management in the Critically Ill Patient. *Curr. Anesthesiol. Rep.* **2021**, *11*, 116–127. [CrossRef] [PubMed]
54. Janz, D.R.; Casey, J.D.; Semler, M.W.; Russell, D.W.; Dargin, J.; Vonderhaar, D.J.; Dischert, K.M.; West, J.R.; Stempek, S.; Wozniak, J.; et al. Effect of a fluid bolus on cardiovascular collapse among critically ill adults undergoing tracheal intubation (PrePARE): A randomised controlled trial. *Lancet Respir. Med.* **2019**, *7*, 1039–1047. [CrossRef] [PubMed]
55. Russell, D.W.; Casey, J.D.; Gibbs, K.W.; Ghamande, S.; Dargin, J.M.; Vonderhaar, D.J.; Joffe, A.M.; Khan, A.; Prekker, M.E.; Brewer, J.M.; et al. Effect of Fluid Bolus Administration on Cardiovascular Collapse Among Critically Ill Patients Undergoing Tracheal Intubation: A Randomized Clinical Trial. *JAMA* **2022**, *328*, 270–279. [CrossRef] [PubMed]
56. Huang, H.B.; Peng, J.M.; Xu, B.; Liu, G.Y.; Du, B. Video Laryngoscopy for Endotracheal Intubation of Critically Ill Adults: A Systemic Review and Meta-Analysis. *Chest* **2017**, *152*, 510–517. [CrossRef]
57. Jiang, J.; Ma, D.; Li, B.; Yue, Y.; Xue, F. Video laryngoscopy does not improve the intubation outcomes in emergency and critical patients—A systematic review and meta-analysis of randomized controlled trials. *Crit. Care* **2017**, *21*, 288. [CrossRef]
58. Lee, D.H.; Lee, B.K.; Jeung, K.W.; Jung, Y.H.; Cho, Y.S.; Youn, C.S.; Min, Y.I. Neuromuscular blockade requirement is associated with good neurologic outcome in cardiac arrest survivors treated with targeted temperature management. *J. Crit. Care* **2017**, *40*, 218–224. [CrossRef] [PubMed]
59. May, T.L.; Riker, R.R.; Fraser, G.L.; Hirsch, K.G.; Agarwal, S.; Duarte, C.; Friberg, H.; Søreide, E.; McPherson, J.; Hand, R.; et al. Variation in sedation and neuromuscular blockade regimens on outcome after cardiac arrest. *Crit. Care Med.* **2018**, *46*, 975–980. [CrossRef] [PubMed]
60. Paul, M.; Bougouin, W.; Dumas, F.; Geri, G.; Champigneulle, B.; Guillemet, L.; Ben Hadj Salem, O.; Legriel, S.; Chiche, J.D.; Charpentier, J.; et al. Comparison of two sedation regimens during targeted temperature management after cardiac arrest. *Resuscitation* **2018**, *128*, 204–210. [CrossRef] [PubMed]

61. Bjelland, T.W.; Dale, O.; Kaisen, K.; Haugen, B.O.; Lydersen, S.; Strand, K.; Klepstad, P. Propofol and remifentanil versus midazolam and fentanyl for sedation during therapeutic hypothermia after cardiac arrest: A randomised trial. *Intensive Care Med.* **2012**, *38*, 959–967. [CrossRef]
62. Dell'Anna, A.M.; Taccone, F.S.; Halenarova, K.; Citerio, G. Sedation after cardiac arrest and during therapeutic hypothermia. *Minerva Anestesiol.* **2014**, *80*, 954–962. [PubMed]
63. Arpino, P.A.; Greer, D.M. Practical pharmacologic aspects of therapeutic hypothermia after cardiac arrest. *Pharmacotherapy* **2008**, *28*, 102–111. [CrossRef] [PubMed]
64. Bjelland, T.W.; Klepstad, P.; Haugen, B.O.; Nilsen, T.; Dale, O. Effects of hypothermia on the disposition of morphine, midazolam, fentanyl, and propofol in intensive care unit patients. *Drug Metab. Dispos.* **2013**, *41*, 214–223. [CrossRef] [PubMed]
65. Tortorici, M.A.; Kochanek, P.M.; Poloyac, S.M. Effects of hypothermia on drug disposition, metabolism, and response: A focus of hypothermia-mediated alterations on the cytochrome P450 enzyme system. *Crit. Care Med.* **2007**, *35*, 2196–2204. [CrossRef]
66. Cronberg, T.; Horn, J.; Kuiper, M.A.; Friberg, H.; Nielsen, N. A structured approach to neurologic prognostication in clinical cardiac arrest trials. *Scand. J. Trauma Resusc. Emerg. Med.* **2013**, *21*, 45. [CrossRef]
67. Amado-Rodríguez, L.; Rodríguez-Garcia, R.; Bellani, G.; Pham, T.; Fan, E.; Madotto, F.; Laffey, J.G.; Albaiceta, G.M.; LUNG SAFE investigators. Mechanical ventilation in patients with cardiogenic pulmonary edema: A sub-analysis of the LUNG SAFE study. *J. Intensive Care* **2022**, *10*, 55. [CrossRef]
68. Serpa Neto, A.; Deliberato, R.O.; Johnson, A.E.W.; Bos, L.D.; Amorim, P.; Pereira, S.M.; Cazati, D.C.; Cordioli, R.L.; Correa, T.D.; Pollard, T.J.; et al. Mechanical power of ventilation is associated with mortality in critically ill patients: An analysis of patients in two observational cohorts. *Intensive Care Med.* **2018**, *44*, 1914–1922. [CrossRef]
69. Nolan, J.P.; Sandroni, C.; Böttiger, B.W.; Cariou, A.; Cronberg, T.; Friberg, H.; Genbrugge, C.; Haywood, K.; Lilja, G.; Moulaert, V.R.M.; et al. European Resuscitation Council and European Society of Intensive Care Medicine Guidelines 2021: Post-resuscitation care. *Resuscitation* **2021**, *161*, 220–269. [CrossRef]
70. Awad, A.; Nordberg, P.; Jonsson, M.; Hofmann, R.; Ringh, M.; Hollenberg, J.; Olson, J.; Joelsson-Alm, E. Hyperoxemia after reperfusion in cardiac arrest patients: A potential dose-response association with 30-day survival. *Crit. Care* **2023**, *27*, 86. [CrossRef]
71. Janz, D.R.; Hollenbeck, R.D.; Pollock, J.S.; McPherson, J.A.; Rice, T.W. Hyperoxia is associated with increased mortality in patients treated with mild therapeutic hypothermia after sudden cardiac arrest. *Crit. Care Med.* **2012**, *40*, 3135–3139. [CrossRef]
72. Roberts, B.W.; Kilgannon, J.H.; Hunter, B.R.; Puskarich, M.A.; Pierce, L.; Donnino, M.; Leary, M.; Kline, J.A.; Jones, A.E.; Shapiro, N.I.; et al. Association Between Early Hyperoxia Exposure After Resuscitation from Cardiac Arrest and Neurological Disability: Prospective Multicenter Protocol-Directed Cohort Study. *Circulation* **2018**, *137*, 2114–2124. [CrossRef] [PubMed]
73. Robba, C.; Badenes, R.; Battaglini, D.; Ball, L.; Sanfilippo, F.; Brunetti, I.; Jakobsen, J.C.; Lilja, G.; Friberg, H.; Wendel-Garcia, P.D.; et al. Oxygen targets and 6-month outcome after out of hospital cardiac arrest: A pre-planned sub-analysis of the targeted hypothermia versus targeted normothermia after Out-of-Hospital Cardiac Arrest (TTM2) trial. *Crit. Care* **2022**, *26*, 323. [CrossRef]
74. Keeley, T.P.; Mann, G.E. Defining Physiological Normoxia for Improved Translation of Cell Physiology to Animal Models and Humans. *Physiol. Rev.* **2019**, *99*, 161–234. [CrossRef] [PubMed]
75. Schödel, J.; Ratcliffe, P.J. Mechanisms of hypoxia signalling: New implications for nephrology. *Nat. Rev. Nephrol.* **2019**, *15*, 641–659. [CrossRef] [PubMed]
76. Chalkias, A.; Xenos, M. Relationship of Effective Circulating Volume with Sublingual Red Blood Cell Velocity and Microvessel Pressure Difference: A Clinical Investigation and Computational Fluid Dynamics Modeling. *J. Clin. Med.* **2022**, *11*, 4885. [CrossRef] [PubMed]
77. Chalkias, A.; Laou, E.; Mermiri, M.; Michou, A.; Ntalarizou, N.; Koutsona, S.; Chasiotis, G.; Garoufalis, G.; Agorogiannis, V.; Kyriakaki, A.; et al. Microcirculation-guided treatment improves tissue perfusion and hemodynamic coherence in surgical patients with septic shock. *Eur. J. Trauma Emerg. Surg.* **2022**, *48*, 4699–4711. [CrossRef] [PubMed]
78. Schmidt, H.; Kjaergaard, J.; Hassager, C.; Mølstrøm, S.; Grand, J.; Borregaard, B.; Roelsgaard Obling, L.E.; Venø, S.; Sarkisian, L.; Mamaev, D.; et al. Oxygen Targets in Comatose Survivors of Cardiac Arrest. *N. Engl. J. Med.* **2022**, *387*, 1467–1476. [CrossRef]
79. McKenzie, N.; Williams, T.A.; Tohira, H.; Ho, K.M.; Finn, J. A systematic review and meta-analysis of the association between arterial carbon dioxide tension and outcomes after cardiac arrest. *Resuscitation* **2017**, *111*, 116–126. [CrossRef]
80. Sitzwohl, C.; Kettner, S.C.; Reinprecht, A.; Dietrich, W.; Klimscha, W.; Fridrich, P.; Sladen, R.N.; Illievich, U.M. The arterial to end-tidal carbon dioxide gradient increases with uncorrected but not with temperature-corrected PaCO2 determination during mild to moderate hypothermia. *Anesth. Analg.* **1998**, *86*, 1131–1136.
81. Lennox, W. The effect on epileptic seizures of varying the composition of the respired air. *J. Clin. Investig.* **1928**, *6*, 23–24.
82. Shoja, M.M.; Tubbs, R.S.; Shokouhi, G.; Loukas, M.; Ghabili, K.; Ansarin, K. The potential role of carbon dioxide in the neuroimmunoendocrine changes following cerebral ischemia. *Life Sci.* **2008**, *83*, 381–387. [CrossRef]
83. Schneider, A.G.; Eastwood, G.M.; Bellomo, R.; Bailey, M.; Lipcsey, M.; Pilcher, D.; Young, P.; Stow, P.; Santamaria, J.; Stachowski, E.; et al. Arterial carbon dioxide tension and outcome in patients admitted to the intensive care unit after cardiac arrest. *Resuscitation* **2013**, *84*, 927–934. [CrossRef] [PubMed]

84. Helmerhorst, H.J.; Roos-Blom, M.J.; van Westerloo, D.J.; Abu-Hanna, A.; de Keizer, N.F.; de Jonge, E. Associations of arterial carbon dioxide and arterial oxygen concentrations with hospital mortality after resuscitation from cardiac arrest. *Crit. Care* **2015**, *19*, 348. [CrossRef] [PubMed]
85. Okada, N.; Matsuyama, T.; Okada, Y.; Okada, A.; Kandori, K.; Nakajima, S.; Kitamura, T.; Ohta, B. Post-Resuscitation Partial Pressure of Arterial Carbon Dioxide and Outcome in Patients with Out-of-Hospital Cardiac Arrest: A Multicenter Retrospective Cohort Study. *J. Clin. Med.* **2022**, *11*, 1523. [CrossRef] [PubMed]
86. Chalkias, A.; Mongardon, N.; Boboshko, V.; Cerny, V.; Constant, A.L.; De Roux, Q.; Finco, G.; Fumagalli, F.; Gkamprela, E.; Legriel, S.; et al. Clinical practice recommendations on the management of perioperative cardiac arrest: A report from the PERIOPCA Consortium. *Crit. Care* **2021**, *25*, 265. [CrossRef]
87. Bro-Jeppesen, J.; Hassager, C.; Wanscher, M.; Østergaard, M.; Nielsen, N.; Erlinge, D.; Friberg, H.; Køber, L.; Kjaergaard, J. Targeted temperature management at 33 °C versus 36 °C and impact on systemic vascular resistance and myocardial function after out-of-hospital cardiac arrest: A sub-study of the Target Temperature Management Trial. *Circ. Cardiovasc. Interv.* **2014**, *7*, 663–672. [CrossRef]
88. Bro-Jeppesen, J.; Annborn, M.; Hassager, C.; Wise, M.P.; Pelosi, P.; Nielsen, N.; Erlinge, D.; Wanscher, M.; Friberg, H.; Kjaergaard, J.; et al. Hemodynamics and vasopressor support during targeted temperature management at 33 °C versus 36 °C after out-of-hospital cardiac arrest: A post hoc study of the target temperature management trial. *Crit. Care Med.* **2015**, *43*, 318–327. [CrossRef]
89. Gaieski, D.F.; Band, R.A.; Abella, B.S.; Neumar, R.W.; Fuchs, B.D.; Kolansky, D.M.; Merchant, R.M.; Carr, B.G.; Becker, L.B.; Maguire, C.; et al. Early goal-directed hemodynamic optimization combined with therapeutic hypothermia in comatose survivors of out-of-hospital cardiac arrest. *Resuscitation* **2009**, *80*, 418–424. [CrossRef]
90. Ko, J.I.; Kim, K.S.; Suh, G.J.; Kim, K.; Kwon, W.Y.; Shin, J.; Jo, Y.H.; Jung, Y.S.; Kim, T.; Shin, S.M. Relative tachycardia is associated with poor outcomes in post-cardiac arrest patients regardless of therapeutic hypothermia. *Am. J. Emerg. Med.* **2019**, *37*, 590–595. [CrossRef]
91. Skrifvars, M.B.; Pettilä, V.; Rosenberg, P.H.; Castrén, M. A multiple logistic regression analysis of in-hospital factors related to survival at six months in patients resuscitated from out-of-hospital ventricular fibrillation. *Resuscitation* **2003**, *59*, 319–328. [CrossRef]
92. Oh, V.M.; Kaye, C.M.; Warrington, S.J.; Taylor, E.A.; Wadsworth, J. Studies of cardioselectivity and partial agonist activity in beta-adrenoceptor blockade comparing effects on heart rate and peak expiratory flow rate during exercise. *Br. J. Clin. Pharmacol.* **1978**, *5*, 107–120. [CrossRef] [PubMed]
93. Lonjaret, L.; Lairez, O.; Minville, V.; Geeraerts, T. Optimal perioperative management of arterial blood pressure. *Integr. Blood Press Control* **2014**, *7*, 49–59. [CrossRef] [PubMed]
94. Bruning, R.; Dykes, H.; Jones, T.W.; Wayne, N.B.; Sikora Newsome, A. Beta-Adrenergic Blockade in Critical Illness. *Front. Pharmacol.* **2021**, *12*, 735841. [CrossRef]
95. Oyama, Y.; Blaskowsky, J.; Eckle, T. Dose-dependent Effects of Esmolol-epinephrine Combination Therapy in Myocardial Ischemia and Reperfusion Injury. *Curr. Pharm. Des.* **2019**, *25*, 2199–2206. [CrossRef] [PubMed]
96. Krumpl, G.; Ulč, I.; Trebs, M.; Kadlecová, P.; Hodisch, J.; Maurer, G.; Husch, B. Pharmacodynamic and -kinetic Behavior of Low-, Intermediate-, and High-Dose Landiolol During Long-Term Infusion in Whites. *J. Cardiovasc. Pharmacol.* **2017**, *70*, 42–51. [CrossRef]
97. Krumpl, G.; Ulc, I.; Trebs, M.; Kadlecová, P.; Hodisch, J. Bolus application of landiolol and esmolol: Comparison of the pharmacokinetic and pharmacodynamic profiles in a healthy Caucasian group. *Eur. J. Clin. Pharmacol.* **2017**, *73*, 417–428. [CrossRef]
98. Matsui, Y.; Suzuki, A.; Shiga, T.; Arai, K.; Hagiwara, N. Effects of Intravenous Landiolol on Heart Rate and Outcomes in Patients with Atrial Tachyarrhythmias and Acute Decompensated Heart Failure: A Single-Center Experience. *Drugs Real World Outcomes* **2019**, *6*, 19–26. [CrossRef]
99. Morisaki, A.; Hosono, M.; Sasaki, Y.; Hirai, H.; Sakaguchi, M.; Nakahira, A.; Seo, H.; Suehiro, S. Very-low-dose continuous drip infusion of landiolol hydrochloride for postoperative atrial tachyarrhythmia in patients with poor left ventricular function. *Gen Thorac. Cardiovasc. Surg.* **2012**, *60*, 386–390. [CrossRef]
100. Kobayashi, S.; Susa, T.; Tanaka, T.; Murakami, W.; Fukuta, S.; Okuda, S.; Doi, M.; Wada, Y.; Nao, T.; Yamada, J.; et al. Low-dose β-blocker in combination with milrinone safely improves cardiac function and eliminates pulsus alternans in patients with acute decompensated heart failure. *Circ. J.* **2012**, *76*, 1646–1653. [CrossRef]
101. Hamaguchi, S.; Nagao, M.; Takahashi, Y.; Ikeda, T.; Yamaguchi, S. Low Dose Landiolol Combined with Catecholamine Can Decrease Heart Rate without Suppression of Cardiac Contraction after Cardiopulmonary Bypass. *Dokkyo J. Med. Sci.* **2014**, *41*, 27–33.
102. Kobayashi, S.; Murakami, W.; Myoren, T.; Tateishi, H.; Okuda, S.; Doi, M.; Nao, T.; Wada, Y.; Matsuzaki, M.; Yano, M. A low-dose β1-blocker effectively and safely slows the heart rate in patients with acute decompensated heart failure and rapid atrial fibrillation. *Cardiology* **2014**, *127*, 105–113. [CrossRef] [PubMed]
103. Nitta, D.; Kinugawa, K.; Imamura, T.; Endo, M.; Amiya, E.; Inaba, T.; Maki, H.; Hatano, M.; Komuro, I. An Experience of Landiolol Use for an Advanced Heart Failure Patient with Severe Hypotension. *Int. Heart J.* **2015**, *56*, 564–567. [CrossRef] [PubMed]

104. Ditali, V.; Garatti, L.; Morici, N.; Villanova, L.; Colombo, C.; Oliva, F.; Sacco, A. Effect of landiolol in patients with tachyarrhythmias and acute decompensated heart failure (ADHF): A case series. *ESC Heart Fail.* **2022**, *9*, 766–770. [CrossRef] [PubMed]
105. Hindricks, G.; Potpara, T.; Dagres, N.; Arbelo, E.; Bax, J.J.; Blomström-Lundqvist, C.; Boriani, G.; Castella, M.; Dan, G.A.; Dilaveris, P.E.; et al. 2020 ESC Guidelines for the diagnosis and management of atrial fibrillation developed in collaboration with the European Association for Cardio-Thoracic Surgery (EACTS): The Task Force for the diagnosis and management of atrial fibrillation of the European Society of Cardiology (ESC) Developed with the special contribution of the European Heart Rhythm Association (EHRA) of the ESC. *Eur. Heart J.* **2021**, *42*, 373–498.
106. Chalkias, A.; Arnaoutoglou, E.; Xanthos, T. Personalized physiology-guided resuscitation in highly monitored patients with cardiac arrest-the PERSEUS resuscitation protocol. *Heart Fail. Rev.* **2019**, *24*, 473–480. [CrossRef]
107. Sakai, M.; Jujo, S.; Kobayashi, J.; Ohnishi, Y.; Kamei, M. Use of low-dose β1-blocker for sinus tachycardia in patients with catecholamine support following cardiovascular surgery: A retrospective study. *J. Cardiothorac. Surg.* **2019**, *14*, 145. [CrossRef]
108. Imabayashi, T.; Murayama, H.; Kuroki, C.; Kiyonaga, N.; Oryouji, T.; Tashiro, S.; Yasuda, T.; Kakihana, Y.; Matunaga, A.; Kanmura, Y. Study of hemodynamics in patients treated with landiolol in the ICU. *Crit. Care* **2009**, *13*, P173. [CrossRef]
109. Sakaguchi, M.; Sasaki, Y.; Hirai, H.; Hosono, M.; Nakahira, A.; Seo, H.; Suehiro, S. Efficacy of landiolol hydrochloride for prevention of atrial fibrillation after heart valve surgery. *Int. Heart J.* **2012**, *53*, 359–363. [CrossRef]
110. Yoshida, Y.; Terajima, K.; Sato, C.; Akada, S.; Miyagi, Y.; Hongo, T.; Takeda, S.; Tanaka, K.; Sakamoto, A. Clinical role and efficacy of landiolol in the intensive care unit. *J. Anesth.* **2008**, *22*, 64–69. [CrossRef]
111. Dabrowski, W.; Siwicka-Gieroba, D.; Piasek, E.; Schlegel, T.T.; Jaroszynski, A. Successful Combination of Landiolol and Levosimendan in Patients with Decompensated Heart Failure. *Int. Heart J.* **2020**, *61*, 384–389. [CrossRef]
112. Anifanti, M.; Iona, I.; Tsikritsaki, K.; Chrysikos, S.; Kalogeromitros, A.; Koukoulitsios, G. Landiolol vs Esmolol on hemodynamic response during weaning of post-operative ICU patients with heart failure. *Eur. Respir. J.* **2021**, *58*, PA3320.
113. Levijoki, J.; Pollesello, P.; Kaivola, J.; Tilgmann, C.; Sorsa, T.; Annila, A.; Kilpeläinen, I.; Haikala, H. Further evidence for the cardiac troponin C mediated calcium sensitization by levosimendan: Structure-response and binding analysis with analogs of levosimendan. *J. Mol. Cell Cardiol.* **2000**, *32*, 479–491. [CrossRef]
114. Huang, L.; Weil, M.H.; Tang, W.; Sun, S.; Wang, J. Comparison between dobutamine and levosimendan for management of postresuscitation myocardial dysfunction. *Crit. Care Med.* **2005**, *33*, 487–491. [CrossRef] [PubMed]
115. Kakavas, S.; Chalkias, A.; Xanthos, T. Vasoactive support in the optimization of post-cardiac arrest hemodynamic status: From pharmacology to clinical practice. *Eur. J. Pharmacol.* **2011**, *667*, 32–40. [CrossRef] [PubMed]
116. Kjaergaard, J.; Møller, J.E.; Schmidt, H.; Grand, J.; Mølstrøm, S.; Borregaard, B.; Venø, S.; Sarkisian, L.; Mamaev, D.; Jensen, L.O.; et al. Blood-Pressure Targets in Comatose Survivors of Cardiac Arrest. *N. Engl. J. Med.* **2022**, *387*, 1456–1466. [CrossRef] [PubMed]
117. Mølstrøm, S.; Nielsen, T.H.; Nordstrøm, C.H.; Forsse, A.; Møller, S.; Venø, S.; Mamaev, D.; Tencer, T.; Theódórsdóttir, Á.; Krøigård, T.; et al. A randomized, double-blind trial comparing the effect of two blood pressure targets on global brain metabolism after out-of-hospital cardiac arrest. *Crit. Care* **2023**, *27*, 73. [CrossRef]
118. McGuigan, P.J.; Giallongo, E.; Blackwood, B.; Doidge, J.; Harrison, D.A.; Nichol, A.D.; Rowan, K.M.; Shankar-Hari, M.; Skrifvars, M.B.; Thomas, K.; et al. The effect of blood pressure on mortality following out-of-hospital cardiac arrest: A retrospective cohort study of the United Kingdom Intensive Care National Audit and Research Centre database. *Crit. Care* **2023**, *27*, 4. [CrossRef] [PubMed]
119. Dupont, V.; Bonnet-Lebrun, A.S.; Boileve, A.; Charpentier, J.; Mira, J.P.; Geri, G.; Cariou, A.; Jozwiak, M. Impact of early mean arterial pressure level on severe acute kidney injury occurrence after out-of-hospital cardiac arrest. *Ann. Intensive Care* **2022**, *12*, 69. [CrossRef] [PubMed]
120. Russo, J.J.; Di Santo, P.; Simard, T.; James, T.E.; Hibbert, B.; Couture, E.; Marbach, J.; Osborne, C.; Ramirez, F.D.; Wells, G.A.; et al. Optimal mean arterial pressure in comatose survivors of out-of-hospital cardiac arrest: An analysis of area below blood pressure thresholds. *Resuscitation* **2018**, *128*, 175–180. [CrossRef]
121. Donadello, K.; Su, F.; Annoni, F.; Scolletta, S.; He, X.; Peluso, L.; Gottin, L.; Polati, E.; Creteur, J.; De Witte, O.; et al. The Effects of Temperature Management on Brain Microcirculation, Oxygenation and Metabolism. *Brain Sci.* **2022**, *12*, 1422. [CrossRef] [PubMed]
122. Chalkias, A. Increasing stress volume vs. increasing tissue perfusion in septic patients. *Eur. J. Anaesthesiol.* **2022**, *39*, 390–391. [CrossRef]
123. Koopmans, M.; Kuiper, M.A.; Endeman, H.; Veenstra, G.; Vellinga, N.A.; de Vos, R.; Boerma, E.C. Microcirculatory perfusion and vascular reactivity are altered in post cardiac arrest patients, irrespective of target temperature management to 33 °C vs. 36 °C. *Resuscitation* **2015**, *86*, 14–18. [CrossRef]
124. Han, C.; Lee, J.H.; Korean Hypothermia Network Investigators. Heart rate and diastolic arterial pressure in cardiac arrest patients: A nationwide, multicenter prospective registry. *PLoS ONE* **2022**, *17*, e0274130. [CrossRef]
125. Chalkias, A.; Laou, E.; Papagiannakis, N.; Spyropoulos, V.; Kouskouni, E.; Theodoraki, K.; Xanthos, T. Assessment of Dynamic Changes in Stressed Volume and Venous Return during Hyperdynamic Septic Shock. *J. Pers. Med.* **2022**, *12*, 724. [CrossRef] [PubMed]

126. Joffre, J.; Lloyd, E.; Wong, E.; Chung-Yeh, C.; Nguyen, N.; Xu, F.; Legrand, M.; Hellman, J. Catecholaminergic Vasopressors Reduce Toll-Like Receptor Agonist-Induced Microvascular Endothelial Cell Permeability But Not Cytokine Production. *Crit. Care Med.* **2021**, *49*, e315–e326. [CrossRef] [PubMed]
127. Demiselle, J.; Fage, N.; Radermacher, P.; Asfar, P. Vasopressin and its analogues in shock states: A review. *Ann. Intensive Care* **2020**, *10*, 9. [CrossRef] [PubMed]
128. Landry, D.W.; Levin, H.R.; Gallant, E.M.; Ashton, R.C., Jr.; Seo, S.; D'Alessandro, D.; Oz, M.C.; Oliver, J.A. Vasopressin deficiency contributes to the vasodilation of septic shock. *Circulation* **1997**, *95*, 1122–1125. [CrossRef] [PubMed]
129. McIntyre, W.F.; Um, K.J.; Alhazzani, W.; Lengyel, A.P.; Hajjar, L.; Gordon, A.C.; Lamontagne, F.; Healey, J.S.; Whitlock, R.P.; Belley-Côté, E.P. Association of Vasopressin Plus Catecholamine Vasopressors vs Catecholamines Alone with Atrial Fibrillation in Patients With Distributive Shock: A Systematic Review and Meta-analysis. *JAMA* **2018**, *319*, 1889–1900. [CrossRef] [PubMed]
130. Bellomo, R.; Forni, L.G.; Busse, L.W.; McCurdy, M.T.; Ham, K.R.; Boldt, D.W.; Hästbacka, J.; Khanna, A.K.; Albertson, T.E.; Tumlin, J.; et al. Renin and Survival in Patients Given Angiotensin II for Catecholamine-Resistant Vasodilatory Shock. A Clinical Trial. *Am. J. Respir. Crit. Care Med.* **2020**, *202*, 1253–1261. [CrossRef]
131. Leisman, D.E.; Fernandes, T.D.; Bijol, V.; Abraham, M.N.; Lehman, J.R.; Taylor, M.D.; Capone, C.; Yaipan, O.; Bellomo, R.; Deutschman, C.S. Impaired angiotensin II type 1 receptor signaling contributes to sepsis-induced acute kidney injury. *Kidney Int.* **2021**, *99*, 148–160. [CrossRef] [PubMed]
132. Chalkias, A.; Laou, E.; Papagiannakis, N.; Varvarousi, G.; Ragias, D.; Koutsovasilis, A.; Makris, D.; Varvarousis, D.; Iacovidou, N.; Pantazopoulos, I.; et al. Determinants of venous return in steady-state physiology and asphyxia-induced circulatory shock and arrest: An experimental study. *Intensive Care Med. Exp.* **2022**, *10*, 13. [CrossRef] [PubMed]
133. Grübler, M.R.; Wigger, O.; Berger, D.; Blöchlinger, S. Basic concepts of heart-lung interactions during mechanical ventilation. *Swiss Med. Wkly.* **2017**, *147*, w14491. [CrossRef] [PubMed]
134. Rothe, C.F.; Maass-Moreno, R.; Flanagan, A.D. Effects of hypercapnia and hypoxia on the cardiovascular system: Vascular capacitance and aortic chemoreceptors. *Am. J. Physiol.* **1990**, *259*, H932–H939. [CrossRef] [PubMed]
135. Stegman, B.; Aggarwal, B.; Senapati, A.; Shao, M.; Menon, V. Serial hemodynamic measurements in post-cardiac arrest cardiogenic shock treated with therapeutic hypothermia. *Eur. Heart J. Acute Cardiovasc. Care* **2015**, *4*, 263–269. [CrossRef]
136. Mentzelopoulos, S.D.; Mongardon, N.; Xanthos, T.; Zakynthinos, S.G. Possible significance of hemodynamic and immunomodulatory effects of early stress-dose steroids in cardiac arrest. *Crit. Care* **2016**, *20*, 211. [CrossRef]
137. Mentzelopoulos, S.D.; Malachias, S.; Chamos, C.; Konstantopoulos, D.; Ntaidou, T.; Papastylianou, A.; Kolliantzaki, I.; Theodoridi, M.; Ischaki, H.; Makris, D.; et al. Vasopressin, steroids, and epinephrine and neurologically favorable survival after in-hospital cardiac arrest: A randomized clinical trial. *JAMA* **2013**, *310*, 270–279. [CrossRef]
138. Mentzelopoulos, S.D.; Koliantzaki, I.; Karvouniaris, M.; Vrettou, C.; Mongardon, N.; Karlis, G.; Makris, D.; Zakynthinos, E.; Sourlas, S.; Aloizos, S.; et al. Exposure to Stress-Dose Steroids and Lethal Septic Shock After In-Hospital Cardiac Arrest: Individual Patient Data Reanalysis of Two Prior Randomized Clinical Trials that Evaluated the Vasopressin-Steroids-Epinephrine Combination Versus Epinephrine Alone. *Cardiovasc. Drugs Ther.* **2018**, *32*, 339–351. [CrossRef]
139. Mentzelopoulos, S.D.; Pappa, E.; Malachias, S.; Vrettou, C.S.; Giannopoulos, A.; Karlis, G.; Adamos, G.; Pantazopoulos, I.; Megalou, A.; Louvaris, Z.; et al. Physiologic effects of stress dose corticosteroids in in-hospital cardiac arrest (CORTICA): A randomized clinical trial. *Resusc. Plus* **2022**, *10*, 100252. [CrossRef]
140. Chalkias, A. Letter to the editor: "The emerging concept of fluid tolerance: A position paper". *J. Crit. Care* **2023**, *74*, 154235. [CrossRef]
141. Kattan, E.; Castro, R.; Miralles-Aguiar, F.; Hernández, G.; Rola, P. The emerging concept of fluid tolerance: A position paper. *J. Crit. Care* **2022**, *71*, 154070. [CrossRef]
142. Beaubien-Souligny, W.; Rola, P.; Haycock, K.; Bouchard, J.; Lamarche, Y.; Spiegel, R.; Denault, A.Y. Quantifying systemic congestion with Point-Of-Care ultrasound: Development of the venous excess ultrasound grading system. *Ultrasound J.* **2020**, *12*, 16. [CrossRef]
143. Thiele, H.; Zeymer, U.; Neumann, F.J.; Ferenc, M.; Olbrich, H.G.; Hausleiter, J.; Richardt, G.; Hennersdorf, M.; Empen, K.; Fuernau, G.; et al. Intraaortic balloon support for myocardial infarction with cardiogenic shock. *N. Engl. J. Med.* **2012**, *367*, 1287–1296. [CrossRef] [PubMed]
144. Ortega-Deballon, I.; Hornby, L.; Shemie, S.D.; Bhanji, F.; Guadagno, E. Extracorporeal resuscitation for refractory out-of-hospital cardiac arrest in adults: A systematic review of international practices and outcomes. *Resuscitation* **2016**, *101*, 12–20. [CrossRef] [PubMed]
145. Fjølner, J.; Greisen, J.; Jørgensen, M.R.; Terkelsen, C.J.; Ilkjaer, L.B.; Hansen, T.M.; Eiskjaer, H.; Christensen, S.; Gjedsted, J. Extracorporeal cardiopulmonary resuscitation after out-of-hospital cardiac arrest in a Danish health region. *Acta Anaesthesiol. Scand.* **2017**, *61*, 176–185. [CrossRef] [PubMed]
146. Ouweneel, D.M.; Eriksen, E.; Sjauw, K.D.; van Dongen, I.M.; Hirsch, A.; Packer, E.J.; Vis, M.M.; Wykrzykowska, J.J.; Koch, K.T.; Baan, J.; et al. Percutaneous mechanical circulatory support versus intra-aortic balloon pump in cardiogenic shock after acute myocardial infarction. *J. Am. Coll. Cardiol.* **2017**, *69*, 278–287. [CrossRef]
147. Coba, V.; Jaehne, A.K.; Suarez, A.; Dagher, G.A.; Brown, S.C.; Yang, J.J.; Manteuffel, J.; Rivers, E.P. The incidence and significance of bacteremia in out of hospital cardiac arrest. *Resuscitation* **2014**, *85*, 196–202. [CrossRef] [PubMed]

148. Polderman, K.H.; Herold, I. Therapeutic hypothermia and controlled normothermia in the intensive care unit: Practical considerations, side effects, and cooling methods. *Crit. Care Med.* **2009**, *37*, 1101–1120. [CrossRef]
149. Cueni-Villoz, N.; Devigili, A.; Delodder, F.; Cianferoni, S.; Feihl, F.; Rossetti, A.O.; Eggimann, P.; Vincent, J.L.; Taccone, F.S.; Oddo, M. Increased blood glucose variability during therapeutic hypothermia and outcome after cardiac arrest. *Crit. Care Med.* **2011**, *39*, 2225–2231. [CrossRef]
150. Booth, G.; Stalker, T.J.; Lefer, A.M.; Scalia, R. Elevated ambient glucose induces acute inflammatory events in the microvasculature: Effects of insulin. *Am. J. Physiol. Endocrinol. Metab.* **2001**, *280*, E848–E856. [CrossRef] [PubMed]
151. Efrati, S.; Berman, S.; Hamad, R.A.; Siman-Tov, Y.; Chanimov, M.; Weissgarten, J. Hyperglycaemia emerging during general anaesthesia induces rat acute kidney injury via impaired microcirculation, augmented apoptosis and inhibited cell proliferation. *Nephrology (Carlton)* **2012**, *17*, 111–122. [CrossRef] [PubMed]
152. Gomes, M.B.; Affonso, F.S.; Cailleaux, S.; Almeida, A.L.; Pinto, L.F.; Tibiriçá, E. Glucose levels observed in daily clinical practice induce endothelial dysfunction in the rabbit macro- and microcirculation. *Fundam. Clin. Pharmacol.* **2004**, *18*, 339–346. [CrossRef] [PubMed]
153. See, K.C. Glycemic targets in critically ill adults: A mini-review. *World J. Diabetes* **2021**, *12*, 1719–1730. [CrossRef] [PubMed]
154. Couper, K.; Laloo, R.; Field, R.; Perkins, G.D.; Thomas, M.; Yeung, J. Prophylactic antibiotic use following cardiac arrest: A systematic review and meta-analysis. *Resuscitation* **2019**, *141*, 166–173. [CrossRef] [PubMed]
155. Bernard, S.A.; Gray, T.W.; Buist, M.D.; Jones, B.M.; Silvester, W.; Gutteridge, G.; Smith, K. Treatment of comatose survivors of out-of-hospital cardiac arrest with induced hypothermia. *N. Engl. J. Med.* **2002**, *346*, 557–563. [CrossRef]
156. Hypothermia after Cardiac Arrest Study Group. Mild therapeutic hypothermia to improve the neurologic outcome after cardiac arrest. *N. Engl. J. Med.* **2002**, *346*, 549–556. [CrossRef]
157. Dankiewicz, J.; Cronberg, T.; Lilja, G.; Jakobsen, J.C.; Levin, H.; Ullén, S.; Rylander, C.; Wise, M.P.; Oddo, M.; Cariou, A.; et al. Hypothermia versus Normothermia after Out-of-Hospital Cardiac Arrest. *N. Engl. J. Med.* **2021**, *384*, 2283–2294. [CrossRef]
158. Le May, M.; Osborne, C.; Russo, J.; So, D.; Chong, A.Y.; Dick, A.; Froeschl, M.; Glover, C.; Hibbert, B.; Marquis, J.F.; et al. Effect of Moderate vs Mild Therapeutic Hypothermia on Mortality and Neurologic Outcomes in Comatose Survivors of Out-of-Hospital Cardiac Arrest: The CAPITAL CHILL Randomized Clinical Trial. *JAMA* **2021**, *326*, 1494–1503. [CrossRef]
159. Schwab, S.; Schwarz, S.; Spranger, M.; Keller, E.; Bertram, M.; Hacke, W. Moderate hypothermia in the treatment of patients with severe middle cerebral artery infarction. *Stroke* **1998**, *29*, 2461–2466. [CrossRef]
160. Schwab, S.; Georgiadis, D.; Berrouschot, J.; Schellinger, P.D.; Graffagnino, C.; Mayer, S.A. Feasibility and safety of moderate hypothermia after massive hemispheric infarction. *Stroke* **2001**, *32*, 2033–2035. [CrossRef]
161. Nutma, S.; Tjepkema-Cloostermans, M.C.; Ruijter, B.J.; Tromp, S.C.; van den Bergh, W.M.; Foudraine, N.A.; Kornips, F.H.M.; Drost, G.; Scholten, E.; Strang, A.; et al. Effects of targeted temperature management at 33 °C vs. 36 °C on comatose patients after cardiac arrest stratified by the severity of encephalopathy. *Resuscitation* **2022**, *173*, 147–153. [CrossRef]
162. Sadaka, F.; Veremakis, C. Therapeutic hypothermia for the management of intracranial hypertension in severe traumatic brain injury: A systematic review. *Brain Inj.* **2012**, *26*, 899. [CrossRef] [PubMed]
163. Dunkley, S.; McLeod, A. Therapeutic hypothermia in patients following traumatic brain injury: A systematic review. *Nurs. Crit. Care* **2017**, *22*, 150. [CrossRef] [PubMed]
164. Seule, M.A.; Muroi, C.; Mink, S.; Yonekawa, Y.; Keller, E. Therapeutic hypothermia in patients with aneurysmal subarachnoid hemorrhage, refractory intracranial hypertension, or cerebral vasospasm. *Neurosurgery* **2009**, *64*, 86–93. [CrossRef]
165. Stravitz, R.T.; Larsen, F.S. Therapeutic hypothermia for acute liver failure. *Crit. Care Med.* **2009**, *37*, S258. [CrossRef] [PubMed]
166. Dmello, D.; Cruz-Flores, S.; Matuschak, G.M. Moderate hypothermia with intracranial pressure monitoring as a therapeutic paradigm for the management of acute liver failure: A systematic review. *Intensive Care Med.* **2010**, *36*, 210. [CrossRef] [PubMed]
167. Lascarrou, J.B.; Merdji, H.; Le Gouge, A.; Colin, G.; Grillet, G.; Girardie, P.; Coupez, E.; Dequin, P.F.; Cariou, A.; Boulain, T.; et al. Targeted Temperature Management for Cardiac Arrest with Nonshockable Rhythm. *N. Engl. J. Med.* **2019**, *381*, 2327–2337. [CrossRef] [PubMed]
168. Hassager, C.; Schmidt, H.; Møller, J.E.; Grand, J.; Mølstrøm, S.; Beske, R.P.; Boesgaard, S.; Borregaard, B.; Bekker-Jensen, D.; Dahl, J.S.; et al. Duration of Device-Based Fever Prevention after Cardiac Arrest. *N. Engl. J. Med.* **2023**, *388*, 888–897. [CrossRef] [PubMed]
169. Hachimi-Idrissi, S.; Zizi, M.; Nguyen, D.N.; Schiettecate, J.; Ebinger, G.; Michotte, Y.; Huyghens, L. The evolution of serum astroglial S-100 beta protein in patients with cardiac arrest treated with mild hypothermia. *Resuscitation* **2005**, *64*, 187–192. [CrossRef] [PubMed]
170. Laurent, I.; Adrie, C.; Vinsonneau, C.; Cariou, A.; Chiche, J.D.; Ohanessian, A.; Spaulding, C.; Carli, P.; Dhainaut, J.F.; Monchi, M. High-volume hemofiltration after out-of-hospital cardiac arrest: A randomized study. *J. Am. Coll. Cardiol.* **2005**, *46*, 432–437. [CrossRef]
171. Castrén, M.; Nordberg, P.; Svensson, L.; Taccone, F.; Vincent, J.L.; Desruelles, D.; Eichwede, F.; Mols, P.; Schwab, T.; Vergnion, M.; et al. Intra-arrest transnasal evaporative cooling: A randomized, prehospital, multicenter study (PRINCE: Pre-ROSC IntraNasal Cooling Effectiveness). *Circulation* **2010**, *122*, 729–736. [CrossRef]
172. Bernard, S.A.; Smith, K.; Cameron, P.; Masci, K.; Taylor, D.M.; Cooper, D.J.; Kelly, A.M.; Silvester, W.; Rapid Infusion of Cold Hartmanns (RICH) Investigators. Induction of therapeutic hypothermia by paramedics after resuscitation from out-of-hospital ventricular fibrillation cardiac arrest: A randomized controlled trial. *Circulation* **2010**, *122*, 737–742. [CrossRef] [PubMed]

173. Nielsen, N.; Wetterslev, J.; Cronberg, T.; Erlinge, D.; Gasche, Y.; Hassager, C.; Horn, J.; Hovdenes, J.; Kjaergaard, J.; Kuiper, M.; et al. Targeted temperature management at 33 °C versus 36 °C after cardiac arrest. *N. Engl. J. Med.* **2013**, *369*, 2197–2206. [CrossRef] [PubMed]
174. Lilja, G.; Nielsen, N.; Friberg, H.; Horn, J.; Kjaergaard, J.; Nilsson, F.; Pellis, T.; Wetterslev, J.; Wise, M.P.; Bosch, F.; et al. Cognitive function in survivors of out-of-hospital cardiac arrest after target temperature management at 33 °C versus 36 °C. *Circulation* **2015**, *131*, 1340–1349. [CrossRef] [PubMed]
175. Kim, F.; Nichol, G.; Maynard, C.; Hallstrom, A.; Kudenchuk, P.J.; Rea, T.; Copass, M.K.; Carlbom, D.; Deem, S.; Longstreth, W.T., Jr.; et al. Effect of prehospital induction of mild hypothermia on survival and neurological status among adults with cardiac arrest: A randomized clinical trial. *JAMA* **2014**, *311*, 45–52. [CrossRef]
176. Debaty, G.; Maignan, M.; Savary, D.; Koch, F.X.; Ruckly, S.; Durand, M.; Picard, J.; Escallier, C.; Chouquer, R.; Santre, C.; et al. Impact of intra-arrest therapeutic hypothermia in outcomes of prehospital cardiac arrest: A randomized controlled trial. *Intensive Care Med.* **2014**, *40*, 1832–1842. [CrossRef]
177. Maynard, C.; Longstreth, W.T., Jr.; Nichol, G.; Hallstrom, A.; Kudenchuk, P.J.; Rea, T.; Copass, M.K.; Carlbom, D.; Deem, S.; Olsufka, M.; et al. Effect of prehospital induction of mild hypothermia on 3-month neurological status and 1-year survival among adults with cardiac arrest: Long-term follow-up of a randomized, clinical trial. *J. Am. Heart Assoc.* **2015**, *4*, e001693. [CrossRef]
178. Deye, N.; Cariou, A.; Girardie, P.; Pichon, N.; Megarbane, B.; Midez, P.; Tonnelier, J.M.; Boulain, T.; Outin, H.; Delahaye, A.; et al. Clinical and Economical Impact of Endovascular Cooling in the Management of Cardiac Arrest (ICEREA) Study Group. Endovascular Versus External Targeted Temperature Management for Patients with Out-of-Hospital Cardiac Arrest: A Randomized, Controlled Study. *Circulation* **2015**, *132*, 182–193. [CrossRef]
179. Cronberg, T.; Lilja, G.; Horn, J.; Kjaergaard, J.; Wise, M.P.; Pellis, T.; Hovdenes, J.; Gasche, Y.; Åneman, A.; Stammet, P.; et al. Neurologic Function and Health-Related Quality of Life in Patients Following Targeted Temperature Management at 33 °C vs. 36 °C After Out-of-Hospital Cardiac Arrest: A Randomized Clinical Trial. *JAMA Neurol.* **2015**, *72*, 634–641. [CrossRef]
180. Pang, P.Y.; Wee, G.H.; Hoo, A.E.; Sheriff, I.M.; Lim, S.L.; Tan, T.E.; Loh, Y.J.; Kerk, K.L.; Sin, Y.K.; Lim, C.H. Therapeutic hypothermia in adult patients receiving extracorporeal life support: Early results of a randomized controlled study. *J. Cardiothorac. Surg.* **2016**, *11*, 43. [CrossRef]
181. Bernard, S.A.; Smith, K.; Finn, J.; Hein, C.; Grantham, H.; Bray, J.E.; Deasy, C.; Stephenson, M.; Williams, T.A.; Straney, L.D.; et al. Induction of Therapeutic Hypothermia During Out-of-Hospital Cardiac Arrest Using a Rapid Infusion of Cold Saline: The RINSE Trial (Rapid Infusion of Cold Normal Saline). *Circulation* **2016**, *134*, 797–805. [CrossRef]
182. Scales, D.C.; Cheskes, S.; Verbeek, P.R.; Pinto, R.; Austin, D.; Brooks, S.C.; Dainty, K.N.; Goncharenko, K.; Mamdani, M.; Thorpe, K.E.; et al. Prehospital cooling to improve successful targeted temperature management after cardiac arrest: A randomized controlled trial. *Resuscitation* **2017**, *121*, 187–194. [CrossRef] [PubMed]
183. Look, X.; Li, H.; Ng, M.; Lim, E.T.S.; Pothiawala, S.; Tan, K.B.K.; Sewa, D.W.; Shahidah, N.; Pek, P.P.; Ong, M.E.H. Randomized controlled trial of internal and external targeted temperature management methods in post-cardiac arrest patients. *Am. J. Emerg. Med.* **2018**, *36*, 66–72. [CrossRef] [PubMed]
184. Kirkegaard, H.; Søreide, E.; de Haas, I.; Pettilä, V.; Taccone, F.S.; Arus, U.; Storm, C.; Hassager, C.; Nielsen, J.F.; Sørensen, C.A.; et al. Targeted Temperature Management for 48 vs. 24 Hours and Neurologic Outcome After Out-of-Hospital Cardiac Arrest: A Randomized Clinical Trial. *JAMA* **2017**, *318*, 341–350. [CrossRef] [PubMed]
185. Lopez-de-Sa, E.; Juarez, M.; Armada, E.; Sanchez-Salado, J.C.; Sanchez, P.L.; Loma-Osorio, P.; Sionis, A.; Monedero, M.C.; Martinez-Sellés, M.; Martín-Benitez, J.C.; et al. A multicentre randomized pilot trial on the effectiveness of different levels of cooling in comatose survivors of out-of-hospital cardiac arrest: The FROST-I trial. *Intensive Care Med.* **2018**, *44*, 1807–1815. [CrossRef]
186. Nordberg, P.; Taccone, F.S.; Truhlar, A.; Forsberg, S.; Hollenberg, J.; Jonsson, M.; Cuny, J.; Goldstein, P.; Vermeersch, N.; Higuet, A.; et al. Effect of Trans-Nasal Evaporative Intra-arrest Cooling on Functional Neurologic Outcome in Out-of-Hospital Cardiac Arrest: The PRINCESS Randomized Clinical Trial. *JAMA* **2019**, *321*, 1677–1685. [CrossRef] [PubMed]
187. Glover, G.W.; Thomas, R.M.; Vamvakas, G.; Al-Subaie, N.; Cranshaw, J.; Walden, A.; Wise, M.P.; Ostermann, M.; Thomas-Jones, E.; Cronberg, T.; et al. Intravascular versus surface cooling for targeted temperature management after out-of-hospital cardiac arrest: An analysis of the TTM trial data. *Crit. Care* **2016**, *20*, 381. [CrossRef]
188. Kim, Y.J.; Park, J.M.; Kim, M.S.; Ryoo, S.M.; Park, J.S.; Kim, S.S.; Kim, Y.O.; Kim, W.Y. Independent risk factors for the shivering occurrence during induction period in out-of-hospital cardiac arrest survivors treated with targeted temperature management. *Ther. Hypothermia Temp. Manag.* **2019**, *9*, 70–75. [CrossRef]
189. Bouwes, A.; Robillard, L.B.; Binnekade, J.M.; de Pont, A.C.; Wieske, L.; Hartog, A.W.; Schultz, M.J.; Horn, J. The influence of rewarming after therapeutic hypothermia on outcome after cardiac arrest. *Resuscitation* **2012**, *83*, 996–1000. [CrossRef]
190. Bro-Jeppesen, J.; Hassager, C.; Wanscher, M.; Søholm, H.; Thomsen, J.H.; Lippert, F.K.; Møller, J.E.; Køber, L.; Kjaergaard, J. Post-hypothermia fever is associated with increased mortality after out-of-hospital cardiac arrest. *Resuscitation* **2013**, *84*, 1734–1740. [CrossRef] [PubMed]
191. Elbadawi, A.; Sedhom, R.; Baig, B.; Mahana, I.; Thakker, R.; Gad, M.; Eid, M.; Nair, A.; Kayani, W.; Denktas, A.; et al. Targeted Hypothermia vs Targeted Normothermia in Survivors of Cardiac Arrest: A Systematic Review and Meta-Analysis of Randomized Trials. *Am. J. Med.* **2022**, *135*, 626–633.e4. [CrossRef]

192. Fernando, S.M.; Di Santo, P.; Sadeghirad, B.; Lascarrou, J.B.; Rochwerg, B.; Mathew, R.; Sekhon, M.S.; Munshi, L.; Fan, E.; Brodie, D.; et al. Targeted temperature management following out-of-hospital cardiac arrest: A systematic review and network meta-analysis of temperature targets. *Intensive Care Med.* **2021**, *47*, 1078–1088. [CrossRef] [PubMed]
193. Granfeldt, A.; Holmberg, M.J.; Nolan, J.P.; Soar, J.; Andersen, L.W.; International Liaison Committee on Resuscitation (ILCOR) Advanced Life Support Task Force. Targeted temperature management in adult cardiac arrest: Systematic review and meta-analysis. *Resuscitation* **2021**, *167*, 160–172. [CrossRef] [PubMed]
194. Aneman, A.; Frost, S.; Parr, M.; Skrifvars, M.B. Target temperature management following cardiac arrest: A systematic review and Bayesian meta-analysis. *Crit. Care* **2022**, *26*, 58. [CrossRef] [PubMed]
195. Koren, O.; Rozner, E.; Yosefia, S.; Turgeman, Y. Therapeutic hypothermia after out of hospital cardiac arrest improve 1-year survival rate for selective patients. *PLoS ONE* **2020**, *15*, e0226956. [CrossRef]
196. Paul, M.; Bougouin, W.; Geri, G.; Dumas, F.; Champigneulle, B.; Legriel, S.; Charpentier, J.; Mira, J.P.; Sandroni, C.; Cariou, A. Delayed awakening after cardiac arrest: Prevalence and risk factors in the Parisian registry. *Intensive Care Med.* **2016**, *42*, 1128–1136. [CrossRef]
197. Rey, A.; Rossetti, A.O.; Miroz, J.P.; Eckert, P.; Oddo, M. Late Awakening in Survivors of Postanoxic Coma: Early Neurophysiologic Predictors and Association with ICU and Long-Term Neurologic Recovery. *Crit. Care Med.* **2019**, *47*, 85–92. [CrossRef]
198. Crombez, T.; Hachimi-Idrissi, S. The influence of targeted temperature management on the pharmacokinetics of drugs administered during and after cardiac arrest: A systematic review. *Acta Clin. Belg.* **2017**, *72*, 116–122. [CrossRef]
199. Lemiale, V.; Dumas, F.; Mongardon, N.; Giovanetti, O.; Charpentier, J.; Chiche, J.D.; Carli, P.; Mira, J.P.; Nolan, J.; Cariou, A. Intensive care unit mortality after cardiac arrest: The relative contribution of shock and brain injury in a large cohort. *Intensive Care Med.* **2013**, *39*, 1972–1980. [CrossRef]
200. Dragancea, I.; Wise, M.P.; Al-Subaie, N.; Cranshaw, J.; Friberg, H.; Glover, G.; Pellis, T.; Rylance, R.; Walden, A.; Nielsen, N.; et al. Protocol-driven neurological prognostication and withdrawal of life-sustaining therapy after cardiac arrest and targeted temperature management. *Resuscitation* **2017**, *117*, 50–57. [CrossRef]
201. Sandroni, C.; Dell'anna, A.M.; Tujjar, O.; Geri, G.; Cariou, A.; Taccone, F.S. Acute kidney injury after cardiac arrest: A systematic review and meta-analysis of clinical studies. *Minerva Anestesiol.* **2021**, *82*, 989–999.
202. Taccone, F.; Cronberg, T.; Friberg, H.; Greer, D.; Horn, J.; Oddo, M.; Scolletta, S.; Vincent, J.L. How to assess prognosis after cardiac arrest and therapeutic hypothermia. *Crit. Care* **2014**, *18*, 202. [CrossRef] [PubMed]
203. Stammet, P.; Collignon, O.; Hassager, C.; Wise, M.P.; Hovdenes, J.; Åneman, A.; Horn, J.; Devaux, Y.; Erlinge, D.; Kjaergaard, J.; et al. Neuron-specific enolase as a predictor of death or poor neurological outcome after out-of-hospital cardiac arrest and targeted temperature management at 33 °C and 36 °C. *J. Am. Coll. Cardiol.* **2015**, *65*, 2104–2114. [CrossRef] [PubMed]
204. Streitberger, K.J.; Leithner, C.; Wattenberg, M.; Tonner, P.H.; Hasslacher, J.; Joannidis, M.; Pellis, T.; Di Luca, E.; Födisch, M.; Krannich, A.; et al. Neuronspecific enolase predicts poor outcome after cardiac arrest and targeted temperature management: A multicenter study on 1,053 patients. *Crit. Care Med.* **2017**, *45*, 1145–1151. [CrossRef] [PubMed]
205. Lamartine Monteiro, M.; Taccone, F.S.; Depondt, C.; Lamanna, I.; Gaspard, N.; Ligot, N.; Mavroudakis, N.; Naeije, G.; Vincent, J.L.; Legros, B. The prognostic value of 48-h continuous EEG during therapeutic hypothermia after cardiac arrest. *Neurocrit. Care* **2016**, *24*, 153–162. [CrossRef]
206. Eertmans, W.; Genbrugge, C.; Haesen, J.; Drieskens, C.; Demeestere, J.; Vander Laenen, M.; Boer, W.; Mesotten, D.; Dens, J.; Ernon, L.; et al. The Prognostic Value of Simplified EEG in Out-of-Hospital Cardiac Arrest Patients. *Neurocrit. Care* **2019**, *30*, 139–148. [CrossRef] [PubMed]
207. Alvarez-Fernández, J.A.; Pérez-Quintero, R. Use of transcranial Doppler ultrasound in the management of post-cardiac arrest syndrome. *Resuscitation* **2009**, *80*, 1321–1322. [CrossRef]
208. Lin, J.J.; Hsia, S.H.; Wang, H.S.; Chiang, M.C.; Lin, K.L. Transcranial Doppler ultrasound in therapeutic hypothermia for children after resuscitation. *Resuscitation* **2015**, *89*, 182–187. [CrossRef] [PubMed]
209. Aaslid, R.; Lindegaard, K.F.; Sorteberg, W.; Nornes, H. Cerebral autoregulation dynamics in humans. *Stroke* **1989**, *20*, 45–52. [CrossRef]
210. Lassen, N.A. Cerebral blood flow and oxygen consumption in man. *Physiol. Rev.* **1959**, *39*, 183–238. [CrossRef]
211. Tan, C.O. Defining the characteristic relationship between arterial pressure and cerebral blood flow. *J. Appl. Physiol. (1985)* **2012**, *113*, 1194–1200. [CrossRef]
212. Buunk, G.; van der Hoeven, J.G.; Frölich, M.; Meinders, A.E. Cerebral vasoconstriction in comatose patients resuscitated from a cardiac arrest? *Intensive Care Med.* **1996**, *22*, 1191–1196. [CrossRef] [PubMed]
213. Bisschops, L.L.; Hoedemaekers, C.W.; Simons, K.S.; van der Hoeven, J.G. Preserved metabolic coupling and cerebrovascular reactivity during mild hypothermia after cardiac arrest. *Crit. Care Med.* **2010**, *38*, 1542–1547. [CrossRef] [PubMed]
214. Sundgreen, C.; Larsen, F.S.; Herzog, T.M.; Knudsen, G.M.; Boesgaard, S.; Aldershvile, J. Autoregulation of cerebral blood flow in patients resuscitated from cardiac arrest. *Stroke* **2001**, *32*, 128–132. [CrossRef]
215. Jha, R.M.; Elmer, J. Transcranial dopplers after cardiac arrest: Should we ride this wave? *Resuscitation* **2019**, *141*, 204–206. [CrossRef]
216. Castro, P.; Azevedo, E.; Sorond, F. Cerebral Autoregulation in Stroke. *Curr. Atheroscler. Rep.* **2018**, *20*, 37. [CrossRef]

217. Wessels, T.; Harrer, J.U.; Jacke, C.; Janssens, U.; Klötzsch, C. The prognostic value of early transcranial Doppler ultrasound following cardiopulmonary resuscitation. *Ultrasound Med. Biol.* **2006**, *32*, 1845–1851. [CrossRef] [PubMed]
218. Lemiale, V.; Huet, O.; Vigué, B.; Mathonnet, A.; Spaulding, C.; Mira, J.P.; Carli, P.; Duranteau, J.; Cariou, A. Changes in cerebral blood flow and oxygen extraction during post-resuscitation syndrome. *Resuscitation* **2008**, *76*, 17–24. [CrossRef]
219. Pollock, J.M.; Whitlow, C.T.; Deibler, A.R.; Tan, H.; Burdette, J.H.; Kraft, R.A.; Maldjian, J.A. Anoxic injury-associated cerebral hyperperfusion identified with arterial spin-labeled MR imaging. *AJNR Am. J. Neuroradiol.* **2008**, *29*, 1302–1307. [CrossRef] [PubMed]
220. Iida, K.; Satoh, H.; Arita, K.; Nakahara, T.; Kurisu, K.; Ohtani, M. Delayed hyperemia causing intracranial hypertension after cardiopulmonary resuscitation. *Crit. Care Med.* **1997**, *25*, 971–976. [CrossRef]
221. Rafi, S.; Tadie, J.M.; Gacouin, A.; Leurent, G.; Bedossa, M.; Le Tulzo, Y.; Maamar, A. Doppler sonography of cerebral blood flow for early prognostication after out-of-hospital cardiac arrest: DOTAC study. *Resuscitation* **2019**, *141*, 188–194. [CrossRef]
222. Iordanova, B.; Li, L.; Clark, R.S.B.; Manole, M.D. Alterations in Cerebral Blood Flow after Resuscitation from Cardiac Arrest. *Front. Pediatr.* **2017**, *5*, 174. [CrossRef] [PubMed]
223. de Riva, N.; Budohoski, K.P.; Smielewski, P.; Kasprowicz, M.; Zweifel, C.; Steiner, L.A.; Reinhard, M.; Fábregas, N.; Pickard, J.D.; Czosnyka, M. Transcranial Doppler pulsatility index: What it is and what it isn't. *Neurocrit. Care* **2012**, *17*, 58–66. [CrossRef] [PubMed]
224. Ameloot, K.; Genbrugge, C.; Meex, I.; Jans, F.; Boer, W.; Vander Laenen, M.; Ferdinande, B.; Mullens, W.; Dupont, M.; Dens, J.; et al. An observational near-infrared spectroscopy study on cerebral autoregulation in post-cardiac arrest patients: Time to drop 'one-size-fits-all' hemodynamic targets? *Resuscitation* **2015**, *90*, 121–126. [CrossRef]
225. Balu, R.; Baghshomali, S.; Abella, B.S.; Kofke, W.A. Abstract 12: Cerebrovascular Pressure Reactivity Predicts Outcome in Diffuse Hypoxic-Ischemic Brain Injury. *Circulation* **2018**, *138*, A12. [CrossRef]
226. Caldwell, M.; Scholkmann, F.; Wolf, U.; Wolf, M.; Elwell, C.; Tachtsidis, I. Modelling confounding effects from extracerebral contamination and systemic factors on functional near-infrared spectroscopy. *Neuroimage* **2016**, *143*, 91–105. [CrossRef]
227. Gonella, S.; Basso, I.; Dimonte, V.; Martin, B.; Berchialla, P.; Campagna, S.; Di Giulio, P. Association Between End-of-Life Conversations in Nursing Homes and End-of-Life Care Outcomes: A Systematic Review and Meta-analysis. *J. Am. Med. Dir. Assoc.* **2019**, *20*, 249–261. [CrossRef]
228. Davidson, J.E.; Aslakson, R.A.; Long, A.C.; Puntillo, K.A.; Kross, E.K.; Hart, J.; Cox, C.E.; Wunsch, H.; Wickline, M.A.; Nunnally, M.E.; et al. Guidelines for Family-Centered Care in the Neonatal, Pediatric, and Adult ICU. *Crit. Care Med.* **2017**, *45*, 103–128. [CrossRef]
229. Adelman, R.D.; Tmanova, L.L.; Delgado, D.; Dion, S.; Lachs, M.S. Caregiver burden: A clinical review. *JAMA* **2014**, *311*, 1052–1060. [CrossRef]
230. Chen, C.; Michaels, J.; Meeker, M.A. Family Outcomes and Perceptions of End-of-Life Care in the Intensive Care Unit: A Mixed-Methods Review. *J. Palliat. Care* **2020**, *35*, 143–153. [CrossRef]
231. Lee, H.W.; Park, Y.; Jang, E.J.; Lee, Y.J. Intensive care unit length of stay is reduced by protocolized family support intervention: A systematic review and meta-analysis. *Intensive Care Med.* **2019**, *45*, 1072–1081. [CrossRef]
232. Walczak, A.; Butow, P.N.; Bu, S.; Clayton, J.M. A systematic review of evidence for end-of-life communication interventions: Who do they target, how are they structured and do they work? *Patient Educ. Couns.* **2016**, *99*, 3–16. [CrossRef] [PubMed]
233. Oczkowski, S.J.; Chung, H.O.; Hanvey, L.; Mbuagbaw, L.; You, J.J. Communication tools for end-of-life decision-making in the intensive care unit: A systematic review and meta-analysis. *Crit. Care* **2016**, *20*, 97. [CrossRef] [PubMed]
234. DeSanto-Madeya, S.; Safizadeh, P. Family Satisfaction with End-of-Life Care in the Intensive Care Unit: A Systematic Review of the Literature. *Dimens. Crit. Care Nurs.* **2017**, *36*, 278–283. [CrossRef]
235. You, J.J.; Jayaraman, D.; Swinton, M.; Jiang, X.; Heyland, D.K. Supporting shared decision-making about cardiopulmonary resuscitation using a video-based decision-support intervention in a hospital setting: A multisite before-after pilot study. *CMAJ Open* **2019**, *7*, E630–E637. [CrossRef] [PubMed]
236. Sahgal, S.; Yande, A.; Thompson, B.B.; Chen, E.P.; Fagerlin, A.; Morgenstern, L.B.; Zahuranec, D.B. Surrogate Satisfaction with Decision Making After Intracerebral Hemorrhage. *Neurocrit. Care* **2021**, *34*, 193–200. [CrossRef] [PubMed]
237. Lim, C.E.; Ng, R.W.; Cheng, N.C.; Cigolini, M.; Kwok, C.; Brennan, F. Advance care planning for haemodialysis patients. *Cochrane Database Syst. Rev.* **2016**, *7*, CD010737. [CrossRef]
238. Kavalieratos, D.; Corbelli, J.; Zhang, D.; Dionne-Odom, J.N.; Ernecoff, N.C.; Hanmer, J.; Hoydich, Z.P.; Ikejiani, D.Z.; Klein-Fedyshin, M.; Zimmermann, C.; et al. Association Between Palliative Care and Patient and Caregiver Outcomes: A Systematic Review and Meta-analysis. *JAMA* **2016**, *316*, 2104–2114. [CrossRef]
239. Huber, M.T.; Highland, J.D.; Krishnamoorthi, V.R.; Tang, J.W. Utilizing the Electronic Health Record to Improve Advance Care Planning: A Systematic Review. *Am. J. Hosp. Palliat. Care* **2018**, *35*, 532–541. [CrossRef]
240. Mentzelopoulos, S.D.; Couper, K.; Voorde, P.V.; Druwé, P.; Blom, M.; Perkins, G.D.; Lulic, I.; Djakow, J.; Raffay, V.; Lilja, G.; et al. European Resuscitation Council Guidelines 2021: Ethics of resuscitation and end of life decisions. *Resuscitation* **2021**, *161*, 408–432. [CrossRef]
241. Brinkman-Stoppelenburg, A.; Rietjens, J.A.; van der Heide, A. The effects of advance care planning on end-of-life care: A systematic review. *Palliat. Med.* **2014**, *28*, 1000–1025. [CrossRef]

242. MacKenzie, M.A.; Smith-Howell, E.; Bomba, P.A.; Meghani, S.H. Respecting Choices and Related Models of Advance Care Planning: A Systematic Review of Published Evidence. *Am. J. Hosp. Palliat. Care* **2018**, *35*, 897–907. [CrossRef] [PubMed]
243. Malhotra, C.; Sim, D.; Jaufeerally, F.R.; Hu, M.; Nadkarni, N.; Ng, C.S.H.; Wong, G.; Tan, B.C.; Lim, J.F.; Chuang, C.Y.; et al. Impact of a Formal Advance Care Planning Program on End-of-Life Care for Patients with Heart Failure: Results From a Randomized Controlled Trial. *J. Card. Fail.* **2020**, *26*, 594–598. [CrossRef] [PubMed]
244. Kernick, L.A.; Hogg, K.J.; Millerick, Y.; Murtagh, F.E.M.; Djahit, A.; Johnson, M. Does advance care planning in addition to usual care reduce hospitalisation for patients with advanced heart failure: A systematic review and narrative synthesis. *Palliat. Med.* **2018**, *32*, 1539–1551. [CrossRef]
245. Scarpi, E.; Dall'Agata, M.; Zagonel, V.; Gamucci, T.; Bertè, R.; Sansoni, E.; Amaducci, E.; Broglia, C.M.; Alquati, S.; Garetto, F.; et al. Early Palliative Care Italian Study Group (EPCISG). Systematic vs. on-demand early palliative care in gastric cancer patients: A randomized clinical trial assessing patient and healthcare service outcomes. *Support Care Cancer* **2019**, *27*, 2425–2434. [CrossRef] [PubMed]
246. Mentzelopoulos, S.D.; Slowther, A.M.; Fritz, Z.; Sandroni, C.; Xanthos, T.; Callaway, C.; Perkins, G.D.; Newgard, C.; Ischaki, E.; Greif, R.; et al. Ethical challenges in resuscitation. *Intensive Care Med.* **2018**, *44*, 703–716. [CrossRef] [PubMed]
247. e-End of Life Care for All (e-ELCA) eLearning Programme. Available online: https://www.skillsforcare.org.uk/Developing-your-workforce/Care-topics/End-of-life-care/e-End-of-Life-Care-for-All-e-ELCA-elearning-programme.aspx (accessed on 26 May 2023).

Disclaimer/Publisher's Note: The statements, opinions and data contained in all publications are solely those of the individual author(s) and contributor(s) and not of MDPI and/or the editor(s). MDPI and/or the editor(s) disclaim responsibility for any injury to people or property resulting from any ideas, methods, instructions or products referred to in the content.

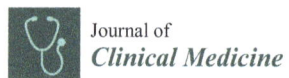

Review

The Techniques of Blood Purification in the Treatment of Sepsis and Other Hyperinflammatory Conditions

Giorgio Berlot [1,2,*], Ariella Tomasini [1], Silvia Zanchi [1] and Edoardo Moro [1]

[1] Department of Anesthesia and Intensive Care, Azienda Sanitaria Universitaria Giuliano Isontina, 34148 Trieste, Italy
[2] UCO Anestesia Rianimazione e Terapia Antalgica, Azienda Sanitaria Universitaria Giuliano Isontina, Strada di Fiume 447, 34149 Trieste, Italy
* Correspondence: berlotg@virgilio.it; Tel.: +039-04039904540; Fax: +039-040912278

Abstract: Even in the absence of strong indications deriving from clinical studies, the removal of mediators is increasingly used in septic shock and in other clinical conditions characterized by a hyperinflammatory response. Despite the different underlying mechanisms of action, they are collectively indicated as blood purification techniques. Their main categories include blood- and plasma processing procedures, which can run in a stand-alone mode or, more commonly, in association with a renal replacement treatment. The different techniques and principles of function, the clinical evidence derived from multiple clinical investigations, and the possible side effects are reviewed and discussed along with the persisting uncertainties about their precise role in the therapeutic armamentarium of these syndromes.

Keywords: septic shock; sepsis mediators; hemofiltration; hemoadsorption

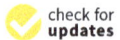

Citation: Berlot, G.; Tomasini, A.; Zanchi, S.; Moro, E. The Techniques of Blood Purification in the Treatment of Sepsis and Other Hyperinflammatory Conditions. *J. Clin. Med.* **2023**, *12*, 1723. https://doi.org/10.3390/jcm12051723

Academic Editor: Spyros D. Mentzelopoulos

Received: 10 January 2023
Revised: 16 February 2023
Accepted: 16 February 2023
Published: 21 February 2023

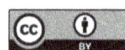

Copyright: © 2023 by the authors. Licensee MDPI, Basel, Switzerland. This article is an open access article distributed under the terms and conditions of the Creative Commons Attribution (CC BY) license (https:// creativecommons.org/licenses/by/ 4.0/).

1. Introduction

Sepsis is defined as a life-threatening organ dysfunction caused by a dysregulated host response to infection [1] that is caused by the release of a huge and only partially known number of mediators produced during the interaction between the infecting germ and the patient's immune system. The possible role of endogenous toxic substances in the pathogenesis of diseases is not a new concept, because since ancient times it was believed that many, if not all, disturbances affecting the humanity were caused by these agents. Consequently, their removal was considered an appropriate therapeutic target; with this aim, bloodletting gained wide popularity, becoming the first procedure of blood purification (BP). However, when in the second half of the 19th century it became clear that an exceedingly high number of microorganisms were responsible for many diseases previously treated with this approach, its use rapidly declined. At present, bloodletting is limited to rather uncommon conditions, including hemochromatosis and polycythemia. The modern era of BP arose in the 1940s, when Kollf et al. started to treat patients with acute or chronic kidney injury (AKI and CKI, respectively) using a cellophane membrane perfused by the patients' blood to remove uremic toxins [2]. It is remarkable that this approach should be unacceptable in the era of evidence-based medicine (EBM) and Ethical Committees, as the first 16 patients died during the procedures or immediately thereafter and only the 17th patient survived and was discharged home [2]. Some decades later, it appeared that the systemic disturbances associated with severe infections, including fever, arterial hypotension, multiple organ failure, etc., could be ascribed more to the interaction between the host's immune system and the infecting agent than to the latter only. Moreover, this reaction appeared to be at least partially determined by circulating factors, as the fluid removed from the bloodstream of septic and trauma patients using a cuprophan membrane was able to induce an intense proteolysis in isolated rat limbs, indicating the presence of a filtrable and transmissible factor able to cause the same muscle alterations observed in critical conditions [3]. From then on, an ever-increasing number of substances with both pro- and anti-inflammatory properties produced in these clinical circumstances have been identified [4], and it was hypothesized that their neutralization could positively influence the clinical course of sepsis and septic shock and/or other clinical conditions characterized by an uncontrolled inflammatory reaction. Conversely, in patients with a prolonged length-of-stay (LoS) in the Intensive Care Unit (ICU), these mediators are replaced or, better to say, are counterbalanced by the action of substances with anti-inflammatory capabilities, making them susceptible to infections sustained by low-virulence strains such as *Acinetobacter baumanii*, and to the reactivation of viruses, including Cytomegalovirus and Herpes viruses.

Aiming to neutralize the pro-inflammatory mediators, two different strategies have been developed. The first consists in the administration of inhibitors of a specific mediator or in the blockade of their cellular receptor; however, the results of many randomized controlled trials (RCTs) in ICU patients were largely below the expectations derived from experimental investigations and small Phase I human studies. However, some subgroup analyses indicated an increased survival of patients with elevated blood levels of the specific mediator targeted by the study substance. The use of inhibitors is advocated in the treatment of clinical conditions characterized by their persistent low-level production, including different rheumatologic and chronic inflammatory intestinal diseases.

The second strategy is based on the extracorporeal elimination of germ-derived substances, such as endotoxin or bloodborne mediators produced by the host via different mechanisms, including (a) their convective removal through an artificial membrane used also in Continuous Renal Replacement Treatments (CRRT) whose cutoff value is compatible with their molecular weight (MW); or (b) their adsorption on the membrane surface (Figure 1).

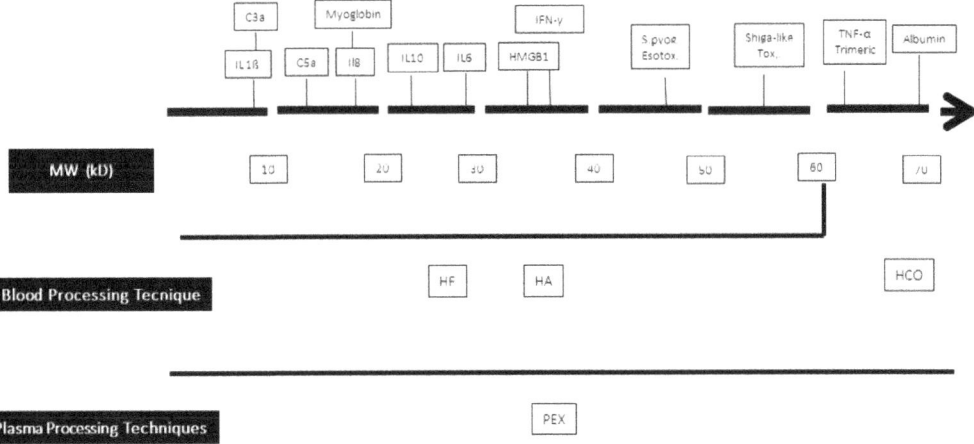

Figure 1. Clearance capabilities of blood purification techniques according to the molecular weight of some bloodborne substances. MW: Molecular Weight; HF: Hemofiltration; HA: hemadsorption; PEX: plasma exchange; HCO: high cut-off membrane. C3a: Activated Complement factor 3; IL: interleukin; HMG 1: High Mobility Group Box 1; IFN-γ: γ Interferon.

The aims of this review are to describe the principles of the different techniques of BP that are currently used, to evaluate the related clinical experiences, and to illustrate the pros and cons of each in the treatment of septic shock and other similar non-infectious clinical conditions caused by an exaggerated production of hyperinflammatory mediators.

2. Rationale of Blood Purification

Different mechanisms have been hypothesized to explain the possible beneficial effects of the elimination of mediators from the bloodstream [5], including:

(a) The lowering of both pro- and anti-inflammatory mediators below a threshold level, thus limiting the associated organ damage [6];
(b) The passage of mediators from the tissues to the blood and their subsequent extracorporeal clearance along a concentration gradient [7];
(c) The restoration of a cytokine gradient between the tissues and the blood, promoting leukocyte chemotaxis [8];
(d) The interaction between the membrane and the immune cells, as demonstrated by the modulation of surface molecules during different BP procedures [9].

It is likely that multiple mechanisms (i.e., a + b), maybe in different time windows, cooperate to achieve the therapeutic effect of BP.

3. Classification and Principles of Function of the BP Techniques

As stated above, different techniques are used to clear the mediators produced during septic shock or other clinical conditions characterized by elevated levels of inflammatory mediators, such as hemophagocytic syndrome (HS). Their removal is related to the characteristic (a) of the mediators, including their MW and the chemico-physical properties; and (b) of the device used, such as the cutoff value of the membrane, its surface of contact with the substrate to be processed, and the affinity for the substance to be cleared.

Thus, BP can be considered an umbrella term covering different techniques that can be primarily subdivided into blood- and plasma-processing procedures (Table 1). The factors influencing the efficacy of the BP differ according to their principle of function. Consequently, as far as the hemofiltration (HF)-based techniques are concerned, in which the mediators are eliminated by convection, the main determinant of removal is the production of ultrafiltrate (Qf), that, in turn, depends on the blood flowing inside the filter (Qb), the size of the pores, the subsequent sieving coefficient, the surface of the membranes used, and their chemico-physical properties. In contrast, only the Qb accounts for the efficacy of the absorption-based procedures [10]. Despite these differences, both families share a more- or less-pronounced time-dependent decay of the clearance capabilities, and their use can last from 2 to 24 h before the exhaustion of the BP effect.

Table 1. Techniques used in BP. Legend: CPFA®: coupled plasma filtration and adsorption.

Substrate	Technique/Brand	Mechanism
Blood	Ultrafiltration	High-volume ultrafiltration High-cutoff membrane
	Hemoadsorption	Toraymixin® oXyris® Cytosorb® Seraph®
Plasma	Plasma exchange Ultrafiltration + plasma adsorption	CPFA®

All BP procedures require a dedicated vascular access using a large-bore catheter and anticoagulation of the extracorporeal circuit using heparin or citrate.

3.1. Blood Processing Techniques

3.1.1. Hemofiltration (HF)

HF's principle of functioning consists in the convective removal of H_2O and solutes, including mediators, from the bloodstream by means of a synthetic membrane with a cutoff value of ~50–60 kDa, which are used also in CRRTs. The ultrafiltrate (UF) produced has the same electrolyte composition as the plasma. In fact, HF is an umbrella term covering multiple strategies that take advantage of the different amounts of UF considering the therapeutic target (see below). More recently, high-cutoff (HCO) membranes have been developed, but their use is associated with high albumin losses [11]; to overcome this problem, HCO membranes can be used in the diffusive rather than the in convective mode, or by slightly reducing their pore size and surfaces [12]. Independent of the characteristics of the membrane used, the volume of UF produced is related either to the aforementioned variables and to the blood flowing over it per unit time (Qb).

3.1.2. Hemoadsorption (HA)

HA consists in the adhesion of the circulating mediators on the surface of a membrane able to capture them. Four HA techniques have been developed so far [5,10,13]. The first takes advantage of an adsorbing column containing multiple polymixin-immobilized fibers (Toraymixin®, Toray Industries, Tokyo, Japan) arrayed into a cartridge to remove the endotoxin molecules from the Qb. Due to this characteristic, its use has been advocated in the treatment of septic shock caused by Gram-negative bacteria only.

The second technique consists in a cartridge containing a synthetic resin constituted by polystyrene and divinylbenzene microbeads (Cytosorb®, Cytosorbents Corporation, Monmouth Junction, NJ, USA; Aferetica s.r.l., Bologna, Italy). The wide adsorptive surface (~40.000 m^2) is able to adsorb hydrophobic pro- and anti-inflammatory mediators with MWs ranging from 5 to 60 kD. Cytosorb® represents an evolution of coupled plasma filtration and adsorption (CPFA; see below), as it uses the same binding resin that is arranged in microtubules instead that in microbeads.

The efficacy of Cytosorb® is concentration-dependent, as substances present in large concentrations are removed more efficiently than those with lower blood levels. Cytosorb® can run in a stand-alone mode or can be associated with a Continuous Renal Replacement Treatment (CRRT) or with an extracorporeal membrane oxygenation (ECMO) apparatus.

The third technique is based on a filter containing a modified AN69 membrane associated with a positively charged polyethyleneimine polymer able to absorb both endotoxin and several different septic mediators (oXiris®, Baxter, Meyzieu, France) from the bloodstream, while simultaneously providing CRRT.

The final technique consists in an HA device (Seraph 100®, ExThera Medical Corp, Martinez, CA, USA) packed with polymer beads covered with covalent end-point heparin ultra-high-MW polyethylene. This design mimics the heparan sulfate attached on the cell surface, allowing the in vitro binding of toxins, bacteria, and Antithrombin III, thus clearing them from the bloodstream [14]. Due to these properties, the US Food and Drug Administration (FDA) recently approved its use for the treatment of COVID-19 patients.

3.2. Plasma Processing Techniques

Three techniques are currently used. They include:

a. Plasmapheresis (PF), which is based on the selective removal of one or more plasma components (lipoproteins, paraproteins, etc.), and is not currently used in the treatment of septic shock;
b. Plasma exchange (PEX), consisting in the removal of one or more volumes of plasma, which is replaced with donors' plasma or albumin. The rationale of PEX consists in the removal of "toxic substances" and the supply of a large amount of plasma components whose absence is considered responsible for the disorder (i.e., ADAMTS 13 for patients with thrombotic thrombocytopenic purpura [15]). Ideally, the best candidate substance for removal by PEX should have a high MW, small volume of distribution, long half-life, and low turnover rate [15];
c. Coupled plasma filtration and adsorption (CPFA), which basically consists in a three-step process: (1) the partial extraction of plasma from the blood via a plasma filter; (2) its processing within a cartridge, where a number of mediators are absorbed by a synthetic resin arranged in microtubules; and (3) reinfusion of the purified plasma

upstream of a second filter used for continuous veno-venous hemodiafiltration in cases of concomitant AKI. The adsorptive capabilities of the resin are exhausted after 10 h, but the CRRT can continue beyond this limit by excluding the plasma processing unit.

4. Clinical Research Evidence

4.1. Hemofiltration

As many clinical investigations have involved only a relatively limited number of patients or are retrospective, the result of prospective RCTs are reported in Table 2 (after).

Table 2. Results of some RCTs of BP in septic shock patients.

Study/Author	BP	Treatment Group N.	Control Group N.	Results
IVOIRE	HVHF	66	71	No difference in hospital mortality
EUPHAS	Toraymixin®	30	34	Improved hemodynamics and survival in the treatment group
ABDOMIX	Toraymixin®	119	113	Non-significant increase in mortality and no improvement in organ failure in the treatment group
EUPHRATES	Toraymixin®	84	78	Toraymixin® compared with sham treatment did not reduce mortality at 28 days
Supady et al. *	Cytosorb®	17	17	Excess mortality in the treatment group
ROMPA	CPFA	19	30	No difference in hospital mortality
COMPACT 1	CPFA	91	93	No difference in hospital mortality
COMPACT 2	CPFA	63	52	Excess mortality in the treatment group

* In COVID-19 patients in association with ECMO.

On the basis of previous investigations, which demonstrated a dose–effect relationship between the UF and survival [16], or reduced need for a vasopressor [17], it has been hypothesized that very elevated UF values per unit time (Qf) could be associated with an improved survival of septic shock patients treated with HF. Indeed, despite some studies demonstrating encouraging results [18], a large RCT using high-volume HF (HVHF) that compared an elevated (70 mL/kg/h) with a normal (35 mL/kg/h) Qf in 137 septic shock patients failed to confirm these findings [19] and this approach has been largely abandoned. Furthermore, the higher Qf reportedly determined a significant loss of antibiotics [20]. An evolution of this technique is the cascade HVHF, which was developed to selectively remove medium molecular weight (MW) molecules while retaining those with lower MW, including vitamins, nutrients, and drugs. The technique combines two different hemofilters with different cutoff values: the first hemofilter, with a larger cut-off, produces an ultrafiltrate containing both large and small MW molecules and flows though another one with a smaller cutoff; then, only medium-MW molecules will be cleared and those with lower MW are reinfused back to the patient as predilution fluid before the first hemofilter [21]. Despite the result of an experimental study that demonstrated a reduction in the need for a vasopressor in a porcine model of sepsis, a recent study of cascade HVHF failed to demonstrate any beneficial effect when compared with standard care in septic shock patients [21,22]. The use of HCO membranes has been associated with the reduction of several inflammatory mediators in some studies [12,23], but another investigation did not confirm these findings [24].

4.2. Hemoperfusion

4.2.1. Endotoxin Adsorption

Whereas this approach is commonly used in Japan on the basis of clinical investigations and clinical registries, in Western countries different RCTs aiming to assess the efficacy of this procedure produced conflicting results. In the Early Use of PolymixinB Hemoperfusion in Abdominal Septic Shock (EUPHAS) study [25], patients treated with this technique demonstrated hemodynamic and respiratory improvements associated with a trend toward a better outcome. However, a subsequent study performed in patients with septic shock due to peritonitis, the ABDOMIX Trial [26], demonstrated a trend of increased mortality in the treatment group. Finally, the Evaluating the Use of Polymixin B Hemoperfusion in the Randomized Controlled of Adults Treated for Endotoxemia and Septic Shock Trial (EUPHRATES) performed in septic shock patients with elevated blood endotoxin levels measured with the Endotoxin Activity Assay (EAA) demonstrated a beneficial effect on different variables, including survival, only in patients with high EAA results [27]. Taken together, it appears that this approach could be effective when the mortality of the control group ranges from 30 to 40%, and/or with elevated blood endotoxin levels. It is also possible that the somewhat divergent findings between Japanese and Western RCTs could be ascribed to different genetic and enzymatic profiles.

4.2.2. Cytosorb®

Although some experimental and clinical investigations demonstrated that the use of Cytosorb® is associated both with the reduction of blood levels of many inflammatory cytokines, with the reduction of the vasopressors and with the improved survival of patients with septic shock [28–31], other studies failed to confirm these findings [32–34]. Recently, Hawchar et al. [35], evaluating 1434 patients with different clinical conditions including 936 cases of septic shock treated with Cytosorb® demonstrated that, although the primary outcome of hospital mortality was higher than that reported in other studies (59% vs. 46.5%, respectively), it was lower than expected according to the APACHE II score (66%). While it is difficult to draw a definite conclusion, it is possible that different variables can account for these contrasting results, including the heterogeneity of patients treated, the intensity of the treatment, and the timeframe of initiation with the clinical course. In fact, in a group of septic shock patients, Berlot et al. demonstrated that in survivors either the amount of blood processed was higher or the interval of time elapsing from the onset of shock and the start of Cytosorb® was shorter than in nonsurvivors [36]. To maximize the effect of Cytosorb®, Bottari et al. [37] advocated the replacement of the cartridge every 12 instead of every 24 h, at least in the initial phase of the treatment, to take full advantage of the adsorptive capabilities of the resin.

4.2.3. oXiris®

Experimentally, this technique was demonstrated to have the same endotoxin-removing capabilities as Toraymixin®, and was similar to Cytosorb® regarding the clearance of mediators. Currently, the clinical experience is limited and basically consists in small case series of patients with septic shock and/or COVID-19, in whom improvements of the hemodynamic conditions, decreases in the blood concentrations of endotoxin and septic mediators, and the decrease of expected mortality was observed [38–40]. However, as stated by Li et al. [41], not dissimilar to what is stated above, the heterogeneity of the patients and the different underlying conditions create background noise and prevent the establishment of the real role of this procedure.

4.2.4. Seraph 100®

In the absence of clinical trials, the role of this device is still uncertain. Recently, Eden et al. [14] demonstrated a rapid resolution of bacteremia in a group of CKI patients undergoing RRT.

5. Plasma Exchange

If the roles of the different HA techniques of HA are not yet clear, even less definite is that of PEX. Besides the time-honored indications in critically ill patients [15], use of PEX in septic shock patients appears somewhat overshadowed by HA. This notwithstanding, a recent RCT involving 40 patients [42] demonstrated a trend for better survival and the improvement of multiple organ failure in patients treated with a single PEX with an exchange volume of >3000 mL of plasma associated with standard treatment ST as compared with the control group which received the ST only; as might be expected, the decrease of sepsis biomarkers and the replenishment of factors supplied with the plasma, including Protein C, Protein S, and ADAMTS 13, were observed in the PEX group, but not in the control group. Moreover, patients in the PEX group were weaned faster from the vasopressors and had a more pronounced decrease of blood lactate levels; similar results were demonstrated by David et al. [43], who observed a decreased need for vasopressors in a group of septic shock patients.

6. Coupled Plasma Filtration and Adsorption

Different investigators reported either the improvement of hemodynamic conditions or better outcomes with CPFA in several relatively small case series of septic shock patients [44–50]. To elucidate this potential role of CPFA in septic shock patients, an initial RCT (COMPACT 1) involving 192 out of 330 pre-planned patients was launched. The trial was suspended when an interim evaluation failed to show any survival benefit in the treatment group; yet, a post hoc analysis demonstrated that survivors had a larger volume of plasma processed (Vp) ($\geq$0.20 L/kg/session) than controls [47]. To evaluate this dose–effect relationship, a second RCT was subsequently started (COMPACT 2) using this value as the threshold Vp for the treatment group. However, this second RCT was also prematurely stopped when an intermediate analysis RCT involving 115 patients demonstrated an increased mortality in patients treated with CPFA [51]. Similar results have been reported by Gimenez-Esparta in another RCT (ROMPA) in 49 septic shock patients treated with CPFA [52]; however, this study was underpowered to draw definite conclusions.

Overall, these results caused the virtual disappearance of CPFA from the therapeutic armamentarium used in critically ill patients. Indeed, the puzzling is question is: why did the RCTs about the use of the CPFA failed to demonstrate any beneficial effect, whereas in single-center studies the outcome was positively influenced by this technique? In other words, has the jury reached the right verdict? As an example, Mariano et al. [53] demonstrated that in a group of severely burned and AKI patients, those treated with the CPFA (n: 39) had a significantly better outcome as compared with those of the control group (n: 87) who were treated with the RRT only (survival rate 51.1% vs. 87.1, respectively, $p < 0.05$). It is conceivable that patients treated in a single ICU take the maximal advantage from the experience of the local ICU staff, while the results of RCTs can be influenced by the co-existence of ICUs with different volumes of procedures.

7. Discussion

Despite several years of use and thousands of patients enrolled in clinical trials with different BP techniques, a number of grey areas persist. The most recent guidelines of the Surviving Sepsis Campaign do not advise for or against leaving centers free to adopt their own policy of BP [54]. Moreover, due to the methodological biases encountered in different investigations, some authors advocate multi-center RCTs that fully satisfy the EBM criteria [55,56]; yet, these studies appear difficult to launch due to the widespread use of these procedures, which makes the implementation of a clinical trial sponsored by the manufacturers or by health authorities unlikely.

The uncertainties concerning the use of BP in septic shock patients and/or in those with severe hyperinflammatory disease are caused by several factors other than infections. These factors can be summarized as follows:

The selection of patients. According to multiple studies, the best candidates are patients with septic shock whose source of sepsis has been identified and/or surgically treated. Due to their costs and inherent risk of iatrogenic complications, the risk/benefit ratio should be considered in every BP candidate.

The timing of initiation. As has been demonstrated with antibiotics, it appears that the early initiation of BP in the hyperinflammatory phase of septic shock is associated with a better outcome. Even in the absence of specific studies, it is reasonable that the same consideration applies in hyperinflammatory conditions other than septic shock [36]. However, there is a lack of clarity regarding their possible role in chronic critically ill patients in whom anti-inflammatory mediators prevail and set the stage for infections with opportunistic germs and viral reactivation.

The intensity of the procedure. It appears that a dose–effect relationship exists for BP. However, the risk of elimination of drugs and nutrients should not be overlooked, especially in the presence of elevated values of Qb or Qf [57]. A U-shaped curve can be hypothesized, in which undesirable effects, such the low removal of mediators and the clearance of antibiotic, are located at the opposed extremities, whereas the beneficial effects lay somewhere in between (Figure 2). As this point is difficult to establish, repeated measurements of the blood concentrations of antibiotics and other drugs are warranted, especially in the initial phase of a BP procedure, when the clearance capabilities are maximal and can impede the rapid achievement of an effective plasma concentration, which is a therapeutic target of pivotal relevance.

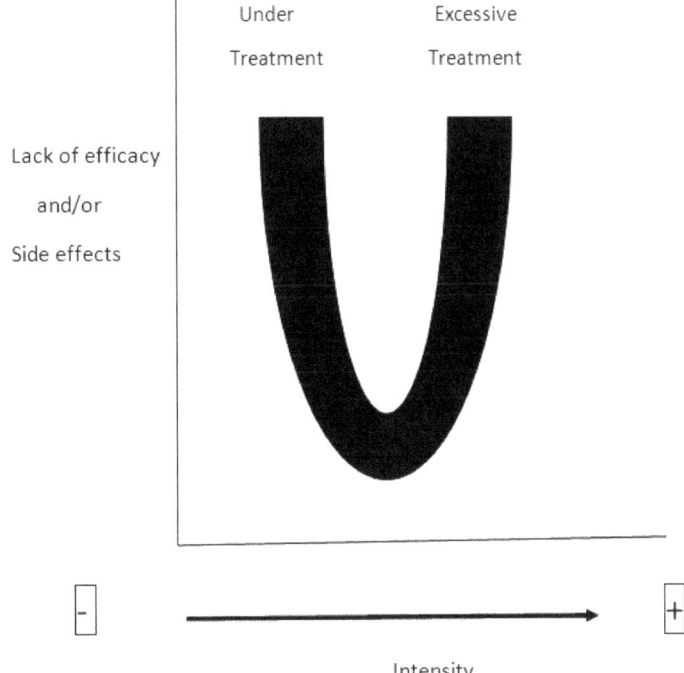

Figure 2. Hypothetical dose–effect relationship between the intensity of the treatment and the occurrence of side effects.

d. The assessment of the efficacy. The outcome of septic shock patients and of patients with non-septic hyperinflammatory conditions can be influenced by factors other than the BP used, including the appropriateness of the antibiotic treatment, the timely and complete drainage of septic foci, underlying conditions, etc. Thus, survival by itself does not represent a reliable marker of the efficacy of BP; consequently, other biological and clinical variables, such as the variation of the blood lactate levels and the changes in the need for vasopressors, can be used as proxies of efficacy [5].

e. The choice of the clinical situation. As stated above, patients with a prolonged LoS in ICU can undergo a biphasic clinical course, the first being characterized by a hyperinflammatory reaction that can be followed by a second one associated with the reduction of the immune capabilities caused by the production of substances with anti-inflammatory properties. These patients are usually old and with several frailties associated with pre-existing irreversible chronic conditions, such as chronic heart failure and obstructive pulmonary disease and worsening of chronic kidney disease. These patients often survive the disease that prompted the ICU admission, but their subsequent clinical course is marked by the occurrence of a number of different complications that make their survival unlikely, including malnutrition, difficulty in weaning from mechanical ventilation, skin ulcers, reinfections, etc. The possible role, if any, of BP in these chronic critically ill patients is not yet clear since most clinical investigations concerning BP treated patients in the initial hyperinflammatory phase and not in the second stage of the disease.

f. Undesired effects other than drug removal. In addition to the iatrogenic risks associated with indwelling large-bore catheters and the need of anticoagulation, all BP procedures can induce an undesired hypothermia due to the extracorporeal circuitry; to overcome this effect, all the currently used devices can warm the blood of the re-entry segment.

g. Lack of precision. BP techniques efficiently clear from the bloodstream all substances with certain chemico-physical properties, independent from their role in that timeframe. In many cases, the rule of "one size fits all" was and is still the rule for BP, and for many other treatments currently used in critically ill septic patients [58]. This is far removed from precision medicine in which the treatment is tailored to the needs of the individual patient. However, this approach is still experimental in critically ill septic patients [59].

8. Conclusions

Multiple factors, including the advancing age of the general population, the widespread use of invasive procedures, the use of immunodepressant drugs, and the ever-increasing occurrence of antibiotic resistance, make it so that the occurrence of septic shock is, and will remain in the future, a highly relevant issue among critically ill patients. Presently, the administration of appropriate antibiotics represents the only undiscussed therapeutic option for its causal treatment. Despite the somewhat conflicting results of many RCTs, BP techniques can be a valid adjunctive measure for these patients, provided that they are applied appropriately and considering their potential scavenging effects on antibiotics and other therapeutic agents.

Author Contributions: Conceptualization, G.B.; writing—original draft preparation, G.B., A.T., S.Z. and E.M. All authors have read and agreed to the published version of the manuscript.

Funding: This research received no external funding.

Institutional Review Board Statement: Not applicable.

Informed Consent Statement: Not applicable.

Data Availability Statement: Not applicable.

Conflicts of Interest: The authors declare no conflict of interest.

References

1. Singer, M.; Deutschman, C.S.; Seymour, C.W.; Shankar-Hari, M.; Annane, D.; Bauer, M.; Bellomo, R.; Bernard, G.R.; Chiche, J.D.; Coopersmith, C.M.; et al. The Third International Consensus Definitions for Sepsis and Septic Shock (Sepsis-3). *JAMA* **2016**, *315*, 801–810. [CrossRef]
2. Wieringa, F.P.; Søndergaard, H.; Ash, S. Father of Artificial Organs—The story of medical pioneer Willem J. Kolff (1911–2009). *Artif. Organs* **2021**, *45*, 1136–1140. [CrossRef]
3. Clowes, G.H., Jr.; George, B.C.; Villee, C.A., Jr.; Saravis, C.A. Muscle proteolysis induced by a circulating peptide in patients with sepsis or trauma. *N. Engl. J. Med.* **1983**, *308*, 545–552. [CrossRef]
4. Wiersinga, W.J.; Leopold, S.J.; Cranendonk, D.R.; van der Poll, T. Host innate immune responses to sepsis. *Virulence* **2014**, *5*, 36–44. [CrossRef] [PubMed]
5. Girardot, T.; Schneider, A.; Rimmelé, T. Blood Purification Techniques for Sepsis and Septic AKI. *Semin. Nephrol.* **2019**, *39*, 505–514. [CrossRef] [PubMed]
6. Ronco, C.; Tetta, C.; Mariano, F.; Wratten, M.L.; Bonello, M.; Bordoni, V.; Cardona, X.; Inguaggiato, P.; Pilotto, L.; d'Intini, V.; et al. Interpreting the mechanisms of continuous renal replacement therapy in sepsis: The peak concentration hypothesis. *Artif. Organs* **2003**, *27*, 792–801. [CrossRef]
7. Lee, P.A.; Matson, J.R.; Pryor, R.W.; Hinshaw, L.B. Continuous arteriovenous hemofiltration therapy for Staphylococcus aureus-induced septicemia in immature swine. *Crit. Care Med.* **1993**, *21*, 914–924. [CrossRef]
8. Rimmelé, T.; Kellum, J.A. Clinical review: Blood purification for sepsis. *Crit. Care* **2011**, *15*, 205. [CrossRef] [PubMed]
9. Ma, S.; Xu, Q.; Deng, B.; Zheng, Y.; Tian, H.; Wang, L.; Ding, F. Granulocyte and monocyte adsorptive apheresis ameliorates sepsis in rats. *Intensive Care Med. Exp.* **2017**, *5*, 18. [CrossRef] [PubMed]
10. Monard, C.; Rimmelé, T.; Ronco, C. Extracorporeal Blood Purification Therapies for Sepsis. *Blood Purif.* **2019**, *47* (Suppl. 3), 1–14. [CrossRef]
11. Morgera, S.; Rocktaschel, J.; Haase, M.; Lehmann, C.; von Heymann, C.; Ziemer, S.; Priem, F.; Hocher, B.; Gohl, H.; Kox, W.J.; et al. Intermittent high permeability hemofiltration in septic patients with acute renal failure. *Intensive Care Med.* **2003**, *29*, 1989–1995. [CrossRef] [PubMed]
12. Villa, G.; Chelazzi, C.; Morettini, E.; Zamidei, L.; Valente, S.; Caldini, A.L.; Zagli, G.; De Gaudio, A.R.; Romagnoli, S. Organ dysfunction during continuous veno-venous high cut-off hemodialysis in patients with septic acute kidney injury: A prospective observational study. *PLoS ONE* **2017**, *12*, e0172039. [CrossRef]
13. Ankawi, G.; Fan, W.; Pomarè Montin, D.; Lorenzin, A.; Neri, M.; Caprara, C.; de Cal, M.; Ronco, C. A New Series of Sorbent Devices for Multiple Clinical Purposes: Current Evidence and Future Directions. *Blood Purif.* **2019**, *47*, 94–100. [CrossRef]
14. Eden, G.; Schmidt, J.J.; Büttner, S.; Kümpers, P.; Hafer, C.; Rovas, A.; Koch, B.F.; Schmidt, B.M.W.; Kielstein, J.T. Safety and efficacy of the Seraph® 100 Microbind® Affinity Blood Filter to remove bacteria from the blood stream: Results of the first in human study. *Crit. Care* **2022**, *17*, 181. [CrossRef] [PubMed]
15. Bauer, P.R.; Ostermann, M.; Russell, L.; Robba, C.; David, S.; Ferreyro, B.L.; Cid, J.; Castro, P.; Juffermans, N.P.; Montini, L.; et al. Investigators. Plasma exchange in the intensive care unit: A narrative review. *Intensive Care Med.* **2022**, *48*, 1382–1396. [CrossRef] [PubMed]
16. Ronco, C.; Bellomo, R.; Homel, P.; Brendolan, A.; Dan, M.; Piccinni, P.; La Greca, G. Effects of different doses in continuous veno-venous haemofiltration on outcomes of acute renal failure: A prospective randomised trial. *Lancet* **2000**, *356*, 26–30. [CrossRef]
17. Cole, L.; Bellomo, R.; Journois, D.; Davenport, P.; Baldwin, I.; Tipping, P. High-volume haemofiltration in human septic shock. *Intensive Care Med.* **2001**, *27*, 978–986. [CrossRef]
18. Rimmelé, T.; Kellum, J.A. High-volume hemofiltration in the intensive care unit: A blood purification therapy. *Anesthesiology* **2012**, *116*, 1377–1387. [CrossRef]
19. Joannes-Boyau, O.; Honore, P.M.; Perez, P.; Bagshaw, S.M.; Grand, H.; Canivet, J.L.; Dewitte, A.; Flamens, C.; Pujol, W.; Grandoulier, A.S.; et al. High-volume versus standard-volume haemofiltration for septic shock patients with acute kidney injury IVOIRE study]: A multicentre randomized controlled trial. *Intensive Care Med.* **2013**, *39*, 1535–1546. [CrossRef]
20. Breilh, D.; Honore, P.M.; De Bels, D.; Roberts, J.A.; Gordien, J.B.; Fleureau, C.; Dewitte, A.; Coquin, J.; Roze, H.; Perez, P.; et al. Pharmacokinetics and Pharmacodynamics of Anti-infective Agents during Continuous Veno-venous Hemofiltration in Critically Ill Patients: Lessons Learned from an Ancillary Study of the IVOIRE Trial. *J. Transl. Intern. Med.* **2019**, *7*, 155–169. [CrossRef]
21. Rimmelé, T.; Hayi-Slayman, D.; Page, M.; Rada, H.; Monchi, M.; Allaouchiche, B. Cascade hemofiltration: Principle, first experimental data. *Ann. Fr. D'anesthesie Reanim.* **2009**, *28*, 249–252. [CrossRef]
22. Coudroy, R.; Payen, D.; Launey, Y.; Lukaszewicz, A.C.; Kaaki, M.; Veber, B.; Collange, O.; Dewitte, A.; Martin-Lefevre, L.; Jabaudon, M.; et al. ABDOMIX group. Modulation by Polymyxin-B Hemoperfusion of Inflammatory Response Related to Severe Peritonitis. *Shock* **2017**, *47*, 93–99. [CrossRef] [PubMed]
23. Atan, R.; Virzi, G.M.; Peck, L.; Ramadas, A.; Brocca, A.; Eastwood, G.; Sood, S.; Ronco, C.; Bellomo, R.; Goehl, H.; et al. High cut-off hemofiltration versus standard hemofiltration: A pilot assessment of effects on indices of apoptosis. *Blood Purif.* **2014**, *37*, 296–303. [CrossRef]

24. Kade, G.; Lubas, A.; Rzeszotarska, A.; Korsak, J.; Niemczyk, S. Effectiveness of High Cut-Off Hemofilters in the Removal of Selected Cytokines in Patients During Septic Shock Accompanied by Acute Kidney Injury-Preliminary Study. *Med. Sci. Monit.* **2016**, *22*, 4338–4344. [CrossRef]
25. Cruz, D.N.; Antonelli, M.; Fumagalli, R.; Foltran, F.; Brienza, N.; Donati, A.; Malcangi, V.; Petrini, F.; Volta, G.; Bobbio Pallavicini, F.M.; et al. Early use of polymyxin B hemoperfusion in abdominal septic shock: The EUPHAS randomized controlled trial. *JAMA* **2009**, *301*, 2445–2452. [CrossRef]
26. Payen, D.; Dupuis, C.; Deckert, V.; Pais de Barros, J.P.; Rérole, A.L.; Lukaszewicz, A.C.; Coudroy, R.; Robert, R.; Lagrost, L. Endotoxin Mass Concentration in Plasma Is Associated with Mortality in a Multicentric Cohort of Peritonitis-Induced Shock. *Front. Med.* **2021**, *8*, 749405. [CrossRef]
27. Dellinger, R.P.; Bagshaw, S.M.; Antonelli, M.; Foster, D.M.; Klein, D.J.; Marshall, J.C.; Palevsky, P.M.; Weisberg, L.S.; Schorr, C.A.; Trzeciak, S.; et al. Effect of Targeted Polymyxin B Hemoperfusion on 28-Day Mortality in Patients with Septic Shock and Elevated Endotoxin Level: The EUPHRATES Randomized Clinical Trial. *JAMA* **2018**, *320*, 1455–1463. [CrossRef] [PubMed]
28. Kogelmann, K.; Jarczak, D.; Scheller, M.; Drüner, M. Hemoadsorption by CytoSorb in septic patients: A case series. *Crit. Care* **2017**, *21*, 74. [CrossRef]
29. Brouwer, W.P.; Duran, S.; Kuijper, M.; Ince, C. Hemoadsorption with CytoSorb shows a decreased observed versus expected 28-day all-cause mortality in ICU patients with septic shock: A propensity-score-weighted retrospective study. *Crit. Care* **2019**, *23*, 317. [CrossRef]
30. Hawchar, F.; László, I.; Öveges, N.; Trásy, D.; Ondrik, Z.; Molnar, Z. Extracorporeal cytokine adsorption in septic shock: A proof of concept randomized, controlled pilot study. *J. Crit. Care* **2019**, *49*, 72–178. [CrossRef] [PubMed]
31. Schultz, P.; Schwier, E.; Eickmeyer, C.; Henzler, D.; Köhler, T. High-dose CytoSorb hemoadsorption is associated with improved survival in patients with septic shock: A retrospective cohort study. *J. Crit. Care* **2021**, *64*, 184–192. [CrossRef] [PubMed]
32. Scharf, C.; Schroeder, I.; Paal, M.; Winkels, M.; Irlbeck, M.; Zoller, M.; Liebchen, U. Can the cytokine adsorber CytoSorb® help to mitigate cytokine storm and reduce mortality in critically ill patients? A propensity score matching analysis. *Ann. Intensive Care* **2021**, *11*, 115. [CrossRef]
33. Wendel Garcia, P.D.; Hilty, M.P.; Held, U.; Kleinert, E.M.; Maggiorini, M. Cytokine adsorption in severe, refractory septic shock. *Intensive Care Med.* **2021**, *47*, 1334–1336. [CrossRef]
34. Supady, A.; Brodie, D.; Wengenmayer, T. Extracorporeal haemoadsorption: Does the evidence support its routine use in critical care? *Lancet Respir. Med.* **2022**, *10*, 307–312. [CrossRef]
35. Hawchar, F.; Tomescu, D.; Träger, K.; Joskowiak, D.; Kogelmann, K.; Soukup, J.; Friesecke, S.; Jacob, D.; Gummert, J.; Faltlhauser, A.; et al. Hemoadsorption in the critically ill-Final results of the International CytoSorb Registry. *PLoS ONE* **2022**, *17*, e0274315. [CrossRef]
36. Berlot, G.; Samola, V.; Barbaresco, I.; Tomasini, A.; di Maso, V.; Bianco, F.; Gerini, U. Effects of the timing and intensity of treatment on septic shock patients treated with CytoSorb®: Clinical experience. *Int. J. Artif. Organs* **2022**, *45*, 249–253. [CrossRef]
37. Bottari, G.; Confalone, V.; Cotugno, N.; Guzzo, I.; Perdichizzi, S.; Manno, E.C.; Stoppa, F.; Cecchetti, C. Efficacy of CytoSorb in a Pediatric Case of Severe Multisystem Infammatory Syndrome (MIS-C): A Clinical Case Report. *Front. Pediatr.* **2021**, *9*, 676298. [CrossRef] [PubMed]
38. Broman, M.E.; Hansson, F.; Vincent, J.L.; Bodelsson, M. Endotoxin and cytokine reducing properties of the oXiris membrane in patients with septic shock: A randomized crossover double-blind study. *PLoS ONE* **2019**, *14*, e0220444. [CrossRef]
39. Turani, F.; Barchetta, R.; Falco, M.; Busatti, S.; Weltert, L. Continuous Renal Replacement Therapy with the Adsorbing Filter oXiris in Septic Patients: A Case Series. *Blood Purif.* **2019**, *47* (Suppl. 3), 1–5. [CrossRef]
40. Schwindenhammer, V.; Girardot, T.; Chaulier, K.; Grégoire, A.; Monard, C.; Huriaux, L.; Illinger, J.; Leray, V.; Uberti, T.; Crozon-Clauzel, J.; et al. oXiris® Use in Septic Shock: Experience of Two French Centres. *Blood Purif.* **2019**, *47* (Suppl. 3), 1–7. [CrossRef] [PubMed]
41. Li, Y.; Sun, P.; Chang, K.; Yang, M.; Deng, N.; Chen, S.; Su, B. Effect of Continuous Renal Replacement Therapy with the oXiris Hemofilter on Critically Ill Patients: A Narrative Review. *J. Clin. Med.* **2022**, *11*, 6719. [CrossRef]
42. Stahl, K.; Wand, P.; Seeliger, B.; Wendel-Garcia, P.D.; Schmidt, J.J.; Schmidt, B.M.W.; Sauer, A.; Lehmann, F.; Budde, U.; Busch, M.; et al. Clinical and biochemical endpoints and predictors of response to plasma exchange in septic shock: Results from a randomized controlled trial. *Crit. Care* **2022**, *26*, 134. [CrossRef] [PubMed]
43. David, S.; Bode, C.; Putensen, C.; Welte, T.; Stahl, K.; EXCHANGE study group. Adjuvant therapeutic plasma exchange in septic shock. *Intensive Care Med.* **2021**, *47*, 352–354. [CrossRef] [PubMed]
44. Ronco, C.; Brendolan, A.; Lonnemann, G.; Bellomo, R.; Piccinni, P.; Digito, A.; Dan, M.; Irone, M.; La Greca, G.; Inguaggiato, P.; et al. A pilot study of coupled plasma filtration with adsorption in septic shock. *Crit. Care Med.* **2002**, *30*, 1250–1255. [CrossRef]
45. Formica, M.; Olivieri, C.; Livigni, S.; Cesano, G.; Vallero, A.; Maio, M.; Tetta, C. Hemodynamic response to coupled plasmafiltration-adsorption in human septic shock. *Intensive Care Med.* **2003**, *29*, 703–708. [CrossRef]
46. Cesano, G.; Livigni, S.; Vallero, A.; Olivieri, C.; Borca, M.; Quarello, F.; Tetta, C.; Formica, M. Trattamento dello shock settico con l'impiego della CPFA (plasmafiltrazione e adsorbimento associate): Impatto sull'emodinamica valutata con sistema PiCCO [Treatment of septic shock with the use of CPFA (associated plasma filtration and adsorption): Impact on hemodynamics monitored with PiCCO]. *G. Ital. Nefrol.* **2003**, *20*, 258–263. (In Italian)
47. Livigni, S.; Bertolini, G.; Rossi, C.; Ferrari, F.; Giardino, M.; Pozzato, M.; Remuzzi, G.; GiViTI: Gruppo Italiano per la Valutazione degli Interventi in Terapia Intensiva (Italian Group for the Evaluation of Interventions in Intensive Care Medicine) is an

independent collaboration network of Italian Intensive Care units. Efficacy of coupled plasma filtration adsorption (CPFA) in patients with septic shock: A multicenter randomised controlled clinical trial. *BMJ Open* **2014**, *4*, e003536. [CrossRef] [PubMed]
48. Hu, D.; Sun, S.; Zhu, B.; Mei, Z.; Wang, L.; Zhu, S.; Zhao, W. Effects of Coupled Plasma Filtration Adsorption on Septic Patients with Multiple Organ Dysfunction Syndrome. *Ren. Fail.* **2012**, *34*, 834–839. [CrossRef]
49. Franchi, M.; Giacalone, M.; Traupe, I.; Rago, R.; Baldi, G.; Giunta, F.; Forfori, F. Coupled plasma filtration adsorption improves hemodynamics in septic shock. *J. Crit. Care* **2016**, *33*, 100–105. [CrossRef]
50. Hazzard, I.; Jones, S.; Quinn, T. Coupled plasma haemofiltration filtration in severe sepsis: Systematic review and meta-analysis. *J. R. Army Med. Corps* **2015**, *161* (Suppl. 1), i17–i22. [CrossRef]
51. Garbero, E.; Livigni, S.; Ferrari, F.; Finazzi, S.; Langer, M.; Malacarne, P.; Meca, M.C.C.; Mosca, S.; Olivieri, C.; Pozzato, M.; et al. High dose coupled plasma filtration and adsorption in septic shock patients. Results of the COMPACT-2: A multicentre, adaptive, randomised clinical trial. *Intensive Care Med.* **2021**, *47*, 1303–1311. [CrossRef] [PubMed]
52. Giménez-Esparza, C.; Portillo-Requena, C.; Colomina-Climent, F.; Allegue-Gallego, J.M.; Galindo-Martínez, M.; Mollà-Jiménez, C.; Antón-Pascual, J.L.; Mármol-Peis, E.; Dólera-Moreno, C.; Rodríguez-Serra, M.; et al. The premature closure of ROMPA clinical trial: Mortality reduction in septic shock by plasma adsorption. *BMJ Open* **2019**, *9*, e030139. [CrossRef] [PubMed]
53. Mariano, F.; Hollo', Z.; Depetris, N.; Malvasio, V.; Mella, A.; Bergamo, D.; Pensa, A.; Berardino, M.; Stella, M.; Biancone, L. Coupled-plasma filtration and adsorption for severe burn patients with septic shock and acute kidney injury treated with renal replacement therapy. *Burns* **2020**, *46*, 190–198. [CrossRef] [PubMed]
54. Evans, L.; Rhodes, A.; Alhazzani, W.; Antonelli, M.; Coopersmith, C.M.; French, C.; Machado, F.R.; Mcintyre, L.; Ostermann, M.; Prescott, H.C.; et al. Surviving sepsis campaign: International guidelines for management of sepsis and septic shock 2021. *Intensive Care Med.* **2021**, *47*, 1181–1247. [CrossRef] [PubMed]
55. Honore, P.M.; Hoste, E.; Molnár, Z.; Jacobs, R.; Joannes-Boyau, O.; Malbrain, M.L.N.G.; Forni, L.G. Cytokine removal in human septic shock: Where are we and where are we going? *Ann. Intensive Care* **2019**, *9*, 56–69. [CrossRef]
56. Putzu, A.; Schorer, R.; Lopez-Delgado, J.C.; Cassina, T.; Landoni, G. Blood Purification and Mortality in Sepsis and Septic Shock: A Systematic Review and Meta-analysis of Randomized Trials. *Anesthesiology* **2019**, *131*, 580–593. [CrossRef]
57. Snow, T.A.C.; Littlewood, S.; Corredor, C.; Singer, M.; Arulkumaran, N. Effect of Extracorporeal Blood Purification on Mortality in Sepsis: A Meta-Analysis and Trial Sequential Analysis. *Blood Purif.* **2021**, *50*, 462–472. [CrossRef] [PubMed]
58. Vincent, J.L. Recent negative clinical trials in septic patients: Maybe a good thing? *Minerva Anestesiol.* **2015**, *81*, 122–124.
59. Vignon, P.; Laterre, P.F.; Daix, T.; François, B. New Agents in Development for Sepsis: Any Reason for Hope? *Drugs* **2020**, *80*, 1751–1761. [CrossRef]

Disclaimer/Publisher's Note: The statements, opinions and data contained in all publications are solely those of the individual author(s) and contributor(s) and not of MDPI and/or the editor(s). MDPI and/or the editor(s) disclaim responsibility for any injury to people or property resulting from any ideas, methods, instructions or products referred to in the content.

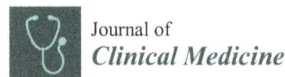

Review

COVID-19-Related ARDS: Key Mechanistic Features and Treatments

John Selickman [1,*], Charikleia S. Vrettou [2], Spyros D. Mentzelopoulos [2,†] and John J. Marini [1,3,†]

1. Department of Pulmonary and Critical Care Medicine, University of Minnesota School of Medicine, Minneapolis, MN 55455, USA
2. First Department of Intensive Care Medicine, National and Kapodistrian University of Athens Medical School, Evaggelismos General Hospital, 10676 Athens, Greece
3. Department of Pulmonary and Critical Care Medicine, Regions Hospital, St. Paul, MN 55101, USA
* Correspondence: selic002@umn.edu
† These authors contributed equally to this work.

Abstract: Acute respiratory distress syndrome (ARDS) is a heterogeneous syndrome historically characterized by the presence of severe hypoxemia, high-permeability pulmonary edema manifesting as diffuse alveolar infiltrate on chest radiograph, and reduced compliance of the integrated respiratory system as a result of widespread compressive atelectasis and fluid-filled alveoli. Coronavirus disease 19 (COVID-19)-associated ARDS (C-ARDS) is a novel etiology caused by severe acute respiratory syndrome coronavirus 2 (SARS-CoV-2) that may present with distinct clinical features as a result of the viral pathobiology unique to SARS-CoV-2. In particular, severe injury to the pulmonary vascular endothelium, accompanied by the presence of diffuse microthrombi in the pulmonary microcirculation, can lead to a clinical presentation in which the severity of impaired gas exchange becomes uncoupled from lung capacity and respiratory mechanics. The purpose of this review is to highlight the key mechanistic features of C-ARDS and to discuss the implications these features have on its treatment. In some patients with C-ARDS, rigid adherence to guidelines derived from clinical trials in the pre-COVID era may not be appropriate.

Keywords: COVID-19; acute respiratory distress syndrome; mechanical ventilation; SARS-CoV-2

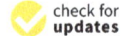

Citation: Selickman, J.; Vrettou, C.S.; Mentzelopoulos, S.D.; Marini, J.J. COVID-19-Related ARDS: Key Mechanistic Features and Treatments. *J. Clin. Med.* **2022**, *11*, 4896. https:// doi.org/10.3390/jcm11164896

Academic Editor: Jesús Villar

Received: 12 July 2022
Accepted: 17 August 2022
Published: 20 August 2022

Publisher's Note: MDPI stays neutral with regard to jurisdictional claims in published maps and institutional affiliations.

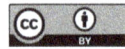

Copyright: © 2022 by the authors. Licensee MDPI, Basel, Switzerland. This article is an open access article distributed under the terms and conditions of the Creative Commons Attribution (CC BY) license (https:// creativecommons.org/licenses/by/ 4.0/).

1. Introduction

Acute respiratory distress syndrome (ARDS), as initially described, defined patients with similar clinical and pathologic findings: refractory hypoxemia; diffuse alveolar infiltrates on chest X-ray; severely reduced lung compliance; and, in those who did not survive, heavy lungs at autopsy, characterized by diffuse alveolar injury with hyaline membranes [1]. As its manifestations appeared superficially similar regardless of etiology, it was reasoned that treatment should be essentially the same, and this quickly became a universally accepted approach [2].

Randomized trials of therapy for such a pathologically and mechanically defined entity, however, might require up to one thousand patients to demonstrate survival benefit. Consequently, the need to establish definitions broad enough to permit sufficient enrollment with smaller numbers became evident [3]. Definitional simplification that excluded such hallmark features of ARDS as low respiratory compliance succeeded in facilitating enrollment for clinical studies, of course, but this came at the expense of specificity. In a recent study, for example, 14% of patients meeting the definition for ARDS had *no identifiable pulmonary lesions* at post mortem examination [4]. As a result, randomized trials incorporating these simplified definitions have included patients with an extraordinary range of respiratory mechanics and severity of illness. Yet, conducting such trials has led to the impression among many clinicians that "ARDS" represents a distinct disease-like entity [5].

Whether all patients with ARDS should be treated similarly and without discrimination regarding etiology is not a new question but rather one with renewed immediacy. The COVID-19 pandemic, caused by severe acute respiratory syndrome coronavirus 2 (SARS-CoV-2), has overwhelmed intensive care units with cases of respiratory failure meeting the broadened diagnostic criteria for ARDS [6]. While the number of patients requiring invasive mechanical ventilation for ARDS secondary to COVID-19 (C-ARDS) has declined over time [7], mortality in this population remains high [8]. Many have argued that C-ARDS should be managed no differently than ARDS of any other etiology, ignoring that the viral pathogenesis of SARS-CoV-2 may lead to a distinct form of ARDS that diverges from "typical" ARDS. For C-ARDS patients requiring mechanical ventilation, current guidelines, derived from studies of ARDS primarily caused by bacterial pneumonia and septic abdominal disease [9], may not be universally appropriate.

The purpose of this review is to describe how the physiology of C-ARDS, generated by the unique viral pathobiology of SARS-CoV-2, may differ from non-COVID ARDS, emphasizing the implications of that difference for both pharmacotherapy and mechanical ventilation. We underline that rigid adherence to all pre-COVID ventilatory guidelines may be ill-advised. Finally, we discuss management of refractory C-ARDS and the role of extracorporeal life support.

2. "Typical" ARDS

ARDS is currently defined by the Berlin Definition (Table 1) [6] and is characterized by high-permeability pulmonary edema and widespread compressive atelectasis. In response to injury, immune cells trigger an inflammatory response that leads to disruption of the alveolar–capillary barrier [10]. Accumulation of protein-rich fluid in alveolar and interstitial spaces inhibits pulmonary surfactant [11] which, along with increased hydrostatic pressures from extravascular lung water, results in collapse of underlying lung units. Physiologically, this manifests as (1) severely impaired gas exchange, with refractory hypoxemia and hypercarbia secondary to intrapulmonary shunt and reduced functioning surface for gas exchange [12–14]; and (2) severely reduced lung compliance. Histologically, this initial phase manifests as "diffuse alveolar damage," a constellation of findings involving damage to the alveolar lining and endothelium, the presence of hyaline membranes, interstitial and alveolar edema, and inflammatory infiltrate [15].

Table 1. Berlin Definition of Acute Respiratory Distress Syndrome. *CXR*, chest X-ray; *CT*, computed tomography; *PaO$_2$/FiO$_2$*, partial pressure of arterial oxygen to fraction of inspired oxygen ratio; *PEEP*, positive end-expiratory pressure; *CPAP*, continuous positive airway pressure.

Timing		Within 1 week of known clinical insult or new or worsening respiratory symptoms
Chest imaging		Bilateral opacities on CXR or CT not fully explained by effusions, lobar/lung collapse, or nodules
Origin of edema		Respiratory failure not fully explained by cardiac failure or fluid overload
Oxygenation	*Mild*	200 mm Hg < PaO$_2$/FiO$_2$ ≤ 300 mm Hg with PEEP or CPAP ≥ 5 cm H$_2$O
	Moderate	100 mm Hg < PaO$_2$/FiO$_2$ ≤ 200 mm Hg with PEEP ≤ 5 cm H$_2$O
	Severe	PaO$_2$/FiO$_2$ ≤ 100 mm Hg with PEEP ≥ 5 cm H$_2$O

Studies using quantitative computerized tomography (CT) have demonstrated that not only is the ARDS lung heterogeneous, with normally aerated units co-existing alongside non-aerated ones [16], but that the location of non-aerated units is strongly influenced by gravity, owing to the compressive forces of overlying edematous lung tissue. For that reason, radiographic densities appear to migrate from the paravertebral region when supine to the parasternal region when prone [17]. These studies have further shown that, in ARDS, compliance of the integrated respiratory system is determined primarily by the number of aerated lung units [18]; in other words, low compliance in ARDS is due in large part to the lungs being "small" not "stiff" [19]. Collectively, these findings gave rise to the concept of the "baby lung", a construct drawing similarity between the volume of aerated tissue in the low-capacity lung of ARDS and the volume of aerated tissue in the lung of a healthy child [20]. As total chest dimensions remain unaltered by ARDS, tissue density inversely parallels the capacity of the baby lung.

This concept has important implications. First, the severity of gas exchange impairment is intrinsically linked to the quantity of non-aerated tissue, with shunt fraction and physiologic dead space increasing, and PaO_2 decreasing, as the percentage of non-aerated lung rises [21]. Therefore, in typical ARDS, oxygenation and compliance are expected to deteriorate in direct proportion to one another. Additionally, the loss of ventilatory capacity means that the entire workload of ventilation is concentrated in an overtaxed baby lung, increasing the risk for progressive injury and further loss of functional lung units [22]. Protective strategies for ventilation have therefore been directed towards expanding the size of the baby lung through alveolar recruitment with the intent of distributing workload among a greater number of functional lung units, while avoiding exposure to (and unnecessary repetition of) tidal cycles that excessively strain vulnerable structural microelements.

While imperfect, as there is significant heterogeneity within the ARDS population, we use the term "typical" to collectively refer to ARDS described in the pre-COVID ARDS literature, which predominantly focused on patients with bacterial pneumonia and intra-abdominal disease.

3. Viral Pathogenesis of SARS-CoV-2

Appreciation for the viral pathogenesis unique to SARS-CoV-2 underpins a solid understanding of physiologic disparities between C-ARDS and non-COVID ARDS. SARS-CoV-2 expresses multiple structural proteins on its viral envelope, including the spike protein, a glycoprotein that mediates binding to host cells [23]. Cellular tropism is determined not only by the expression of angiotensin converting enzyme 2 (ACE2) receptors on the surface of host cells [24], which the spike protein binds to directly, but also the presence of transmembrane serine protease (TMPRSS2), which cleaves spike protein and facilitates viral uptake [25]. Following the release of the viral ribonucleoprotein into the cytoplasm, viral replicases use endoplasmic reticulum membranes to form double membrane vesicles for "protected" viral RNA transcription (termed replication factories) [26,27].

ACE2 receptors are expressed widely throughout the body, but their concentration is especially high in the pulmonary vascular endothelium and respiratory tract. As a result, the cells first targeted by SARS-CoV-2 following inhalation are those located in the nasopharynx and upper airway (e.g., multiciliated cells or sustentacular cells of the olfactory mucosa) [28,29]. When host immunity fails to clear SARS-CoV-2 infection, it spreads to the lower respiratory tract, either by aspiration of viral particles from the oropharynx or gradual progression throughout the tracheobronchial tree; in some cases, it may bypass the upper respiratory tract altogether [30]. Upon reaching the alveoli, SARS-CoV-2 primarily affects alveolar type 2 (AT2) cells which, in health, are tasked with both production of pulmonary surfactant and regeneration of AT1 cells (which constitute the majority of the alveolar epithelium) [31].

Following infection, host cells initially attempt to control viral spread through innate immunity. Cytoplasmic pattern recognition proteins detect RNA fragments of SARS-CoV-2, triggering the release of interferons, pro-inflammatory cytokines and leukocyte recruitment [32]; additional cytokine release occurs when damage-associated molecular patterns in host cells are released in response to injury [33]. If the innate immune response is dysfunctional, infection will spread, increasing the risk for severe COVID-19; alternatively, if the adaptive B and T cell responses to innate cytokine and chemokine release are absent, uncontrolled inflammation may ensue [34].

Alveolar cell injury or death causes disruption of the alveolar epithelium, thereby setting off an imbalance between coagulation activation and fibrinolysis [26,35]. Fibrin-rich alveolar exudates form hyaline membranes, which prevent further fluid accumulation into the injured alveoli but also hinder the alveolar–capillary oxygen transport [26,36]. Diffuse alveolar damage is followed by small-vessel endothelial activation and injury secondary to hypoxia, cytokines, chemokines, damage-associated molecular patterns, and direct infection by the virus [26,37,38]. Diffuse endotheliitis with inflammatory cell infiltrates may induce widespread endothelial cell apoptosis, pyroptosis, and microcirculatory dysfunction contributing to C-ARDS and also promoting extrapulmonary organ/system failure [26,37]. Release of the endothelial tissue factor can activate the extrinsic coagulation pathway [39]. Extracellular RNA, DNA, and exposed collagen can also activate factor XII and the intrinsic coagulation pathway [40]. Concurrently, platelets seal off the area of endothelial damage to prevent vascular leakage and secrete coagulation-sustaining factors [41] (Figure 1).

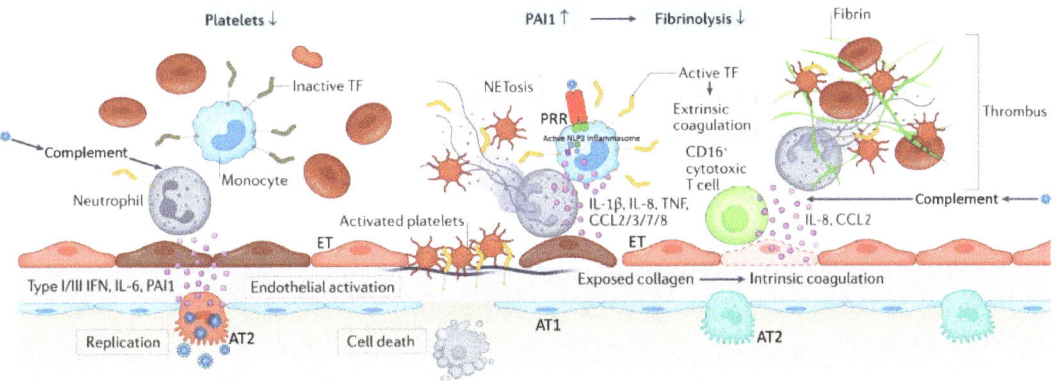

Figure 1. Severe coronavirus disease 19 is characterized by immune cell-mediated hypercoagulability and hypofibrinolysis. Hypoxia, cytokines, chemokines, damage-associated molecular patterns, and direct infection by the virus contribute to alveolar and endothelial cell death, and disruption of the alveolar–capillary barrier. Exposed extracellular matrix can trigger both the extrinsic coagulation (via tissue factor (TF)) and the intrinsic coagulation (via collagen/RNA). Recruited monocytes (with virus-activated NLP3 inflammasomes) and neutrophils amplify the inflammatory response, as well as the activation of coagulation by expressing active tissue factor (TF) and releasing neutrophil extracellular traps (NETs), respectively. Complement activation by the virus promotes active TF expression by neutrophils, and differentiation of cytotoxic CD-16⁺ T cells. NETs recruit platelets, which are subsequently activated by NET histones and the C3a and C5a complement fragments; this results in platelet release of cytokines. Activated platelets secrete coagulation-sustaining factors. The immunothrombotic process leads to diffuse small-vessel thromboses and thrombocytopenia. Concurrently, increased expression of plasminogen activator inhibitor (PA1) attenuates fibrinolysis. *AT1*, alveolar type 1 cell; *AT2*, alveolar type 2 cell; *ET*, endothelial cell; *PRR*, pattern recognition receptor; *IL*, interleukin; *CCL*, CC chemokine ligand; *IFN*, interferon. Reproduced in part with permission from [26]; copyright (2022) by Springer Nature.

In the context of COVID-19 immunothrombosis (Figure 1), recognition of SARS-CoV-2 through pattern recognition receptors of monocytes results in the release of activated tissue factor at sites of virus localization [26,42]. SARS-CoV-2 stimulates the NLPR3 inflammasome, with consequent production of interleukin (IL) 1 beta (IL-1-β) and IL-18 [42,43]. Concurrently, there is increased release of IL-6 from the alveolar epithelium, which in turn stimulates the production of clotting factors in the liver and tissue factor in the endothelium [26]. Complement activation by SARS-CoV-2 results in (1) upregulated expression of tissue factor by neutrophils [26,44]; and (2) differentiation of a CD-16 expressing T cell subpopulation, promoting immune complex-induced degranulation, microvascular endothelial cell injury, and release of IL-8 and chemokines [26,45]. Activated neutrophils release neutrophil extracellular traps (NETs), which directly activate factor XII and bind von Willebrand factor to promote recruitment of platelets [42]. NET histones, and complement fragments C3a and C5a, activate platelets, while neutrophil elastase and myeloperoxidase inactivate anticoagulants such as tissue factor pathway inhibitor [42]. NET-associated platelets activate the intrinsic coagulation pathway and release large amounts of pro-inflammatory cytokines [42]. Immune-activated platelets (through pattern recognition receptors) also propagate the innate immune response and immunothrombosis by releasing platelet factor 4 and high-mobility group box 1 protein, as well as platelet-derived extracellular vesicles [46]. Immunothrombotic mechanisms are further enhanced by hypofibrinolyis secondary to increased expression of plasminogen activator inhibitor [26,47] (Figure 1).

Systemic hyperinflammation is the *sine qua non* of C-ARDS and may be especially prominent in subsets of patients with (1) risk factors such as age, obesity, cardio-respiratory comorbidity, diabetes, and immunosuppression [26,48,49]; (2) genetic predisposition (e.g., variants at chemokine receptor genes or genes involved in interferon induction and amplification) [26,50–54]; and (3) autoantibodies against type I interferons [55,56]. Besides C-ARDS, severe and potentially lethal COVID-19 may also have extrapulmonary manifestations including gastrointestinal symptoms, acute cardiac, renal, and liver injury, rhabdomyolysis, coagulopathy, cardiac arrhythmias, and circulatory failure [26,57]. Lastly, while some studies have demonstrated systemic inflammation in C-ARDS to be less robust than non-COVID ARDS [58,59], pro-inflammatory responses are tightly linked to injury of the pulmonary vascular endothelium and immunothrombosis, both of which are distinct pathophysiologic features of C-ARDS in terms of their severity and ubiquity [30].

4. Pharmacologic Interventions

Despite hypercoagulability, full therapeutic anticoagulation did not prove superior to prophylactic anticoagulation in an international randomized controlled trial (RCT) of severe COVID-19 [60]. In contrast, treatments focusing on the inflammatory component of COVID-19 thrombosis have been repeatedly associated with improved patient outcomes. Indeed, "general inhibition" of inflammatory processes with dexamethasone or hydrocortisone resulted in a 30–36% reduction in the odds for in-hospital death of critically ill COVID-19 patients [61,62].

Despite initially discouraging findings [63], a meta-analysis of 19 RCTs reported a 17% reduction in the odds for in-hospital mortality with the IL-6 antagonist tocilizumab compared to usual care or placebo [64]. When compared to usual care, the addition of baracitinib, a janus kinase inhibitor, also resulted in shorter recovery time [65], reduced mortality [66], and lower frequency of adverse events [67]; furthermore, in a meta-analysis of four RCTs, baracitinib was associated with a 31% reduction in the odds for in-hospital death [68]. Guided by soluble urokinase plasminogen receptor plasma levels, treatment with IL-1 alpha and IL-1 beta antagonists also resulted in a 64% reduction in clinically worsened status at day 28, less organ dysfunction at day 7, and lower in-hospital mortality [69].

Collectively, these results highlight not only the clinical relevance of inhibiting key inflammatory processes that contribute to widespread endothelial dysfunction, diffuse small-vessel thromboses, and multiorgan failure, but also a broader theme—the treatment of C-ARDS, whether it be pharmacologic or otherwise, diverges from the treatment of non-COVID ARDS.

5. Blood Purification Interventions

In septic shock, extracorporeal cytokine removal with Cytosorb has been associated with lower IL-6 levels [70], reduced norepinephrine requirements [71], and lower observed vs. expected, 28-day, all-cause mortality [70,72]. These data, along with the recently proven efficacy of immunomodulating agents and the potentially beneficial effects reported by COVID-19 case series [73,74], supported the hypothesis that cytokine adsorption might improve severe COVID-19 outcomes [75,76]. However, in a small RCT of severe C-ARDS requiring extracorporeal membrane oxygenation (ECMO), patients treated with Cytosorb for 72 h had similar IL-6 concentrations and higher 30-day mortality compared to control [75]. Furthermore, in a second RCT of COVID-19 patients with vasoplegic shock, Cytosorb treatment for 3–7 days did not expedite shock reversal, and had no significant effect on markers of inflammation, vasopressor requirements, and 90-day mortality [76]. Notably, these findings are consistent with the results of two prior, small RCTs in septic or cardiac surgery patients [77,78]. Collectively, Cytosorb RCTs have failed to demonstrate any clinically meaningful difference between intervention and control groups [75]. Any previously observed cytokine lowering and hemodynamic stabilization are likely attributable to the natural course of the disease and adjunctive therapy rather than non-specific cytokine adsorption [75]. Alternative approaches to extracorporeal blood purification such as heparin-functionalized adsorbents are currently under evaluation with respect to their efficacy in depleting pathogens and mediators of immunothrombosis [46].

6. Distinct Pathologic Features of C-ARDS

Substantial clinical and biologic heterogeneity exists within the ARDS population [79]. Subphenotypes with distinct clinical features and responses to therapy have been identified with respect to the initial site of injury (pulmonary or extrapulmonary) [80] and biologic markers of inflammation (hypo- or hyperinflammatory) [81]. It should thus come as little surprise that properties unique to the SARS-CoV-2 virus itself might result in a form of ARDS with distinctive pathophysiology, or that even amongst patients with ARDS of a single etiology (e.g., C-ARDS), there might be a significant diversity of findings and responses to treatment (Table 2).

Table 2. Comparative presentation of major characteristic features of typical ARDS and C-ARDS. *ARDS*, acute respiratory distress syndrome; *C-ARDS*, coronavirus disease (COVID) 19-related ARDS; *SARS-CoV-2*, severe acute, respiratory syndrome coronavirus 2; *PaO$_2$/FiO$_2$*, oxygen arterial partial pressure-to-fraction of inspired oxygen fraction ratio; *PEEP*, positive end-expiratory pressure; *ECMO*, extracorporeal membrane oxygenation. * May predispose to early, profound hypoxemia and the conceptual risk of pre-intubation, patient self-inflicted lung injury.

	Typical ARDS	C-ARDS
Etiology	Diverse, pulmonary or extrapulmonary (e.g., bacterial or viral pneumonia, severe trauma, aspiration, sepsis, etc.)	SARS-CoV-2 infection of alveolar type 2 cells (primarily)
Hypoxemia (PaO$_2$/FiO$_2$ ≤ 300 mmHg at a PEEP level of ≥ 5 cmH$_2$O)	Acute onset (e.g., within <48 h after the clinical insult), or progressive onset (i.e., within 7 days after the clinical insult)	Progressive onset (i.e., within 7 or more days after the onset of COVID-19 symptoms) *
Lung compliance at hypoxemia onset	Usually low (e.g., <40 cmH$_2$O/L)	Usually high (e.g., >40 cmH$_2$O/L)
Recruitment potential	Low or high, depending on the extent/nature of lung unit involvement and associated atelectasis	Initially low—may increase with disease progression and development of edema and atelectasis
Functional-to-anatomical shunt ratio/hyperperfusion of gasless tissue *	Usually 0.5–2.0/no	Usually > 2.0/yes
Alveolar capillary microthrombosis/new vessel growth	Present/present	Diffuse (~9 times more prevalent)/marked (2.7 times higher)
Clinical benefit from lung-protective ventilation	Proven	Highly likely
Clinical benefit from prone positioning	Proven	Highly likely
Clinical benefit from corticosteroids	Likely; more high-quality evidence needed	Proven
Clinical benefit from targeted anti-inflammatory interventions	Uncertain; lack of intervention-specific evidence	Proven
Clinical benefit from ECMO	Likely	Possible; high-quality evidence still needed

Reports comparing the pathologic features of C-ARDS to other forms of viral or non-viral ARDS are fraught with conflicting results, as accounting for the stage of disease and evolution of practice patterns over time is challenging. One theme that has consistently emerged, however, is the near-universal presence of pulmonary vascular abnormalities in patients with C-ARDS [82].

Though often present, pulmonary vascular lesions are not a dominant histopathologic feature of usual ARDS and are seldom widespread in post mortem lung specimens [15,83]. In patients with C-ARDS, however, they not only occur commonly [84,85] but are extensive, occupying greater than 25% of the lung parenchyma in over half of the patients examined at autopsy in one study [86]. While microvascular thrombi may be a shared histologic finding among all patients with ARDS caused by pulmonary viruses, including influenza A and SARS-CoV-1 [82], the extent of microthrombosis appears to be far greater in patients with C-ARDS [38]. This prevalence tends to uncouple gas exchange from mechanical properties, calling into question the specifics of ventilation management guidelines developed from clinical trials in the non-C-ARDS setting. Furthermore, the thrombotic burden is not confined to the microcirculation; the incidence of large-vessel pulmonary emboli is higher in patients with C-ARDS than in those of ARDS secondary to other viral and non-viral etiologies [87,88]. Other pulmonary vascular derangements observed at autopsy include severe endothelial injury [37,38] and the presence of dilated/engorged capillaries [89].

Studies incorporating dual-energy computerized tomographic angiography (CTA), digital subtraction CTA, and high-resolution CT have further extended these findings. Pulmonary vascular abnormalities on CT, most notably vessel enlargement, are common in patients with COVID-19 and may even be present prior to the development of C-ARDS [90]. Enlarged vessels suggestive of vasodilatation can be frequently observed within an area of ground glass or consolidation [91], contrary to the expected physiologic response to regional hypoxia (i.e., vasoconstriction). Perfusion imaging confirms that a considerable fraction of opacified lung parenchyma demonstrates increased uptake (indicating blood flow) in spite of diminished or even absent ventilation [92]. Perfusion abnormalities, on the other hand, are detected in areas of *normal lung density* [90], with one study of mechanically ventilated C-ARDS patients reporting that perfusion defects were not only present in every patient studied, but that the median extent of vascular abnormality approached 50% [93].

7. Respiratory Mechanics and Gas Exchange in C-ARDS

Early in the pandemic, Gattinoni and colleagues reported novel findings in their first 16 patients with C-ARDS; these patients had a relatively *high* tidal compliance (averaging 50.2 mL/cm H_2O) associated with significantly elevated shunt fraction (0.50) [94]; furthermore, in the eight patients they evaluated using quantitative CT, the ratio of shunt fraction to gasless tissue was markedly higher (roughly 2.5 times) than those observed in usual ARDS [95], consistent with hyperperfusion of gasless tissue.

Chiumello and colleagues performed similar quantitative CT analysis in 32 consecutive C-ARDS patients receiving mechanical ventilation and compared gas exchange, respiratory mechanics, and CT variables to those of two historical cohorts of usual ARDS: one matched 1:1 for PaO_2/FiO_2 (P/F) and one matched 1:1 for compliance [96]. Compared to the C-ARDS cohort, the historical ARDS cohort matched for P/F had significantly lower compliance values (39.9 versus 49.4 mL/cmH_2O) and gas volumes on CT (930 mL versus 1670 mL). The historical ARDS cohort matched for compliance, on the other hand, had a higher P/F when compared to the C-ARDS cohort (160 versus 106.5 mmHg).

These findings are well explained by the pulmonary vasculopathy and diffuse, inflammation-triggered microthrombosis observed in COVID-related lung disease. In typical ARDS, airspace flooding, collapse, and consolidation tend to parallel the severity of oxygenation impairment and fall in compliance. C-ARDS challenges this conceptual framework; specifically, lung compliance may be well preserved in the early and mild stages of C-ARDS (at least in a major fraction of these patients), with severe hypoxemia not occurring primarily as a result of airspace filling and lung unit drop-out, but as the consequence of increased perfusion to non-ventilated lung units [89,97–100]. Over time, however, progression of C-ARDS fundamentally alters the lung's mechanical properties. In late phase ARDS, regardless of the cause, lung capacity becomes severely reduced and is characterized by high dead space, limited recruitability, and low compliance [101].

As might be expected from the loosely defined and oxygenation-based criteria for ARDS and the evolving nature of COVID-related lung injury, there is wide overlap between the mechanics of C-ARDS and usual ARDS; indeed, several studies evaluating their comparative mechanical properties did not identify distinctive mean differences between cohorts [102,103], which may in part be a function of the stage of illness in which such observations were made [104,105].

8. Mechanical Ventilation in C-ARDS

The goals of invasive mechanical ventilation in C-ARDS are to relieve excessive work of breathing, improve gas exchange, and avoid aggravation of existing lung injury. Repeated exposure to tidal cycles that cause excessive, fracturing strain of structural microelements is believed to be the proximate mechanical stimulus for ventilator-induced lung injury (VILI) [106]; in recent years, a better understanding of the biophysical causes of VILI has shifted our traditional focus from the inflation pattern of a single tidal cycle toward avoiding exposure to damaging levels of tidal energy and power [107]. At the bedside, however, the focus remains on attempting to restrain tidal plateau and driving pressures below defined numerical thresholds. Unfortunately, this well-intentioned objective is often pursued through application of inflexible ventilatory targets and without consideration of the stage of disease.

In many patients with C-ARDS, ventilator strategies shown to be beneficial in clinical trials of unselected patients with ARDS will be appropriate; for others, however, they may not apply. The body of C-ARDS literature has expanded at a remarkable pace throughout the pandemic, providing guidance in certain areas regarding optimal ventilator management. Knowledge gained through physiologic studies preceding the C-ARDS era must be applied judiciously in order to provide individualized care for patients with ARDS of any etiology—including those with COVID-19.

8.1. Tidal Volume in C-ARDS

Twenty years ago, the ARMA trial [9] demonstrated a 9% absolute reduction in mortality among mechanically ventilated ARDS patients randomized to an initial tidal volume of 6 mL/kg predicted body weight, forming the basis for what has become a standard of care codified in most ARDS guidelines [108,109]. While large tidal volumes that lead to excessive strain are undoubtedly misguided in any acutely injured lung [110], several points are worth noting with respect to tidal volume selection in C-ARDS:

(1) Data from the ARMA trial, derived primarily from patients with ARDS secondary to bacterial pneumonia and sepsis, may not be wholly translatable to patients with ARDS secondary to novel forms of viral pneumonia with unique pathologic features, such as C-ARDS.
(2) Even in the ARMA trial, tidal volumes could be liberalized if necessary to facilitate patient comfort and adequate ventilation.
(3) In three large randomized trials that preceded the ARMA trial, no differences were found between patients treated with means of 7.2 mL/kg versus 10.6 mL/kg predicted body weight [111]; 7.2 mL/kg versus 10.4 mL/kg dry body weight [112]; and 7.3 mL/kg versus 10.2 mL/kg predicted body weight [113].

In the subpopulation of C-ARDS patients with less alveolar injury and relatively preserved compliance, larger tidal volumes of 7–8 mL/kg predicted body weight may result in tolerable strain and energy input without the risk of VILI [107]. In such patients, enforcing low tidal volumes can unnecessarily increase dead space [114], lead to reabsorption atelectasis from hypoventilation, and necessitate additional sedation to facilitate breathing comfort. However, as the severity of disease progresses and compliance declines, lower tidal volumes may be required to prevent the generation of strain that exceeds critical thresholds of injury.

8.2. Application of PEEP in C-ARDS

Since the severity of gas exchange impairment and loss of compliance in the baby lung of ARDS reflect the reduced number of lung units available to accept ventilation, it is logical that interventions leading to an increase in the number of functional lung units should improve hypoxemia, reduce dead space, and increase compliance. Positive end-expiratory pressure (PEEP) is applied with the intent of achieving these goals by preventing collapse of unstable alveoli and thereby stabilizing "recruitment." Expanding the ventilatory capacity in this manner additionally serves to distribute energy across a greater number of lung units, perhaps decreasing the quantity of damaging tidal energy transferred to the parenchymal matrix and reducing the risk of VILI [19].

Employing PEEP for the purposes of alveolar recruitment, however, hinges on the assumptions that compromised gas exchange is due primarily to loss of otherwise functional lung units and that these collapsed, or fluid-filled, units will regain function in response to the application of end-expiratory pressure. In C-ARDS, these assumptions may not hold true, and if they do, may be strongly dependent on the timing of the intervention [115].

Within the baby lung, the regional effects of PEEP are highly variable, as both recruitment and overdistension occur simultaneously as the lung expands. The net benefit of PEEP depends on whether recruitment of functional lung units outweighs overdistension within those that were already functional. When overdistension prevails, gas exchange is adversely affected as blood flow is directed away from overdistended lung units that previously participated in gas exchange, resulting in increased dead space and encouraging hypercarbia. The effects of net overdistension on oxygenation, on the other hand, are variable. Oxygenation may initially improve in response to increased PEEP despite net overdistension, especially if decreased cardiac output leads to reduction in blood flow through areas of intrapulmonary shunt, making the P/F ratio a poor surrogate for recruitment [116,117].

When PEEP results in significant net recruitment, respiratory compliance (a correlate of baby lung size) will improve. However, when PEEP results in significant net overdistension, compliance will fall as open lung units are shifted past the upper inflection point of their pressure–volume curve. Under these conditions, the increased energy input associated with higher PEEP serves only to increase the risk of VILI and hemodynamic perturbations [118].

In recent decades, lung-protective strategies have focused on not only the use of low tidal volumes for ventilation, but also the application of higher PEEP [108]. "PEEP tables," in which PEEP is increased in a stepwise fashion with respect to the inspired oxygen requirement, assume that impaired oxygenation is secondary to the loss of functional lung units. Based on their use in clinical trials, such tables are commonly used by clinicians managing ARDS to select PEEP [119]. In many centers, this practice resulted in the early use of PEEP levels exceeding 14 cmH$_2$O for C-ARDS [120]. In C-ARDS, however, impaired oxygen exchange is often strongly influenced by vascular dysfunction—not loss of functional lung units—in which case high levels of PEEP are not beneficial. In one study of mechanically ventilated patients with C-ARDS, partitioned respiratory mechanics were measured at low and high levels of PEEP [121]. Compared to 5 cmH$_2$O, a PEEP of 15 cmH$_2$O resulted in reduced lung compliance, increased lung strain, and an increased ventilatory ratio (i.e., a surrogate of physiological dead space defined as the quotient of measured over predicted product of minute ventilation and PaCO$_2$ [122]). Had PEEP in that study [121] been set in accordance with the P/F table used in a recent clinical trial [123], it would have been 18 cmH$_2$O.

While response to PEEP varies significantly among individual patients with C-ARDS [100], functional recruitment appears to be diminished relative to usual ARDS [96] and likely is influenced by the stage of disease and timing of observation [124]. Studies incorporating quantitative CT have either demonstrated minimal recruitment of additional lung units at higher levels of PEEP [125] or recruitment without simultaneous improvement in PaCO$_2$, suggesting that recruited units are not functional/participating in gas exchange [126]. Indeed, higher levels of PEEP in C-ARDS have been reported to have deleterious effects on both gas exchange [121,127] and respiratory mechanics [121,125,127–129], consistent with net overdistension. In the advanced stages of C-ARDS when consolidation is extensive, even PEEP levels as low as 5 cmH$_2$O may be associated with markedly elevated airway plateau and driving pressures [101].

These data serve to underscore the importance of tailoring PEEP to the patient's individual physiology. To minimize the hemodynamic and mechanical risks associated with PEEP, it should only be increased if doing so leads to demonstrable recruitment of functional lung units. While all methods of PEEP titration are imperfect, targeting optimal compliance is a reasonable strategy. If an increase in PEEP results in improved system compliance (while tidal volume is held constant), aeratable lung capacity has increased and recruitment has occurred. Recruitment of functional lung units is additionally associated with reduced PaCO$_2$ for a given minute ventilation as a result of decreased dead space ventilation and increased surface area for gas exchange; while physiologic dead space is not routinely measured in clinical settings, the ventilatory ratio correlates reasonably well [122], is easily measured, and can be tracked following adjustments in PEEP. Similarly, the recruitment to inflation (R/I) ratio is a bedside test that has been used to estimate lung recruitability in response to changes in PEEP [130].

8.3. Body Positioning

Lung tissue mass is not distributed evenly, with 60% being located in the dependent (dorsal) half of the sterno-vertebral axis when supine [131]. In ARDS, the dorsal lung is predisposed to compressive atelectasis when supine due to the weight of overlying edematous tissue. External compression of lower lung units by the abdominal contents and of medial lung units by the weight of the overlying heart may also occur [132,133]. Atelectasis results in relatively well-perfused but reversibly non-ventilated alveoli [134]. The ventral lung, on the other hand, is predisposed to overdistension during passive ventilation, not only because it receives a greater proportion of that ventilation, but also due to the increased regional compliance of the anterior chest wall (relative to the posterior chest wall), which permits a greater degree of end-tidal distension of adjacent lung units [135].

In the prone position, previously compressed dorsal and medial lung units are recruited, and previously gas-filled ventral lung units become less distended or collapse altogether. Despite this tendency for collapse of ventral lung units, there is typically net recruitment, as the loss of ventral lung units is outweighed by recruitment of units in the dorsal region, which contains a greater mass of lung tissue [136]. Prone positioning further results in better anatomical matching of the lung and chest wall shapes and compliance along the vertical axis, leading to less variation in size of individual pulmonary units [135] (Figure 2). Since the distribution of lung perfusion remains virtually unchanged in the prone position, these changes result in more homogenous ventilation, with decreases in both venous admixture and dead space. Proning may also result in reduced lung stress (i.e., transpulmonary pressure) and strain (i.e., the tidal volume-to-end-expiratory lung volume ratio) [137], decreasing the risk of VILI.

The use of prone positioning has increased significantly during the COVID pandemic, with 77% of mechanically ventilated C-ARDS patients with a P/F < 100 being placed in the prone position [139] compared to only 16% of ARDS patients with a P/F < 100 during the pre-COVID era [140]. It remains one of the few interventions in severe ARDS associated with survival benefit, as demonstrated by a landmark study showing significant mortality reduction when patients with ARDS and a P/F < 150 were placed the prone position for least 16 h daily [141]. While that trial preceded the advent of COVID, recent investigations performed in C-ARDS patients also suggest a survival benefit, with one retrospective study demonstrating a small but statistically significant reduction in the risk of death when C-ARDS patients with a P/F < 200 were proned within the first 2 days of ICU admission [142].

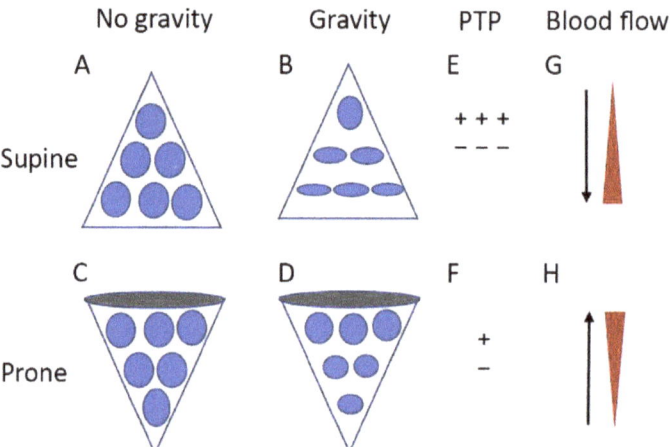

Figure 2. Diagrammatic presentation of physiological mechanisms associated with pronation in acute respiratory distress syndrome (ARDS). (**A,C**) show the shape of lung units (i.e., alveoli) without the effect of gravity. (**B**) In the supine position, the volume of dorsal lung units is significantly smaller than the volume of ventral lung units, as a result of gravity and pleural pressure; thus, ventral lung units are more prone to overdistention and dorsal lung units are more prone to compression atelectasis. (**D**) In the prone position, gravity and pleural pressure result in a decrease in the volume of the ventral lung units and an increase in the volume of the dorsal lung units. (**E**) In the supine position, the ventral transpulmonary pressure (PTP) may substantially exceed the dorsal PTP (**F**) Prone positioning reduces the ventral-to-dorsal PTP gradient thereby augmenting the homogeneity of ventilation. (**G**) The reopening, dorsal lung units continue to receive most of the blood flow. (**H**) The ventral lung units may exhibit a greater tendency to collapse, but are still relatively underperfused. Reproduced in concordance with the Creative Commons Attribution License (CC-BY) from [138].

Studies that have investigated the physiologic effects of prone positioning in C-ARDS patients have generally reported improved oxygenation, with P/F increasing ≥ 20 mmHg in approximately 75% of patients [139]. Responses to proning are heterogeneous though, and available data suggest that the mechanisms responsible for improved oxygenation may differ from those in usual ARDS.

Unlike typical ARDS, net recruitment of C-ARDS lungs following placement in the prone position is relatively modest and often negligible [143]. Improved system compliance, typically present when significant net recruitment occurs, has not been observed in most studies [139,143–146]. While measurements of partitioned respiratory mechanics would be needed to conclude with certainty that the lack of improvement in system compliance is not the result of decreased chest wall compliance in the prone position, counterbalancing a simultaneous increase in compliance of newly recruited lung, an absence of significant recruitment is suggested by other findings as well.

CO_2 exchange often improves in the prone position as a result of decreased dead space and recruitment of additional lung units. Most studies that have evaluated gas exchange in the prone position in C-ARDS patients, however, have reported little change in the $PaCO_2$ (or ventilatory ratio) [139,143,145,146]. Compared to typical ARDS, the changes in both respiratory system compliance and $PaCO_2$ following prone positioning are significantly less in patients with C-ARDS [99]. In the absence of recruitment, the most plausible mechanism to explain improved oxygenation is better matching of ventilation/perfusion ratios of vaso-dysregulated tissue [136].

Timing may also play a significant role in response to prone positioning [99,143]. In unresolving ARDS, atelectasis and edema may evolve into significant dorsal consolidation and diffuse fibrosis; in this setting, there is minimal recruitment of dorsal tissue in the prone position—only increased ventral atelectasis. A significant percentage of such patients either experience worsened P/F ratio in the prone position or fail to meet the accepted criteria for "responsiveness" (improvement in P/F ≥ 20 mmHg) [145].

9. Extracorporeal Life Support for C-ARDS

Extracorporeal life support (ECLS) refers to supplemental gas exchange via an external circuit. ECMO provides sufficient blood flow rates for either respiratory gas exchange support alone (venovenous (VV) ECMO) or complemented by circulatory support (venoarterial (VA) ECMO). Extracorporeal carbon dioxide removal (ECCO$_2$R) requires lower blood flow rates than ECMO and yet efficiently clears carbon dioxide (CO$_2$). However, unlike ECMO, ECCO$_2$R does not effectively re-oxygenate the mixed venous blood. ECMO requires the placement of a central venous cannula, attached to a circuit that pumps blood under negative pressure and delivers it to an "oxygenator" or "membrane lung" (i.e., a gas exchange device). Oxygen passing through the device's hollow and gas-permeable fibers then transfers across them into the diverted venous blood flow, while CO$_2$ is removed by diffusing from blood into the unidirectional stream of "sweep" gas passing through the fiber lumens. The membrane-oxygenated blood is then pumped back into the patient via a second intravascular cannula inserted so that its tip is placed close to the right atrium, or via the return channel of a dual-lumen cannula. Both types of external circuit require anticoagulation. Compared to ECMO, ECCO$_2$R can be achieved using smaller catheters, thereby reducing the risk of cannulation-related complications. Such cannulation is usually percutaneous, using a modified Seldinger technique with imaging guidance. As the application of ECLS is clinically demanding, current evidence suggests that it should be performed in selected centers with adequate experience [147].

VV-ECMO has proven effective in patients with hypoxemia refractory to optimized mechanical ventilation settings and adjunctive therapies, including prone positioning [148,149]. Current criteria for initiating ECMO in C-ARDS are those previously used in the ECMO to Rescue Lung Injury in Severe ARDS (EOLIA) trial, and comprise: a P/F of <80 mmHg for >6 h; a P/F of <50 mmHg for >3 h; or an arterial pH of <7.25 with PaCO$_2$ ≥ 60 mmHg for >6 h [147,148]. In the EOLIA trial, patients with the abovementioned criteria were randomized either to receive VV-ECMO or to continue treatment with conventional mechanical ventilation [150]. Although the study did not show a statistically significant difference in 60-day mortality between the two groups, the effect estimate favored the intervention group (relative risk, 0.76; 95% confidence interval, 0.55–1.04; P = 0.09). In addition, 28% of patients of the control group were crossed over to VV-ECMO for refractory hypoxemia. These facts could still imply a likely VV-ECMO mortality benefit. Notably, enrolled patients had to be on mechanical ventilation for < 7 days while other adjunctive therapies, including inhaled nitric oxide, recruitment maneuvers, high-frequency oscillatory ventilation, and infusion of almitrine were also allowed [150]. While the majority of the patients had ARDS caused by pneumonia, bacterial (45%) or viral (18%), approximately 37% of the study population had ARDS of other etiology.

In accordance with current guidelines, major contraindications to VV-ECMO could include prolonged (i.e., >10 days) mechanical ventilation, morbid obesity or advanced age (e.g., >75 years), chronic respiratory failure, heart failure requiring VA-ECMO, heparin-induced thrombocytopenia, cancer with life expectancy of <5 years, a moribund condition or a Simplified Acute Physiology Score II of >90, non-drug-induced coma after cardiac arrest, irreversible neurologic injury, the presence of a treatment limitation decision, patient/surrogate decline of blood products, expected difficulty with vascular cannulation, and unavailability of adequate specialized staff and ECMO equipment [150,151]. Current recommendations do not advise any deviations from conventional ECMO practices applied to ARDS patients without COVID-19, including anticoagulation [151].

The initial goal of ECMO is to maintain adequate oxygenation. However, the primary mechanism of benefit may be a decreased risk of VILI, the result of membrane CO$_2$ clearance, lower driving and plateau pressures, and reduced tidal volumes and inflation power used during ECMO [149]. Additional clinical goals of ECMO might include minimization of sedation, early weaning from mechanical ventilation, and patient mobilization. However, in C-ARDS, discontinuation of sedation could be potentially followed by extreme patient respiratory effort and risk P-SILI [152] There currently is insufficient evidence to support or refute early mobilization or extubation with awake ECMO in this setting [151].

Except for very severe ARDS, where hypoxemia is the major concern, there is a rationale for lowering ventilation volumes and pressures beyond standard values to reduce further the risk of VILI. As doing so may lead to hypercapnic acidosis, $ECCO_2R$ can be used to avoid impermissible hypercapnia [153]. In April 2020, emergency authorization was issued for the use of an $ECCO_2R$ device in patients with C-ARDS, with or without mechanical ventilation [154]. This approach is not only physiologically sound, but also can be less costly and technically easier to apply than ECMO. Nevertheless, in a multicenter RCT of typical ARDS, the use of $ECCO_2R$ was not associated with a reduction in 90-day mortality [155].

The effect of ECMO on outcomes of C-ARDS patients has been evolving and repeatedly evaluated during the pandemic. In a 2021 systematic review of 22 observational studies, ECMO outcomes of C-ARDS were similar to those of non-COVID-19 patients [156]. However, subsequent studies and meta-analyses reported rises of up to 15% in the mortality rates during the second wave as well as after the first year of the pandemic [157–159]. This finding has been attributed to (1) the evolving viral strains of SARS-CoV-2; (2) the evolution of pharmacological treatment during the later phases of the pandemic (e.g., the addition of immunomodulatory therapies); and (3) the broader and longer use of non-invasive ventilation in the C-ARDS population [158]. Changes in COVID-19 treatment strategies may have contributed to the selection of patients with refractory disease and/or more severe P-SILI for ECMO treatment [157]. The main risk factors for mortality reported in the literature for C-ARDS patients on ECMO include older age, the presence of multiple comorbidities and systemic acidosis, the need for renal replacement therapy and high vasopressor infusion rates, and finally the occurrence of bleeding complications [156,160]. Other frequent complications include thromboembolic events, infections, ventilator-associated pneumonia, bacteremia, and ECMO circuit-related mechanical problems [157,158]. The occurrence of neurological complications and in particular of intracranial hemorrhage, although rare, affecting 6–12% of the patients, has been associated with a mortality rate of 90%, implying that C-ARDS patients on ECMO could benefit from early non-invasive neuromonitoring protocols [161].

Despite the similar guidelines for patient selection and implementation of ECMO in C-ARDS and typical ARDS, there are some significant differences between these two groups. There are more practical difficulties affecting the medical and nursing teams caused by the risk of transmission and the use of personal protective equipment during C-ARDS ECMO. C-ARDS patients have a higher risk of thrombosis and a higher prevalence of right ventricular failure [162]. The use of immunomodulatory and/or immunosuppressive therapies is also more frequent in C-ARDS, and a *longer* duration of support is likely to be necessary for these patients [163]. It is currently acknowledged that successful lung recovery is possible after prolonged VV-ECMO (>28 days) [164]. Distinct clinical courses of C-ARDS ECMO have been described. Some patients with C-ARDS achieve lung recovery shortly after the initiation of ECMO (i.e., within a few days), while others require prolonged ECMO, posing unique clinical challenges. While a delayed lung recovery may be possible in such patients on prolonged ECMO, alternative trajectories such as lung transplantation, or transition to comfort-based care, may need to be considered [151,165].

The combination of prone positioning and ECMO (PP-ECMO) may also be considered [166,167]. In a physiological study of C-ARDS, PP-ECMO was associated with higher P/F ratio, better respiratory system compliance, and lower driving pressure and mechanical power of ventilation; improvements in respiratory mechanics persisted after supine repositioning [168]. In a retrospective, multicenter, cohort study of C-ARDS patients featuring propensity score matching, PP-ECMO was associated with improved oxygenation, reduced intrapulmonary shunt, tolerance of longer ECMO duration, and lower in-hospital mortality [169]. Further high-quality research is still needed to determine the potential clinical usefulness of PP-ECMO in C-ARDS. Table 3 summarizes currently available therapeutic options for C-ARDS.

Table 3. Evidence-based treatments for coronavirus disease 19 (COVID-19)-related acute respiratory distress syndrome (ARDS). PaO_2/FiO_2, oxygen arterial partial pressure-to-inspired oxygen fraction ratio; PEEP, positive end-expiratory pressure. * Time interval corresponds to the maximum recommended duration of therapy. † To be reduced to 2 mg if estimated glomerular filtration rate is 60 mL/min or less.

Intervention	Mechanism of Action	Evidence for Efficacy
Remdesivir day 1: 200 mg IV days 2–10: 100 mg IV	Inhibition of the viral RNA-dependent, RNA polymerase	Shortens the time to recovery in hospitalized COVID-19 patients
Dexamethasone days 1–10 *: 6 mg IV	Anti-inflammator linked to the activation of the glucocorticoid receptor	Reduces the probability of in-hospital death in critically ill COVID-19 patients
Tocilizumab single dose: 8 mg/kg IV (max. 800 mg)	Interleukin 6 antagonism	Reduces the probability of in-hospital death in critically ill COVID-19 patients
Baracitinib days 1–14 *: 4 mg † oral or enteral	Janus kinase inhibition	Reduces the probability of in-hospital death in critically ill COVID-19 patients
Anakinra days 1–10 *: 100 mg subcutaneously	Interleukin 1 alpha/beta antagonism	Reduces the probability of in-hospital death in critically ill COVID-19 patients
Prone positioning for at least 16 h per day until $PaO_2/FiO_2 \geq 150$ mmHg at PEEP ≤ 10 cmH$_2$O and FiO$_2 \leq 0.6$	Attenuation of lung stress and strain Reversal of compression atelectasis Increased homogeneity of ventilation Improved ventilation/perfusion matching	Reduces the probability of in-hospital death in moderate to severe ARDS
Extracorporeal membrane oxygenation	Minimization of lung stress and strain ("lung rest") with very low tidal volumes and ventilation pressures	Possible mortality benefit in severe ARDS

10. Conclusions

Typical ARDS is characterized by high-permeability edema, widespread atelectasis, and a loss of compliance that relates directly to the reduced capacity of aerated lung units. COVID-19, a novel etiology of ARDS, has distinct pathologic findings consistent with severe injury to—and dysfunction of—the pulmonary vasculature as a result of SARS-CoV-2-induced endothelial injury and immunothrombosis. The lungs of patients with C-ARDS may be more likely to overdistend than to recruit in response to customary levels of PEEP. A subpopulation of patients with C-ARDS may present with severely deranged gas exchange that is uncoupled from the comparatively mild parenchymal injury. Just as typical ARDS encompasses a broad range of clinical findings, so too does C-ARDS, often transitioning in its more advanced stages to a form indistinguishable from typical ARDS. Some have argued that all patients with ARDS, regardless of etiology, should be treated identically. This approach, however, ignores the physiologic variability that not only exists between patients, but also within individual patients depending on the phase of the disease.

Randomized trials in ARDS have identified several interventions that lead to improved outcomes. These studies have enrolled patients with significant heterogeneity though and as such, a significant degree of heterogeneity in treatment effect is to be expected [170]. They report the mean intervention effects observed in a population, but with regard to benefit, wide individual variability exists. Randomized trials have provided safe starting points from which to approach mechanical ventilation in the individual, but such rules are not inviolable. A more holistic approach, taking into consideration the unique physiology of individual patients, is warranted—as exemplified by C-ARDS.

Author Contributions: Conceptualization by J.S., C.S.V., S.D.M. and J.J.M.; writing—original draft preparation by J.S., C.S.V. and S.D.M.; writing—review and editing by J.S., C.S.V., S.D.M. and J.J.M. All authors have read and agreed to the published version of the manuscript.

Funding: This research received no external funding.

Conflicts of Interest: The authors declare no conflict of interest.

References

1. Ashbaugh, D.G.; Bigelow, D.B.; Petty, T.L.; Levine, B.E. Acute respiratory distress in adults. *Lancet* **1967**, *2*, 319–323. [CrossRef]
2. Gattinoni, L.; Marini, J.J. Isn't it time to abandon ARDS? The COVID-19 lesson. *Crit. Care* **2021**, *25*, 326. [CrossRef] [PubMed]
3. Bernard, G.R. Acute respiratory distress syndrome: A historical perspective. *Am. J. Respir. Crit. Care Med.* **2005**, *172*, 798–806. [CrossRef] [PubMed]
4. Thille, A.W.; Esteban, A.; Fernandez-Segoviano, P.; Rodriguez, J.M.; Aramburu, J.A.; Penuelas, O.; Cortes-Puch, I.; Cardinal-Fernandez, P.; Lorente, J.A.; Frutos-Vivar, F. Comparison of the Berlin definition for acute respiratory distress syndrome with autopsy. *Am. J. Respir. Crit. Care Med.* **2013**, *187*, 761–767. [CrossRef]
5. Marini, J.J. Limitations of clinical trials in acute lung injury and acute respiratory distress syndrome. *Curr. Opin. Crit. Care* **2006**, *12*, 25–31. [CrossRef] [PubMed]
6. Force, A.D.T.; Ranieri, V.M.; Rubenfeld, G.D.; Thompson, B.T.; Ferguson, N.D.; Caldwell, E.; Fan, E.; Camporota, L.; Slutsky, A.S. Acute respiratory distress syndrome: The Berlin Definition. *JAMA* **2012**, *307*, 2526–2533. [CrossRef]
7. Iuliano, A.D.; Brunkard, J.M.; Boehmer, T.K.; Peterson, E.; Adjei, S.; Binder, A.M.; Cobb, S.; Graff, P.; Hidalgo, P.; Panaggio, M.J.; et al. Trends in Disease Severity and Health Care Utilization During the Early Omicron Variant Period Compared with Previous SARS-CoV-2 High Transmission Periods—United States, December 2020–January 2022. *MMWR Morb. Mortal. Wkly. Rep.* **2022**, *71*, 146–152. [CrossRef]
8. Lim, Z.J.; Subramaniam, A.; Ponnapa Reddy, M.; Blecher, G.; Kadam, U.; Afroz, A.; Billah, B.; Ashwin, S.; Kubicki, M.; Bilotta, F.; et al. Case Fatality Rates for Patients with COVID-19 Requiring Invasive Mechanical Ventilation. A Meta-analysis. *Am. J. Respir. Crit. Care Med.* **2021**, *203*, 54–66. [CrossRef]
9. Acute Respiratory Distress Syndrome Network; Brower, R.G.; Matthay, M.A.; Morris, A.; Schoenfeld, D.; Thompson, B.T.; Wheeler, A. Ventilation with lower tidal volumes as compared with traditional tidal volumes for acute lung injury and the acute respiratory distress syndrome. *N. Engl. J. Med.* **2000**, *342*, 1301–1308. [CrossRef]
10. Thompson, B.T.; Chambers, R.C.; Liu, K.D. Acute Respiratory Distress Syndrome. *N. Engl. J. Med.* **2017**, *377*, 1904–1905. [CrossRef]
11. Holm, B.A.; Matalon, S. Role of pulmonary surfactant in the development and treatment of adult respiratory distress syndrome. *Anesth. Analg.* **1989**, *69*, 805–818. [CrossRef] [PubMed]
12. Niklason, L.; Eckerstrom, J.; Jonson, B. The influence of venous admixture on alveolar dead space and carbon dioxide exchange in acute respiratory distress syndrome: Computer modelling. *Crit. Care* **2008**, *12*, R53. [CrossRef] [PubMed]
13. Radermacher, P.; Maggiore, S.M.; Mercat, A. Fifty Years of Research in ARDS. Gas Exchange in Acute Respiratory Distress Syndrome. *Am. J. Respir. Crit. Care Med.* **2017**, *196*, 964–984. [CrossRef] [PubMed]
14. Robertson, H.T.; Swenson, E.R. What do dead-space measurements tell us about the lung with acute respiratory distress syndrome? *Respir. Care* **2004**, *49*, 1006–1007.
15. Katzenstein, A.L.; Bloor, C.M.; Leibow, A.A. Diffuse alveolar damage—The role of oxygen, shock, and related factors. A review. *Am. J. Pathol.* **1976**, *85*, 209–228.
16. Gattinoni, L.; Mascheroni, D.; Torresin, A.; Marcolin, R.; Fumagalli, R.; Vesconi, S.; Rossi, G.P.; Rossi, F.; Baglioni, S.; Bassi, F.; et al. Morphological response to positive end expiratory pressure in acute respiratory failure. Computerized tomography study. *Intensive Care Med.* **1986**, *12*, 137–142. [CrossRef]
17. Gattinoni, L.; Pelosi, P.; Vitale, G.; Pesenti, A.; D'Andrea, L.; Mascheroni, D. Body position changes redistribute lung computed-tomographic density in patients with acute respiratory failure. *Anesthesiology* **1991**, *74*, 15–23. [CrossRef]
18. Gattinoni, L.; Pesenti, A.; Avalli, L.; Rossi, F.; Bombino, M. Pressure-volume curve of total respiratory system in acute respiratory failure. Computed tomographic scan study. *Am. Rev. Respir. Dis.* **1987**, *136*, 730–736. [CrossRef]
19. Gattinoni, L.; Marini, J.J.; Pesenti, A.; Quintel, M.; Mancebo, J.; Brochard, L. The "baby lung" became an adult. *Intensive Care Med.* **2016**, *42*, 663–673. [CrossRef]
20. Gattinoni, L.; Pesenti, A. The concept of "baby lung". *Intensive Care Med.* **2005**, *31*, 776–784. [CrossRef]
21. Gattinoni, L.; Pesenti, A.; Bombino, M.; Baglioni, S.; Rivolta, M.; Rossi, F.; Rossi, G.; Fumagalli, R.; Marcolin, R.; Mascheroni, D.; et al. Relationships between lung computed tomographic density, gas exchange, and PEEP in acute respiratory failure. *Anesthesiology* **1988**, *69*, 824–832. [CrossRef] [PubMed]
22. Marini, J.J.; Gattinoni, L. Time Course of Evolving Ventilator-Induced Lung Injury: The "Shrinking Baby Lung". *Crit. Care Med.* **2020**, *48*, 1203–1209. [CrossRef] [PubMed]
23. Wiersinga, W.J.; Rhodes, A.; Cheng, A.C.; Peacock, S.J.; Prescott, H.C. Pathophysiology, Transmission, Diagnosis, and Treatment of Coronavirus Disease 2019 (COVID-19): A Review. *JAMA* **2020**, *324*, 782–793. [CrossRef] [PubMed]
24. Zhou, P.; Yang, X.L.; Wang, X.G.; Hu, B.; Zhang, L.; Zhang, W.; Si, H.R.; Zhu, Y.; Li, B.; Huang, C.L.; et al. A pneumonia outbreak associated with a new coronavirus of probable bat origin. *Nature* **2020**, *579*, 270–273. [CrossRef]
25. Hoffmann, M.; Kleine-Weber, H.; Schroeder, S.; Kruger, N.; Herrler, T.; Erichsen, S.; Schiergens, T.S.; Herrler, G.; Wu, N.H.; Nitsche, A.; et al. SARS-CoV-2 Cell Entry Depends on ACE2 and TMPRSS2 and Is Blocked by a Clinically Proven Protease Inhibitor. *Cell* **2020**, *181*, 271–280.e278. [CrossRef]
26. Lamers, M.M.; Haagmans, B.L. SARS-CoV-2 pathogenesis. *Nat. Rev. Microbiol.* **2022**, *20*, 270–284. [CrossRef]

27. Ogando, N.S.; Dalebout, T.J.; Zevenhoven-Dobbe, J.C.; Limpens, R.; van der Meer, Y.; Caly, L.; Druce, J.; de Vries, J.J.C.; Kikkert, M.; Barcena, M.; et al. SARS-coronavirus-2 replication in Vero E6 cells: Replication kinetics, rapid adaptation and cytopathology. *J. Gen. Virol.* **2020**, *101*, 925–940. [CrossRef]
28. Khan, M.; Yoo, S.J.; Clijsters, M.; Backaert, W.; Vanstapel, A.; Speleman, K.; Lietaer, C.; Choi, S.; Hether, T.D.; Marcelis, L.; et al. Visualizing in deceased COVID-19 patients how SARS-CoV-2 attacks the respiratory and olfactory mucosae but spares the olfactory bulb. *Cell* **2021**, *184*, 5932–5949.e5915. [CrossRef]
29. Hou, Y.J.; Okuda, K.; Edwards, C.E.; Martinez, D.R.; Asakura, T.; Dinnon, K.H., 3rd; Kato, T.; Lee, R.E.; Yount, B.L.; Mascenik, T.M.; et al. SARS-CoV-2 Reverse Genetics Reveals a Variable Infection Gradient in the Respiratory Tract. *Cell* **2020**, *182*, 429–446.e414. [CrossRef]
30. Osuchowski, M.F.; Winkler, M.S.; Skirecki, T.; Cajander, S.; Shankar-Hari, M.; Lachmann, G.; Monneret, G.; Venet, F.; Bauer, M.; Brunkhorst, F.M.; et al. The COVID-19 puzzle: Deciphering pathophysiology and phenotypes of a new disease entity. *Lancet Respir. Med.* **2021**, *9*, 622–642. [CrossRef]
31. Barkauskas, C.E.; Cronce, M.J.; Rackley, C.R.; Bowie, E.J.; Keene, D.R.; Stripp, B.R.; Randell, S.H.; Noble, P.W.; Hogan, B.L. Type 2 alveolar cells are stem cells in adult lung. *J. Clin. Investig.* **2013**, *123*, 3025–3036. [CrossRef] [PubMed]
32. Carty, M.; Guy, C.; Bowie, A.G. Detection of Viral Infections by Innate Immunity. *Biochem. Pharmacol.* **2021**, *183*, 114316. [CrossRef] [PubMed]
33. Land, W.G. Role of DAMPs in respiratory virus-induced acute respiratory distress syndrome-with a preliminary reference to SARS-CoV-2 pneumonia. *Genes Immun.* **2021**, *22*, 141–160. [CrossRef]
34. Hernandez Acosta, R.A.; Esquer Garrigos, Z.; Marcelin, J.R.; Vijayvargiya, P. COVID-19 Pathogenesis and Clinical Manifestations. *Infect. Dis. Clin. N. Am.* **2022**, *36*, 231–249. [CrossRef] [PubMed]
35. Sebag, S.C.; Bastarache, J.A.; Ware, L.B. Therapeutic modulation of coagulation and fibrinolysis in acute lung injury and the acute respiratory distress syndrome. *Curr. Pharm. Biotechnol.* **2011**, *12*, 1481–1496. [CrossRef]
36. Iba, T.; Levy, J.H.; Levi, M.; Thachil, J. Coagulopathy in COVID-19. *J. Thromb. Haemost.* **2020**, *18*, 2103–2109. [CrossRef]
37. Varga, Z.; Flammer, A.J.; Steiger, P.; Haberecker, M.; Andermatt, R.; Zinkernagel, A.S.; Mehra, M.R.; Schuepbach, R.A.; Ruschitzka, F.; Moch, H. Endothelial cell infection and endotheliitis in COVID-19. *Lancet* **2020**, *395*, 1417–1418. [CrossRef]
38. Ackermann, M.; Verleden, S.E.; Kuehnel, M.; Haverich, A.; Welte, T.; Laenger, F.; Vanstapel, A.; Werlein, C.; Stark, H.; Tzankov, A.; et al. Pulmonary Vascular Endothelialitis, Thrombosis, and Angiogenesis in Covid-19. *N. Engl. J. Med.* **2020**, *383*, 120–128. [CrossRef]
39. Owens, A.P., 3rd; Mackman, N. Tissue factor and thrombosis: The clot starts here. *Thromb. Haemost.* **2010**, *104*, 432–439. [CrossRef]
40. Kenawy, H.I.; Boral, I.; Bevington, A. Complement-Coagulation Cross-Talk: A Potential Mediator of the Physiological Activation of Complement by Low pH. *Front. Immunol.* **2015**, *6*, 215. [CrossRef]
41. Swieringa, F.; Spronk, H.M.H.; Heemskerk, J.W.M.; van der Meijden, P.E.J. Integrating platelet and coagulation activation in fibrin clot formation. *Res. Pract. Thromb. Haemost.* **2018**, *2*, 450–460. [CrossRef] [PubMed]
42. Bonaventura, A.; Vecchie, A.; Dagna, L.; Martinod, K.; Dixon, D.L.; Van Tassell, B.W.; Dentali, F.; Montecucco, F.; Massberg, S.; Levi, M.; et al. Endothelial dysfunction and immunothrombosis as key pathogenic mechanisms in COVID-19. *Nat. Rev. Immunol.* **2021**, *21*, 319–329. [CrossRef] [PubMed]
43. Rodrigues, T.S.; de Sa, K.S.G.; Ishimoto, A.Y.; Becerra, A.; Oliveira, S.; Almeida, L.; Goncalves, A.V.; Perucello, D.B.; Andrade, W.A.; Castro, R.; et al. Inflammasomes are activated in response to SARS-CoV-2 infection and are associated with COVID-19 severity in patients. *J. Exp. Med.* **2021**, *218*, e20201707. [CrossRef]
44. Kambas, K.; Markiewski, M.M.; Pneumatikos, I.A.; Rafail, S.S.; Theodorou, V.; Konstantonis, D.; Kourtzelis, I.; Doumas, M.N.; Magotti, P.; Deangelis, R.A.; et al. C5a and TNF-alpha up-regulate the expression of tissue factor in intra-alveolar neutrophils of patients with the acute respiratory distress syndrome. *J. Immunol.* **2008**, *180*, 7368–7375. [CrossRef] [PubMed]
45. Georg, P.; Astaburuaga-Garcia, R.; Bonaguro, L.; Brumhard, S.; Michalick, L.; Lippert, L.J.; Kostevc, T.; Gabel, C.; Schneider, M.; Streitz, M.; et al. Complement activation induces excessive T cell cytotoxicity in severe COVID-19. *Cell* **2022**, *185*, 493–512.e425. [CrossRef]
46. Ebeyer-Masotta, M.; Eichhorn, T.; Weiss, R.; Laukova, L.; Weber, V. Activated Platelets and Platelet-Derived Extracellular Vesicles Mediate COVID-19-Associated Immunothrombosis. *Front. Cell Dev. Biol.* **2022**, *10*, 914891. [CrossRef]
47. Mackman, N.; Antoniak, S.; Wolberg, A.S.; Kasthuri, R.; Key, N.S. Coagulation Abnormalities and Thrombosis in Patients Infected With SARS-CoV-2 and Other Pandemic Viruses. *Arterioscler. Thromb. Vasc. Biol.* **2020**, *40*, 2033–2044. [CrossRef]
48. Williamson, E.J.; Walker, A.J.; Bhaskaran, K.; Bacon, S.; Bates, C.; Morton, C.E.; Curtis, H.J.; Mehrkar, A.; Evans, D.; Inglesby, P.; et al. Factors associated with COVID-19-related death using OpenSAFELY. *Nature* **2020**, *584*, 430–436. [CrossRef]
49. O'Driscoll, M.; Ribeiro Dos Santos, G.; Wang, L.; Cummings, D.A.T.; Azman, A.S.; Paireau, J.; Fontanet, A.; Cauchemez, S.; Salje, H. Age-specific mortality and immunity patterns of SARS-CoV-2. *Nature* **2021**, *590*, 140–145. [CrossRef]
50. Zhang, Q.; Bastard, P.; Liu, Z.; Le Pen, J.; Moncada-Velez, M.; Chen, J.; Ogishi, M.; Sabli, I.K.D.; Hodeib, S.; Korol, C.; et al. Inborn errors of type I IFN immunity in patients with life-threatening COVID-19. *Science* **2020**, *370*, eabd4570. [CrossRef]
51. Severe Covid, G.G.; Ellinghaus, D.; Degenhardt, F.; Bujanda, L.; Buti, M.; Albillos, A.; Invernizzi, P.; Fernandez, J.; Prati, D.; Baselli, G.; et al. Genomewide Association Study of Severe Covid-19 with Respiratory Failure. *N. Engl. J. Med.* **2020**, *383*, 1522–1534. [CrossRef]
52. Pairo-Castineira, E.; Clohisey, S.; Klaric, L.; Bretherick, A.D.; Rawlik, K.; Pasko, D.; Walker, S.; Parkinson, N.; Fourman, M.H.; Russell, C.D.; et al. Genetic mechanisms of critical illness in COVID-19. *Nature* **2021**, *591*, 92–98. [CrossRef]

53. Initiative, C.-H.G. Mapping the human genetic architecture of COVID-19. *Nature* **2021**, *600*, 472–477. [CrossRef] [PubMed]
54. Asano, T.; Boisson, B.; Onodi, F.; Matuozzo, D.; Moncada-Velez, M.; Maglorius Renkilaraj, M.R.L.; Zhang, P.; Meertens, L.; Bolze, A.; Materna, M.; et al. X-linked recessive TLR7 deficiency in ~1% of men under 60 years old with life-threatening COVID-19. *Sci. Immunol.* **2021**, *6*, eabl4348. [CrossRef] [PubMed]
55. Koning, R.; Bastard, P.; Casanova, J.L.; Brouwer, M.C.; van de Beek, D.; Amsterdam, U.M.C. COVID-19 Biobank Investigators. Autoantibodies against type I interferons are associated with multi-organ failure in COVID-19 patients. *Intensive Care Med.* **2021**, *47*, 704–706. [CrossRef]
56. Bastard, P.; Rosen, L.B.; Zhang, Q.; Michailidis, E.; Hoffmann, H.H.; Zhang, Y.; Dorgham, K.; Philippot, Q.; Rosain, J.; Beziat, V.; et al. Autoantibodies against type I IFNs in patients with life-threatening COVID-19. *Science* **2020**, *370*, eabd4585. [CrossRef]
57. Berlin, D.A.; Gulick, R.M.; Martinez, F.J. Severe Covid-19. *N. Engl. J. Med.* **2020**, *383*, 2451–2460. [CrossRef]
58. Kox, M.; Waalders, N.J.B.; Kooistra, E.J.; Gerretsen, J.; Pickkers, P. Cytokine Levels in Critically Ill Patients With COVID-19 and Other Conditions. *JAMA* **2020**, *234*, 1565–1567. [CrossRef]
59. Leisman, D.E.; Ronner, L.; Pinotti, R.; Taylor, M.D.; Sinha, P.; Calfee, C.S.; Hirayama, A.V.; Mastroiani, F.; Turtle, C.J.; Harhay, M.O.; et al. Cytokine elevation in severe and critical COVID-19: A rapid systematic review, meta-analysis, and comparison with other inflammatory syndromes. *Lancet Respir. Med.* **2020**, *8*, 1233–1244. [CrossRef]
60. The REMAP-CAP; ACTIV-4a; ATTACC Investigators; Goligher, E.C.; Bradbury, C.A.; McVerry, B.J.; Lawler, P.R.; Berger, J.S.; Gong, M.N.; Carrier, M.; et al. Therapeutic Anticoagulation with Heparin in Critically Ill Patients with COVID-19. *N. Engl. J. Med.* **2021**, *385*, 777–789. [CrossRef]
61. Group, R.C.; Horby, P.; Lim, W.S.; Emberson, J.R.; Mafham, M.; Bell, J.L.; Linsell, L.; Staplin, N.; Brightling, C.; Ustianowski, A.; et al. Dexamethasone in Hospitalized Patients with COVID-19. *N. Engl. J. Med.* **2021**, *384*, 693–704. [CrossRef]
62. The WHO Rapid Evidence Appraisal for COVID-19 Therapies (REACT) Working Group; Sterne, J.A.C.; Murthy, S.; Diaz, J.V.; Slutsky, A.S.; Villar, J.; Angus, D.C.; Annane, D.; Azevedo, L.C.P.; Berwanger, O.; et al. Association Between Administration of Systemic Corticosteroids and Mortality Among Critically Ill Patients With COVID-19: A Meta-analysis. *JAMA* **2020**, *324*, 1330–1341. [CrossRef] [PubMed]
63. Stone, J.H.; Frigault, M.J.; Serling-Boyd, N.J.; Fernandes, A.D.; Harvey, L.; Foulkes, A.S.; Horick, N.K.; Healy, B.C.; Shah, R.; Bensaci, A.M.; et al. Efficacy of Tocilizumab in Patients Hospitalized with Covid-19. *N. Engl. J. Med.* **2020**, *383*, 2333–2344. [CrossRef] [PubMed]
64. The WHO Rapid Evidence Appraisal for COVID-19 Therapies (REACT) Working Group; Shankar-Hari, M.; Vale, C.L.; Godolphin, P.J.; Fisher, D.; Higgins, J.P.T.; Spiga, F.; Savovic, J.; Tierney, J.; Baron, G.; et al. Association Between Administration of IL-6 Antagonists and Mortality Among Patients Hospitalized for COVID-19: A Meta-analysis. *JAMA* **2021**, *326*, 499–518. [CrossRef]
65. Kalil, A.C.; Patterson, T.F.; Mehta, A.K.; Tomashek, K.M.; Wolfe, C.R.; Ghazaryan, V.; Marconi, V.C.; Ruiz-Palacios, G.M.; Hsieh, L.; Kline, S.; et al. Baricitinib plus Remdesivir for Hospitalized Adults with Covid-19. *N. Engl. J. Med.* **2021**, *384*, 795–807. [CrossRef]
66. Marconi, V.C.; Ramanan, A.V.; de Bono, S.; Kartman, C.E.; Krishnan, V.; Liao, R.; Piruzeli, M.L.B.; Goldman, J.D.; Alatorre-Alexander, J.; de Cassia Pellegrini, R.; et al. Efficacy and safety of baricitinib for the treatment of hospitalised adults with COVID-19 (COV-BARRIER): A randomised, double-blind, parallel-group, placebo-controlled phase 3 trial. *Lancet Respir. Med.* **2021**, *9*, 1407–1418. [CrossRef]
67. Wolfe, C.R.; Tomashek, K.M.; Patterson, T.F.; Gomez, C.A.; Marconi, V.C.; Jain, M.K.; Yang, O.O.; Paules, C.I.; Palacios, G.M.R.; Grossberg, R.; et al. Baricitinib versus dexamethasone for adults hospitalised with COVID-19 (ACTT-4): A randomised, double-blind, double placebo-controlled trial. *Lancet Respir. Med.* **2022**. [CrossRef]
68. Selvaraj, V.; Finn, A.; Lal, A.; Khan, M.S.; Dapaah-Afriyie, K.; Carino, G.P. Baricitinib in hospitalised patients with COVID-19: A meta-analysis of randomised controlled trials. *EClinicalMedicine* **2022**, *49*, 101489. [CrossRef]
69. Kyriazopoulou, E.; Poulakou, G.; Milionis, H.; Metallidis, S.; Adamis, G.; Tsiakos, K.; Fragkou, A.; Rapti, A.; Damoulari, C.; Fantoni, M.; et al. Early treatment of COVID-19 with anakinra guided by soluble urokinase plasminogen receptor plasma levels: A double-blind, randomized controlled phase 3 trial. *Nat. Med.* **2021**, *27*, 1752–1760. [CrossRef]
70. Friesecke, S.; Trager, K.; Schittek, G.A.; Molnar, Z.; Bach, F.; Kogelmann, K.; Bogdanski, R.; Weyland, A.; Nierhaus, A.; Nestler, F.; et al. International registry on the use of the CytoSorb(R) adsorber in ICU patients: Study protocol and preliminary results. *Med. Klin. Intensivmed. Notfmed.* **2019**, *114*, 699–707. [CrossRef]
71. Hawchar, F.; Laszlo, I.; Oveges, N.; Trasy, D.; Ondrik, Z.; Molnar, Z. Extracorporeal cytokine adsorption in septic shock: A proof of concept randomized, controlled pilot study. *J. Crit. Care* **2019**, *49*, 172–178. [CrossRef]
72. Brouwer, W.P.; Duran, S.; Kuijper, M.; Ince, C. Hemoadsorption with CytoSorb shows a decreased observed versus expected 28-day all-cause mortality in ICU patients with septic shock: A propensity-score-weighted retrospective study. *Crit. Care* **2019**, *23*, 317. [CrossRef] [PubMed]
73. Rieder, M.; Wengenmayer, T.; Staudacher, D.; Duerschmied, D.; Supady, A. Cytokine adsorption in patients with severe COVID-19 pneumonia requiring extracorporeal membrane oxygenation. *Crit. Care* **2020**, *24*, 435. [CrossRef] [PubMed]
74. Alharthy, A.; Faqihi, F.; Memish, Z.A.; Balhamar, A.; Nasim, N.; Shahzad, A.; Tamim, H.; Alqahtani, S.A.; Brindley, P.G.; Karakitsos, D. Continuous renal replacement therapy with the addition of CytoSorb cartridge in critically ill patients with COVID-19 plus acute kidney injury: A case-series. *Artif. Organs* **2021**, *45*, E101–E112. [CrossRef] [PubMed]

75. Stockmann, H.; Thelen, P.; Stroben, F.; Pigorsch, M.; Keller, T.; Krannich, A.; Spies, C.; Treskatsch, S.; Ocken, M.; Kunz, J.V.; et al. CytoSorb Rescue for COVID-19 Patients with Vasoplegic Shock and Multiple Organ Failure: A Prospective, Open-Label, Randomized Controlled Pilot Study. *Crit. Care Med.* **2022**, *50*, 964–976. [CrossRef] [PubMed]
76. Supady, A.; Weber, E.; Rieder, M.; Lother, A.; Niklaus, T.; Zahn, T.; Frech, F.; Muller, S.; Kuhl, M.; Benk, C.; et al. Cytokine adsorption in patients with severe COVID-19 pneumonia requiring extracorporeal membrane oxygenation (CYCOV): A single centre, open-label, randomised, controlled trial. *Lancet Respir. Med.* **2021**, *9*, 755–762. [CrossRef]
77. Schadler, D.; Pausch, C.; Heise, D.; Meier-Hellmann, A.; Brederlau, J.; Weiler, N.; Marx, G.; Putensen, C.; Spies, C.; Jorres, A.; et al. The effect of a novel extracorporeal cytokine hemoadsorption device on IL-6 elimination in septic patients: A randomized controlled trial. *PLoS ONE* **2017**, *12*, e0187015. [CrossRef]
78. Poli, E.C.; Alberio, L.; Bauer-Doerries, A.; Marcucci, C.; Roumy, A.; Kirsch, M.; De Stefano, E.; Liaudet, L.; Schneider, A.G. Cytokine clearance with CytoSorb(R) during cardiac surgery: A pilot randomized controlled trial. *Crit. Care* **2019**, *23*, 108. [CrossRef]
79. Wilson, J.G.; Calfee, C.S. ARDS Subphenotypes: Understanding a Heterogeneous Syndrome. *Crit. Care* **2020**, *24*, 102. [CrossRef]
80. Gattinoni, L.; Pelosi, P.; Suter, P.M.; Pedoto, A.; Vercesi, P.; Lissoni, A. Acute respiratory distress syndrome caused by pulmonary and extrapulmonary disease. Different syndromes? *Am. J. Respir. Crit. Care Med.* **1998**, *158*, 3–11. [CrossRef]
81. Calfee, C.S.; Delucchi, K.; Parsons, P.E.; Thompson, B.T.; Ware, L.B.; Matthay, M.A.; Network, N.A. Subphenotypes in acute respiratory distress syndrome: Latent class analysis of data from two randomised controlled trials. *Lancet Respir. Med.* **2014**, *2*, 611–620. [CrossRef]
82. Satturwar, S.; Fowkes, M.; Farver, C.; Wilson, A.M.; Eccher, A.; Girolami, I.; Pujadas, E.; Bryce, C.; Salem, F.; El Jamal, S.M.; et al. Postmortem Findings Associated with SARS-CoV-2: Systematic Review and Meta-analysis. *Am. J. Surg. Pathol.* **2021**, *45*, 587–603. [CrossRef] [PubMed]
83. Tomashefski, J.F., Jr.; Davies, P.; Boggis, C.; Greene, R.; Zapol, W.M.; Reid, L.M. The pulmonary vascular lesions of the adult respiratory distress syndrome. *Am. J. Pathol.* **1983**, *112*, 112–126. [PubMed]
84. Hariri, L.P.; North, C.M.; Shih, A.R.; Israel, R.A.; Maley, J.H.; Villalba, J.A.; Vinarsky, V.; Rubin, J.; Okin, D.A.; Sclafani, A.; et al. Lung Histopathology in Coronavirus Disease 2019 as Compared With Severe Acute Respiratory Sydrome and H1N1 Influenza: A Systematic Review. *Chest* **2021**, *159*, 73–84. [CrossRef] [PubMed]
85. Milross, L.; Majo, J.; Cooper, N.; Kaye, P.M.; Bayraktar, O.; Filby, A.; Fisher, A.J. Post-mortem lung tissue: The fossil record of the pathophysiology and immunopathology of severe COVID-19. *Lancet Respir. Med.* **2022**, *10*, 95–106. [CrossRef]
86. Carsana, L.; Sonzogni, A.; Nasr, A.; Rossi, R.S.; Pellegrinelli, A.; Zerbi, P.; Rech, R.; Colombo, R.; Antinori, S.; Corbellino, M.; et al. Pulmonary post-mortem findings in a series of COVID-19 cases from northern Italy: A two-centre descriptive study. *Lancet Infect. Dis.* **2020**, *20*, 1135–1140. [CrossRef]
87. Poissy, J.; Goutay, J.; Caplan, M.; Parmentier, E.; Duburcq, T.; Lassalle, F.; Jeanpierre, E.; Rauch, A.; Labreuche, J.; Susen, S.; et al. Pulmonary Embolism in Patients With COVID-19: Awareness of an Increased Prevalence. *Circulation* **2020**, *142*, 184–186. [CrossRef]
88. Helms, J.; Tacquard, C.; Severac, F.; Leonard-Lorant, I.; Ohana, M.; Delabranche, X.; Merdji, H.; Clere-Jehl, R.; Schenck, M.; Fagot Gandet, F.; et al. High risk of thrombosis in patients with severe SARS-CoV-2 infection: A multicenter prospective cohort study. *Intensive Care Med.* **2020**, *46*, 1089–1098. [CrossRef]
89. Villalba, J.A.; Hilburn, C.F.; Garlin, M.A.; Elliott, G.A.; Li, Y.; Kunitoki, K.; Poli, S.; Alba, G.A.; Madrigal, E.; Taso, M.; et al. Vasculopathy and Increased Vascular Congestion in Fatal COVID-19 and ARDS. *Am. J. Respir. Crit. Care Med.* **2022**. [CrossRef]
90. Santamarina, M.G.; Boisier Riscal, D.; Beddings, I.; Contreras, R.; Baque, M.; Volpacchio, M.; Martinez Lomakin, F. COVID-19: What Iodine Maps From Perfusion CT can reveal-A Prospective Cohort Study. *Crit. Care* **2020**, *24*, 619. [CrossRef]
91. Li, Q.; Huang, X.T.; Li, C.H.; Liu, D.; Lv, F.J. CT features of coronavirus disease 2019 (COVID-19) with an emphasis on the vascular enlargement pattern. *Eur. J. Radiol.* **2021**, *134*, 109442. [CrossRef] [PubMed]
92. Poschenrieder, F.; Meiler, S.; Lubnow, M.; Zeman, F.; Rennert, J.; Scharf, G.; Schaible, J.; Stroszczynski, C.; Pfeifer, M.; Hamer, O.W. Severe COVID-19 pneumonia: Perfusion analysis in correlation with pulmonary embolism and vessel enlargement using dual-energy CT data. *PLoS ONE* **2021**, *16*, e0252478. [CrossRef] [PubMed]
93. Patel, B.V.; Arachchillage, D.J.; Ridge, C.A.; Bianchi, P.; Doyle, J.F.; Garfield, B.; Ledot, S.; Morgan, C.; Passariello, M.; Price, S.; et al. Pulmonary Angiopathy in Severe COVID-19: Physiologic, Imaging, and Hematologic Observations. *Am. J. Respir. Crit. Care Med.* **2020**, *202*, 690–699. [CrossRef] [PubMed]
94. Gattinoni, L.; Coppola, S.; Cressoni, M.; Busana, M.; Rossi, S.; Chiumello, D. COVID-19 Does Not Lead to a "Typical" Acute Respiratory Distress Syndrome. *Am. J. Respir. Crit. Care Med.* **2020**, *201*, 1299–1300. [CrossRef] [PubMed]
95. Cressoni, M.; Caironi, P.; Polli, F.; Carlesso, E.; Chiumello, D.; Cadringher, P.; Quintel, M.; Ranieri, V.M.; Bugedo, G.; Gattinoni, L. Anatomical and functional intrapulmonary shunt in acute respiratory distress syndrome. *Crit. Care Med.* **2008**, *36*, 669–675. [CrossRef]
96. Chiumello, D.; Busana, M.; Coppola, S.; Romitti, F.; Formenti, P.; Bonifazi, M.; Pozzi, T.; Palumbo, M.M.; Cressoni, M.; Herrmann, P.; et al. Physiological and quantitative CT-scan characterization of COVID-19 and typical ARDS: A matched cohort study. *Intensive Care Med.* **2020**, *46*, 2187–2196. [CrossRef]
97. Barbeta, E.; Motos, A.; Torres, A.; Ceccato, A.; Ferrer, M.; Cilloniz, C.; Bueno, L.; Badia, J.R.; Castro, P.; Ferrando, C.; et al. SARS-CoV-2-induced Acute Respiratory Distress Syndrome: Pulmonary Mechanics and Gas-Exchange Abnormalities. *Ann. Am. Thorac. Soc.* **2020**, *17*, 1164–1168. [CrossRef]

98. Vasques, F.; Sanderson, B.; Formenti, F.; Shankar-Hari, M.; Camporota, L. Physiological dead space ventilation, disease severity and outcome in ventilated patients with hypoxaemic respiratory failure due to coronavirus disease 2019. *Intensive Care Med.* **2020**, *46*, 2092–2093. [CrossRef]
99. Camporota, L.; Sanderson, B.; Chiumello, D.; Terzi, N.; Argaud, L.; Rimmele, T.; Metuor, R.; Verstraete, A.; Cour, M.; Bohe, J.; et al. Prone Position in COVID-19 and -COVID-19 Acute Respiratory Distress Syndrome: An International Multicenter Observational Comparative Study. *Crit. Care Med.* **2022**, *50*, 633–643. [CrossRef]
100. Grieco, D.L.; Bongiovanni, F.; Chen, L.; Menga, L.S.; Cutuli, S.L.; Pintaudi, G.; Carelli, S.; Michi, T.; Torrini, F.; Lombardi, G.; et al. Respiratory physiology of COVID-19-induced respiratory failure compared to ARDS of other etiologies. *Crit. Care* **2020**, *24*, 529. [CrossRef]
101. Kummer, R.L.; Shapiro, R.S.; Marini, J.J.; Huelster, J.S.; Leatherman, J.W. Paradoxically Improved Respiratory Compliance With Abdominal Compression in COVID-19 ARDS. *Chest* **2021**, *160*, 1739–1742. [CrossRef] [PubMed]
102. Haudebourg, A.F.; Perier, F.; Tuffet, S.; de Prost, N.; Razazi, K.; Mekontso Dessap, A.; Carteaux, G. Respiratory Mechanics of COVID-19- versus Non-COVID-19-associated Acute Respiratory Distress Syndrome. *Am. J. Respir. Crit. Care Med.* **2020**, *202*, 287–290. [CrossRef] [PubMed]
103. Panwar, R.; Madotto, F.; Laffey, J.G.; van Haren, F.M.P. Compliance Phenotypes in Early Acute Respiratory Distress Syndrome before the COVID-19 Pandemic. *Am. J. Respir. Crit. Care Med.* **2020**, *202*, 1244–1252. [CrossRef] [PubMed]
104. Beloncle, F.; Studer, A.; Seegers, V.; Richard, J.C.; Desprez, C.; Fage, N.; Merdji, H.; Pavlovsky, B.; Helms, J.; Cunat, S.; et al. Longitudinal changes in compliance, oxygenation and ventilatory ratio in COVID-19 versus non-COVID-19 pulmonary acute respiratory distress syndrome. *Crit. Care* **2021**, *25*, 248. [CrossRef] [PubMed]
105. Gattinoni, L.; Coppola, S.; Cressoni, M.; Busana, M.; Rossi, S.; Chiumello, D. Reply by Gattinoni et al. to Hedenstierna et al., to Maley et al., to Fowler et al., to Bhatia and Mohammed, to Bos, to Koumbourlis and Motoyama, and to Haouzi et al. *Am. J. Respir. Crit. Care Med.* **2020**, *202*, 628–630. [CrossRef]
106. Marini, J.J.; Gattinoni, L. Energetics and the Root Mechanical Cause for Ventilator-induced Lung Injury. *Anesthesiology* **2018**, *128*, 1062–1064. [CrossRef]
107. Marini, J.J.; Rocco, P.R.M.; Gattinoni, L. Static and Dynamic Contributors to Ventilator-induced Lung Injury in Clinical Practice. Pressure, Energy, and Power. *Am. J. Respir. Crit. Care Med.* **2020**, *201*, 767–774. [CrossRef]
108. Fan, E.; Del Sorbo, L.; Goligher, E.C.; Hodgson, C.L.; Munshi, L.; Walkey, A.J.; Adhikari, N.K.J.; Amato, M.B.P.; Branson, R.; Brower, R.G.; et al. An Official American Thoracic Society/European Society of Intensive Care Med.icine/Society of Critical Care Medicine Clinical Practice Guideline: Mechanical Ventilation in Adult Patients with Acute Respiratory Distress Syndrome. *Am. J. Respir. Crit. Care Med.* **2017**, *195*, 1253–1263. [CrossRef]
109. Alhazzani, W.; Moller, M.H.; Arabi, Y.M.; Loeb, M.; Gong, M.N.; Fan, E.; Oczkowski, S.; Levy, M.M.; Derde, L.; Dzierba, A.; et al. Surviving Sepsis Campaign: Guidelines on the Management of Critically Ill Adults with Coronavirus Disease 2019 (COVID-19). *Crit. Care Med.* **2020**, *48*, e440–e469. [CrossRef]
110. Dreyfuss, D.; Saumon, G. Ventilator-induced lung injury: Lessons from experimental studies. *Am. J. Respir. Crit. Care Med.* **1998**, *157*, 294–323. [CrossRef]
111. Stewart, T.E.; Meade, M.O.; Cook, D.J.; Granton, J.T.; Hodder, R.V.; Lapinsky, S.E.; Mazer, C.D.; McLean, R.F.; Rogovein, T.S.; Schouten, B.D.; et al. Evaluation of a ventilation strategy to prevent barotrauma in patients at high risk for acute respiratory distress syndrome. Pressure- and Volume-Limited Ventilation Strategy Group. *N. Engl. J. Med.* **1998**, *338*, 355–361. [CrossRef] [PubMed]
112. Brochard, L.; Roudot-Thoraval, F.; Roupie, E.; Delclaux, C.; Chastre, J.; Fernandez-Mondejar, E.; Clementi, E.; Mancebo, J.; Factor, P.; Matamis, D.; et al. Tidal volume reduction for prevention of ventilator-induced lung injury in acute respiratory distress syndrome. The Multicenter Trail Group on Tidal Volume reduction in ARDS. *Am. J. Respir. Crit. Care Med.* **1998**, *158*, 1831–1838. [CrossRef] [PubMed]
113. Brower, R.G.; Shanholtz, C.B.; Fessler, H.E.; Shade, D.M.; White, P., Jr.; Wiener, C.M.; Teeter, J.G.; Dodd-o, J.M.; Almog, Y.; Piantadosi, S. Prospective, randomized, controlled clinical trial comparing traditional versus reduced tidal volume ventilation in acute respiratory distress syndrome patients. *Crit. Care Med.* **1999**, *27*, 1492–1498. [CrossRef] [PubMed]
114. Liu, X.; Liu, X.; Xu, Y.; Xu, Z.; Huang, Y.; Chen, S.; Li, S.; Liu, D.; Lin, Z.; Li, Y. Ventilatory Ratio in Hypercapnic Mechanically Ventilated Patients with COVID-19-associated Acute Respiratory Distress Syndrome. *Am. J. Respir. Crit. Care Med.* **2020**, *201*, 1297–1299. [CrossRef] [PubMed]
115. Marini, J.J.; Gattinoni, L. Management of COVID-19 Respiratory Distress. *JAMA* **2020**, *323*, 2329–2330. [CrossRef]
116. Gattinoni, L.; Marini, J.J. In search of the Holy Grail: Identifying the best PEEP in ventilated patients. *Intensive Care Med.* **2022**, *48*, 728–731. [CrossRef]
117. Barthelemy, R.; Beaucote, V.; Bordier, R.; Collet, M.; Le Gall, A.; Hong, A.; de Roquetaillade, C.; Gayat, E.; Mebazaa, A.; Chousterman, B.G. Haemodynamic impact of positive end-expiratory pressure in SARS-CoV-2 acute respiratory distress syndrome: Oxygenation versus oxygen delivery. *Br. J. Anaesth.* **2021**, *126*, e70–e72. [CrossRef]
118. Suter, P.M.; Fairley, B.; Isenberg, M.D. Optimum end-expiratory airway pressure in patients with acute pulmonary failure. *N. Engl. J. Med.* **1975**, *292*, 284–289. [CrossRef]

119. Dickel, S.; Grimm, C.; Popp, M.; Struwe, C.; Sachkova, A.; Golinski, M.; Seeber, C.; Fichtner, F.; Heise, D.; Kranke, P.; et al. A Nationwide Cross-Sectional Online Survey on the Treatment of COVID-19-ARDS: High Variance in Standard of Care in German ICUs. *J. Clin. Med.* **2021**, *10*, 3363. [CrossRef]
120. Grasselli, G.; Zangrillo, A.; Zanella, A.; Antonelli, M.; Cabrini, L.; Castelli, A.; Cereda, D.; Coluccello, A.; Foti, G.; Fumagalli, R.; et al. Baseline Characteristics and Outcomes of 1591 Patients Infected With SARS-CoV-2 Admitted to ICUs of the Lombardy Region, Italy. *JAMA* **2020**, *323*, 1574–1581. [CrossRef]
121. Chiumello, D.; Bonifazi, M.; Pozzi, T.; Formenti, P.; Papa, G.F.S.; Zuanetti, G.; Coppola, S. Positive end-expiratory pressure in COVID-19 acute respiratory distress syndrome: The heterogeneous effects. *Crit. Care* **2021**, *25*, 431. [CrossRef] [PubMed]
122. Sinha, P.; Calfee, C.S.; Beitler, J.R.; Soni, N.; Ho, K.; Matthay, M.A.; Kallet, R.H. Physiologic Analysis and Clinical Performance of the Ventilatory Ratio in Acute Respiratory Distress Syndrome. *Am. J. Respir. Crit. Care Med.* **2019**, *199*, 333–341. [CrossRef] [PubMed]
123. Beitler, J.R.; Sarge, T.; Banner-Goodspeed, V.M.; Gong, M.N.; Cook, D.; Novack, V.; Loring, S.H.; Talmor, D.; Group, E.P.-S. Effect of Titrating Positive End-Expiratory Pressure (PEEP) With an Esophageal Pressure-Guided Strategy vs an Empirical High PEEP-Fio2 Strategy on Death and Days Free from Mechanical Ventilation Among Patients With Acute Respiratory Distress Syndrome: A Randomized Clinical Trial. *JAMA* **2019**, *321*, 846–857. [CrossRef]
124. Pan, C.; Chen, L.; Lu, C.; Zhang, W.; Xia, J.A.; Sklar, M.C.; Du, B.; Brochard, L.; Qiu, H. Lung Recruitability in COVID-19-associated Acute Respiratory Distress Syndrome: A Single-Center Observational Study. *Am. J. Respir. Crit. Care Med.* **2020**, *201*, 1294–1297. [CrossRef]
125. Ball, L.; Robba, C.; Maiello, L.; Herrmann, J.; Gerard, S.E.; Xin, Y.; Battaglini, D.; Brunetti, I.; Minetti, G.; Seitun, S.; et al. Computed tomography assessment of PEEP-induced alveolar recruitment in patients with severe COVID-19 pneumonia. *Crit. Care* **2021**, *25*, 81. [CrossRef] [PubMed]
126. Protti, A.; Santini, A.; Pennati, F.; Chiurazzi, C.; Cressoni, M.; Ferrari, M.; Iapichino, G.E.; Carenzo, L.; Lanza, E.; Picardo, G.; et al. Lung Response to a Higher Positive End-Expiratory Pressure in Mechanically Ventilated Patients With COVID-19. *Chest* **2022**, *161*, 979–988. [CrossRef] [PubMed]
127. Roesthuis, L.; van den Berg, M.; van der Hoeven, H. Advanced respiratory monitoring in COVID-19 patients: Use less PEEP! *Crit. Care* **2020**, *24*, 230. [CrossRef]
128. Perier, F.; Tuffet, S.; Maraffi, T.; Alcala, G.; Victor, M.; Haudebourg, A.F.; De Prost, N.; Amato, M.; Carteaux, G.; Mekontso Dessap, A. Effect of Positive End-Expiratory Pressure and Proning on Ventilation and Perfusion in COVID-19 Acute Respiratory Distress Syndrome. *Am. J. Respir. Crit. Care Med.* **2020**, *202*, 1713–1717. [CrossRef]
129. Mauri, T.; Spinelli, E.; Scotti, E.; Colussi, G.; Basile, M.C.; Crotti, S.; Tubiolo, D.; Tagliabue, P.; Zanella, A.; Grasselli, G.; et al. Potential for Lung Recruitment and Ventilation-Perfusion Mismatch in Patients With the Acute Respiratory Distress Syndrome From Coronavirus Disease 2019. *Crit. Care Med.* **2020**, *48*, 1129–1134. [CrossRef]
130. Chen, L.; Del Sorbo, L.; Grieco, D.L.; Junhasavasdikul, D.; Rittayamai, N.; Soliman, I.; Sklar, M.C.; Rauseo, M.; Ferguson, N.D.; Fan, E.; et al. Potential for Lung Recruitment Estimated by the Recruitment-to-Inflation Ratio in Acute Respiratory Distress Syndrome. A Clinical Trial. *Am. J. Respir. Crit. Care Med.* **2020**, *201*, 178–187. [CrossRef]
131. Gattinoni, L.; Camporota, L.; Marini, J.J. Prone Position and COVID-19: Mechanisms and Effects. *Crit. Care Med.* **2022**, *50*, 873–875. [CrossRef] [PubMed]
132. Rouby, J.J.; Puybasset, L.; Nieszkowska, A.; Lu, Q. Acute respiratory distress syndrome: Lessons from computed tomography of the whole lung. *Crit. Care Med.* **2003**, *31*, S285–S295. [CrossRef] [PubMed]
133. Albert, R.K.; Hubmayr, R.D. The prone position eliminates compression of the lungs by the heart. *Am. J. Respir. Crit. Care Med.* **2000**, *161*, 1660–1665. [CrossRef]
134. Pelosi, P.; D'Andrea, L.; Vitale, G.; Pesenti, A.; Gattinoni, L. Vertical gradient of regional lung inflation in adult respiratory distress syndrome. *Am. J. Respir. Crit. Care Med.* **1994**, *149*, 8–13. [CrossRef] [PubMed]
135. Gattinoni, L.; Taccone, P.; Carlesso, E.; Marini, J.J. Prone position in acute respiratory distress syndrome. Rationale, indications, and limits. *Am. J. Respir. Crit. Care Med.* **2013**, *188*, 1286–1293. [CrossRef] [PubMed]
136. Guerin, C.; Albert, R.K.; Beitler, J.; Gattinoni, L.; Jaber, S.; Marini, J.J.; Munshi, L.; Papazian, L.; Pesenti, A.; Vieillard-Baron, A.; et al. Prone position in ARDS patients: Why, when, how and for whom. *Intensive Care Med.* **2020**, *46*, 2385–2396. [CrossRef]
137. Mentzelopoulos, S.D.; Roussos, C.; Zakynthinos, S.G. Prone position reduces lung stress and strain in severe acute respiratory distress syndrome. *Eur. Respir. J.* **2005**, *25*, 534–544. [CrossRef]
138. Chen, L.; Zhang, Y.; Li, Y.; Song, C.; Lin, F.; Pan, P. The Application of Awake-Prone Positioning Among Non-intubated Patients With COVID-19-Related ARDS: A Narrative Review. *Front. Med. (Lausanne)* **2022**, *9*, 817689. [CrossRef]
139. Langer, T.; Brioni, M.; Guzzardella, A.; Carlesso, E.; Cabrini, L.; Castelli, G.; Dalla Corte, F.; De Robertis, E.; Favarato, M.; Forastieri, A.; et al. Prone position in intubated, mechanically ventilated patients with COVID-19: A multi-centric study of more than 1000 patients. *Crit. Care* **2021**, *25*, 128. [CrossRef]
140. Bellani, G.; Laffey, J.G.; Pham, T.; Fan, E. The LUNG SAFE study: A presentation of the prevalence of ARDS according to the Berlin Definition! *Crit. Care* **2016**, *20*, 268. [CrossRef]
141. Guerin, C.; Reignier, J.; Richard, J.C.; Beuret, P.; Gacouin, A.; Boulain, T.; Mercier, E.; Badet, M.; Mercat, A.; Baudin, O.; et al. Prone positioning in severe acute respiratory distress syndrome. *N. Engl. J. Med.* **2013**, *368*, 2159–2168. [CrossRef] [PubMed]

142. Mathews, K.S.; Soh, H.; Shaefi, S.; Wang, W.; Bose, S.; Coca, S.; Gupta, S.; Hayek, S.S.; Srivastava, A.; Brenner, S.K.; et al. Prone Positioning and Survival in Mechanically Ventilated Patients With Coronavirus Disease 2019-Related Respiratory Failure. *Crit. Care Med.* **2021**, *49*, 1026–1037. [CrossRef] [PubMed]
143. Fossali, T.; Pavlovsky, B.; Ottolina, D.; Colombo, R.; Basile, M.C.; Castelli, A.; Rech, R.; Borghi, B.; Ianniello, A.; Flor, N.; et al. Effects of Prone Position on Lung Recruitment and Ventilation-Perfusion Matching in Patients With COVID-19 Acute Respiratory Distress Syndrome: A Combined CT Scan/Electrical Impedance Tomography Study. *Crit. Care Med.* **2022**, *50*, 723–732. [CrossRef] [PubMed]
144. Zarantonello, F.; Sella, N.; Pettenuzzo, T.; Andreatta, G.; Calore, A.; Dotto, D.; De Cassai, A.; Calabrese, F.; Boscolo, A.; Navalesi, P. Early physiological effects of prone positioning in COVID-19 Acute Respiratory Distress Syndrome. *Anesthesiology* **2022**. Online ahead of print. [CrossRef]
145. Rossi, S.; Palumbo, M.M.; Sverzellati, N.; Busana, M.; Malchiodi, L.; Bresciani, P.; Ceccarelli, P.; Sani, E.; Romitti, F.; Bonifazi, M.; et al. Mechanisms of oxygenation responses to proning and recruitment in COVID-19 pneumonia. *Intensive Care Med.* **2022**, *48*, 56–66. [CrossRef]
146. Protti, A.; Santini, A.; Pennati, F.; Chiurazzi, C.; Ferrari, M.; Iapichino, G.E.; Carenzo, L.; Dalla Corte, F.; Lanza, E.; Martinetti, N.; et al. Lung response to prone positioning in mechanically-ventilated patients with COVID-19. *Crit. Care* **2022**, *26*, 127. [CrossRef]
147. Brodie, D.; Slutsky, A.S.; Combes, A. Extracorporeal Life Support for Adults with Respiratory Failure and Related Indications: A Review. *JAMA* **2019**, *322*, 557–568. [CrossRef]
148. Fernando, S.M.; Qureshi, D.; Tanuseputro, P.; Fan, E.; Munshi, L.; Rochwerg, B.; Talarico, R.; Scales, D.C.; Brodie, D.; Dhanani, S.; et al. Mortality and costs following extracorporeal membrane oxygenation in critically ill adults: A population-based cohort study. *Intensive Care Med.* **2019**, *45*, 1580–1589. [CrossRef]
149. Nesseler, N.; Fadel, G.; Mansour, A.; Para, M.; Falcoz, P.E.; Mongardon, N.; Porto, A.; Bertier, A.; Levy, B.; Cadoz, C.; et al. Extracorporeal Membrane Oxygenation for Respiratory Failure Related to COVID-19: A Nationwide Cohort Study. *Anesthesiology* **2022**, *136*, 732–748. [CrossRef]
150. Combes, A.; Hajage, D.; Capellier, G.; Demoule, A.; Lavoue, S.; Guervilly, C.; Da Silva, D.; Zafrani, L.; Tirot, P.; Veber, B.; et al. Extracorporeal Membrane Oxygenation for Severe Acute Respiratory Distress Syndrome. *N. Engl. J. Med.* **2018**, *378*, 1965–1975. [CrossRef]
151. Badulak, J.; Antonini, M.V.; Stead, C.M.; Shekerdemian, L.; Raman, L.; Paden, M.L.; Agerstrand, C.; Bartlett, R.H.; Barrett, N.; Combes, A.; et al. Extracorporeal Membrane Oxygenation for COVID-19: Updated 2021 Guidelines from the Extracorporeal Life Support Organization. *ASAIO J.* **2021**, *67*, 485–495. [CrossRef]
152. Gattinoni, L.; Gattarello, S.; Steinberg, I.; Busana, M.; Palermo, P.; Lazzari, S.; Romitti, F.; Quintel, M.; Meissner, K.; Marini, J.J.; et al. COVID-19 pneumonia: Pathophysiology and management. *Eur. Respir. Rev.* **2021**, *30*, 210138. [CrossRef] [PubMed]
153. Bain, W.; Yang, H.; Shah, F.A.; Suber, T.; Drohan, C.; Al-Yousif, N.; DeSensi, R.S.; Bensen, N.; Schaefer, C.; Rosborough, B.R.; et al. COVID-19 versus Non-COVID-19 Acute Respiratory Distress Syndrome: Comparison of Demographics, Physiologic Parameters, Inflammatory Biomarkers, and Clinical Outcomes. *Ann. Am. Thorac. Soc.* **2021**, *18*, 1202–1210. [CrossRef] [PubMed]
154. Dalia, A.A.; Convissar, D.; Crowley, J.; Raz, Y.; Funamoto, M.; Wiener-Kronish, J.; Shelton, K. The role of extracorporeal membrane oxygenation in COVID-19. *J. Cardiothorac. Vasc. Anesth.* **2022**, *36*, 3668–3675. [CrossRef] [PubMed]
155. McNamee, J.J.; Gillies, M.A.; Barrett, N.A.; Perkins, G.D.; Tunnicliffe, W.; Young, D.; Bentley, A.; Harrison, D.A.; Brodie, D.; Boyle, A.J.; et al. Effect of Lower Tidal Volume Ventilation Facilitated by Extracorporeal Carbon Dioxide Removal vs Standard Care Ventilation on 90-Day Mortality in Patients with Acute Hypoxemic Respiratory Failure: The REST Randomized Clinical Trial. *JAMA* **2021**, *326*, 1013–1023. [CrossRef]
156. Ramanathan, K.; Shekar, K.; Ling, R.R.; Barbaro, R.P.; Wong, S.N.; Tan, C.S.; Rochwerg, B.; Fernando, S.M.; Takeda, S.; MacLaren, G.; et al. Extracorporeal membrane oxygenation for COVID-19: A systematic review and meta-analysis. *Crit. Care* **2021**, *25*, 211. [CrossRef]
157. Ling, R.R.; Ramanathan, K.; Sim, J.J.L.; Wong, S.N.; Chen, Y.; Amin, F.; Fernando, S.M.; Rochwerg, B.; Fan, E.; Barbaro, R.P.; et al. Evolving outcomes of extracorporeal membrane oxygenation during the first 2 years of the COVID-19 pandemic: A systematic review and meta-analysis. *Crit. Care* **2022**, *26*, 147. [CrossRef]
158. Barbaro, R.P.; MacLaren, G.; Boonstra, P.S.; Combes, A.; Agerstrand, C.; Annich, G.; Diaz, R.; Fan, E.; Hryniewicz, K.; Lorusso, R.; et al. Extracorporeal membrane oxygenation for COVID-19: Evolving outcomes from the international Extracorporeal Life Support Organization Registry. *Lancet* **2021**, *398*, 1230–1238. [CrossRef]
159. Broman, L.M.; Eksborg, S.; Lo Coco, V.; De Piero, M.E.; Belohlavek, J.; Lorusso, R.; Euro, E.C.-W.G.; Euro, E.S.C. Extracorporeal membrane oxygenation for COVID-19 during first and second waves. *Lancet Respir. Med.* **2021**, *9*, e80–e81. [CrossRef]
160. Chong, W.H.; Saha, B.K.; Medarov, B.I. Clinical Characteristics Between Survivors and Nonsurvivors of COVID-19 Patients Requiring Extracorporeal Membrane Oxygenation (ECMO) Support: A Systematic Review and Meta-Analysis. *J. Intensive Care Med.* **2022**, *37*, 304–318. [CrossRef]
161. Kannapadi, N.V.; Jami, M.; Premraj, L.; Etchill, E.W.; Giuliano, K.; Bush, E.L.; Kim, B.S.; Seal, S.; Whitman, G.; Cho, S.M. Neurological Complications in COVID-19 Patients With ECMO Support: A Systematic Review and Meta-Analysis. *Heart Lung Circ.* **2022**, *31*, 292–298. [CrossRef] [PubMed]

162. Paternoster, G.; Bertini, P.; Innelli, P.; Trambaiolo, P.; Landoni, G.; Franchi, F.; Scolletta, S.; Guarracino, F. Right Ventricular Dysfunction in Patients With COVID-19: A Systematic Review and Meta-analysis. *J. Cardiothorac. Vasc. Anesth.* **2021**, *35*, 3319–3324. [CrossRef] [PubMed]
163. Li, X.; Guo, Z.; Li, B.; Zhang, X.; Tian, R.; Wu, W.; Zhang, Z.; Lu, Y.; Chen, N.; Clifford, S.P.; et al. Extracorporeal Membrane Oxygenation for Coronavirus Disease 2019 in Shanghai, China. *ASAIO J.* **2020**, *66*, 475–481. [CrossRef] [PubMed]
164. Dreier, E.; Malfertheiner, M.V.; Dienemann, T.; Fisser, C.; Foltan, M.; Geismann, F.; Graf, B.; Lunz, D.; Maier, L.S.; Muller, T.; et al. ECMO in COVID-19-prolonged therapy needed? A retrospective analysis of outcome and prognostic factors. *Perfusion* **2021**, *36*, 582–591. [CrossRef]
165. Cypel, M.; Keshavjee, S. When to consider lung transplantation for COVID-19. *Lancet Respir. Med.* **2020**, *8*, 944–946. [CrossRef]
166. Giani, M.; Rezoagli, E.; Guervilly, C.; Rilinger, J.; Duburcq, T.; Petit, M.; Textoris, L.; Garcia, B.; Wengenmayer, T.; Grasselli, G.; et al. Prone positioning during venovenous extracorporeal membrane oxygenation for acute respiratory distress syndrome: A pooled individual patient data analysis. *Crit. Care* **2022**, *26*, 8. [CrossRef] [PubMed]
167. Poon, W.H.; Ramanathan, K.; Ling, R.R.; Yang, I.X.; Tan, C.S.; Schmidt, M.; Shekar, K. Prone positioning during venovenous extracorporeal membrane oxygenation for acute respiratory distress syndrome: A systematic review and meta-analysis. *Crit. Care* **2021**, *25*, 292. [CrossRef]
168. Laghlam, D.; Charpentier, J.; Hamou, Z.A.; Nguyen, L.S.; Pene, F.; Cariou, A.; Mira, J.P.; Jozwiak, M. Effects of Prone Positioning on Respiratory Mechanics and Oxygenation in Critically Ill Patients With COVID-19 Requiring Venovenous Extracorporeal Membrane Oxygenation. *Front. Med.* **2021**, *8*, 810393. [CrossRef]
169. Giani, M.; Martucci, G.; Madotto, F.; Belliato, M.; Fanelli, V.; Garofalo, E.; Forlini, C.; Lucchini, A.; Panarello, G.; Bottino, N.; et al. Prone Positioning during Venovenous Extracorporeal Membrane Oxygenation in Acute Respiratory Distress Syndrome. A Multicenter Cohort Study and Propensity-matched Analysis. *Ann. Am. Thorac. Soc.* **2021**, *18*, 495–501. [CrossRef]
170. Iwashyna, T.J.; Burke, J.F.; Sussman, J.B.; Prescott, H.C.; Hayward, R.A.; Angus, D.C. Implications of Heterogeneity of Treatment Effect for Reporting and Analysis of Randomized Trials in Critical Care. *Am. J. Respir. Crit. Care Med.* **2015**, *192*, 1045–1051. [CrossRef]

Review

Second- and Third-Tier Therapies for Severe Traumatic Brain Injury

Charikleia S. Vrettou * and Spyros D. Mentzelopoulos

First Department of Intensive Care Medicine, Evaggelismos General Hospital, National and Kapodistrian University of Athens Medical School, 10676 Athens, Greece
* Correspondence: vrettou@hotmail.com

Abstract: Intracranial hypertension is a common finding in patients with severe traumatic brain injury. These patients need treatment in the intensive care unit, where intracranial pressure monitoring and, whenever possible, multimodal neuromonitoring can be applied. A three-tier approach is suggested in current recommendations, in which higher-tier therapies have more significant side effects. In this review, we explain the rationale for this approach, and analyze the benefits and risks of each therapeutic modality. Finally, we discuss, based on the most recent recommendations, how this approach can be adapted in low- and middle-income countries, where available resources are limited.

Keywords: brain trauma; intracranial hypertension; neuromonitoring

1. Introduction

Traumatic brain injury (TBI) is defined as "an alteration in brain function, or other evidence of brain pathology caused by an external force", while severe TBI is specified by a score of ≤ 8 in the Glasgow Coma Scale (GCS) [1]. Severe TBI is a multifaceted condition, rather than a single disease. According to a recent, large, prospective study, the most common mechanisms for severe TBI are falls in very-high-income countries, and road traffic accidents elsewhere [2]. Pathological findings may be focal or global. Focal findings include extradural, subdural and intracerebral hematomas, as well as contusions. Global findings include diffuse axonal injury, brain swelling and ischemia, and post-traumatic hydrocephalus [3]. A common characteristic of severe TBI is intracranial hypertension (ICH), which ranges, in different cohorts, from 50 to 80% of the cases [4].

ICH is considered an important component of TBI pathophysiology because it is related to significant morbidity and mortality, and carries the risk of cerebral herniation [5–7]. The latest recommendations by the Brain Trauma Foundation advise to maintain intracranial pressure (ICP) at ≤ 22 mmHg and cerebral perfusion pressure (CPP) at ≥ 60 mmHg. An escalating approach has been adopted for the treatment of ICH [3,8–13], according to which different treatment modalities are prioritized on the basis of their efficacy and relative risks of their application [8,9,11,13–15]. Treatments with more severe side effects are classified as higher tier, while safer treatments, such as analgesia, sedation, and hyperosmolar therapy, are considered lower tier. It is expected that refractory ICH will eventually require higher-tier therapies that carry higher risk of complications. The concept of separate tiers serves two important purposes. Firstly, it alerts physicians to the increased risks associated with escalation of treatment. Before taking those risks, it is advised that a thorough examination and repeated imaging be performed, as appropriate. Medical imaging, in particular computerized tomography (CT) of the brain, may reveal evolving lesions, such as contusions and hematomas that demand surgical evacuation, rather than escalation of medical treatment [8,10–12,15–17]. A detailed medical and neurological evaluation, on the other hand, may identify extracranial causes of ICP elevation, such as infections, respiratory deterioration, and sodium disturbances [3,8–12,18,19]. Secondly, a tiered design allows for flexible choices among the modalities of each tier, or even for skipping a tier, if considered advantageous to the patient. In order to apply the tier concept effectively, clinicians need to be familiar with the treatments involved and to be aware of their side effects. They also need to formulate a treatment and escalation strategy that is tailored to the clinical presentation and therapeutic needs of each patient.

The purpose of this review is to focus on treatments that carry significant side effects, the so called second- and third-tier therapies [8] in patients with blunt traumatic brain injury. A prerequisite for the safe management of these patients is their admission to the intensive care unit (ICU), where the required interventions can be applied in the safest possible way. Basic support measures applied in the ICU are considered tier zero therapies, while initial treatments targeting the ICH are classified into tier one (Figure 1) [8].

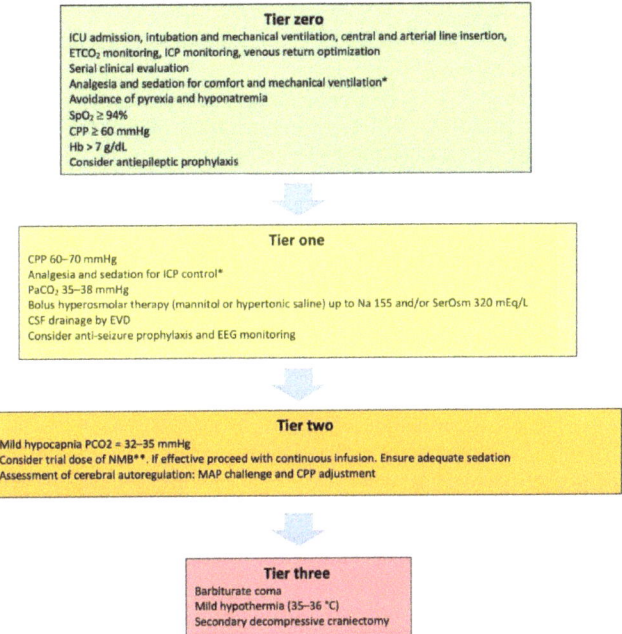

Figure 1. Treatment modalities included in the tiered approach for the management of intracranial hypertension. ICU: intensive care unit; ETCO$_2$: end-tidal carbon dioxide partial pressure; ICP: intracranial pressure; SpO$_2$: oxygen saturation; CPP: cerebral perfusion pressure; Hb: hemoglobin concentration; SerOsm: serum osmolality; CSF: cerebrospinal fluid; EVD: external ventricular drain; EEG: electroencephalography; NMB: neuromuscular blocker; MAP: mean arterial pressure. * Propofol and midazolam are the most commonly used anesthetic agents. Morphine, fentanyl, sulfentanil and remifentanil are the most commonly used analgesics [20]. ** Non-depolarizing agents are considered as safer than succinylcholine [21].

As shown in Figure 1, tier one therapies targeting at lowering the ICP include escalation of analgesia and sedation, normocapnia, the use of an external ventricular drain (EVD) to drain cerebrospinal fluid (CSF), and hyperosmolar therapy. Both mannitol 20% and hypertonic sodium chloride solutions can be used as hyperosmolar agents. Common side effects include derangements of the fluid and electrolyte balance, and for this reason, ICP-guided (rather than scheduled) administration is advised [22]. In cases with significant brain edema, the placement of an EVD can be technically difficult, with higher risk of hemorrhage and misplacement, because the ventricular system may be compressed [23]. Furthermore, the presence of an EVD carries a small but significant risk of infection [24]. Even though tier one interventions are not free of complications, treatments beyond this level have recently been related to an additional negative effect on survival [14,19]. For this reason, tier-two and -three therapies require increased caution and clinical experience for their safe application [15].

2. Tier-Two Therapies

2.1. Mild Hypocapnia (PaCO$_2$ 32–35 mmHg)

Mild hypocapnia, targeting a PaCO$_2$ of 32–35 mmHg, is among the second-tier choices. Mild hyperventilation is an effective and rapid way to reduce the ICP by inducing cerebral vasoconstriction and reducing cerebral blood flow [25]. However, it carries the risk of cerebral ischemia. A study in brain injured patients and normal controls, using multimodal neuromonitoring and positron emission tomography (PET) of the brain, showed that mild hypocapnia significantly reduced the ICP, but also increased the volume of ischemic brain tissue in both perilesional and normal regions of the brain, compared to normocapnia levels and to normal controls [26]. Interestingly, ischemic brain volume increased even when jugular venous saturation (SjO$_2$) measurements, used for the assessment of global brain oxygen demands, were within the acceptable range. More recent studies report acceptable cerebral oxygenation and blood flow parameters during mild hyperventilation [27–30]. A practical approach, based on current evidence, is the application of mild hyperventilation with concomitant use of multimodal neuromonitoring, including methods for the focal and global assessment of the cerebral oxygenation adequacy [8,10,31]. Such modalities are the perfusion computerized tomography (CTP), the transcranial color duplex ultrasonography (TCD), as well as the SjO$_2$ and the brain parenchymal oxygenation (PbrO$_2$) monitoring. In practice, these techniques are not always available in general ICUs, thus limiting the application of mild hypocapnia as a potentially useful intervention. In view of such restrictions, and based on the current limited evidence, mild hyperventilation is considered an acceptable measure before escalating to higher tiers. In any case, close monitoring of the PaCO$_2$ is important to avoid an accidental reduction in the PaCO$_2$ below 30 mmHg [32].

In addition to the risk of brain ischemia, lowering the PCO$_2$ may pose additional problems to trauma patients. The subsequent rise of the pH carries the risk of reduced blood flow to other body organs and has been related to tissue hypoxia, cardiac arrythmias, hypokalemia, hypocalcemia, hypophosphatemia, and lower epileptic threshold [31]. Moreover, increased tidal volumes may be necessary for mild hypocapnia, and this may render mechanical ventilation traumatizing to the lung [33]. Since blood flow to the brain is known to be reduced during the first 24 h after brain trauma, it is reasonable to avoid mild hypocapnia during this time period [34]. Finally, hypocapnia below 30 mmHg had better be kept as a temporizing measure for cases of extremes in ICH, when signs of critical neuroworsening (Figure 2) or impending herniation, such as the Cushing's reflex (i.e., increased blood pressure, bradycardia, and irregular breathing if the patient is not already deeply sedated and mechanically ventilated) are present. Acute hypocapnia can be applied as a bridge to higher-tier therapies, for a limited period of time, until other, longer acting measures are in place. Subsequently, a gradual return to normocapnia is advised, in order to avoid rebound ICH [11].

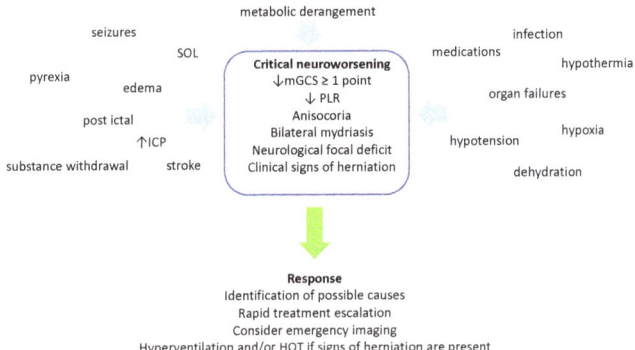

Figure 2. Definition, causes, and management of critical neuroworsening. mGCS: motor Glasgow Coma Score; PLR: pupillary light reflex; SOL: space-occupying lesion; ICP: intracranial pressure; HOT: hyperosmolar therapy.

2.2. Neuromuscular Blockade (NMB)

Neuromuscular blockers, mostly non-depolarizing ones, such as cis-atracurium, have been used in the past as a tier zero therapy in patients with brain trauma [14]. There is, however, limited evidence for the effect of NMB on ICH. It has been described that paralysis may lower the ICP by 2–3 mmHg [21]. Theoretically, lowering ventilation pressures and limiting ventilator asynchrony can improve venous outflow to the main vessels of the chest [35]. Even though this has a likely beneficial effect, NMB should be applied with caution, and for short periods.

In one study that included TBI patients, increased rates of ventilator associated pneumonia and prolonged ICU stay was reported in patients who received NMB for >12 h compared to those who did not [36]. Another concern is the effect of NMB on the long-term outcomes. Prolonged use of NMB is associated with ICU-acquired neuromuscular weakness, also known as ICU neuromyopathy [37,38]. This entity can significantly affect the quality of life of the patients and is related to the post-intensive care syndrome, which affects more than 60% of ICU survivors [39]. Prolonged immobilization, steroid and aminoglycoside use have also been shown to contribute to ICU neuromyopathy [40,41].

NMB may be indicated for trauma patients who, in addition to brain injury, also have lung contusions, acute respiratory distress syndrome (ARDS) or abdominal compartment syndrome [35,42]. NMB is also justified during stimulating procedures, such as tracheal suction and bronchoscopy, in patients who are deeply sedated [43], and can be necessary during the application of cooling measures to lower body temperature. Since muscular activity significantly contributes to CO_2 production, NMB can assist CO_2 control [44]. A trial for NMB is currently suggested for patients in whom ICH is not controlled with tier one measures, with continued infusion reserved for those who show a favorable response, or for patients who need NMB for other reasons, as previously described [21].

2.3. Assessment of Static Autoregulation—The Mean Arterial Pressure (MAP) Challenge

Cerebral pressure autoregulation, both static and dynamic, can be severely impaired following TBI [45]. The assessment of dynamic pressure autoregulation requires special equipment that may not be available to most ICUs. Static pressure autoregulation (sPAR), on the other hand, can be evaluated at the patient's bedside [46,47]. In some cases, there may be hints that sPAR is intact. For example, the ICP may rise acutely following a MAP drop, and may recede when the MAP is restored with the administration of fluids or vasopressors. The consensus working group in the recent guidelines, suggest Rosenthal's method for evaluating sPAR by using the MAP challenge [48,49]. In cases where autoregulation is preserved, and the baseline CPP is above the lower breakpoint of sPAR, a further rise of the CPP will result in vasoconstriction. Vasoconstriction will lead to decreased cerebral blood flow (CBF) and cerebral blood volume, and to a drop in the ICP. To perform the assessment, clinicians need to maintain vasopressor and sedatives infusions, as well as ventilation parameters stable. After recording the baseline MAP and CPP, the vasopressors are titrated to a MAP rise of 10 mmHg, and the patient's response is observed for a maximum of 20 min. The ideal positive response comprises an ICP drop in response to the MAP rise [45,50]. Subsequently, the MAP and CPP need to be adjusted accordingly.

The assessment of sPAR can be associated with several clinical problems. Clinical experience is required to treat a possible spike of the ICP caused by the rising MAP in cases where the sPAR is disrupted. Furthermore, adjusting the MAP/CPP, is a separate clinical decision that needs to take into account the relative risks of increasing the vasopressor infusion rate. This may be difficult in trauma patients who require high vasopressor dose and/or have concurrent ARDS or cardiac dysfunction [51]. Finally, the sPAR status may not be stable over the clinical course of the patient, and may require frequent reassessment [50]. Several additional tools have been proposed in the assessment of CBF and sPAR, such as transcranial color duplex ultrasonography, near-infrared spectroscopy, and brain perfusion imaging [46,47,52,53].

3. Tier-Three Therapies

3.1. Therapeutic Hypothermia

For many years, therapeutic hypothermia was used for the management of ICH in TBI based on favorable findings derived mainly from experimental studies of ischemic models, according to which hypothermia has significant neuroprotective effects [54]. Lowering the body temperature, and in particular the brain temperature, below 36 °C, decreases the metabolic demands of the brain tissue, hence decreases the CBF, the cerebral blood volume, and the ICP. At the cellular level, hypothermia mitigates calcium induced neurotoxicity, neuronal apoptosis, inflammatory response, and cytotoxic edema [55]. Nevertheless, these experimental findings did not translate to positive clinical outcomes. In a meta-analysis of 18 trials published in 2016, no decrease in mortality was observed, while hypothermia was related to increased risk of pneumonia and cardiovascular complications [54,56]. The EUROTHERM study, a randomized trial that finally included 387 TBI patients, was discontinued due to safety concerns, because of worse outcomes in the hypothermia arm that were attributed to adverse reactions during the rewarming period. Interestingly, the control arm received higher-tier therapies and more barbiturates than the patients treated with hypothermia [57]. The POLAR study, another randomized trial using early, sustained prophylactic hypothermia in patients with severe TBI, did not show any improvement in outcomes, either. However, there were deviations from the cooling protocol that may have masked a possible beneficial effect of hypothermia [58]. Based on these results, current recommendations suggest the use of mild hypothermia, targeting core body temperatures of 35–36 °C as a tier-three intervention. Temperatures of < 35 °C are not recommended, due to increased risk for systemic complications [48]. In view of these facts, the term "targeted temperature management" (TTM), that reflects the currently recommended practice for post-cardiac arrest patients, would also be appropriate for TBI [55].

When considering TTM, the overall patient's condition needs to be evaluated in view of anticipated side effects. The latter may include impaired cardiac contractility, coagulation and platelet dysfunction, increased risk for arrhythmias and infections, and significant fluid and electrolyte shifts [59]. These complications have been reported mainly in patients cooled down to 32–35 °C, and are more pronounced during the rewarming phase [57]. The targeted temperatures can be achieved with the use of external cooling measures. Cooling blankets or other devices with feedback control are appropriate when available, in order to avoid unwanted temperature shifts or body temperature below the desired level [59]. Notably, some patients are spontaneously hypothermic following TBI [60]. While there are no recommendations on temperature correction in this setting, maintaining temperatures at 35–36 °C and avoiding rewarming beyond this point seems reasonable [60]. Compared to other tier-three treatments, temperature management may be more suitable for patients without active bleeding and signs of shock, who are not candidates for surgical decompression.

3.2. Metabolic Suppression with Barbiturates

Pentobarbital and thiopentone are the most commonly used barbiturates for ICH in TBI. Both drugs are potent sedatives that can induce greater metabolic suppression than midazolam or propofol, and also have antiepileptic properties. By depressing brain function, oxygen consumption and metabolism, barbiturates also reduce the CBF and the ICP [3]. Barbiturates bind to neuronal γ-aminobutyric acid alpha (GABA$_A$) receptors and cause neuronal hyperpolarization and inhibition of the action potential [61]. In addition, it has been shown that they reduce lactate and pyruvate production in the brain and inhibit lipid peroxidation mediated by free radicals [62]. These findings imply that barbiturates may also possess significant neuroprotective effects. Nevertheless, there is no evidence to support improvement in clinical outcomes with their use [63].

A plausible argument for this discrepancy is the association of barbiturates with significant side effects, the most prominent being hemodynamic compromise presenting as hypotension and myocardial depression. Consequently, the use of barbiturates in trauma patients with shock or myocardial injury is limited, since they may further increase vasopressor requirements for the maintenance of adequate CPP [64,65]. Other side effects are immunosuppression, hepatic and renal dysfunction, suppression of gut motility, and dyskalemias, which usually appear as hypokalemia during the loading phase and hyperkalemia during withdrawal. The latter may require renal replacement therapy in some cases [66,67]. At increased doses, barbiturates suppress the pupillary light reflex, in which case patient monitoring relies mainly on invasive measures or imaging. Finally, barbiturate use can lead to prolonged sedation due to drug accumulation, and consequently to prolonged need for mechanical ventilation [68–72].

When metabolic suppression with barbiturates is planned, it is advised to administer a test dose and record the patient's response. A favorable response is characterized by ICP drop and concurrent maintenance of adequate CPP. If this is achieved, then loading doses can be administered, e.g., thiopental 250 mg boluses up to a total dose of 3–5 g, and then continuous infusion of 3–8 mg/kg/h. The endpoint of barbiturate administration is the control of the ICP with the minimum effective dose, in order to minimize side effects. This is achieved with the application of electroencephalographic monitoring and titration of the barbiturate infusion rate to a suppression–burst pattern of >>50%, since a further increase in barbiturate dose is unlikely to affect the ICP [73,74]. Other concurrent therapeutic goals include the maintenance of euvolemia and of the CPP [58]. Once ICH is treated and barbiturates are to be withdrawn, a gradual reduction over a few days is advised to avoid hyperkalemia and a rebound rise of the ICP.

While barbiturate use for metabolic suppression of the brain is suggested by guidelines, the so called low-dose (e.g., 2 mg/kg/h) barbiturate use has been adopted by many hospitals [68]. Adding low-dose barbiturates to other sedatives, such as midazolam and propofol, carries the risk of additive cardiovascular depression, but may also improve neuroprotection and reduce the time to drug elimination. Nevertheless, this practice is not supported by evidence and is not recommended by most experts in recent consensus guidelines [7]. A suppression burst pattern can also be induced by propofol and, in a small number of cases, by midazolam infusion, but none of these agents lowers the ICP as effectively as barbiturates. This is attributed to the profound suppression of cerebral rate of oxygen consumption during barbiturate induced suppression burst [43,75]. On the other hand, propofol carries significant risks when used in high doses and for prolonged periods (>5 mg/kg/h, >48 h). Cardiovascular depression, that may affect the MAP and CPP is commonly reported. Other side effects include the elevation of pancreatic enzymes, pancreatitis, lipemia, increased caloric administration due to the lipid formulation of the infused drug, and the propofol infusion syndrome (PRIS). PRIS is characterized by lactic acidosis, electrocardiographic changes, such as J-point and ST-segment elevation and T-wave inversion, hepatomegaly, and elevated transaminases. It can progress to rhabdomyolysis, renal failure, hyperkalemia, malignant arrhythmias, and cardiovascular collapse. Although PRIS is rare, the reported mortality rate is high (48–52%). The exact pathophysiology of PRIS is unclear, but possible mechanisms involve interaction of propofol with mitochondrial function and lipid metabolism [76].

3.3. Decompressive Craniectomy

The last modality in tier three is the physiologically most effective one, i.e., the surgical opening of the cranial cavity. Decompressive craniectomy lowers the ICP, and this has been confirmed by two randomized trials, the DECRA, published in 2011 and the RESCUE-ICP, published in 2016. There are many differences between these two studies. Patients in the DECRA trial were recruited early, within 72 h of TBI, and had a lower ICP threshold and lower-tier treatments applied [77]. Patients in the RESCUE ICP trial had an ICP of >25 mmHg, not responding to maximum medical therapy, including hypothermia, but not barbiturate coma [78]. In the DECRA trial, similar mortality was observed in the two study groups, with higher rates of unfavorable outcomes in the craniectomy group. In the RESCUE-ICP trial, there was a survival advantage in the intervention group. While there were higher rates of unfavorable outcomes among survivors at six-month follow-up, there were also statistically significant higher rates of favorable outcomes at 12 months [78].

Complications of decompressive craniectomy include infections, intracranial hemorrhage, seizures, transcranial herniation, formation of subdural hygromas, and hydrocephalus. These, combined with the risks of cranioplasty [49] and of a poor neurological outcome, may hinder the decision for craniectomy. The risks described, as well as the probable need for long-term care, have to be thoroughly explained to the patients' families before the procedure. Patients with acute subdural hematomas often have concomitant underlying intraparenchymal hematomas and contusions [79]. In many cases where subdural hematomas warrant evacuation, the brain bulges beyond the table of the skull postoperatively, and there is a surgical option for primary craniectomy, i.e., "to leave the bone flap out". While there is limited evidence in support of primary craniectomy in this setting, there are some studies that show better outcomes with this strategy [80,81] and a relevant randomized trial is ongoing [82]. In the meantime, decompressive craniectomy remains a tier-three therapy, from which previously fit patients with unilateral pathology, and adequate medical and social support are more likely to benefit. Decompressive craniectomy also remains a rescue option for patients not responding to conservative treatments [49].

4. Second- and Third-Tier Therapies in Low- and Middle-Income Countries (LMICs)

The management of ICH in TBI patients is even more challenging in developing countries. Surgical procedures may have a more central role in the management of ICH, because available resources for neuromonitoring are limited, as opposed to the capacity for surgical decompression. Following the BEST TRIP (the Benchmark Evidence from South American Trials: Treatment of Intracranial Pressure) trial [83], protocols such as the CREVICHE (Consensus REVised ICE algorithm) have appeared, which give directions on the application of tiered therapies in this setting, based on clinical examination and brain CT findings [84]. Figure 3 depicts a simplified version of the protocols suggested in low-income countries setting, when ICP monitoring is not applied. Scheduled hyperosmolar therapy as well as continuous infusion of 3% hypertonic saline are allowed in this setting, and decompressive craniectomy remains a tier-three intervention [84]. While most craniectomies performed in low/middle-income countries are primary procedures, the clinical decisions, particularly for secondary craniectomies, may be difficult, due to the limited capability for long-term support and rehabilitation, that may compromise neurological outcomes. The proposed surgical techniques are also discussed in the relevant literature. Floating or hinged bone flaps have been suggested to avoid the need for reconstructive cranioplasty, but there are no recommendations to support this practice. Current guidelines advise that these procedures should be performed by neurosurgeons or at least neurosurgical trainees that are adequately trained, and that decisions should be made in the context of local knowledge, medical resources, capacity for long-term care, and cultural beliefs [79,85].

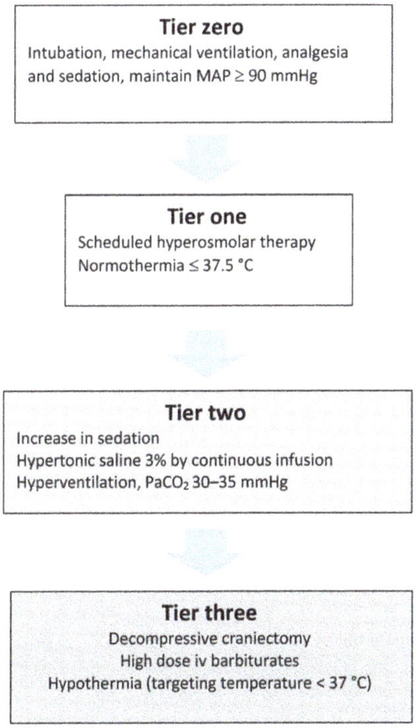

Tier zero
Intubation, mechanical ventilation, analgesia and sedation, maintain MAP ≥ 90 mmHg

↓

Tier one
Scheduled hyperosmolar therapy
Normothermia ≤ 37.5 °C

↓

Tier two
Increase in sedation
Hypertonic saline 3% by continuous infusion
Hyperventilation, $PaCO_2$ 30–35 mmHg

↓

Tier three
Decompressive craniectomy
High dose iv barbiturates
Hypothermia (targeting temperature < 37 °C)

Figure 3. A simplified version of the three-tier therapy protocol proposed for the treatment of suspected intracranial hypertension when intracranial pressure monitoring is not employed. Decisions on escalation and de-escalation are based on serial clinical examination and computerized tomography imaging. MAP: mean arterial pressure; $PaCO_2$: partial arterial pressure of carbon dioxide.

5. Conclusions

Tier-two and -three therapies for ICH in TBI are associated with significant adverse effects and complications, and are applied when ICH poses a bigger threat to the patient. The tier concept allows for flexibility in the therapeutic choices and for patient-tailored strategies in different resource settings. Individualized approaches can be achieved by the use of advanced imaging and neuromonitoring modalities. Future research is oriented towards strengthening the existing evidence and identifying the specific patient profiles that can benefit from each separate therapeutic modality.

Author Contributions: All authors (C.S.V. and S.D.M.) were involved in the conceptualization, writing, revision, and critical review of this manuscript. All authors have read and agreed to the published version of the manuscript.

Funding: This research received no external funding.

Institutional Review Board Statement: Not applicable.

Informed Consent Statement: Not applicable.

Conflicts of Interest: The authors declare no conflict of interest.

References

1. Menon, D.K.; Schwab, K.; Wright, D.W.; Maas, A.I. Position Statement: Definition of Traumatic Brain Injury. *Arch. Phys. Med. Rehabil.* **2010**, *91*, 1637–1640. [CrossRef] [PubMed]
2. Clark, D.; Joannides, A.; Adeleye, A.O.; Bajamal, A.H.; Bashford, T.; Biluts, H.; Budohoski, K.; Ercole, A.; Fernández-Méndez, R.; Figaji, A.; et al. Casemix, Management, and Mortality of Patients Receiving Emergency Neurosurgery for Traumatic Brain Injury in the Global Neurotrauma Outcomes Study: A Prospective Observational Cohort Study. *Lancet Neurol.* **2022**, *21*, 438–449. [CrossRef]
3. Menon, D.K.; Ercole, A. Critical Care Management of Traumatic Brain Injury. In *Handbook of Clinical Neurology*; Elsevier B.V.: Amsterdam, The Netherlands, 2017; Volume 140, pp. 239–274.
4. Maas, A.I.R.; Menon, D.K.; David Adelson, P.D.; Andelic, N.; Bell, M.J.; Belli, A.; Bragge, P.; Brazinova, A.; Büki, A.; Chesnut, R.M.; et al. Traumatic Brain Injury: Integrated Approaches to Improve Prevention, Clinical Care, and Research. *Lancet Neurol.* **2017**, *16*, 987–1048. [CrossRef]
5. Vik, A.; Nag, T.; Fredriksli, O.A.; Skandsen, T.; Moen, K.G.; Schirmer-Mikalsen, K.; Manley, G.T. Relationship of "Dose" of Intracranial Hypertension to Outcome in Severe Traumatic Brain Injury. *J. Neurosurg.* **2008**, *109*, 678–684. [CrossRef] [PubMed]
6. Kahraman, S.; Dutton, R.P.; Hu, P.; Xiao, Y.; Aarabi, B.; Stein, D.M.; Scalea, T.M. Automated Measurement of "Pressure Times Time Dose" of Intracranial Hypertension Best Predicts Outcome after Severe Traumatic Brain Injury. *J. Trauma-Inj. Infect. Crit. Care* **2010**, *69*, 110–118. [CrossRef]
7. Güiza, F.; Depreitere, B.; Piper, I.; Citerio, G.; Chambers, I.; Jones, P.A.; Lo, T.Y.M.; Enblad, P.; Nillson, P.; Feyen, B.; et al. Visualizing the Pressure and Time Burden of Intracranial Hypertension in Adult and Paediatric Traumatic Brain Injury. *Intensive Care Med.* **2015**, *41*, 1067–1076. [CrossRef]
8. Hawryluk, G.W.J.; Aguilera, S.; Buki, A.; Bulger, E.; Citerio, G.; Cooper, D.J.; Arrastia, R.D.; Diringer, M.; Figaji, A.; Gao, G.; et al. A Management Algorithm for Patients with Intracranial Pressure Monitoring: The Seattle International Severe Traumatic Brain Injury Consensus Conference (SIBICC). *Intensive Care Med.* **2019**, *45*, 1783–1794. [CrossRef]
9. Stocchetti, N.; Maas, A.I.R. Traumatic Intracranial Hypertension. *N. Engl. J. Med.* **2014**, *370*, 2121–2130. [CrossRef]
10. Meyfroidt, G.; Bouzat, P.; Casaer, M.P.; Chesnut, R.; Hamada, S.R.; Helbok, R.; Hutchinson, P.; Maas, A.I.R.; Manley, G.; Menon, D.K.; et al. Management of Moderate to Severe Traumatic Brain Injury: An Update for the Intensivist. *Intensive Care Med.* **2022**, *48*, 649–666. [CrossRef]
11. Stocchetti, N.; Carbonara, M.; Citerio, G.; Ercole, A.; Skrifvars, M.B.; Smielewski, P.; Zoerle, T.; Menon, D.K. Severe Traumatic Brain Injury: Targeted Management in the Intensive Care Unit. *Lancet Neurol.* **2017**, *16*, 452–464. [CrossRef]
12. Stocchetti, N.; Zoerle, T.; Carbonara, M. Intracranial Pressure Management in Patients with Traumatic Brain Injury: An Update. *Curr. Opin. Crit. Care* **2017**, *23*, 110–114. [CrossRef] [PubMed]
13. Carney, N.; Totten, A.M.; O'Reilly, C.; Ullman, J.S.; Hawryluk, G.W.J.; Bell, M.J.; Bratton, S.L.; Chesnut, R.; Harris, O.A.; Kissoon, N.; et al. Guidelines for the Management of Severe Traumatic Brain Injury, Fourth Edition. *Neurosurgery* **2017**, *80*, 6–15. [CrossRef] [PubMed]
14. Huijben, J.A.; Dixit, A.; Stocchetti, N.; Maas, A.I.R.; Lingsma, H.F.; van der Jagt, M.; Nelson, D.; Citerio, G.; Wilson, L.; Menon, D.K.; et al. Use and Impact of High Intensity Treatments in Patients with Traumatic Brain Injury across Europe: A CENTER-TBI Analysis. *Crit. Care* **2021**, *25*, 78. [CrossRef] [PubMed]
15. Gelormini, C.; Caricato, A. "Tier-Three" Therapies in Intracranial Hypertension: Is It Worthwhile? *Minerva Anestesiol.* **2021**, *87*, 1287–1289. [CrossRef] [PubMed]
16. Robba, C.; Iannuzzi, F.; Taccone, F.S. Tier-Three Therapies for Refractory Intracranial Hypertension in Adult Head Trauma. *Minerva Anestesiol.* **2021**, *87*, 1359–1366. [CrossRef]
17. Adatia, K.; Newcombe, V.F.J.; Menon, D.K. Contusion Progression Following Traumatic Brain Injury: A Review of Clinical and Radiological Predictors, and Influence on Outcome. *Neurocrit. Care* **2021**, *34*, 312–324. [CrossRef]
18. Iaccarino, C.; Lippa, L.; Munari, M.; Castioni, C.A.; Robba, C.; Caricato, A.; Pompucci, A.; Signoretti, S.; Zona, G.; Rasulo, F.A.; et al. Management of Intracranial Hypertension Following Traumatic Brain Injury: A Best Clinical Practice Adoption Proposal for Intracranial Pressure Monitoring and Decompressive Craniectomy: Joint Statements by the Traumatic Brain Injury Section of the Italian Society of Neurosurgery (SINch) and the Neuroanesthesia and Neurocritical Care Study Group of the Italian Society of Anesthesia, Analgesia, Resuscitation and Intensive Care (SIAARTI). *J. Neurosurg. Sci.* **2021**, *65*, 219–238.
19. Cnossen, M.C.; Huijben, J.A.; van der Jagt, M.; Volovici, V.; van Essen, T.; Polinder, S.; Nelson, D.; Ercole, A.; Stocchetti, N.; Citerio, G.; et al. Variation in Monitoring and Treatment Policies for Intracranial Hypertension in Traumatic Brain Injury: A Survey in 66 Neurotrauma Centers Participating in the CENTER-TBI Study. *Crit. Care* **2017**, *21*, 233. [CrossRef]
20. Roberts, D.J.; Hall, R.I.; Kramer, A.H.; Robertson, H.L.; Gallagher, C.N.; Zygun, D.A. Sedation for Critically Ill Adults with Severe Traumatic Brain Injury: A Systematic Review of Randomized Controlled Trials. *Crit. Care Med.* **2011**, *39*, 2743–2751. [CrossRef]
21. Sanfilippo, F.; Santonocito, C.; Veenith, T.; Astuto, M.; Maybauer, M.O. The Role of Neuromuscular Blockade in Patients with Traumatic Brain Injury: A Systematic Review. *Neurocrit. Care* **2015**, *22*, 325–334. [CrossRef]
22. Brain Trauma Foundation; American Association of Neurological Surgeons; Congress of Neurological Surgeons. Guidelines for the management of severe traumatic brain injury. *J. Neurotrauma.* **2007**, *24* (Suppl. S1), S1–S106, Erratum in *J. Neurotrauma* **2008**, *25*, 276–278. [CrossRef]

23. AlAzri, A.; Mok, K.; Chankowsky, J.; Mullah, M.; Marcoux, J. Placement Accuracy of External Ventricular Drain When Comparing Freehand Insertion to Neuronavigation Guidance in Severe Traumatic Brain Injury. *Acta Neurochir.* **2017**, *159*, 1399–1411. [CrossRef] [PubMed]
24. Ramanan, M.; Lipman, J.; Shorr, A.; Shankar, A. A Meta-Analysis of Ventriculostomy-Associated Cerebrospinal Fluid Infections. *BMC Infect. Dis.* **2015**, *15*, 3. [CrossRef]
25. Godoy, D.A.; Seifi, A.; Garza, D.; Lubillo-Montenegro, S.; Murillo-Cabezas, F. Hyperventilation Therapy for Control of Posttraumatic Intracranial Hypertension. *Front. Neurol.* **2017**, *8*, 250. [CrossRef] [PubMed]
26. Coles, J.P.; Fryer, T.D.; Coleman, M.R.; Smielewski, P.; Gupta, A.K.; Minhas, P.S.; Aigbirhio, F.; Chatfield, D.A.; Williams, G.B.; Boniface, S.; et al. Hyperventilation Following Head Injury: Effect on Ischemic Burden and Cerebral Oxidative Metabolism. *Crit. Care Med.* **2007**, *35*, 568–578. [CrossRef]
27. Beqiri, E.; Czosnyka, M.; Lalou, A.D.; Zeiler, F.A.; Fedriga, M.; Steiner, L.A.; Chieregato, A.; Smielewski, P. Influence of Mild-Moderate Hypocapnia on Intracranial Pressure Slow Waves Activity in TBI. *Acta Neurochir.* **2020**, *162*, 345–356. [CrossRef]
28. Geeraerts, T. Moderate Hypocapnia for Intracranial Pressure Control after Traumatic Brain Injury: A Common Practice Requiring Further Investigations. *Intensive Care Med.* **2021**, *47*, 1009–1010. [CrossRef]
29. Godoy, D.A.; Badenes, R.; Robba, C.; Murillo Cabezas, F. Hyperventilation in Severe Traumatic Brain Injury Has Something Changed in the Last Decade or Uncertainty Continues? A Brief Review. *Front. Neurol.* **2021**, *12*, 573237. [CrossRef]
30. Brandi, G.; Stocchetti, N.; Pagnamenta, A.; Stretti, F.; Steiger, P.; Klinzing, S. Cerebral Metabolism Is Not Affected by Moderate Hyperventilation in Patients with Traumatic Brain Injury. *Crit. Care* **2019**, *23*, 45. [CrossRef]
31. Gouvea Bogossian, E.; Peluso, L.; Creteur, J.; Taccone, F.S. Hyperventilation in Adult TBI Patients: How to Approach It? *Front. Neurol.* **2021**, *11*, 580859. [CrossRef]
32. Imberti, R.; Bellinzona, G.; Langer, M. Cerebral tissue PO_2 and $SjvO_2$ changes during moderate hyperventilation in patients with severe traumatic brain injury. *J. Neurosurg.* **2002**, *96*, 97–102. [CrossRef]
33. Meyer, N.J.; Gattinoni, L.; Calfee, C.S. Acute Respiratory Distress Syndrome. *Lancet* **2021**, *398*, 622–637. [CrossRef]
34. Cai, G.; Zhang, X.; Ou, Q.; Zhou, Y.; Huang, L.; Chen, S.; Zeng, H.; Jiang, W.; Wen, M. Optimal Targets of the First 24-h Partial Pressure of Carbon Dioxide in Patients with Cerebral Injury: Data from the MIMIC-III and IV Database. *Neurocrit. Care* **2022**, *36*, 412–420. [CrossRef] [PubMed]
35. Papazian, L.; Forel, J.-M.; Gacouin, A.; Penot-Ragon, C.; Perrin, G.; Loundou, A.; Jaber, S.; Arnal, J.-M.; Perez, D.; Seghboyan, J.-M.; et al. Neuromuscular Blockers in Early Acute Respiratory Distress Syndrome. *N. Engl. J. Med.* **2010**, *363*, 1107–1116. [CrossRef]
36. Hsiang, J.K.; Chesnut, R.M.; Crisp, C.B.; Klauber, M.R.; Blunt, B.A.; Marshall, L.F. Early, routine paralysis for intracranial pressure control in severe head injury: Is it necessary? *Crit. Care Med.* **1994**, *22*, 1471–1476. [CrossRef] [PubMed]
37. Murray, M.J.; Deblock, H.; Erstad, B.; Gray, A.; Jacobi, J.; Jordan, C.; McGee, W.; McManus, C.; Meade, M.; Nix, S.; et al. Clinical Practice Guidelines for Sustained Neuromuscular Blockade in the Adult Critically Ill Patient. *Crit. Care Med.* **2016**, *44*, 2079–2103. [CrossRef]
38. Hermans, G.; van den Berghe, G. Clinical Review: Intensive Care Unit Acquired Weakness. *Crit. Care* **2015**, *19*, 274. [CrossRef]
39. Inoue, S.; Hatakeyama, J.; Kondo, Y.; Hifumi, T.; Sakuramoto, H.; Kawasaki, T.; Taito, S.; Nakamura, K.; Unoki, T.; Kawai, Y.; et al. Post-intensive Care Syndrome: Its Pathophysiology, Prevention, and Future Directions. *Acute Med. Surg.* **2019**, *6*, 233–246. [CrossRef]
40. Lee, M.; Kang, J.; Jeong, Y.J. Risk Factors for Post–Intensive Care Syndrome: A Systematic Review and Meta-Analysis. *Aust. Crit. Care* **2020**, *33*, 287–294. [CrossRef]
41. Price, D.R.; Mikkelsen, M.E.; Umscheid, C.A.; Armstrong, E.J. Neuromuscular Blocking Agents and Neuromuscular Dysfunction Acquired in Critical Illness: A Systematic Review and Meta-Analysis. *Crit. Care Med.* **2016**, *44*, 2070–2078. [CrossRef]
42. De Laet, I.; Hoste, E.; Verholen, E.; de Waele, J.J. The Effect of Neuromuscular Blockers in Patients with Intra-Abdominal Hypertension. *Intensive Care Med.* **2007**, *33*, 1811–1814. [CrossRef] [PubMed]
43. Oddo, M.; Crippa, I.A.; Mehta, S.; Menon, D.; Payen, J.F.; Taccone, F.S.; Citerio, G. Optimizing Sedation in Patients with Acute Brain Injury. *Crit. Care* **2016**, *20*, 128. [CrossRef]
44. Mccall, M.; Jeejeebhoy, K.; Pencharz, P.; Moulton, R. Effect of Neuromuscular Blockade on Energy Expenditure in Patients With Severe Head Injury. *J. Parenter. Enteral Nutr.* **2003**, *27*, 27–35. [CrossRef] [PubMed]
45. Rangel-Castilla, L.; Gasco, J.; Nauta, H.J.W.; Okonkwo, D.O.; Robertson, C.S. Cerebral Pressure Autoregulation in Traumatic Brain Injury. *Neurosurg. Focus* **2008**, *25*, E7. [CrossRef] [PubMed]
46. Donnelly, J.; Czosnyka, M.; Adams, H.; Robba, C.; Steiner, L.A.; Cardim, D.; Cabella, B.; Liu, X.; Ercole, A.; Hutchinson, P.J.; et al. Individualizing Thresholds of Cerebral Perfusion Pressure Using Estimated Limits of Autoregulation. *Crit. Care Med.* **2017**, *45*, 1464–1471. [CrossRef]
47. Robba, C.; Cardim, D.; Sekhon, M.; Budohoski, K.; Czosnyka, M. Transcranial Doppler: A Stethoscope for the Brain-Neurocritical Care Use. *J. Neurosci. Res.* **2018**, *96*, 720–730. [CrossRef]
48. Rosenthal, G.; Sanchez-Mejia, R.O.; Phan, N.; Hemphill, J.C.; Martin, C.; Manley, G.T. Incorporating a Parenchymal Thermal Diffusion Cerebral Blood Flow Probe in Bedside Assessment of Cerebral Autoregulation and Vasoreactivity in Patients with Severe Traumatic Brain Injury: Clinical Article. *J. Neurosurg.* **2011**, *114*, 62–70. [CrossRef]

49. Hawryluk, G.W.J.; Rubiano, A.M.; Totten, A.M.; O'Reilly, C.; Ullman, J.S.; Bratton, S.L.; Chesnut, R.; Harris, O.A.; Kissoon, N.; Shutter, L.; et al. Guidelines for the Management of Severe Traumatic Brain Injury: 2020 Update of the Decompressive Craniectomy Recommendations. *Neurosurgery* **2020**, *87*, 427–434. [CrossRef]
50. Lang, E.W.; Chesnut, R.M. A Bedside Method for Investigating the Integrity and Critical Thresholds of Cerebral Pressure Autoregulation in Severe Traumatic Brain Injury Patients. *Br. J. Neurosurg.* **2000**, *14*, 117–126.
51. Annane, D.; Ouanes-Besbes, L.; de Backer, D.; Gordon, A.C.; Hernández, G.; Olsen, K.M.; Osborn, T.M.; Russell, J.A.; Zanotti Cavazzoni, S.; Peake, S.; et al. A Global Perspective on Vasoactive Agents in Shock. *Intensive Care Med.* **2018**, *44*, 833–846. [CrossRef]
52. Depreitere, B.; Citerio, G.; Smith, M.; Adelson, P.D.; Aries, M.J.; Bleck, T.P.; Bouzat, P.; Chesnut, R.; de Sloovere, V.; Diringer, M.; et al. Cerebrovascular Autoregulation Monitoring in the Management of Adult Severe Traumatic Brain Injury: A Delphi Consensus of Clinicians. *Neurocrit. Care* **2021**, *34*, 731–738. [CrossRef] [PubMed]
53. Moerman, A.; de Hert, S. Why and How to Assess Cerebral Autoregulation? *Best Pract. Res. Clin. Anaesthesiol.* **2019**, *33*, 211–220. [CrossRef]
54. Hirst, T.C.; Klasen, M.G.; Rhodes, J.K.; MacLeod, M.R.; Andrews, P.J.D. A Systematic Review and Meta-Analysis of Hypothermia in Experimental Traumatic Brain Injury: Why Have Promising Animal Studies Not Been Replicated in Pragmatic Clinical Trials? *J. Neurotrauma* **2020**, *37*, 2057–2068. [CrossRef]
55. Ceulemans, A.G.; Zgavc, T.; Kooijman, R.; Hachimi-Idrissi, S.; Sarre, S.; Michotte, Y. The Dual Role of the Neuroinflammatory Response after Ischemic Stroke: Modulatory Effects of Hypothermia. *J. Neuroinflamm.* **2010**, *7*, 74. [CrossRef]
56. Zhu, Y.; Yin, H.; Zhang, R.; Ye, X.; Wei, J. Therapeutic Hypothermia versus Normothermia in Adult Patients with Traumatic Brain Injury: A Meta-Analysis. *Springerplus* **2016**, *5*, 801. [CrossRef]
57. Andrews, P.J.D.; Sinclair, H.L.; Rodriguez, A.; Harris, B.A.; Battison, C.G.; Rhodes, J.K.J.; Murray, G.D. Hypothermia for Intracranial Hypertension after Traumatic Brain Injury. *N. Engl. J. Med.* **2015**, *373*, 2403–2412. [CrossRef]
58. Cooper, D.J.; Nichol, A.D.; Bailey, M.; Bernard, S.; Cameron, P.A.; Pili-Floury, S.; Forbes, A.; Gantner, D.; Higgins, A.M.; Huet, O.; et al. Effect of Early Sustained Prophylactic Hypothermia on Neurologic Outcomes among Patients with Severe Traumatic Brain Injury. *JAMA-J. Am. Med. Assoc.* **2018**, *320*, 2211–2220. [CrossRef]
59. Polderman, K.H. Application of Therapeutic Hypothermia in the Intensive Care Unit: Opportunities and Pitfalls of a Promising Treatment Modality-Part 2: Practical Aspects and Side Effects. *Intensive Care Med.* **2004**, *30*, 757–769. [CrossRef]
60. Rubiano, A.M.; Sanchez, A.I.; Estebanez, G.; Peitzman, A.; Sperry, J.; Puyana, J.C. The Effect of Admission Spontaneous Hypothermia on Patients with Severe Traumatic Brain Injury. *Injury* **2013**, *44*, 1219–1225. [CrossRef]
61. Zwerus, R.; Absalom, A. Update on Anesthetic Neuroprotection. *Curr. Opin. Anaesthesiol.* **2015**, *28*, 424–430. [CrossRef]
62. Almaas, R.; Saugstad, O.D.; Pleasure, D.; Rootwelt, T. Effect of Barbiturates on Hydroxyl Radicals, Lipid Peroxidation, and Hypoxic Cell Death in Human NT2-N Neurons. *Anesthesiology* **2000**, *92*, 764–774. [CrossRef]
63. Léger, M.; Frasca, D.; Roquilly, A.; Seguin, P.; Cinotti, R.; Dahyot-Fizelier, C.; Asehnoune, K.; le Borgne, F.; Gaillard, T.; Foucher, Y.; et al. Early Use of Barbiturates Is Associated with Increased Mortality in Traumatic Brain Injury Patients from a Propensity Score-Based Analysis of a Prospective Cohort. *PLoS ONE* **2022**, *17*, e0268013. [CrossRef]
64. Majdan, M.; Mauritz, W.; Wilbacher, I.; Brazinova, A.; Rusnak, M.; Leitgeb, J. Barbiturates Use and Its Effects in Patients with Severe Traumatic Brain Injury in Five European Countries. *J. Neurotrauma* **2013**, *30*, 23–29. [CrossRef] [PubMed]
65. Roberts, I.; Sydenham, E. Barbiturates for Acute Traumatic Brain Injury. *Cochrane Database Syst. Rev.* **2012**, *2012*, CD000033. [CrossRef]
66. Cairns, C.J.; Thomas, B.; Fletcher, S.; Parr, M.J.; Finfer, S.R. Life-Threatening Hyperkalaemia Following Therapeutic Barbiturate Coma. *Intensive Care Med.* **2002**, *28*, 1357–1360. [CrossRef]
67. Aytuluk, H.G.; Topcu, H. Severe Hypokalemia and Rebound Hyperkalemia during Barbiturate Coma in Patients with Severe Traumatic Brain Injury. *Neurocirugia* **2020**, *31*, 216–222. [CrossRef]
68. Stover, J.F.; Stocker, R. PHARMACODYNAMICS Barbiturate Coma May Promote Reversible Bone Marrow Suppression in Patients with Severe Isolated Traumatic Brain Injury. *Eur. J. Clin. Pharmacol.* **1998**, *54*, 529–534. [CrossRef]
69. Stover, J.F.; Lenzlinger, P.M.; Stocker, R.; Morganti-Kossmann, M.C.; Imhof, H.G.; Trentz, O.; Kossmann, T. Thiopental in CSF and Serum Correlates with Prolonged Loss of Cortical Activity. *Eur. Neurol.* **1998**, *39*, 223–228. [CrossRef]
70. Wheeler, D.W.; Thompson, A.J.; Corletto, F.; Reckless, J.; Loke, J.C.T.; Lapaque, N.; Grant, A.J.; Mastroeni, P.; Grainger, D.J.; Padgett, C.L.; et al. Anaesthetic Impairment of Immune Function Is Mediated via GABAA Receptors. *PLoS ONE* **2011**, *6*, e17152. [CrossRef]
71. Loop, T.; Humar, M.; Pischke, S.; Hoetzel, A.; Schmidt, R.; Pahl, H.L.; Geiger, K.K.; Pannen, B.H.J. Thiopental Inhibits Tumor Necrosis Factor-Induced Activation of Nuclear Factor B through Suppression of IB Kinase Activity. *Anesthesiology* **2003**, *99*, 360–367. [CrossRef]
72. Andrefsky, J.C.; Frank, J.I.; Chyatte, D. The ciliospinal reflex in pentobarbital coma. *J. Neurosurg.* **1999**, *90*, 644–646. [CrossRef]
73. Ellington, A.L. Electroencephalographic pattern of burst suppression in a case of barbiturate coma. *Electroencephalogr. Clin. Neurophysiol.* **1968**, *25*, 491–493. [CrossRef]
74. Zeiler, F.A.; Akoth, E.; Gillman, L.M.; West, M. Burst Suppression for ICP Control: A Systematic Review. *J. Intensive Care Med.* **2017**, *32*, 130–139. [CrossRef] [PubMed]

75. Wechsler, R.L.; Dripps, R.D.; Kety, S.S. Blood flow and oxygen consumption of the human brain during anesthesia produced by thiopental. *Anesthesiology* **1951**, *12*, 308–314. [CrossRef] [PubMed]
76. Hemphill, S.; McMenamin, L.; Bellamy, M.C.; Hopkins, P.M. Propofol Infusion Syndrome: A Structured Literature Review and Analysis of Published Case Reports. *Br. J. Anaesth.* **2019**, *122*, 448–459. [CrossRef]
77. Cooper, D.J.; Rosenfeld, J.V.; Murray, L.; Arabi, Y.M.; Davies, A.R.; D'Urso, P.; Kossmann, T.; Ponsford, J.; Seppelt, I.; Reilly, P.; et al. Decompressive Craniectomy in Diffuse Traumatic Brain Injury. *N. Engl. J. Med.* **2011**, *364*, 1493–1502. [CrossRef]
78. Hutchinson, P.J.; Kolias, A.G.; Timofeev, I.S.; Corteen, E.A.; Czosnyka, M.; Timothy, J.; Anderson, I.; Bulters, D.O.; Belli, A.; Eynon, C.A.; et al. Trial of Decompressive Craniectomy for Traumatic Intracranial Hypertension. *N. Engl. J. Med.* **2016**, *375*, 1119–1130. [CrossRef]
79. Hutchinson, P.J.; Kolias, A.G.; Tajsic, T.; Adeleye, A.; Aklilu, A.T.; Apriawan, T.; Bajamal, A.H.; Barthélemy, E.J.; Devi, B.I.; Bhat, D.; et al. Consensus Statement from the International Consensus Meeting on the Role of Decompressive Craniectomy in the Management of Traumatic Brain Injury: Consensus Statement. *Acta Neurochir.* **2019**, *161*, 1261–1274. [CrossRef]
80. Hartings, J.A.; Vidgeon, S.; Strong, A.J.; Zacko, C.; Vagal, A.; Andaluz, N.; Ridder, T.; Stanger, R.; Fabricius, M.; Mathern, B.; et al. Surgical Management of Traumatic Brain Injury: A Comparative-Effectiveness Study of 2 Centers: Clinical Article. *J. Neurosurg.* **2014**, *120*, 434–446. [CrossRef]
81. Li, L.M.; Kolias, A.G.; Guilfoyle, M.R.; Timofeev, I.; Corteen, E.A.; Pickard, J.D.; Menon, D.K.; Kirkpatrick, P.J.; Hutchinson, P.J. Outcome Following Evacuation of Acute Subdural Haematomas: A Comparison of Craniotomy with Decompressive Craniectomy. *Acta Neurochir.* **2012**, *154*, 1555–1561. [CrossRef]
82. Kolias, A.G.; Adams, H.; Timofeev, I.; Czosnyka, M.; Corteen, E.A.; Pickard, J.D.; Turner, C.; Gregson, B.A.; Kirkpatrick, P.J.; Murray, G.D.; et al. Decompressive Craniectomy Following Traumatic Brain Injury: Developing the Evidence Base. *Br. J. Neurosurg.* **2016**, *30*, 246–250. [CrossRef] [PubMed]
83. Chesnut, R.M.; Temkin, N.; Carney, N.; Dikmen, S.; Rondina, C.; Videtta, W.; Petroni, G.; Lujan, S.; Pridgeon, J.; Barber, J.; et al. A Trial of Intracranial-Pressure Monitoring in Traumatic Brain Injury. *N. Engl. J. Med.* **2012**, *367*, 2471–2481. [CrossRef] [PubMed]
84. Chesnut, R.M.; Temkin, N.; Dikmen, S.; Rondina, C.; Videtta, W.; Petroni, G.; Lujan, S.; Alanis, V.; Falcao, A.; de La Fuenta, G.; et al. A Method of Managing Severe Traumatic Brain Injury in the Absence of Intracranial Pressure Monitoring: The Imaging and Clinical Examination Protocol. *J. Neurotrauma* **2018**, *35*, 54–63. [CrossRef]
85. Kolias, A.G.; Viaroli, E.; Rubiano, A.M.; Adams, H.; Khan, T.; Gupta, D.; Adeleye, A.; Iaccarino, C.; Servadei, F.; Devi, B.I.; et al. The Current Status of Decompressive Craniectomy in Traumatic Brain Injury. *Curr. Trauma Rep.* **2018**, *4*, 326–332. [CrossRef]

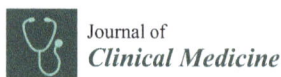

Review

Fungal Infections in Critically Ill COVID-19 Patients: Inevitabile Malum

Nikoletta Rovina *, Evangelia Koukaki, Vasiliki Romanou, Sevasti Ampelioti, Konstantinos Loverdos, Vasiliki Chantziara, Antonia Koutsoukou and George Dimopoulos

1st Department of Respiratory Medicine, Medical School, National and Kapodistrian University of Athens and "Sotiria" Chest Disease Hospital, 152 Mesogeion Ave, 11527 Athens, Greece; e.koukaki@yahoo.gr (E.K.); vassoromanou@gmail.com (V.R.); sevi.ampelioti@gmail.com (S.A.); kloverdos@yahoo.com (K.L.); vchantziara@yahoo.gr (V.C.); koutsoukou@yahoo.gr (A.K.); gdimop@med.uoa.gr (G.D.)
* Correspondence: nikrovina@med.uoa.gr; Tel.: +30-210-7763650

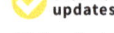

Citation: Rovina, N.; Koukaki, E.; Romanou, V.; Ampelioti, S.; Loverdos, K.; Chantziara, V.; Koutsoukou, A.; Dimopoulos, G. Fungal Infections in Critically Ill COVID-19 Patients: Inevitabile Malum. *J. Clin. Med.* **2022**, *11*, 2017. https://doi.org/10.3390/jcm11072017

Academic Editor: Spyros D. Mentzelopoulos

Received: 10 March 2022
Accepted: 31 March 2022
Published: 4 April 2022

Publisher's Note: MDPI stays neutral with regard to jurisdictional claims in published maps and institutional affiliations.

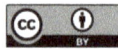

Copyright: © 2022 by the authors. Licensee MDPI, Basel, Switzerland. This article is an open access article distributed under the terms and conditions of the Creative Commons Attribution (CC BY) license (https://creativecommons.org/licenses/by/4.0/).

Abstract: Patients with severe COVID-19 belong to a population at high risk of invasive fungal infections (IFIs), with a reported incidence of IFIs in critically ill COVID-19 patients ranging between 5% and 26.7%. Common factors in these patients, such as multiple organ failure, immunomodulating/immunocompromising treatments, the longer time on mechanical ventilation, renal replacement therapy or extracorporeal membrane oxygenation, make them vulnerable candidates for fungal infections. In addition to that, SARS-CoV2 itself is associated with significant dysfunction in the patient's immune system involving both innate and acquired immunity, with reduction in both $CD4^+$ T and $CD8^+$ T lymphocyte counts and cytokine storm. The emerging question is whether SARS-CoV-2 inherently predisposes critically ill patients to fungal infections or the immunosuppressive therapy constitutes the igniting factor for invasive mycoses. To approach the dilemma, one must consider the unique pathogenicity of SARS-CoV-2 with the deranged immune response it provokes, review the well-known effects of immunosuppressants and finally refer to current literature to probe possible causal relationships, synergistic effects or independent risk factors. In this review, we aimed to identify the prevalence, risk factors and mortality associated with IFIs in mechanically ventilated patients with COVID-19.

Keywords: fungal infections; critically ill; CAPA; COVID-19; CAM; CAC

1. Introduction

COVID-19, caused by SARS-CoV2, made its appearance at the end of 2019 in Wuhan (China) and rapidly spread worldwide, evolving to an emergency global public health event. This is justified by the fact that, to date, over 250 million people have been infected worldwide, and more than 5 million have died [1]. By the beginning of March 2020, the World Health Organization (WHO) officially labeled the disease as a pandemic [2]. The disease has a wide range of symptoms; patients may present asymptomatic, with mild symptoms such as fever and cough or worse, such as severe cases developing dyspnea and hypoxia [3,4]. Like in severe acute respiratory syndrome coronavirus (SARS-CoV) and Middle East respiratory syndrome (MERS), SARS-CoV2 may induce a hyper-inflammatory response (cytokine storm) and a pneumonia complicated by Acute Respiratory Distress Syndrome (ARDS), severe alveolar damage and inflammatory exudation [5,6].

In COVID-19, primary coinfections are rare [7,8]; however, critically ill patients (which represent around 20% of all patients) and especially those who are finally admitted to the Intensive Care Unit (ICU) (around 5%) are more vulnerable to develop secondary infections on the basis of multiple organ failure, prolonged time on mechanical ventilation and dependence on renal replacement therapy or extracorporeal membrane oxygenation [9,10]. In addition, SARS-CoV2 itself is associated with significant dysfunction in the patient's immune system involving both innate and acquired immunity, with reduction in both

CD4$^+$ T and CD8$^+$ T lymphocyte counts. A cytokine storm takes place, which is characterized by excessively increased pro-inflammatory molecules, inhibition of natural killer cells and cytotoxic lymphocytes [11,12]. On this ground, secondary infections as a complication of viral respiratory diseases are not uncommon, and they have been described in previous pandemics.

Infections in these patients need to be identified early because they affect the management, and more significantly, the outcome. Fungal infections are especially associated with a higher mortality rate in critically ill patients admitted to the ICU, raising a considerable concern about invasive fungal infections in COVID-19 patients. Interestingly, in an Italian ICU, the incidence of secondary blood stream infections (BSIs) in COVID-19 patients was almost 20 times higher than the incidence reported in European ICUs in non COVID-19 patients [13]. According to authors, this finding could be attributed to factors such as the dysregulated immune system in severe COVID-19, the extensive use of antimicrobials in these patients, as well as, the worse adherence to the infection control and prevention measures due to the overwhelming pandemic wave in Italy at that time.

In this review, we provide an up to date insight on the epidemiology and the risk factors for invasive fungal infections, as well as, the current view on the potential role of drugs which modulate and/or compromise immune response in increasing the prevalence of fungal co-infections in critically ill COVID-19 patients.

2. Pathophysiology and Risk Factors

The emergence of fungal co-infections in COVID-19 patients is not that unexpected considering the MERS and SARS outbreaks [14]. The variety of fungal co-infections (most commonly pulmonary or tracheobronchial aspergillosis—CAPA, CAC and CAM) and their relatively high incidence, as described above, especially in critically ill patients, have posed questions on what the underlying pathogenetic mechanisms are of such an occurrence and whether any risk factors could be identified [15].

The SARS-CoV2 spike protein binds to angiotensin converting enzyme 2 (ACE2) receptor of epithelial cells and type 2 pneumocytes, thus allowing viral entry. The release of danger-associated molecular patterns (DAMPs) by dying or damaged cells ignites an immune response and a cascade of inflammation, which in turn leads to tissue damage [16–18]. This extensive lung damage may lead to higher vulnerability to invasive fungal infections such as pulmonary aspergillosis [14]. DAMPs have been implicated in the regulation of inflammation of fungal diseases, and host inflammation may favor the transition of fungal colonization to fungal infection [19]. This could explain in part why patients with hyperinflammatory response (such as COVID-19 critically ill patients) are more vulnerable to fungal infections, Figure 1.

On the other side of the immunologic spectrum, COVID-19 interferes toward impaired local immune response, dysfunctional mucociliary activity and disruption of epithelial barriers [17,20]. In the case of *Aspergillus*, conidia in the airways are cleared poorly, enabling bronchial inflammation and invasion and possibly leading to CAPA [20]. The high prevalence of CAPA but with low blood galactomannan detection may indicate less frequent angioinvasion compared to usual invasive aspergillosis and maybe local disease [21]. Lymphopenia—also a common lab characteristic of COVID-19 infection—and, consequently, possibly T-cell lymphocyte population decline may lead to a favorable environment for invasive fungal infections [16]. The effect of immunomodulation is under debate, and it will be discussed separately.

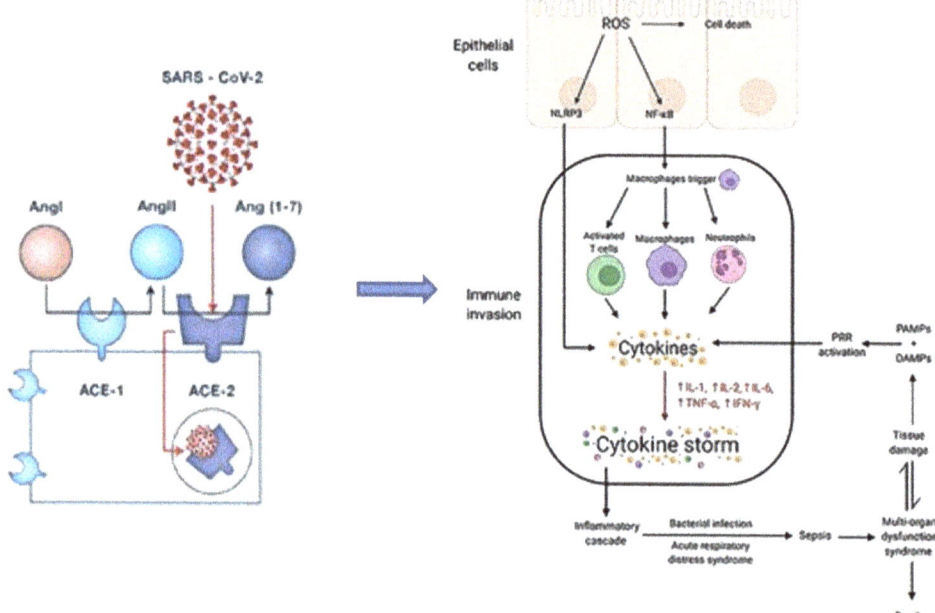

Figure 1. SARS-CoV2 spike protein binds to angiotensin converting enzyme 2 (ACE2) receptor of epithelial cells and type 2 pneumocytes, thus allowing viral entry. The release of danger-associated molecular patterns (DAMPs) by dying or damaged cells ignites an immune response and a cascade of inflammation, which in turn leads to tissue damage. This extensive lung damage may lead to higher vulnerability to invasive fungal infections.

In general, it could be hypothesized that the high incidence of aspergillosis and candidemia in COVID-19 patients could be related to high rates of invasive procedures, such as intubation, which may predispose to fungal colonization and proliferation; prolonged/high corticosteroid or other immunomodulatory treatment regimens; underlying (or developing due to COVID-19) pulmonary disease; dysregulation of the immunity caused by COVID-19; and empiric antimicrobial therapy changing the flora/microbiota of the respiratory tract [14,17].

The risk factors can be divided into the following categories.

2.1. Host Factors

Initially, for patients with severe COVID-19, it could be hypothesized that increased fungal co-infections correspond to an increased prevalence of pre-existing risk factors for fungal infections (as they are defined by European Organization for Research and Treatment of Cancer and the Mycoses Study Group Education and Research Consortium—EORTC/MSGERC) [15]. However, it seems that only a minority of patients have such risk factors [14,21]. Even though, in general, critically ill patients with COVID-19 are usually older or have more comorbidities, a strong correlation with specific characteristics that might predispose to vulnerability to fungal infections (e.g., disease, gender) has not been documented [14,17]. Structural lung diseases might be of importance for the development of CAPA [14,16], as some studies identify a higher incidence in patients with COPD or asthma [22]. In addition, in India, diabetes and diabetic ketoacidosis have been correlated with increased likelihood of mucormycosis in COVID-19 patients, but not in patients with CAPA [14,21]. Finally, from a small series in Hungary, patients with CAPA seemed to be preferably older males and in need of oxygen support, suggesting that critical illness might be a risk factor [23].

2.2. Healthcare Associated Factors

As with other medical reasons, admission to hospital or ICU increases the incidence of infections. Mechanical ventilation/intubation, ICU length of stay and presence of indwelling catheters have been implicated in the emergence of secondary infections in ICU patients. In addition, empiric antibiotic treatment may shift the microbiota towards increased prevalence of fungal species. In literature, fungal infections seem to be correlated with hospital admission and intubation [17], even though CAPA has been described in patients with various respiratory support [22], such as invasive or non-invasive ventilation. There is also a correlation of length of ICU stay with the development of CAPA [22]. Although renal failure seems not to be a risk factor, renal replacement therapy seems to be associated with the development of fungal infections, such as CAPA, in critically ill COVID-19 patients [22]. To our knowledge, there are no case reports for outpatients with COVID-19 CAPA or CAC.

There is a debate in the literature on whether corticosteroids favor fungal infections or not [21], and this will be discussed further, separately. It is a fact that critically ill patients may have more risk factors independent of COVID-19 that may confound the correlations. Table 1.

Table 1. Risk factors for fungal infections.

CAPA/Invasive *Aspergillus* Tracheobronchitis
1. High/long dose of corticosteroids; 2. Underlying structural lung disease; 3. Host factors, such as neutropenia, allogeneic stem cell transplant, immunosuppression, inherited severe immunodeficiency; 4. Intubation and mechanical ventilation; 5. Cancer/chemotherapy; 6. Azithromycin (PMID: 33316401)/broad spectrum antibiotics; 7. Severe lung damage due to COVID-19.
CAC
1. Prolonged hospital stay; 2. Mechanical ventilation; 3. Central venous catheters; 4. Surgical procedures; 5. Broad-spectrum antibiotics.
MAC
1. Diabetes, diabetic ketoacidosis

CAPA: COVID-19-associated pulmonary aspergillosis; CAC: COVID-19-associated candidemia; MAC: Mycobacterium Avium Complex.

3. Prevalence of Invasive Fungal Infections in Critically Ill COVID-19 Patients

The reported incidence of invasive fungal infections in critically ill COVID-19 patients ranges between 5% and 26.7% [24–31]. Fekkar et al. found an overall incidence of fungal respiratory complications at 4.8% [24]. Chong et al., in their review of 49 studies on secondary pulmonary infections in COVID-19 cases, noted a 6.4% incidence of fungal infections [25]. In a descriptive study of 99 COVID-19 patients, Chen et al. reported fungal co-infections in 5% of the patients [26]. Moreover, among 52 critically ill patients, Yang et al. noted 3 (5.8%) with fungal infections [27], while Musuuza et al. in their meta-analysis reported a pooled prevalence of fungal co-infections in 4% and fungal superinfections in 8% [28]. Furthermore, in a retrospective study of 140 ICU patients, Bardi et al. reported fungal infections in 15% of them [29]. In this line, White et al. reported a far higher prevalence of 26.7% of invasive fungal infections in critically ill COVID-19 patients [30]. On the other hand, in a meta-analysis of 426 COVID-19 patients who were admitted to the ICU, the overall pooled proportion of fungal co-infection was 0.12 [31] (Table 2).

3.1. Candidiasis

The risk of invasive candidiasis is high in patients receiving antibacterials, hemodialysis, parenteral nutrition, undergoing mechanical ventilation and having central venous catheters. All these factors are common in the COVID-19 critical-care patient [32,33]. COVID-19-associated candidiasis (CAC) mostly presents as candidaemia, with *Candida albicans* and *Candida glabrata* being the most frequent pathogens. Candidemia in COVID-19 patients has been increasingly described in the literature. In a US hospital, among patients with COVID-19 admitted to the ICU, 8.9% developed candidemia [34]. A single-hospital study in Brazil reported candidemia incidence during the pandemic to be nearly five times higher than before the pandemic [35]. Seagle et al. studied 251 patients with candidemia, of which 25.5% were positive for SARS-CoV2 [36]. Outbreaks of the multidrug-resistant *Candida auris* have also been reported [37] (Table 2).

3.2. Aspergillosis

Back from 2018, Schauwvlieghe et al. developed the modified AspICU criteria to help diagnose influenza associated pulmonary aspergillosis (IAPA), which (in the absence of histology) essentially relies on mycological evidence of *Aspergillus* spp. in the form of a positive bronchoalveolar lavage (BAL) culture or positive galactomannan in serum/BAL [38]. In a retrospective observational study of critically ill COVID-19 patients, although the rate of fungal antigenemia was high (around 50%), *Aspergillus* was not identified in any specimens by culturing. This was associated with the prophylactic antifungal therapy the patients were receiving [39]. Despite differences in the pathogenicity of COVID-19 and influenza, obviously a similar manifestation appeared in the critically ill COVID-19 patients. Not long ago, a panel of experts proposed criteria for a new clinical entity called CAPA (COVID-19-Associated Pulmonary Aspergillosis), a superinfection with high incidence and high mortality. In Koehler et al.'s study of 94 cases, the overall incidence was 22.6% [40]. Studies in France [16,41] identified a similar incidence of CAPA (30%). However, other studies showed lower incidence and variation in prevalence, indicating that further investigation is needed [42] (Table 2).

3.3. Mucormycosis

Another significant complication of COVID-19 infection is COVID-19 associated mucormycosis (CAM), mostly in patients with uncontrolled diabetes mellitus or in geographical regions with higher incidences of mucormycosis (e.g., India) [43]. CAM includes patients with acute invasive fungal rhino-orbital mucormycosis, or cavitary pulmonary mucormycosis [44,45]. Meawed et al. isolated Mucor in 8.2% of 197 critically ill COVID-19 patients under mechanical ventilation who developed VAP [46]. Selarka et al., in India, characterized mucormycosis in patients with COVID-19 as an epidemic within a pandemic, as from the 2567 COVID-19 patients admitted to 3 tertiary centers, 47 (1.8%) were diagnosed with mucormycosis [47] (Table 2).

3.4. Pneumocystis

Pneumonocystis jirovencii infections have been reported in low numbers and mainly in patients with other underlying conditions (e.g., HIV, hematologic malignancy) [48]. COVID-19 and *Pneumocystis* share numerous overlapping characteristics, such as radiological, clinical and laboratory findings. As a result, there is a great possibility of misdiagnosis [49]. Alanio et al. studied samples from 108 HIV-negative COVID-19 patients. *P. jirovencii* was postitive in 9.3% [50] of the patients. Blaize et al. also explored the incidence of *Pneumocystis* in pulmonary specimens obtained from severe COVID-19 patients and found it around 1.4% [51]. In March 2021, the first case of *Pneumocystis* confirmed through autopsy was published in a 52-year-old male, who was diagnosed with COVID-19 posthumously [52].

Other rare invasive fungal diseases that have been diagnosed in COVID-19 patients, include *Rhodotorula fungaemia*, *Fusarium* and *Trichosporon* infections [53,54]. *Cryptococcus* should be considered in high-risk patients [55]. Endemic fungal species such as *Histoplasma*, *Coccidioides* or *Blastomyces* should be considered in specific geographical areas (Table 2).

Table 2. Prevalence of Invasive Fungal Infections in critically ill COVID-19 patients.

Literature	Trial Design/Population	Type of IFI	Incidence
Fekkar A. et al. [24]	R, SC, n = 145 COVID-19 ICU MV pts screened for fungal superinfection; 54% on ECMO	prob/putat IFI (1 *Fusarium* case)	4.8%
Chong W.H. et al. [25]	Literature review; 28 O studies, 21 cr/s	Secondary FI	6.4%
Chen N. et al. [26]	R, SC, 99 hospital pts	Secondary FI	5%
Yang X. et al. [27]	R, SC, O, 52 ICU pts		5.8%
Musuuza J.S. et al. [28]	MA of 118 studies	Fungal co- and superinfections	4% and 8%, respect
Bardi T. et al. [29]	R, SC, 140 ICU pts	FI	15%
White et al. [30]	MC, P, 137 ICU pts screened for IFI	IFI	26.7%
Peng J. et al. [31]	SRMA of 9 studies	IFI	0.12 (opp)
Bishburg E. et al. [34]	SC, R, 89 COVID-19 ICU pts	CAC	8.9%
Nucci M. et al. [35]	SC	CAC	×5 comp to prepandemic
Seagle E.E. et al. [36]	Surveillance data	candidemia	Among 251 candidemia pts, 25.5% were SARS-CoV-2
Gouzien L. et al. [42]	R, O, COVID-19 ICU pts	CAPA	1.5%
Hoenigl M. et al. [43]	Review of 80 CAM cases	CAM	0.3–0.8% prevalence in COVID-19 ICU pts
Meawed T.E. et al. [46]	Cross-sectional study of 197 critically-ill MV COVID-19 pts	Fungal VAP	16.4% *Aspergillus* 8.2% mucor
Selarka L. et al. [47]	P, O, MC	CAM	1.8%
Alanio et al. [50]	O, 108 critically-ill COVID-19 pts	PJP	9.3%
Blaize et al. [51]	PCR assays on severe COVID-19 pts	PJP	1.4%

CAC: COVID-19-associated candidemia, CAM: COVID-19-associated mucormycosis, CAPA: COVID-19-associated pulmonary aspergillosis, Comp to: compared to, Cr/s: case reports/series, (I)FI: (Invasive) fungal infection, MA: metanalysis, MC: multicenter, MV: mechanically ventilated, O: observational, opp: overall pooled proportion, P: prospective, prob: probable, pts: patients, put: putative, R: retrospective, respect: respectively, SC: single center, SRMA: Systematic review and metanalysis.

4. Immunosuppressive Therapy as Risk Factor for Fungal Infections in Critically Ill COVID-19 Patients

The emerging question is whether SARS-CoV-2 inherently predisposes to fungal infections in the critically ill patients or the immunosuppressive therapy constitutes the igniting factor for invasive mycoses. To approach the dilemma, one must consider the unique pathogenicity of SARS-CoV-2 with the deranged immune response it provokes, review the well-known effects of immunosuppressants and finally refer to current literature to probe possible causal relationships, synergistic effects or independent risk factors.

As mentioned above, SARS-CoV-2 binds to ACE2 receptors and invades the respiratory epithelium causing mucociliary clearance dysfunction and extensive disruption in mucosal integrity. Moreover, in severely ill patients, the immune response to SARS-CoV-2 is totally dysregulated with defective monocytes and neutrophils, diminished IFN I and III production [56] and a DAMP-driven [57] explosive release of pro-inflammatory cytokines (IL-6, IL-1, IL-2, TNF, MCPI) that further damage the lung [58,59], Figure 1. In addition, the adaptive immunity dysfunction is expressed with lymphocytopenia, which correlates with COVID-19 severity, CD8$^+$ and CD4$^+$ exhaustion and alterations in Th1 and Th2 responses [60,61].

Current treatment guidelines for critically ill COVID-19 patients target the immune aberration and cytokine storm with corticosteroids and other immunomodulators, such as tocilizumab, Janus kinase (baricitinib) and anakinra [62–64]. Glucocorticosteroids (GCS) interfere with virtually total human immunome through transcriptional changes after binding to their intracellular receptors [65]. High doses and long-term use of corticosteroids are known to predispose to bacterial and fungal infections [66]. Tocilizumab, a humanized monoclonal antibody against soluble and membrane IL-6 receptors, used since the mid-1990s in rheumatoid arthritis patients is implicated in a small but significant increase in the risk of infection [67], especially of the respiratory system via the inhibition of Th17 proliferation [68].

All in all, anatomical disruption and immune impairment by SARS-CoV-2 itself together with immunomodulatory therapeutic modalities compose the perfect environment allowing fungi to become invasive [31,69]. Molds and yeasts rarely become pathogenic in immunocompetent hosts. They mostly behave as opportunistic agents [70]. GCS increase susceptibility to invasive aspergillosis by inhibiting macrophage from phagocytosing molds, which in turn germinate quickly into hyphae [71]. IFN type I defects, PMN dysfunction and lymphopenia leave *Aspergillus* uncontrolled to invade damaged respiratory epithelium and cause tracheobronchitis [60,72]. Additional in vitro experiments show that *A. fumigatus* and *A. flavus* thrive in GCS-rich environments [73]. Yeast infections, such as candidaemia—a mostly healthcare-associated infection—are also favored by GCS effects on TNFa, monocytes, macrophages, PMNs and T-lymphocytes [74–77] and possibly by the decreased expression of human leukocyte antigen DR on the membrane of circulating monocytes [61]. Similarly, GCS are implicated in zygomycosis possibly through phagocyte dysfunction and hyperglycaemia [78,79]. GCS, albeit indispensable in treating *Pneumocystis Jirovecii* pneumonia (PJP) with hypoxemia, constitute a well-recognized risk factor for PJP manifestation, especially during GCS tapering [80,81].

4.1. Glucocorticosteroids

Moreover, in the critical care setting, GCS treatment consists of a common predisposing factor for invasive pulmonary Aspergillosis (IPA), as is shown by several observational studies. In a US cohort, 77% of IPA ICU patients received steroids [82]. In the Spanish ICU cohort by Garnacho-Montero et al. [83], steroid treatment (prednisone 20 mg equivalent dose for 3 weeks) was a major predisposing factor for *Aspergillus* colonization and infection. In the ICU special environment, several other factors apart from GCS use predispose to yeast infections: total parenteral nutrition, antibiotic use, intravascular catheters, acute kidney injury, renal replacement therapy, heart disease, mechanical ventilation, prior septic shock, other immunosuppressive medication and underlying comorbidities, such as COPD and diabetes [84,85]. Interestingly, gene polymorphism in ICU population may further increase fungal susceptibility [81,86].

In the COVID-19 era, multiple studies, mostly small, retrospective and observational, highlight an association between GCS and COVID associated Pulmonary Aspergillosis (CAPA) [87–91]. White et al. [30] in one of the largest trials from the UK with prospective screening of 135 PCR-confirmed COVID-19 patients for invasive fungal disease concluded that GCS increased the likelihood of aspergillosis in COVID-19 patients. They implied that negative events in GCS-treated patients could be potentially attributable to CAPA rather than COVID-19 and urged for active surveillance for aspergillosis. Delliere et al. [92], in their French cohort of COVID-19 ICU patients who deteriorated clinically, highlighted a trend with high dose dexamethasone and invasive aspergillosis (11.5 vs. 28.6%, $p = 0.08$, cumulative dose of dexamethasone $\geq$100 mg OR 3.7, 95% CI 1.0–9.7). The association did not reach significance, probably because of insufficient statistical power. Fekkar et al. [24], in their multicenter trial, emphasized a low incidence of fungal respiratory complications (4.8%) in a population of COVID-19 ICU patients who received GCS less often (16.7%)

than in other series. In the multivariate model analysis, GCS were related to invasive pulmonary mold infection (OR 8.55; IQR 6.8–10.3; p = 0.01). It is important to note that this correlation referred to GCS received in dose >0.3 mg/kg/day, for >6 weeks, before COVID-19 diagnosis for underlying disease. No patient on GCS, mostly dexamethasone 20 mg/d for 10 days, for COVID-19 developed invasive mycosis. Marr et al. [20] noted that GCS, systemic or inhalational, were the most common immunosuppressive agent among their 20 patients with CAPA. Of note, Meijer et al. [93] compared the incidence of invasive aspergillosis between the first and second wave and correlated the increased incidence of CAPA to the universal introduction of GCS. The significant decrease in the rates of patients needing mechanical ventilation in the second wave (p < 0.01) was counterbalanced by a higher percentage of CAPA diagnoses (24.2% vs. 15.2%, second and first wave, respectively, p = 0.36). All CAPA patients in their single center series had received dexamethasone. Similarly, Fortarezza et al. [94] published autopsy results from 45 confirmed COVID-19 pts with unusual clinical course; 20% proved to have CAPA (20%). Interestingly, most were patients from the second wave, when GCS were mainstay of treatment.

In the context of Candida infections in COVID-19 patients, Obata et al. [95] in their retrospective chart review of COVID-19 patients compared the incidence of secondary infections between patients who received GCS and those who did not and found a statistically significant increase in fungal infections in patients receiving GCS (12.7% vs. 0.7%, p < 0.001). No *Candida* infections vs. 7% incidence were noted among the no-GCS and GCS arms, respectively. In the Brazilian multicenter cohort by Riche et al. [96], comparison between candidemia rates in patients with COVID-19 and non-COVID-19 patients revealed a 10-fold increase in the former group, mainly in those hospitalized in the ICU. Of note, all cases of COVID-related candidemia had received high dose GCS for severe COVID-19. A very well-structured comparison of candidemia in COVID-19 and non-COVID-19 patients [36] found that systemic GCS administration was twice that of non-COVID-19 patients before *Candida* diagnosis. Their data showed that candidemia in patients with COVID-19 appears later than in non-COVID-19 patients, which made them deduce that healthcare practices associated with severe COVID-19, such as immunomodulating treatments, are likely major contributors to candidemia. Steroid use, among others, was mentioned as a risk factor for *Candida auris* bloodstream infection in certain case series [97].

On the contrary, Ho et al. [98] in their multicenter study show similar rates of blood culture positivity for *Candida* in hospitalized COVID-19 patients between GCS and no-GCS groups. Rutsaert et al. observed high incidence of CAPA despite the absence of systemic corticosteroid use [99]. Van Biesen [100] noted a 22% incidence of CAPA in patients not exposed to GCS. Likewise, Wang et al. [101] in their early study showed that treatment with GCS was not an independent risk factor for IPA in COVID-19 ICU patients, as opposed to older age, initial antibiotic usage of β-lactamase inhibitor combination, mechanical ventilation and COPD. Comparably, Janssen et al., in their multinational observational study [102], did not find a correlation between GCS and CAPA.

Concerning infections by *Zygomycetes* in COVID-19 patients, (COVID-19-Associated Mucormycosis, CAM), the cohorts come mainly from the Indian sub-continent. Patel et al. point out that 32.6% of CAM patients had no underlying factor other than SARS-CoV-2 infection, while improper GCS use (higher dose or prolonged administration) was independently associated with the "black fungus disease" [103]. As for tocilizumab, only 2.7% of the CAM patients in the aforementioned study received tocilizumab. Not unexpectedly, the predominant risk factor for mucormycosis was found to be diabetes. The authors suggested that their data should be compared to data from Western countries, where the main predisposing factor for mucormycosis are hematological malignances and organ transplantation, apart from diabetes mellitus. Several other cohorts reported the frequency of GCS use among CAM patients as high as 60% [104,105], over 85% [106,107] and 100% [107]. With regards to *Pneumocystis jirovecii* Pneumonia (PJP), Chong et al. [108], in their excellent review of PJP-SARS-CoV-2 co-infection case reports, conclude that the virus may predispose to this fungal entity through lymphocytopenia and macrophage dysfunction. Although 10 out of

12 co-infected patients received steroids for COVID-19 management, they mention that a safe conclusion as to the predisposing factors could not be made.

4.2. Tocilizumab

As for tocilizumab, there are no data from the Pre-COVID era, since there was no indication for ICU patients. In the COVID-era, there are several studies showing the high prevalence of CAPA among tocilizumab-treated patients. Lamoth et al. [109] raised the suspicion of tocilizumab contributing to IPA since the three patients with pulmonary aspergillosis in their cohort of COVID-19 ICU patients had received tocilizumab, as was the case for the non-IPA patients. Kimming et al. [110], in their retrospective study of critically ill COVID-19 patients, showed that receiving tocilizumab was associated with a higher risk of secondary fungal infections (5.6 vs. 0%; $p = 0.112$); of note, more patients in the tocilizumb group received corticosteroids as well. Importantly, the large multinational cohort by Prattes et al. comparing CAPA to non-CAPA COVID-19 critically ill patients [111] demonstrated tocilizumab, and not GCS, as a risk factor for CAPA. Tocilizumab in this study was mostly used in the dose of 8 mg/kg BW.

Reviewing tocilizumab and *Candida* infections, Antinori [112] reported a 6.9% incidence of candidemia among 43 severe COVID-19 patients hospitalized in ward and ICU. All candidemic patients had received TPN and tocilizumab (8 mg/kg repeated within 12 h), while the interval between administration of tocilizumab's last dose to candidemia was 13 days (median). Seagle et al. examined the receipt of tocilizumab in candidemic patients with and without COVID-19 [36] and found it to be 30 times more common in COVID-19-Associated Candidemia (18.8% vs. 0.5% without COVID-19; $p \leq 0.0001$). Guaraldi et al. [113] also showed that tocilizumab increases the incidence of candidemia and IFIs. In a Spanish cohort, treatment with tocilizumab alone or in combination with GCS increased the risk of systemic candidiasis (p-value = 0.05; 0.010, respectively [114]).

These findings are opposed to several smaller case series. Xu et al. [115] traced no secondary fungal infections in a small series of 21 severe and critically ill COVID-19 patients treated with tocilizumab. Obata et al. [95] in the abovementioned trial made a subgroup analysis for tocilizumab treatment together with GCS and revealed no significant difference in fungal infections between patients who received tocilizumab or not. Likewise, Hermine et al. [116], in their prospective, randomized, open-label trial comparing tocilizumab to usual care, found no fungal sepsis cases in the tocilizumab group vs. 2 out of 67 in the usual care group. Recent literature features influenza as independently associated with invasive pulmonary aspergillosis [38]. The same is not, still, the case for COVID-19. The debate is still ongoing whether SARS-CoV-2 predisposes to fungal infections and, if yes, to what extent and how it interacts with the immune modulation by current treatment modalities.

Table 3 summarizes the studies on invasive Aspergillosis in COVID-19 patients.

Table 4 summarizes the studies on Candida infections in COVID-19 patients treated with steroids.

Table 3. Invasive Aspergillosis in COVID-19 patients (case reports and hematology patient case series excluded).

Literature	Trial Design and Population	Diagnostic Criteria Used	CS Used	CS Length	Other IST	Comorbidities	IA Incidence	Time to IA Dx	Mortality
Alanio A. et al. [87] France	P, O, n = 27 ICU pts, 9/27 CAPA, med age 63 [IQR 56–71]	EORTC-MSGERC or IAPA + ser β-D-glucan and qPCR (serum or pulm specimens)	6/9 pts: dexa IV 20 mg/d (D1–5) then 10 mg/d (D6–10). 2/9 pts on prev GCS	10 ds	NM	HPN more frequent in IPA (7/9 vs. 6/18, $p = 0.046$)	Probable IPAs: (4%) putative IPAs: 30%	NM	4/9
van Arkel A.E. et al. [88] Netherlands	O, n = 31 ICU pts on MV	*A. fumigatus* 5/6, A. Ag GM (+) BAL fluid: 3/6	3/6 pts: CS before IPA Dx, dose < 0.3 mg/kg/d	<3 wks	No	3/6 Pre-existing lung disease	6/31 (19.35%) presumed IPA	Sx onset—IPA: med 11.5 ds (8–42), ICU admis–IPA: med 5 ds (3–28)	66.7% died, med 12 ICU ds (11–20)
Bartoletti et al. [89] Italy	P, MC, n = 822	CAPA	MP 1 mg/kg	5–7 ds	TOCI		27.7%	Intub-CAPA: med 4ds (2–8). sx onset-CAPA: med 14ds (11–22)	↑↑ ICU mortality after adj for age, RRT, admis severity scores
Benedetti et al. [90] Argentina	n = 5 ICU pts	IAPA or EORTC-MSGERC serum markers, or AspICU	5/5 CS (<0.3 mg/kg)	<3wks	No	1/5 hematologic malignancy 2/5 diabetes		Sx onset-CAPA: 22 ds (13–52). ICU admis-CAPA: med 12 ds	1/5 died (rest still on MV)
Delliere et al. [92] France	R, O, MC, n = 360 ICU pts; 108 pts sampled on deterioration. 1 SOT. 1 myeloma	EORTC/MSGERC CAPA	NM	NM	Sarilumab 1 pt, eculizumab 6 pts, toci 4 pts	Azithromycin (>3 ds) and prob IPA (OR 3.1, 95% CI, 1.1–8.5, $p = 0.02$). HD dexa and IPA: 11.5% vs. 28.6%, ($p = 0.08$), cumul dose ≥100 mg and IPA (OR 3.7, 95% CI 1.0–9.7).	5.7% in ICU pts 8.5% in MV pts 19.4% in deteriorated pts	Sx onset–IPA: 16 ds (10–23) ICU admis—IPA: 6 ds (1–15)	IPA pts vs. non-IPA: 71.4% vs. 36.8%, $p < 0.01$).

Table 3. Cont.

Literature	Trial Design and Population	Diagnostic Criteria Used	CS Used	CS Length	Other IST	Comorbidities	IA Incidence	Time to IA Dx	Mortality
Dupont et al. [91] France	R, 153 ICU pts screened for fungi; 106 PCR SARS-Co-V2 (+)	AspICU + serum/BAL GM	37% CS	short time	NM	HTN 36.8%, DM 36.8%, TB/COPD/asthma 36.8%	17.9% putative IPA	MV-CAPA: 6 ds	42%
Fekkar A. et al. [24] France	R, SC, n = 145 COVID-19 ICU MV pts screened for fungal superinfection; 54% on ECMO	EORTC/MSGERC, Mycology lab (microscopy, cultures, PCR respir samples and serum for Aspergillus, PJP, mucorales, GMI, β-D-glucan	Long-term (>3 wks) CS before COVID-19 and IFI (OR, 8.55; IQR, 6.8–10.3; $p = 0.01$), CS for COVID-19 (dexa 20 mg/d × 10 ds) no IFI	10 ds	6 Toci 3 saril 1 antiIL1	100% MV, 68% ↑BW, 57% HTN, 32% DM, 14% preexisting immunosuppression	4.8% prob/putat IFI (1 fusarium case), 17.2% colonization	ICU admis-IFI: med 7 ds (IQR, 2–56)	Survival 74.5%
Fortarezza et al. [94] Italy	n = 45 COVID-19 autopsies	Histology	CS: 88% of CAPA vs. 54% non-CAPA CS: 12/28 pts 1st wave vs. 16/17 pts 2nd wave	NM	No Toci No antiIL-1	7/9 ICU 7/9 HTN 3/9 COPD	20% proven CAPA, 1st wave 2/28 vs. 2nd wave 7/17	NM	NA
Janssen et al. [102] Belgium, Netherlands, France	O, MC, 2 ICU cohorts: N1 = 512 N2 = 304	ECCM/ISHAM	CS use not more prevalent in CAPA groups vs. non-CAPA	NM	Other IST < 90 ds before ICU admis	CAPA vs. nonCAPA: COPD 19% vs. 8% ($p = 0.042$). HIV (AIDS) 7% vs. 0.4% ($p = 0.011$)	10–15%	ICU admis to CAPA: 6 ds (IQR 3–9)	43–52%
Lamoth et al. [109] Switzerland	n = 80 ICU MV pts	IAPA	NM	NA	Toci—IPA Dx: 4 ds	No pt had any predisposing factors acc to EORTC/MSG	3.8% 1 probable 2 putative	COVID dx- IPA: med 9 ds, ICU admis-IPA: 6 ds, MV start-IPA: med 5 ds	1/3 died

Table 3. Cont.

Literature	Trial Design and Population	Diagnostic Criteria Used	CS Used	CS Length	Other IST	Comorbidities	IA Incidence	Time to IA Dx	Mortality
Marr et al. [20] Spain, USA	R, MC $n = 20$ CAPA	*Aspergillus* recovery in BAS, sputum, BAL or GMI ≥ 1, imaging	NM Systemic and inh CS most common IST associated with CAPA	NM	NM	Age HTN Pulm dis underlying immunosuppressive disease/drugs	NA	Sx onset-CAPA: med 11 ds, ICU admis-CAPA: 9 ds	NM
Meijer et al. [93] Netherlands	SC, P, 1st wave: 33 MV ICU pts vs. 2nd wave: 33 MV ICU pts	2020 ECMM/ISHAM	All CAPA pts in 2nd wave on CS: Dexa 6 mg	10 ds	no	CVD 4/13 DM 3/13 HTN 2/13 COPD 1/13 ARF 1/13	1st vs. 2nd wave poss and prob CAPA: 15.2% vs. 25% ($p = 0.36$) In total: 19.7%	NM	40–50% mortality in both groups
Obata R. et al. [95] USA	R, 226 COVID-19 hosp pts, 57 on CS vs. 169 no-CS	NM	Dexa (48/57), P (6/57), MP (1/57), MP + P 1/57, HC 1/57	Max 10ds	20/57 Toci	NM	CAPA in CS vs. no-CS: 5.3% vs. 0.6% CAPA in toci vs. no-toci: 5% vs. 5.4%	NM	NM
Prattes et al. [111] Europe, USA	MC, P, MN 592 COVID-19 ICU pts	2020 ECMM/ISHAM	Majority on GCS	NM	Toci	Age MV Toci	Proven 1.9%, Prob 13.5% poss: 3% No-CAPA: 81.6%	ICU admis-CAPA: 8 ds (0–31)	Survival in CAPA pts vs. non-CAPA: 29% vs. 57%
Rutsaert et al. [99] Belgium	$n = 20$ MV pts med 66 yo (56–77)	AspICU	1/7 CS (pemphigus)	NM	NM	4/7 DL 2/7 obesity 3/7 DM 3/7 HTN	7/20 (35%) proven IPA	Sx onset—IPA: 11–23 ds	4/7 died

Table 3. Cont.

Literature	Trial Design and Population	Diagnostic Criteria Used	CS Used	CS Length	Other IST	Comorbidities	IA Incidence	Time to IA Dx	Mortality
Van Biesen et al. [100] Netherlands	42 MV ICU pts (9 IPA vs. 33 non-IPA)	AspICU + GMI ≥ 1	No CS	NA	NM	1/9 SOT COPD and asthma more common in IPA group	9/42	NM	22% IPA vs. 15.1% non-IPA ($p = 0.6$)
White et al. [30] UK	$n = 137$ ICU pts screened for IFI	AspICU, IAPA, CAPA	12/25 different CS	N/M	no	12/25 CRD 8/25 HTN 6/25 DM 6/25 obesity 5/25 CA	14.1% CAPA	ICU admiss- (+) Aspergillus tests: 8 ds (0–35)	CAPA mortality 57.9% depending on appropriate Tx

admis = admission, ARF = Acute Renal Failure, BAS = Bronchial aspirate, BSI = Blood-stream infections, BW = body weight, CFR = Case Fatality Rate, CS = corticosteroids, CRD = Chronic Respiratory Disease, cumul = cumulative, CVD = cardiovascular disease, DL = dyslipidemia, Ds = days, dexa = dexamethasone, DM = diabetes mellitus, Dx = diagnosis, ECMO = Extra-corporeal membrane oxygenation, GM = galactomannan, GMI = galactomannan index, HD = high dose, HTN = Hypertension, IA = Invasive Aspergillosis, IFI = invasive fungal infection, intub = intubation, IST = immunosuppressive therapy, MC = Multicenter, med = median, MN = multi-national, MP = methylprednisolone, MV = mechanically ventilated, m = median, n = number of patients, NA = not applicable, NM = not mentioned, O = observational, OR = odds Ratio, P = Prospective, prev = previous, prob = probable, put = putative, R = Retrospective, resp sampl on deterior = respiratory sampling on deterioration, ROM = Rhino-orbital mucormycosis, saril = sarilumab, SC = single center, Sx = symptom, Toci = tocilizumab, unclass = unclassified.

Table 4. *Candida* infections in COVID-19 patients treated with steroids.

Literature	Trial Design	CS Used	CS Length	Other IST	Comorbidities/ Risk Factors	Candida Infection Incidence	Time to CAC Dx	Mortality
Antinori et al. [112] Italy	$n = 43$ severe COVID-19 pts; 3/43 candidemia	NM	NM	Toci	TPN (3/3), antibiotics (2/3), toci (3/3)	6.9% BSI	Toci last dose—CAC: med 13 ds	Still hospitalized on publication
Chowdhary et al. [97] India	$n = 596$ COVID-19 ICU pts, 420 MV, 15 *Candida* BSI	NM	NM	NM	↑ICU LOS, HTN, DM, CKD, CS (10/15)	2.5% BSI	Admis-CAC: 10–12 ds	53% (60% for *C. auris*)
Ho et al. [98] USA	$n = 4313$ hospitalised, 574 (13.3%) received CS R, O,	MP > P > dexa	6.34–9.53 ds	Toci	HTN 35.4% DM23.4% CKD 13%	BSI	NM	

Table 4. Cont.

Literature	Trial Design	CS Used	CS Length	Other IST	Comorbidities/Risk Factors	Candida Infection Incidence	Time to CAC Dx	Mortality
Obata et al. [95] USA	R, 226 COVID-19 hosp pts, 57 on CS vs. 169 no-CS	See Table 1	Max 10ds	20/57 Toci	NM	CAC in CS vs. no-CS: 7% vs. 0% CAC in toci vs. no-toci: 15% vs. 2.7%	NM	NM
Riche et al. [96] Brazil	R, candidemia incidence between COVID and non-COVID inpatients	MP > dexa > P	2–13 ds	No	HD CS CVC 90.9% ICU pts (72.7%)	×10 increase in candidemia	ICU admis-CAC: 0–22 ds	72.7% following CS use
Seagle et al. [36] USA	Candidemia in COVID-19 and non-COVID-19 pts, surveillance data	NM	NM	Toci more likely among pts with COVID-19 compared to non-COVID-19 pts	Candidemia RF in non-COVID pts: LD, malignancy, prior surgeries CAC each >1.3 times more common: ICU, MV, CVC, CS, IST. Common RF in COVID-19 pts: DM, obesity.	CS within 30 ds of CAC: ×2 vs. non-COVID-19 pts	SARS-CoV-2 (+) test-*Candida* culture: med 15 ds ([IQR]: 8–21 days)	CAC: ×2 mortality (62.5%) vs. candidemia in non-COVID-19 pts (32.1%)
Segrelles-Calvo [114] et al. Spain	O, P, n = 218 ICU pts	MP	1–10 ds	Toci-CAC: RR 1.378, p = 0.05. Toci + MP/dexa (p = 0.01)	Malignancies more common in COVID-19 with candida co-infection. ICU, TPN, CVC, ↑LO ICU stay	14.4% (+) Candida tests		

N = number, admis = admission, ARF = Acute Renal Failure, BAS = Bronchial aspirate, BSI = Blood-stream infections, BW = body weight, CFR = Case Fatality Rate, CS = corticosteroids, CRD = Chronic Respiratory Disease, cumul = cumulative, CVD = cardiovascular disease, DL = dyslipidemia, Ds = days, dexa = dexamethasone, DM = diabetes mellitus, Dx = diagnosis, ECMO = Extra-corporeal membrane oxygenation, GM = galactomannan, GMI = Galactomannan index, HD = high dose, HTN = Hypertension, IA = Invasive Aspergillosis, IFI = invasive fungal infection, intub = intubation, IST = immunosuppressive therapy, MC = Multicenter, med = median, MN = multi-national, MP = methylprednisolone, MV = mechanically ventilated, m = median, n = number of patients, NA = not applicable, NM = not mentioned, O = observational, OR = odds Ratio, P = Prospective, prev = previous, prob = probable, put = putative, R = Retrospective, resp sampl = respiratory sampling on deterior = respiratory sampling on deterioration, ROM = Rhino-orbital mucormycosis, saril = sarilumab, SC = single center, Sx = symptom, Toci = tocilizumab, unclass = unclassified.

5. Mortality and Fungal Infections in Critically Ill COVID-19 Patients

The available data clearly suggest that IFI identification in a critically ill COVID-19 patient confers a highly dismal prognosis, regardless of the causative fungal agent. However, as IFIs tend to occur more frequently to the most seriously affected patients, it is, as of yet, less clear whether this excess mortality associated with IFI diagnosis is attributable to IFI per se, the severity of the underlying disease or, most probably, a combination of both. Unfortunately, a further increase in IFI-driven mortality must be awaited as multi-drug-resistant species, such as *Candida auris*, rapidly spread around the world.

Invasive pulmonary aspergillosis has repeatedly been shown to be associated with increased mortality in critically ill patients with COVID-19 [116]. In an early landmark study, Bartoletti et al. [89] prospectively applied a CAPA screening protocol consisting of consecutive bronchoalveolar lavage (BAL) sampling for galactomannan (GM) measurement in all COVID-19 ICU patients requiring invasive mechanical ventilation (on admission, at day 7 of mechanical ventilation and in case of respiratory deterioration). CAPA was diagnosed in 30 out of 108 enrollees. Mortality was twice as high in CAPA patients compared with their non-CAPA counterparts, and both CAPA diagnosis and higher initial BAL GM levels were identified as independent risk factors for mortality even after adjusting for age, underlying disease severity on ICU admission and need for renal replacement therapy. Although not statistically significant, a trend towards better outcomes was shown in CAPA patients who received treatment with voriconazole. In another prospective study, White and colleagues corroborated the favorable effect of antifungal treatment administration on survival in patients with CAPA [30]. In their CAPA cohort, the clear majority of patients who did not receive appropriate antifungal treatment died, while mortality fell to 46.7% in those properly managed with antifungals. The larger study on CAPA to date was a multinational observational study conducted by the European Confederation of Medical Mycology (ECMM) [111]. 109 ICU patients with histologically proven, probable and possible CAPA according to ECMM/ISHAM diagnostic criteria [30] were analyzed and compared with 483 non-CAPA COVID-19 patients. Length of ICU stay and 90-day mortality were significantly higher in CAPA than in non-CAPA patients (56% versus 41%), and CAPA diagnosis continued to be an independent predictor of mortality after adjusting for age, study center and comorbidities. Collectively, these data strongly support the idea that CAPA may constitute a major contributor to excess mortality in critically ill COVID-19 patients. On the other hand, several reports have described patients diagnosed with CAPA who survived despite lack of appropriate antifungal treatment administration [20,86,117]. Furthermore, in a recently published study on Aspergillus test profiles of 58 patients with CAPA, 30-day ICU mortality was not significantly higher in CAPA patients treated with antifungal agents compared with those left untreated [118]. The authors also failed to show a significant effect of BAL GM positivity or levels on patient outcome, with only serum biomarkers having prognostic value. These findings are directly contradictory to those of earlier studies and may imply that increased fatality rates observed in critically ill patients with CAPA may, at least in part, be attributable to the co-existence of other risk factors for mortality [119].

Candidemia is a usually fatal secondary infection in COVID-19 patients. A case–control study conducted during the first wave of the pandemic showed an extremely high all-cause mortality rate (72.5 versus 26.9%) in COVID-19 ICU patients with candidemia compared with non-candidemic controls matched with CAC cases according to length of hospitalization before candidemia occurrence [120]. Moreover, candidemia appears to be more lethal in critically ill COVID-19 patients in comparison with their non-COVID-19 counterparts. Using data from a nationwide surveillance program in the US, Seagle and colleagues studied 251 patients with candidemia, one quarter of which had been diagnosed with COVID-19 [36]. Hospital all-cause mortality was twice as high in patients with CAC compared with patients without COVID-19 (62.5 vs. 32.1%). In another large study, all patients admitted to the ICUs of a single reference hospital in Turkey during a period of two years extending both before and after the SARS-CoV 2 outbreak were included, and those with

Candida species isolated in blood cultures were analyzed [121]. Mortality was exceptionally high in both COVID-19 and non-COVID-19 groups, but candidemia-associated fatalities were significantly more common in the former (92.5 vs. 79.4%). A delay in pre-emptive antifungal treatment administration in deteriorating septic patients may have contributed to these overwhelmingly high mortality rates, as one-third of all patients with candidemia included in the study never actually received any antifungal, and this was more common in the COVID-19 group. The same study provides insights into possible risk factors for mortality in CAC. In multivariate logistic regression analysis older age (>65 years), prior corticosteroid administration and presence of sepsis were recognized as potential predictors of adverse outcomes in patients with CAC. In line with the reports, smaller observational studies and case series have consistently documented CAC fatality rates exceeding 50% [122].

An issue of concern with an anticipated effect on mortality is the emergence and rapid spread of resistant *Candida* strains, most notably of the *Candida auris* species, which has preceded the outbreak of SARS-CoV2 but may have been accelerated by the pandemic [123]. Although the only rarely resistant *Candida albicans* remains the most commonly isolated Candida species in candidemic non-COVID-19 and COVID-19 patients alike, occasionally, non-susceptible strains of non-*albicans Candida* species (including *Candida glabrata*, *Candida parapsilosis* and *Candia kruzei*) are increasingly reported and may constitute most bloodstream *Candida* infections in some instances [122,124]. *Candida auris* was originally described in 2009 in a Japanese patient with external otitis and has, thenceforth, been isolated in an ever-growing number of countries across the world [123]. *Candida auris* possesses a unique combination of worrisome features, due to which it has been declared an "urgent threat" by the US Centers for Disease Control and Prevention (CDC) [125]. *Candida auris* is characterized by high rates of resistance to azoles and amphotericin B (85% and 33%, respectively, according to recent CDC data), and pan-resistant strains with additional lack of susceptibility to echinocandins have rarely but increasingly been isolated from patients without prior echinocandin exposure [126]. Furthermore, *Candida auris* can form biofilms, presents difficulties in laboratory identification, is more resilient to commonly used disinfectants and, importantly, can remain on most of the surfaces of the health-care environment in viable forms for long periods of time, the latter facilitating transmission between patients and outbreaks, especially in intensive and long-term care units [123]. Secondary *Candida auris* infections have regularly been reported worldwide during the SARS-CoV-2 pandemic [96,125,127–129]. Although the specific effect of *Candida auris* infection on mortality of critically ill COVID-19 patients has not been formally addressed, in one of the first CAC documentations coming from India, mortality was higher in candidemic COVID-19 patients with *Candida auris* compared with those with non-*auris* species [96].

Like other IFIs, mucormycosis is associated with considerable mortality in COVID-19 patients, which is heavily dependent on the site of infection. Additionally, major long-term sequelae are frequently reserved for survivors. In the largest study published so far, the investigators retrospectively analyzed the outcomes of 187 hospitalized patients with CAM in India [102]. A 3-month case fatality rate of 45.7% was estimated, which was not significantly different from that of another group of non-COVID patients diagnosed with mucormycosis during the same period. In a multivariate logistic regression analysis performed in the entire study population, older age, pulmonary mucormycosis, cerebral dissemination of rhino-orbital infection and ICU stay were all identified as risk factors for mortality. On the other hand, sequential antifungal combination treatment with amphotericin B plus a triazole (posaconazole or isavouconazole), although not recommended by current guidelines [130], was independently linked with a better prognosis. Recently, an international group of experts initiated by ECMM and ISHAM studied 80 published and unpublished cases of CAM from 18 countries [131]. A very similar all-cause mortality rate of 48.8% was found. Mortality was relentlessly high in those with pulmonary and disseminated mucormycosis (81% versus only 24.3% in isolated rhino-orbital disease). Again, central nervous system involvement in patients with rhino-orbital mucormycosis was shown to confer worse prognosis (59.1% mortality in this subgroup) and long-term disability in the form of vision loss in survivors (46.3% among survivors, all with cerebral involvement). Surgical therapy in combination with antifungals was demonstrated to improve survival in patients with isolated rhino-orbital infection. A high level of clinical suspicion allowing early identification of possible mucormycosis and timely initiation of amphotericin combined with aggressive surgical resection and debridement, when feasible, remain the mainstay of mucormycosis management, irrespective of COVID-19 status [130].

6. Conclusions

There is increasing evidence for the association between COVID-19 and IFIs. Emerging data demonstrate that the clinical course of COVID-19 can be complicated by a variety of fungal super-infections leading to unfavorable outcomes. It must be noted that critically ill COVID-19 patients have a number of risk factors predisposing them to fungal infections. The unique pathogenicity of SARS-CoV-2 with the deranged immune response it provokes, the well-known effects of immunosuppressant treatments and finally the causal relationships, synergistic effects or independent risk factors of critical illness compose the canvas of vulnerability for IFIs. The burden of fungal infections is largely not estimated. Studies based on histopathological confirmation are needed to improve our knowledge on the extent of the problem.

Author Contributions: Conceptualization, N.R. and G.D.; Methodology, N.R. and G.D.; Writing—original draft preparation, N.R., E.K., V.R., S.A., K.L. and V.C.; writing—review and editing, N.R., A.K. and G.D.; Supervision, N.R., A.K. and G.D. All authors have read and agreed to the published version of the manuscript.

Funding: This research received no external funding.

Informed Consent Statement: Not applicable.

Data Availability Statement: Not applicable.

Conflicts of Interest: The authors declare no conflict of interest.

References

1. Live Updates COVID-19—World Health Organization—who.int. Available online: https://www.worldometers.info/coronavirus/ (accessed on 6 November 2021).
2. WHO Coronavirus (COVID-19) Dashboard. Available online: https://covid19.who.int (accessed on 6 November 2021).
3. Michelen, M.; Jones, N.; Stavropoulou, C. In Patients of COVID-19, What Are the Symptoms and Clinical Features of Mild and Moderate Cases? Available online: https://www.cebm.net/covid-19/in-patients-of-covid-19-what-are-the-symptoms-and-clinical-features-of-mild-and-moderate-case/CEBM (accessed on 20 November 2021).
4. Atzrodt, C.L.; Maknojia, I.; McCarthy, R.D.; Oldfield, T.M.; Po, J.; Ta, K.T.; Stepp, H.E.; Clements, T.P. A Guide to COVID-19: A global pandemic caused by the novel coronavirus SARS-CoV-2. *FEBS J.* **2020**, *287*, 3633–3650. [CrossRef] [PubMed]
5. Wang, Y.; Wang, Y.; Chen, Y.; Qin, Q. Unique epidemiological and clinical features of the emerging 2019 novel coron- avirus pneumonia (COVID-19) implicate special control measures. *J. Med. Virol.* **2020**, *6*, 568–576. [CrossRef] [PubMed]
6. Yang, W.; Cao, Q.; Qin, L.; Wang, X.; Cheng, Z.; Pan, A.; Dai, J.; Sun, Q.; Zhao, F.; Qu, J.; et al. Clinical characteristics and imaging manifestations of the 2019 novel coronavirus disease (COVID-19): A multi-center study in Wenzhou city, Zhejiang, China. *J. Infect.* **2020**, *80*, 388–393. [CrossRef] [PubMed]
7. Hughes, S.; Troise, O.; Donaldson, H.; Mughal, N.; Moore, L.S.P. Bacterial and fungal coinfection among hospitalized patients with COVID-19: A retrospective cohort study in a UK secondary-care setting. *Clin. Microbiol. Infect.* **2020**, *26*, 1395–1399. [CrossRef]
8. Karaba, S.M.; Jones, G.; Helsel, T.; Smith, L.L.; Avery, R.; Dzintars, K.; Salinas, A.B.; Keller, S.C.; Townsend, J.L.; Klein, E.; et al. Prevalence of Co-infection at the Time of Hospital Admission in COVID-19 Patients. A Multicenter Study. *Open Forum Infect. Dis.* **2020**, *8*, ofaa578. [CrossRef]
9. Grasselli, G.; Greco, M.; Zanella, A.; Albano, G.; Antonelli, M.; Bellani, G.; Bonanomi, E.; Cabrini, L.; Carlesso, E.; Castelli, G.; et al. Risk Factors Associated with Mortality Among Patients With COVID-19 in Intensive Care Units in Lombardy, Italy. *JAMA Intern. Med.* **2020**, *180*, 1345–1355. [CrossRef]
10. Schmidt, M.; Hajage, D.; Demoule, A.; Pham, T.; Combes, A.; Dres, M.; Lebbah, S.; Kimmoun, A.; Mercat, A.; Beduneau, G.; et al. Clinical characteristics and day-90 outcomes of 4244 critically ill adults with COVID-19: A prospective cohort study. *Intensive Care Med.* **2021**, *47*, 60–73.

11. Qin, C.; Zhou, L.; Hu, Z.; Zhang, S.; Yang, S.; Tao, Y.; Xie, C.; Ma, K.; Shang, K.; Wang, W.; et al. Dysregulation of Immune Response in Patients with Coronavirus 2019 (COVID-19) in Wuhan, China. *Clin. Infect. Dis.* **2020**, *71*, 762–768. [CrossRef]
12. Mehta, P.; McAuley, D.F.; Brown, M.; Sanchez, E.; Tattersall, R.S.; Manson, J.J. COVID-19: Consider cytokine storm syndromes and immunosuppression. *Lancet* **2020**, *395*, 1033–1034. [CrossRef]
13. Cataldo, M.A.; Tetaj, N.; Selleri, M.; Marchioni, L.; Capone, A.; Caraffa, E.; Di Caro, A.; Petrosillo, N. Incidence of bacterial and fungal bloodstream infections in COVID-19 patients in intensive care: An alarming "collateral effect". *J. Glob. Antimicrob. Resist.* **2020**, *23*, 290–291. [CrossRef]
14. Chiurlo, M.; Mastrangelo, A.; Ripa, M.; Scarpellini, P. Invasive fungal infections in patients with COVID-19: A review on pathogenesis, epidemiology, clinical features, treatment, and outcomes. *New Microbiol.* **2021**, *44*, 71–83.
15. De Pauw, B.; Walsh, T.J.; Donnelly, J.P.; Stevens, D.A.; Edwards, J.E.; Calandra, T.; Pappas, P.G.; Maertens, J.; Lortholary, O.; Kauffman, C.A.; et al. Revised Definitions of Invasive Fungal Disease from the European Organization for Research and Treatment of Cancer/Invasive Fungal Infections Cooperative Group and the National Institute of Allergy and Infectious Diseases Mycoses Study Group (EORTC/MSG) Consensus Group. *Clin. Infect. Dis.* **2008**, *46*, 1813–1821. [CrossRef]
16. Arastehfar, A.; Carvalho, A.; Van De Veerdonk, F.L.; Jenks, J.D.; Koehler, P.; Krause, R.; Cornely, O.A.; Perlin, D.S.; Lass-Flörl, C.; Hoenigl, M. COVID-19 Associated Pulmonary Aspergillosis (CAPA)—From Immunology to Treatment. *J. Fungi* **2020**, *6*, 91. [CrossRef]
17. Ezeokoli, O.; Gcilitshana, O.; Pohl, C. Risk Factors for Fungal Co-Infections in Critically Ill COVID-19 Patients, with a Focus on Immunosuppressants. *J. Fungi* **2021**, *7*, 545, PMID:34356924. PMCID:PMC8304654. [CrossRef]
18. Martu, M.A.; Maftei, G.A.; Sufaru, I.G.; Jelihovschi, I.; Luchian, I.; Hurjui, L.; Martu, I.; Pasarin, L. COVID-19 and periodontal disease: Etiopathogenic and clinical immplications. *Rom. J. Oral Rehabil.* **2020**, *12*, 116–124.
19. Cunha, C.; Carvalho, A.; Esposito, A.; Esposito, F.; Bistoni, F.; Romani, L. DAMP signaling in fungal infections and diseases. *Front. Immunol.* **2012**, *3*, 286. [CrossRef]
20. Marr, K.A.; Platt, A.; Tornheim, J.A.; Zhang, S.X.; Datta, K.; Cardozo, C.; Garcia-Vidal, C. Aspergillosis Complicating Severe Coronavirus Disease. *Emerg. Infect. Dis.* **2021**, *27*, 18–25. [CrossRef]
21. Verweij, P.E.; Brüggemann, R.J.M.; Azoulay, E.; Bassetti, M.; Blot, S.; Buil, J.B.; Calandra, T.; Chiller, T.; Clancy, C.J.; Cornely, O.A.; et al. Taskforce report on the diagnosis and clinical management of COVID-19 associated pulmonary aspergillosis. *Intensive Care Med.* **2021**, *47*, 819–834. [CrossRef]
22. Montrucchio, G.; Lupia, T.; Lombardo, D.; Stroffolini, G.; Corcione, S.; De Rosa, F.G.; Brazzi, L. Risk factors for invasive aspergillosis in ICU patients with COVID-19: Current insights and new key elements. *Ann. Intensive Care* **2021**, *11*, 136. [CrossRef]
23. Szabo, B.G.; Lakatos, B.; Bobek, I.; Szabo, E.; Szlavik, J.; Vályi-Nagy, I. Invasive fungal infections among critically ill adult COVID-19 patients: First experiences from the national centre in Hungary. *J. Med. Mycol.* **2021**, *31*, 101198. [CrossRef]
24. Fekkar, A.; Lampros, A.; Mayaux, J.; Poignon, C.; Demeret, S.; Constantin, J.-M.; Marcelin, A.-G.; Monsel, A.; Luyt, C.-E.; Blaize, M. Occurrence of Invasive Pulmonary Fungal Infections in Patients with Severe COVID-19 Admitted to the ICU. *Am. J. Respir. Crit. Care Med.* **2021**, *203*, 307–317. [CrossRef]
25. Chong, W.H.; Saha, B.K.; Ramani, A.; Chopra, A. State-of-the-art review of secondary pulmonary infections in patients with COVID-19 pneumonia. *Infection* **2021**, *49*, 591–605. [CrossRef]
26. Chen, N.; Zhou, M.; Dong, X.; Qu, J.; Gong, F.; Han, Y.; Qiu, Y.; Wang, J.; Liu, Y.; Wei, Y.; et al. Epidemiological and clinical characteristics of 99 cases of 2019 novel coronavirus pneumonia in Wuhan, China: A descriptive study. *Lancet* **2020**, *395*, 507–513. [CrossRef]
27. Yang, X.; Yu, Y.; Xu, J.; Shu, H.; Xia, J.; Liu, H.; Wu, Y.; Zhang, L.; Yu, Z.; Fang, M.; et al. Clinical course and outcomes of critically ill patients with SARS-CoV-2 pneumonia in Wuhan, China: A single-centered, retrospective, observational study. *Lancet Respir. Med.* **2020**, *8*, 475–481, Erratum in *Lancet Respir. Med.* **2020**, *8*, e26. [CrossRef]
28. Musuuza, J.S.; Watson, L.; Parmasad, V.; Putman-Buehler, N.; Christensen, L.; Safdar, N. Prevalence and outcomes of co-infection and superinfection with SARS-CoV-2 and other pathogens: A systematic review and meta-analysis. *PLoS ONE* **2021**, *16*, e0251170. [CrossRef]
29. Bardi, T.; Pintado, V.; Gomez-Rojo, M.; Escudero-Sanchez, R.; Lopez, A.A.; Diez-Remesal, Y.; Castro, N.M.; Ruiz-Garbajosa, P.; Pestaña, D. Nosocomial infections associated to COVID-19 in the intensive care unit: Clinical characteristics and outcome. *Eur. J. Clin. Microbiol.* **2021**, *40*, 495–502. [CrossRef]
30. White, P.L.; Dhillon, R.; Cordey, A.; Hughes, H.; Faggian, F.; Soni, S.; Pandey, M.; Whitaker, H.; May, A.; Morgan, M.; et al. A National Strategy to Diagnose Coronavirus Disease 2019–Associated Invasive Fungal Disease in the Intensive Care Unit. *Clin. Infect. Dis.* **2020**, *73*, e1634–e1644. [CrossRef]
31. Peng, J.; Wang, Q.; Mei, H.; Zheng, H.; Liang, G.; She, X.; Liu, W. Fungal co-infection in COVID-19 patients: Evidence from a systematic review and meta-analysis. *Aging* **2021**, *13*, 7745–7757. [CrossRef]
32. White, P.L. Diagnosis of invasive fungal disease in coronavirus disease 2019: Approaches and pitfalls. *Curr. Opin. Infect. Dis.* **2021**, *34*, 573–580. [CrossRef]
33. Calandra, T.; Roberts, J.A.; Antonelli, M.; Bassetti, M.; Vincent, J.-L. Diagnosis and management of invasive candidiasis in the ICU: An updated approach to an old enemy. *Crit. Care* **2016**, *20*, 125. [CrossRef]
34. Bishburg, E.; Okoh, A.; Nagarakanti, S.R.; Lindner, M.; Migliore, C.; Patel, P. Fungemia in COVID-19 ICU patients, a single medical center experience. *J. Med. Virol.* **2021**, *93*, 2810–2814. [CrossRef] [PubMed]

35. Nucci, M.; Barreiros, G.; Guimarães, L.F.; Deriquehem, V.A.; Castiñeiras, A.C.; Nouér, S.A. Increased incidence of candidemia in a tertiary care hospital with the COVID-19 pandemic. *Mycoses* **2020**, *64*, 152–156. [CrossRef] [PubMed]
36. Seagle, E.E.; Jackson, B.R.; Lockhart, S.R.; Georgacopoulos, O.; Nunnally, N.S.; Roland, J.; Barter, D.M.; Johnston, H.L.; Czaja, C.A.; Kayalioglu, H.; et al. The Landscape of Candidemia During the Coronavirus Disease 2019 (COVID-19) Pandemic. *Clin. Infect. Dis.* **2021**, *74*, 802–811. [CrossRef] [PubMed]
37. Prestel, C.; Anderson, E.; Forsberg, K.; Lyman, M.; de Perio, M.A.; Kuhar, D.; Edwards, K.; Rivera, M.; Shugart, A.; Walters, M.; et al. *Candida auris* outbreak in a COVID-19 specialty care unit—Florida, July–August 2020. *MMWR Morb. Mortal. Wkly. Rep.* **2021**, *70*, 56–57. [CrossRef]
38. Schauwvlieghe, A.F.A.D.; Rijnders, B.J.A.; Philips, N.; Verwijs, R.; Vanderbeke, L.; Van Tienen, C.; Lagrou, K.; Verweij, P.E.; Van De Veerdonk, F.L.; Gommers, D.; et al. Invasive aspergillosis in patients admitted to the intensive care unit with severe influenza: A retrospective cohort study. *Lancet Respir. Med.* **2018**, *6*, 782–792. [CrossRef]
39. Yang, S.; Hua, M.; Liu, X.; Du, C.; Pu, L.; Xiang, P.; Wang, L.; Liu, J. Bacterial and fungal co-infections among COVID-19 patients in intensive care unit. *Microbes Infect.* **2021**, *23*, 104806. [CrossRef]
40. Koehler, P.; Bassetti, M.; Chakrabarti, A.; Chen, S.C.A.; Colombo, A.L.; Hoenigl, M.; Klimko, N.; Lass-Flörl, C.; Oladele, R.O.; Vinh, D.C.; et al. Defining and managing COVID-19-associated pulmonary aspergillosis: The 2020 ECMM/ISHAM consensus criteria for research and clinical guidance. *Lancet Infect. Dis.* **2021**, *21*, e149–e162. [CrossRef]
41. Brown, L.-A.K.; Ellis, J.; Gorton, R.; De, S.; Stone, N. Surveillance for COVID-19-associated pulmonary aspergillosis. *Lancet Microbe* **2020**, *1*, e152. [CrossRef]
42. Gouzien, L.; Cocherie, T.; Eloy, O.; Legriel, S.; Bedos, J.-P.; Simon, C.; Marque-Juillet, S.; Ferré, A.; Bruneel, F. Invasive Aspergillosis associated with Covid-19: A word of caution. *Infect. Dis. Now* **2021**, *51*, 383–386. [CrossRef]
43. Hoenigl, M.; Seidel, D.; Carvalho, A.; Rudramurthy, S.M.; Arastehfar, A.; Gangneux, J.P.; Nasir, N.; Bonifaz, A.; Araiza, J.; Klimko, N.; et al. The emergence of COVID-19- & associated mucormycosis: Analysis of cases from 18 countries. *Lancet Microbe* 2022. [CrossRef]
44. Khan, N.; Gutierrez, C.G.; Martinez, D.V.; Proud, K.C. A case report of COVID-19 associated pulmonary mucormycosis. *Arch. Clin. Cases* **2020**, *07*, 46–51. [CrossRef]
45. Pasero, D.; Sanna, S.; Liperi, C.; Piredda, D.; Branca, G.P.; Casadio, L.; Simeo, R.; Buselli, A.; Rizzo, D.; Bussu, F.; et al. A challenging complication following SARS-CoV-2 infection: A case of pulmonary mucormycosis. *Infection* **2020**, *49*, 1055–1060. [CrossRef]
46. Meawed, T.E.; Ahmed, S.M.; Mowafy, S.M.; Samir, G.M.; Anis, R.H. Bacterial and fungal ventilator associated pneumonia in critically ill COVID-19 patients during the second wave. *J. Infect. Public Health* **2021**, *14*, 1375–1380. [CrossRef]
47. Selarka, L.; Sharma, S.; Saini, D.; Sharma, S.; Batra, A.; Waghmare, V.T.; Dileep, P.; Patel, S.; Shah, M.; Parikh, T.; et al. Mucormycosis and COVID-19: An epidemic within a pandemic in India. *Mycoses* **2021**, *64*, 1253–1260. [CrossRef]
48. Rubiano, C.; Tompkins, K.; Sellers, S.A.; Bramson, B.; Eron, J.; Parr, J.B.; Schranz, A.J. Pneumocystis and Severe Acute Respiratory Syndrome Coronavirus 2 Coinfection: A Case Report and Review of an Emerging Diagnostic Dilemma. *Open Forum Infect. Dis.* **2020**, *8*, ofaa633. [CrossRef]
49. Choy, C.Y.; Wong, C.S. It's not all about COVID-19: Pneumocystis pneumonia in the era of a respiratory outbreak. *J. Int. AIDS Soc.* **2020**, *23*, e25533. [CrossRef]
50. Alanio, A.; Dellière, S.; Voicu, S.; Bretagne, S.; Mégarbane, B. The presence of *Pneumocystis jirovecii* in critically ill patients with COVID-19. *J. Infect.* **2020**, *82*, 84–123. [CrossRef]
51. Blaize, M.; Mayaux, J.; Luyt, C.-E.; Lampros, A.; Fekkar, A. COVID-19–related Respiratory Failure and Lymphopenia Do Not Seem Associated with Pneumocystosis. *Am. J. Respir. Crit. Care Med.* **2020**, *202*, 1734–1736. [CrossRef]
52. Jeican, I.I.; Inisca, P.; Gheban, D.; Tăbăran, F.; Aluaș, M.; Trombitas, V.; Cristea, V.; Crivii, C.; Junie, L.M.; Albu, S. COVID-19 and *Pneumocystis jirovecii* Pulmonary Coinfection-The First Case Confirmed through Autopsy. *Medicina* **2021**, *57*, 302. [CrossRef]
53. Poignon, C.; Blaize, M.; Vezinet, C.; Lampros, A.; Monsel, A.; Fekkar, A. Invasive pulmonary fusariosis in an immunocompetent critically ill patient with severe COVID-19. *Clin. Microbiol. Infect.* **2020**, *26*, 1582–1584. [CrossRef]
54. Nobrega de Almeida, J., Jr.; Moreno, L.; Francisco, E.C.; Noronha Marques, G.; Mendes, A.V.; Barberino, M.G.; Colombo, A.L. *Trichosporon asahii* superinfections in critically ill COVID-19 patients overexposed to antimicro- bials and corticosteroids. *Mycoses* **2021**, *64*, 817–822. [CrossRef]
55. Khatib, M.Y.; Ahmed, A.A.; Shaat, S.B.; Mohamed, A.S.; Nashwan, A.J. Cryptococcemia in a patient with COVID-19: A case report. *Clin. Case Rep.* **2020**, *9*, 853–855. [CrossRef]
56. Blanco-Melo, D.; Nilsson-Payant, B.E.; Liu, W.C.; Uhl, S.; Hoagland, D.; Møller, R.; Jordan, T.X.; Oishi, K.; Panis, M.; Sachs, D.; et al. Imbalanced Host Response to SARS-CoV-2 Drives Development of COVID-19. *Cell* **2020**, *181*, 1036–1045.e9. [CrossRef]
57. Land, W.G. Role of DAMPs in respiratory virus-induced acute respiratory distress syndrome—With a preliminary reference to SARS-CoV-2 pneumonia. *Genes Immun.* **2021**, *22*, 141–160. [CrossRef]
58. Galani, I.-E.; Rovina, N.; Lampropoulou, V.; Triantafyllia, V.; Manioudaki, M.; Pavlos, E.; Koukaki, E.; Fragkou, P.C.; Panou, V.; Rapti, V.; et al. Untuned antiviral immunity in COVID-19 revealed by temporal type I/III interferon patterns and flu comparison. *Nat. Immunol.* **2020**, *22*, 32–40. [CrossRef]
59. Chen, G.; Wu, D.; Guo, W.; Cao, Y.; Huang, D.; Wang, H.; Wang, T.; Zhang, X.; Chen, H.; Yu, H.; et al. Clinical and immunological features of severe and moderate coronavirus disease 2019. *J. Clin. Investig.* **2020**, *130*, 2620–2629. [CrossRef]
60. Moore, J.B.; June, C.H. Cytokine release syndrome in severe COVID-19. *Science* **2020**, *368*, 473–474. [CrossRef]

61. Tavakolpour, S.; Rakhshandehroo, T.; Wei, E.X.; Rashidian, M. Lymphopenia during the COVID-19 infection: What it shows and what can be learned. *Immunol. Lett.* **2020**, *225*, 31–32. [CrossRef]
62. Giamarellos-Bourboulis, E.J.; Netea, M.G.; Rovina, N.; Akinosoglou, K.; Antoniadou, A.; Antonakos, N.; Damoraki, G.; Gkavogianni, T.; Adami, M.-E.; Katsaounou, P.; et al. Complex Immune Dysregulation in COVID-19 Patients with Severe Respiratory Failure. *Cell Host Microbe* **2020**, *27*, 992–1000.e3. [CrossRef]
63. World Health Organization Clinical Management of COVID-19. 2020. Available online: https://apps.who.int/iris/rest/bitstreams/1278777/retrieve (accessed on 1 April 2021).
64. IDSA Guidelines on the Treatment and Management of Patients with COVID-19. Available online: https://www.idsociety.org/practice-guideline/covid-19-guideline-treatment-and-management (accessed on 15 December 2021).
65. COVID-19 Rapid Guideline: Managing COVID-19. Available online: https://www.guidelines.co.uk/infection/nice-covid-19-management (accessed on 15 December 2021).
66. Olnes, M.J.; Kotliarov, Y.; Biancotto, A.; Cheung, F.; Chen, J.; Shi, R.; Zhou, H.; Wang, E.; Tsang, J.S.; Nussenblatt, R. Effects of Systemically Administered Hydrocortisone on the Human Immunome. *Sci. Rep.* **2016**, *6*, 23002. [CrossRef]
67. Romanou, V.; Koukaki, E.; Chantziara, V.; Stamou, P.; Kote, A.; Vasileiadis, I.; Koutsoukou, A.; Rovina, N. Dexamethasone in the treatment of COVID-19: Primus inter pares? *J. Pers. Med.* **2021**, *11*, 556. [CrossRef] [PubMed]
68. Campbell, L.; Chen, C.; Bhagat, S.S.; Parker, R.A.; Östör, A.J.K. Risk of adverse events including serious infections in rheumatoid arthritis patients treated with tocilizumab: A systematic literature review and meta-analysis of randomized controlled trials. *Rheumatology* **2010**, *50*, 552–562. [CrossRef] [PubMed]
69. Conti, H.R.; Gaffen, S.L. IL-17–Mediated Immunity to the Opportunistic Fungal Pathogen *Candida albicans*. *J. Immunol.* **2015**, *195*, 780–788. [CrossRef] [PubMed]
70. Schaffner, A.; Douglas, H.; Braude, A. Selective protection against conidia by mononuclear and against mycelia by polymorphonuclear phagocytes in resistance to *Aspergillus*. Observations on these two lines of defense in vivo and in vitro with human and mouse phagocytes. *J. Clin. Investig.* **1982**, *69*, 617–631. [CrossRef]
71. Patterson, T.F.; Kirkpatrick, W.R.; White, M.; Hiemenz, J.W.; Wingard, J.R.; Dupont, B.; Rinaldi, M.G.; Stevens, D.A.; Graybill, J.R. Invasive aspergillosis. Disease spectrum, treatment practices, and outcomes. *Medicine* **2000**, *79*, 250–260. [CrossRef]
72. Luvanda, M.; Posch, W.; Vosper, J.; Zaderer, V.; Noureen, A.; Lass-Flörl, C.; Wilflingseder, D. Dexamethasone Promotes *Aspergillus fumigatus* Growth in Macrophages by Triggering M2 Repolarization via Targeting PKM2. *J. Fungi* **2021**, *7*, 70. [CrossRef]
73. Clemons, K.V.; Calich, V.L.G.; Burger, E.; Filler, S.G.; Graziutti, M.; Murphy, J.; Roilides, E.; Campa, A.; Dias, M.R.; Edwards, J.E.; et al. Pathogenesis I: Interactions of host cells and fungi. *Med. Mycol.* **2000**, *38* (Suppl. 1), 99–111. [CrossRef]
74. Ng, T.T.C.; Robson, G.D.; Denning, D.W. Hydrocortisone-enhanced growth of *Aspergillus* spp.: Implications for pathogenesis. *Microbiology* **1994**, *140*, 2475–2479. [CrossRef]
75. Schaffner, A. Therapeutic concentrations of glucocorticoids suppress the antimicrobial activity of human macrophages without impairing their responsiveness to gamma interferon. *J. Clin. Investig.* **1985**, *76*, 1755–1764. [CrossRef]
76. Antinori, S.; Milazzo, L.; Sollima, S.; Galli, M.; Corbellino, M. Candidemia and invasive candidiasis in adults: A narrative review. *Eur. J. Intern. Med.* **2016**, *34*, 21–28. [CrossRef]
77. Lionakis, M.S.; Netea, M.G. Candida and Host Determinants of Susceptibility to Invasive Candidiasis. *PLOS Pathog.* **2013**, *9*, e1003079. [CrossRef]
78. Kontoyiannis, D.P.; Wessel, V.C.; Bodey, G.P.; Rolston, K.V. Zygomycosis in the 1990s in a tertiary-care cancer center. *Clin. Infect. Dis.* **2000**, *30*, 851–856. [CrossRef]
79. Ibrahim, A.S.; Spellberg, B.; Walsh, T.J.; Kontoyiannis, D.P. Pathogenesis of mucormycosis. *Clin. Infect. Dis.* **2012**, *54* (Suppl. 1), S16–S22. [CrossRef]
80. Slivka, A.; Wen, P.Y.; Shea, W.; Loeffler, J.S. *Pneumocystis carinii* pneumonia during steroid taper in patients with primary brain tumors. *Am. J. Med.* **1993**, *94*, 216–219. [CrossRef]
81. Youssef, J.; Novosad, S.A.; Winthrop, K.L. Infection Risk and Safety of Corticosteroid Use. *Rheum. Dis. Clin. N. Am.* **2016**, *42*, 157–176. [CrossRef]
82. Baddley, J.W.; Stephens, J.M.; Ji, X.; Gao, X.; Schlamm, H.T.; Tarallo, M. Aspergillosis in Intensive Care Unit (ICU) patients: Epidemiology and economic outcomes. *BMC Infect. Dis.* **2013**, *13*, 29. [CrossRef]
83. Garnacho-Montero, J.; Amaya-Villar, R.; Ortiz-Leyba, C.; León, C.; Alvarez-Lerma, F.; Nolla-Salas, J.; Iruretagoyena, J.R.; Barcenilla, F. Isolation of *Aspergillus* spp. from the respiratory tract in critically ill patients: Risk factors, clinical presentation and outcome. *Crit. Care* **2005**, *9*, R191–R199. [CrossRef]
84. Pappas, P.G.; Kauffman, C.A.; Andes, D.; Benjamin, D.K., Jr.; Calandra, T.F.; Edwards, J.E., Jr.; Filler, S.G.; Fisher, J.F.; Kullberg, B.J.; Ostrosky-Zeichner, L.; et al. Clinical Practice Guidelines for the Management of Candidiasis: 2009 Update by the Infectious Diseases Society of America. *Clin. Infect. Dis.* **2009**, *48*, 503–535. [CrossRef]
85. Poissy, J.; Funginos, T.; Damonti, L.; Bignon, A.; Khanna, N.; Von Kietzell, M.; Boggian, K.; Neofytos, D.; Vuotto, F.; Coiteux, V.; et al. Risk factors for candidemia: A prospective matched case-control study. *Crit. Care* **2020**, *24*, 1–11. [CrossRef]
86. Lionakis, M.S.; Swamydas, M.; Fischer, B.G.; Plantinga, T.S.; Johnson, M.D.; Jaeger, M.; Green, N.M.; Masedunskas, A.; Weigert, R.; Mikelis, C.; et al. CX3CR1-dependent renal macrophage survival promotes *Candida* control and host survival. *J. Clin. Investig.* **2013**, *123*, 5035–5051. [CrossRef]

87. Alanio, A.; Dellière, S.; Fodil, S.; Bretagne, S.; Mégarbane, B. Prevalence of putative invasive pulmonary aspergillosis in critically ill patients with COVID-19. *Lancet Respir. Med.* **2020**, *8*, e48–e49. [CrossRef]
88. Van Arkel, A.L.E.; Rijpstra, T.A.; Belderbos, H.N.A.; Van Wijngaarden, P.; Verweij, P.E.; Bentvelsen, R.G. COVID-19-associated Pulmonary Aspergillosis. *Am. J. Respir. Crit. Care Med.* **2020**, *202*, 132–135. [CrossRef]
89. Bartoletti, M.; Pascale, R.; Cricca, M.; Rinaldi, M.; Maccaro, A.; Bussini, L.; Fornaro, G.; Tonetti, T.; Pizzilli, G.; Francalanci, E.; et al. Epidemiology of invasive pulmonary aspergillosis among COVID-19 intubated patients: A prospective study. *Clin. Infect. Dis.* **2021**, *73*, e3606–e3614. [CrossRef]
90. Benedetti, M.F.; Alava, K.H.; Sagardia, J.; Cadena, R.C.; Laplume, D.; Capece, P.; Posse, G.; Nusblat, A.D.; Cuestas, M.L. COVID-19 associated pulmonary aspergillosis in ICU patients: Report of five cases from Argentina. *Med. Mycol. Case Rep.* **2020**, *31*, 24–28. [CrossRef]
91. Dupont, D.; Menotti, J.; Turc, J.; Miossec, C.; Wallet, F.; Richard, J.C.; Argaud, L.; Paulus, S.; Wallon, M.; Ader, F.; et al. Pulmonary aspergillosis in critically ill patients with Coronavirus Disease 2019 (COVID-19). *Med. Mycol.* **2021**, *59*, 110–114. [CrossRef]
92. Dellière, S.; Dudoignon, E.; Fodil, S.; Voicu, S.; Collet, M.; Oillic, P.-A.; Salmona, M.; Dépret, F.; Ghelfenstein-Ferreira, T.; Plaud, B.; et al. Risk factors associated with COVID-19-associated pulmonary aspergillosis in ICU patients: A French multicentric retrospective cohort. *Clin. Microbiol. Infect.* **2020**, *27*, 790.e1–790.e5. [CrossRef]
93. Meijer, E.F.J.; Dofferhoff, A.S.M.; Hoiting, O.; Meis, J.F. COVID-19-associated pulmonary aspergillosis: A prospective single-center dual case series. *Mycoses* **2021**, *64*, 457–464. [CrossRef]
94. Fortarezza, F.; Boscolo, A.; Pezzuto, F.; Lunardi, F.; Acosta, M.J.; Giraudo, C.; Del Vecchio, C.; Sella, N.; Tiberio, I.; Godi, I.; et al. Proven COVID-19–associated pulmonary aspergillosis in patients with severe respiratory failure. *Mycoses* **2021**, *64*, 1223–1229. [CrossRef]
95. Obata, R.; Maeda, T.; Rizk, D.; Kuno, T. Increased Secondary Infection in COVID-19 Patients Treated with Steroids in New York City. *Jpn. J. Infect. Dis.* **2021**, *74*, 307–315. [CrossRef]
96. Riche, C.V.W.; Cassol, R.; Pasqualotto, A.C. Is the Frequency of Candidemia Increasing in COVID-19 Patients Receiving Corticosteroids? *J. Fungi* **2020**, *6*, 286. [CrossRef]
97. Chowdhary, A.; Tarai, B.; Singh, A.; Sharma, A. Multidrug-Resistant Candida auris Infections in Critically Ill Coronavirus Disease Patients, India, April–July 2020. *Emerg. Infect. Dis.* **2020**, *26*, 2694–2696. [CrossRef] [PubMed]
98. Ho, K.S.; Narasimhan, B.; Difabrizio, L.; Rogers, L.; Bose, S.; Li, L.; Chen, R.; Sheehan, J.; El-Halabi, M.A.; Sarosky, K.; et al. Impact of corticosteroids in hospitalised COVID-19 patients. *BMJ Open Respir. Res.* **2021**, *8*, e000766. [CrossRef] [PubMed]
99. Rutsaert, L.; Steinfort, N.; Van Hunsel, T.; Bomans, P.; Naesens, R.; Mertes, H.; Dits, H.; Van Regenmortel, N. COVID-19-associated invasive pulmonary aspergillosis. *Ann. Intensive Care* **2020**, *10*, 71. [CrossRef] [PubMed]
100. Van Biesen, S.; Kwa, D.; Bosman, R.J.; Juffermans, N.P. Detection of Invasive Pulmonary Aspergillosis in COVID-19 with Non-directed Bronchoalveolar Lavage. *Am. J. Respir. Crit. Care Med.* **2020**, *202*, 1171–1173. [CrossRef]
101. Wang, J.; Yang, Q.; Zhang, P.; Sheng, J.; Zhou, J.; Qu, T. Clinical characteristics of invasive pulmonary aspergillosis in patients with COVID-19 in Zhejiang, China: A retrospective case series. *Crit. Care* **2020**, *24*, 299. [CrossRef]
102. Janssen, N.A.; Nyga, R.; Vanderbeke, L.; Jacobs, C.; Ergün, M.; Buil, J.B.; van Dijk, K.; Altenburg, J.; Bouman, C.S.; van der Spoel, H.I.; et al. Multinational Observational Cohort Study of COVID-19–Associated Pulmonary Aspergillosis1. *Emerg. Infect. Dis.* **2021**, *27*, 2892–2898. [CrossRef]
103. Patel, A.; Agarwal, R.; Rudramurthy, S.M.; Shevkani, M.; Xess, I.; Sharma, R.; Savio, J.; Sethuraman, N.; Madan, S.; Shastri, P.; et al. Multicenter Epidemiologic Study of Coronavirus Disease-Associated Mucormycosis, India. *Emerg. Infect. Dis.* **2021**, *27*, 2349–2359. [CrossRef]
104. Mishra, N.; Mutya, V.S.S.; Thomas, A.; Rai, G.; Reddy, B.; Mohanan, A.A.; Ray, S.; Thiruvengadem, A.V.; Siddini, V.; Hegde, R. A case series of invasive mucormycosis in patients with COVID-19 infection. *Int. J. Otorhinolaryngol. Head Neck Surg.* **2021**, *7*, 867–870. [CrossRef]
105. Meher, R.; Wadhwa, V.; Kumar, V.; Phanbuh, D.S.; Sharma, R.; Singh, I.; Rathore, P.K.; Goel, R.; Arora, R.; Garg, S.; et al. COVID associated mucormycosis: A preliminary study from a dedicated COVID Hospital in Delhi. *Am. J. Otolaryngol.* **2021**, *43*, 103220. [CrossRef]
106. Moorthy, A.; Gaikwad, R.; Krishna, S.; Hegde, R.; Tripathi, K.K.; Kale, P.G.; Rao, P.S.; Haldipur, D.; Bonanthaya, K. SARS-CoV-2, Uncontrolled Diabetes and Corticosteroids-An Unholy Trinity in Invasive Fungal Infections of the Maxillofacial Region? A Retrospective, Multi-centric Analysis. *J. Maxillofac. Oral Surg.* **2021**, *20*, 418–425. [CrossRef]
107. Sen, M.; Honavar, S.G.; Bansal, R.; Sengupta, S.; Rao, R.; Kim, U.; Sharma, M.; Sachdev, M.; Grover, A.K.; Surve, A.; et al. Epidemiology, clinical profile, management, and outcome of COVID-19-associated rhino-orbital-cerebral mucormycosis in 2826 patients in India—Collaborative OPAI-IJO Study on Mucormycosis in COVID-19 (COSMIC), Report 1. *Indian J. Ophthalmol.* **2021**, *69*, 1670.
108. Chong, W.H.; Saha, B.K.; Chopra, A. Narrative review of the relationship between COVID-19 and PJP: Does it represent coinfection or colonization? *Infection* **2021**, *49*, 1079–1090. [CrossRef]
109. Lamoth, F.; Glampedakis, E.; Boillat-Blanco, N.; Oddo, M.; Pagani, J.-L. Incidence of invasive pulmonary aspergillosis among critically ill COVID-19 patients. *Clin. Microbiol. Infect.* **2020**, *26*, 1706–1708. [CrossRef]
110. Kimmig, L.M.; Wu, D.; Gold, M.; Pettit, N.N.; Pitrak, D.; Mueller, J.; Husain, A.N.; Mutlu, E.A.; Mutlu, G.M. IL-6 Inhibition in Critically Ill COVID-19 Patients Is Associated with Increased Secondary Infections. *Front. Med.* **2020**, *7*, 583897. [CrossRef]

111. Prattes, J.; Wauters, J.; Giacobbe, D.R.; Salmanton-García, J.; Maertens, J.; Bourgeois, M.; Reynders, M.; Rutsaert, L.; Van Regenmortel, N.; Lormans, P.; et al. Risk factors and outcome of pulmonary aspergillosis in critically ill coronavirus disease 2019 patients—A multinational observational study by the European Confederation of Medical Mycology. *Clin. Microbiol. Infect.* **2021**, *28*, 580–587. [CrossRef]
112. Antinori, S.; Bonazzetti, C.; Gubertini, G.; Capetti, A.; Pagani, C.; Morena, V.; Rimoldi, S.; Galimberti, L.; Sarzi-Puttini, P.; Ridolfo, A.L. Tocilizumab for cytokine storm syndrome in COVID-19 pneumonia: An increased risk for candidemia? *Autoimmun. Rev.* **2020**, *19*, 102564. [CrossRef]
113. Guaraldi, G.; Meschiari, M.; Cozzi-Lepri, A.; Milic, J.; Tonelli, R.; Menozzi, M.; Franceschini, E.; Cuomo, G.; Orlando, G.; Borghi, V.; et al. Tocilizumab in patients with severe COVID-19: A retrospective cohort study. *Lancet Rheumatol.* **2020**, *2*, e474–e484. [CrossRef]
114. Segrelles-Calvo, G.; de SAraújo, G.R.; Llopis-Pastor, E.; Carrillo, J.; Hernández-Hernández, M.; Rey, L.; Melean, N.R.; Escribano, I.; Antón, E.; Zamarro, C.; et al. *Candida* spp. co-infection in COVID-19 patients with severe pneumonia: Prevalence study and associated risk factors. *Respir. Med.* **2021**, *188*, 106619. [CrossRef]
115. Xu, X.; Han, M.; Li, T.; Sun, W.; Wang, D.; Fu, B.; Zhou, Y.; Zheng, X.; Yang, Y.; Li, X.; et al. Effective treatment of severe COVID-19 patients with tocilizumab. *Proc. Natl. Acad. Sci. USA* **2020**, *117*, 10970–10975. [CrossRef]
116. Hermine, O.; Mariette, X.; Tharaux, P.L.; Resche-Rigon, M.; Porcher, R.; Ravaud, P.; Bureau, S.; Dougados, M.; Tibi, A.; Azoulay, E.; et al. Effect of Tocilizumab vs Usual Care in Adults Hospitalized With COVID-19 and Moderate or Severe Pneumonia: A Randomized Clinical Trial. *JAMA Intern. Med.* **2021**, *181*, 32–40. [CrossRef]
117. Dimopoulos, G.; Almyroudi, M.-P.; Myrianthefs, P.; Rello, J. COVID-19-Associated Pulmonary Aspergillosis (CAPA). *J. Intensiv. Med.* **2021**, *1*, 71–80. [CrossRef]
118. Permpalung, N.; Chiang, T.P.; Massie, A.B.; Zhang, S.X.; Avery, R.K.; Nematollahi, S.; Ostrander, D.; Segev, D.L.; Marr, K.A. COVID-19 Associated Pulmonary Aspergillosis in Mechanically Ventilated Patients. *Clin. Infect. Dis.* **2021**, *74*, 83–91. [CrossRef]
119. Ergün, M.; Brüggemann, R.J.M.; Alanio, A.; Dellière, S.; van Arkel, A.; Bentvelsen, R.G.; Rijpstra, T.; Brugge, S.V.D.S.-V.D.; Lagrou, K.; Janssen, N.A.F.; et al. Aspergillus Test Profiles and Mortality in Critically Ill COVID-19 Patients. *J. Clin. Microbiol.* **2021**, *59*, e0122921. [CrossRef]
120. Paramythiotou, E.; Dimopoulos, G.; Koliakos, N.; Siopi, M.; Vourli, S.; Pournaras, S.; Meletiadis, J. Epidemiology and Incidence of COVID-19-Associated Pulmonary Aspergillosis (CAPA) in a Greek Tertiary Care Academic Reference Hospital. *Infect. Dis. Ther.* **2021**, *10*, 1779–1792. [CrossRef]
121. Omrani, A.S.; Koleri, J.; Ben Abid, F.; Daghfal, J.; Odaippurath, T.; Peediyakkal, M.Z.; Baiou, A.; Sarsak, E.; Elayana, M.; Kaleeckal, A.; et al. Clinical characteristics and risk factors for COVID-19-associated Candidemia. *Med. Mycol.* **2021**, *59*, 1262–1266. [CrossRef]
122. Kayaaslan, B.; Eser, F.; Kaya Kalem, A.; Bilgic, Z.; Asilturk, D.; Hasanoglu, I.; Ayhan, M.; Tezer Tekce, Y.; Erdem, D.; Turan, S.; et al. Characteristics of candidemia in COVID-19 patients; Increased incidence, earlier occurrence and higher mortality rates compared to non-COVID-19 patients. *Mycoses* **2021**, *64*, 1083–1091. [CrossRef]
123. Casalini, G.; Giacomelli, A.; Ridolfo, A.; Gervasoni, C.; Antinori, S. Invasive Fungal Infections Complicating COVID-19: A Narrative Review. *J. Fungi* **2021**, *7*, 921. [CrossRef]
124. Garcia-Bustos, V.; Cabanero-Navalon, M.D.; Ruiz-Saurí, A.; Ruiz-Gaitán, A.C.; Salavert, M.; Tormo, M.Á.; Pemán, J. What Do We Know about *Candida auris*? State of the Art, Knowledge Gaps, and Future Directions. *Microorganisms* **2021**, *9*, 2177. [CrossRef] [PubMed]
125. Macauley, P.; Epelbaum, O. Epidemiology and Mycology of Candidaemia in non-oncological medical intensive care unit patients in a tertiary center in the United States: Overall analysis and comparison between non-COVID-19 and COVID-19 cases. *Mycoses* **2021**, *64*, 634–640. [CrossRef] [PubMed]
126. Hanson, B.M.; Dinh, A.Q.; Tran, T.T.; Arenas, S.; Pronty, D.; Gershengorn, H.B.; Ferreira, T.; Arias, C.A.; Shukla, B.S. *Candida auris* Invasive Infections during a COVID-19 Case Surge. *Antimicrob. Agents Chemother.* **2021**, *65*, e0114621. [CrossRef] [PubMed]
127. Lyman, M.; Forsberg, K.; Reuben, J.; Dang, T.; Free, R.; Seagle, E.E.; Sexton, D.J.; Soda, E.; Jones, H.; Hawkins, D.; et al. Notes from the Field: Transmission of Pan-Resistant and Echinocandin-Resistant *Candida auris* in Health Care Facilities—Texas and the District of Columbia, January–April 2021. *MMWR. Morb. Mortal. Wkly. Rep.* **2021**, *70*, 1022–1023. [CrossRef]
128. Allaw, F.; Zahreddine, N.K.; Ibrahim, A.; Tannous, J.; Taleb, H.; Bizri, A.; Dbaibo, G.; Kanj, S. First *Candida auris* Outbreak during a COVID-19 Pandemic in a Tertiary-Care Center in Lebanon. *Pathogens* **2021**, *10*, 157. [CrossRef]
129. Almeida, J.N.D.; Francisco, E.C.; Hagen, F.; Brandão, I.B.; Pereira, F.M.; Presta Dias, P.H.; de Miranda Costa, M.M.; de Souza Jordão, R.T.; de Groot, T.; Colombo, A.L. Emergence of *Candida auris* in Brazil in a COVID-19 Intensive Care Unit. *J. Fungi* **2021**, *7*, 220. [CrossRef]
130. Villanueva-Lozano, H.; Treviño-Rangel, R.D.J.; González, G.M.; Ramírez-Elizondo, M.T.; Lara-Medrano, R.; Aleman-Bocanegra, M.C.; Guajardo-Lara, C.E.; Gaona-Chávez, N.; Castilleja-Leal, F.; Torre-Amione, G.; et al. Outbreak of *Candida auris* infection in a COVID-19 hospital in Mexico. *Clin. Microbiol. Infect.* **2021**, *27*, 813–816. [CrossRef]
131. Rudramurthy, S.M.; Hoenigl, M.; Meis, J.F.; Cornely, O.A.; Muthu, V.; Gangneux, J.P.; Perfect, J.; Chakrabarti, A.; Isham, E.A. ECMM/ISHAM recommendations for clinical management of COVID-19 associated mucormycosis in low- and middle-income countries. *Mycoses* **2021**, *64*, 1028–1037. [CrossRef]

Brief Report

A Trend towards Diaphragmatic Muscle Waste after Invasive Mechanical Ventilation in Multiple Trauma Patients—What to Expect?

Liliana Mirea [1,2], Cristian Cobilinschi [1,2,*], Raluca Ungureanu [1,2,*], Ana-Maria Cotae [1,2], Raluca Darie [1], Radu Tincu [1,3], Oana Avram [1,3], Sorin Constantinescu [4,5], Costin Minoiu [4,6], Alexandru Baetu [2,7] and Ioana Marina Grintescu [1,2]

1. Department of Anesthesiology and Intensive Care, Clinical Emergency Hospital Bucharest, 014461 Bucharest, Romania
2. Department of Anesthesiology and Intensive Care II, Carol Davila University of Medicine and Pharmacy, 050474 Bucharest, Romania
3. Department of Clinical Toxicology, Carol Davila University of Medicine and Pharmacy, 050474 Bucharest, Romania
4. Department of Radiology, Carol Davila University of Medicine and Pharmacy, 050474 Bucharest, Romania
5. Department of Radiology, Victor Atanasiu National Aviation and Space Medicine Institute, 010825 Bucharest, Romania
6. Department of Radiology, Clinical Emergency Hospital Bucharest, 014461 Bucharest, Romania
7. Department of Anesthesiology and Intensive Care, Grigore Alexandrescu Clinical Emergency Hospital for Children, 011743 Bucharest, Romania
* Correspondence: cristian.cobilinschi@umfcd.ro (C.C.); ralucaung@yahoo.com (R.U.); Tel.: +40-765018776 (C.C.); +40-744821993 (R.U.)

Abstract: Considering the prioritization of life-threatening injuries in trauma care, secondary dysfunctions such as ventilator-induced diaphragmatic dysfunction (VIDD) are often overlooked. VIDD is an entity induced by muscle inactivity during invasive mechanical ventilation, associated with a profound loss of diaphragm muscle mass. In order to assess the incidence of VIDD in polytrauma patients, we performed an observational, retrospective, longitudinal study that included 24 polytraumatized patients. All included patients were mechanically ventilated for at least 48 h and underwent two chest CT scans during their ICU stay. Diaphragmatic thickness was measured by two independent radiologists on coronal and axial images at the level of celiac plexus. The thickness of the diaphragm was significantly decreased on both the left and right sides (left side: -0.82 mm axial $p = 0.034$; -0.79 mm coronal $p = 0.05$; right side: -0.94 mm axial $p = 0.016$, -0.91 coronal $p = 0.013$). In addition, we obtained a positive correlation between the number of days of mechanical ventilation and the difference between the two measurements of the diaphragm thickness on both sides ($r = 0.5$; $p = 0.02$). There was no statistically significant correlation between the body mass indexes on admission, the use of vitamin C or N-acetyl cysteine, and the differences in diaphragmatic thickness.

Keywords: multiple trauma; thoracic trauma; mechanical ventilation; diaphragmatic muscle; diaphragmatic dysfunction; ventilator-induced diaphragmatic dysfunction

1. Introduction

Multiple trauma continues to be a global health problem, as it is so far the leading cause of death and disability [1]. Although real progress achieved through the development of advanced trauma life support principles, the morbidity associated with multiple trauma and mortality is still high [1,2].

Trauma-related respiratory failure may occur as a consequence of pulmonary contusion following blunt thoracic trauma but may also be induced indirectly by extrapulmonary factors such as associated traumatic brain injury, transfusions, fat embolism, and a systemic inflammatory response [3]. Acute respiratory distress syndrome (ARDS) after trauma may occur in more than 25% of cases with a variable onset depending on the severity of injuries [4]. Taking into account the multitude of risk factors for respiratory distress, mechanical ventilation is generally required for the management of multiple trauma patients [4].

The use of mechanical ventilation has significantly improved the outcome of multiple trauma patients through oxygenation and ventilation/perfusion ratio improvement [3,5]. However, inadequate mechanical ventilation proved to be more detrimental considering the high risk of ventilator-induced lung injury (VILI) [3]. Moreover, prolonged mechanical ventilation has an increased incidence of ventilator-associated pneumonia, a powerful determinant of increased mortality and prolonged hospital stay [6].

Recent data revealed that diaphragm muscle inactivity during mechanical ventilation might be associated with marked muscle atrophy and, subsequently, prolonged stay in the intensive care unit (ICU), weaning failure, and other unfavorable outcomes [7]. This new entity, called "ventilatory-induced diaphragmatic dysfunction (VIDD)", may be characterized by the loss of both slow-twitch and fast-twitch fibers secondary to increased oxidative stress and exacerbated proteolysis [7,8].

Although VIDD diagnostic may be identified through a variety of imaging tools, very few research papers were dedicated to this topic. As a result, this study aims to evaluate diaphragm muscle dimensions in multiple trauma patients under mechanical ventilation using computed tomography (CT) scan.

2. Materials and Methods

A retrospective analysis of mechanically ventilated multiple trauma patients admitted to the Clinical Emergency Hospital of Bucharest was performed. The main goal of this study was to evaluate early changes in diaphragmatic thickness using CT-scan images ordered for different reasons during the patient's stay in the ICU. Furthermore, the correlation between diaphragmatic measurements and the duration of mechanical ventilation was also determined.

All patients with multiple trauma, as defined by an Injury Severity Score ≥ 16, admitted into our hospital were included in the study group. Other inclusion criteria were mechanical ventilation for at least 48 h, as well as having performed two chest CT scan evaluations for different clinical reasons during their stay in the ICU. Multiple trauma patients with suspected or confirmed diaphragmatic rupture were not included in the final study group. Patients who had a history of invasive mechanical ventilation for more than 48 h in the last three months and comorbidities such as chronic obstructive, pulmonary disease (COPD), neoplasia, severe undernutrition (Body Mass Index (BMI) < 18 kg/m^2), autoimmune (e.g., polymyositis, dermatomyositis, systemic sclerosis) or neurological diseases (e.g., multiple sclerosis, myasthenia gravis) were excluded. Patients under long-term use of glucocorticoids or anabolic hormones were also excluded from the final study group. According to the local protocol and the latest guideline of the European Society for Clinical Nutrition and Metabolism (ESPEN), all patients included in the final study group benefited from enteral nutritional support in the first 48 h [9]. Calorie intake was based on an estimated energy expenditure measured through indirect calorimetry, and a protein intake of 1.3 g/kg body weight was targeted.

Diaphragmatic thickness measurements were performed twice by two independent radiologists using the CT scan images obtained on admission and after day 5. The celiac axis was used as a reference point. At this level, diaphragm muscle thickness was measured on axial as well as coronal images. Mean obtained values and differences between the two sets of measurements were used for the final analysis.

Demographic data and clinical and laboratory parameters, Trauma scores (e.g., Injury severity score—ISS), and ICU predictive scores (e.g., Acute Physiology and Chronic Health Evaluation II—APACHE II) were collected from electronic patient records and analyzed.

The whole study protocol was designed according to STROBE guidelines and was approved by the Institutional Ethics Committee of the Clinical Emergency Hospital in Bucharest.

2.1. Statistical Analysis

Statistical analysis of the database was performed using MeDCalc 14.1. A Bland—Altman concordance analysis between the two sets of measurements made by different radiologists was performed, and a simple linear regression was adjusted for the time interval between the two CT scans. In the linear regression analysis, the F-test derived from the ratio of the mean square regression and the mean square residual was used to evaluate whether the variability of the regression model could be explained by variations in the dependent variable or could be attributed to random chance. In other words, a significant F-test validated the relationship between the independent and the dependent variables.

The Spearman correlation coefficient (r) was also measured in order to describe the relations between the diaphragmatic thickness and other variables. Knowing that the correlation coefficient r ranges between −1 and 1, a negative r value indicates an inversely proportional relationship between variables, while a positive correlation confirms a proportional relation. When the r value is null, no correlation is validated. p value less than 0.05 was considered significant.

Sample Size

In order to establish the correlation between diaphragmatic thickness and the duration of mechanical ventilation, the sample size was estimated using the sample size calculator for correlation coefficients. As a result, 23 patients were needed in order to achieve a study power of 80% (type 1 error alpha with significance level 0.05 and type 2 error beta 0.2) with an estimated correlation coefficient of 0.55.

3. Results

Between 2019 and 2020, 105 multiple trauma patients were admitted into the Intensive Care Unit. Only 63 (66.15%) patients were admitted into our unit per primam, and 42 (44.1%) patients were transferred from other hospitals after variable intervals. After considering the exclusion criteria, the final study group included 24 patients. Details regarding excluded patients are presented in Figure 1.

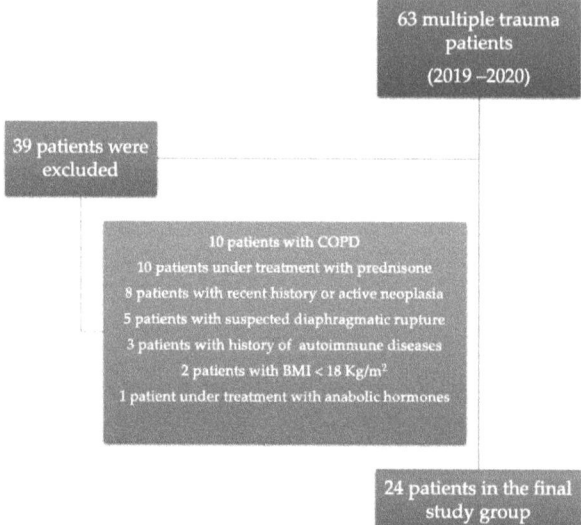

Figure 1. Final study group after the application of exclusion criteria.

The median age in the study group was 59 years (16–81) (Figure 2), and 15 patients (62.5%) were male. Nutritional status evaluation based on BMI calculation indicated a median value of 26 kg/m² (Figure 2).

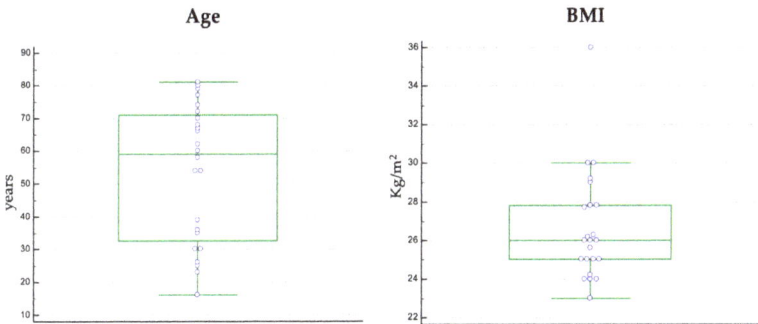

Figure 2. Age and BMI distribution in the final study group.

Trauma severity assessment revealed a median ISS score of 35 (18–57) (Figure 3). A detailed traumatic assessment is presented in Table 1. Disease severity assessment on ICU admission indicated a median APACHE II score of 19 (9–57) (Figure 3) and a median Sequential Organ Failure Assessment (SOFA) score of 7.

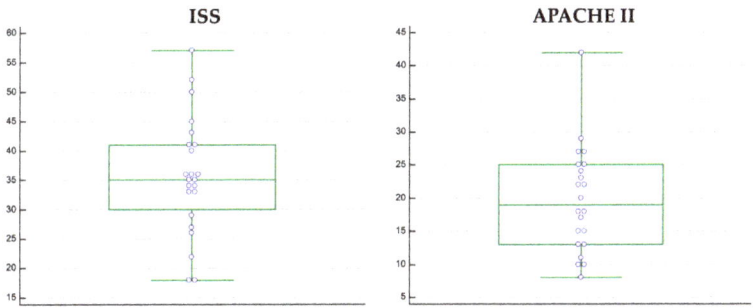

Figure 3. ISS and APACHE II scores distribution in the final study group.

Table 1. Traumatic assessment in the study group.

Body System	Number of Patients
Trauma brain injury	19 (79.1%)
Facial injury	9 (37.5%)
Thoracic trauma	22 (91.6%)
Abdominal trauma	7 (29.1%)
Pelvic injury	9 (37.5%)
Extremity injuries	17 (70.8%)

The mean duration of mechanical ventilation was 16.27 ± 9.1 days (median 16.5, range 28) (Figure 4), and the mean ICU stay was 26 days ± 12 days. Between the CT exams, all patients received only pressure-controlled mechanical ventilation with a mean PEEP value of 6 ± 1.1 cm H_2O. While admitted into the ICU, 18 patients (75%) received therapy with corticosteroids (the equivalent of dexamethasone 8 mg/day for at least 5 days) for different medical reasons, and 11 patients (45.8%) had their treatment supplemented with intravenous vitamin C (750 mg/daily). Antioxidant therapy with N-acetylcysteine (900 mg/daily for at least 5 days) was prescribed for only 6 patients (25%). No patient received muscle relaxants during the analyzed period. Out of the final study group, 18 patients (75%) were successfully extubated, and tracheostomy was necessary for 3 patients (7.2%).

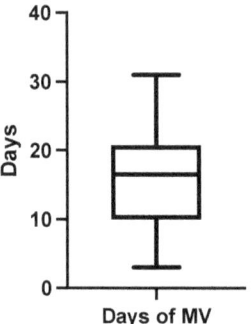

Figure 4. Duration of mechanical ventilation distribution.

To identify systematic biases or trends in the differences between the two radiological measurements, we performed a Bland—Altman concordance analysis (Figure 5). To calculate the measurement biases, the formula A − B/Average was used. The resulting measurement biases obtained were small (−0.02 axial left, 0.05 axial right, 0.08 coronal left, and −0.01 coronal right), and the 95% interval between the limits of agreement concludes that the two main investigators did not have large measurement differences and did not distort the resulted data.

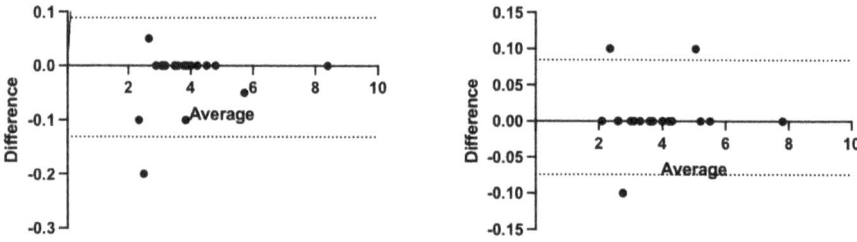

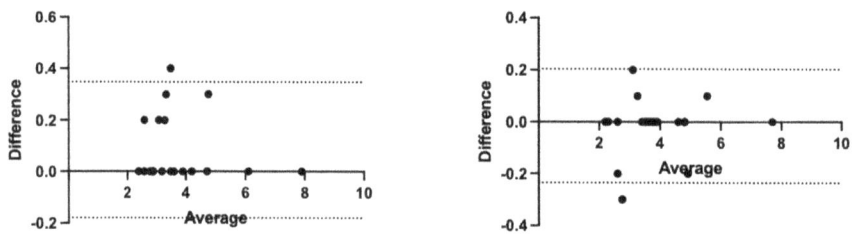

Figure 5. Bland—Altman concordance analysis for the two sets of measurements performed on admission.

All patients underwent at least two chest CT scan evaluations. The mean interval between the two radiological investigations was 6.08 ± 5.8 days. Considering that the second set of measurements could not be performed on exactly the same day for every patient from the study group, a regression analysis adjusted for the interval between the two radiological investigations was performed (Figure 6).

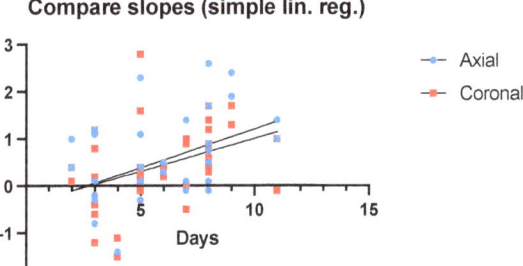

Figure 6. Simple linear regression adjusted for the time interval between the two CT scans.

Time is represented on the OX axis. The difference (in millimeters) between the axial and coronal measurements from the two CT scans is shown on the OY axis. The slope of the line corresponding to axial differences has a value of 0.16, with a Y-intercept of −0.43 and an X-intercept of 2.62. The slope of the coronal line has a value of 0.13 with a Y-intercept of −0.38 and an X-intercept of 2.76. The coronal slope (F = 6.18, p = 0.017) differs significantly from the value of 0 in statistical terms. The axial slope (F = 7.52, p = 0.094) did not meet the significance threshold. Based on these statistical data, a difference of 0.16 mm can be observed each day throughout the duration of mechanical ventilation procedures.

A proportional relationship was found between the diaphragmatic measurements obtained both on axial sections (left: r = 0.48, p = 0.035; right: r = 0.46, p = 0.046) and coronal sections (left: r = 0.62, p= 0.004; right: r = 0.46, p = 0.04), on the one hand, and the duration of mechanical ventilation (Figure 7), on the other hand, suggesting that prolonged mechanical ventilation is directly associated with diaphragmatic thinning.

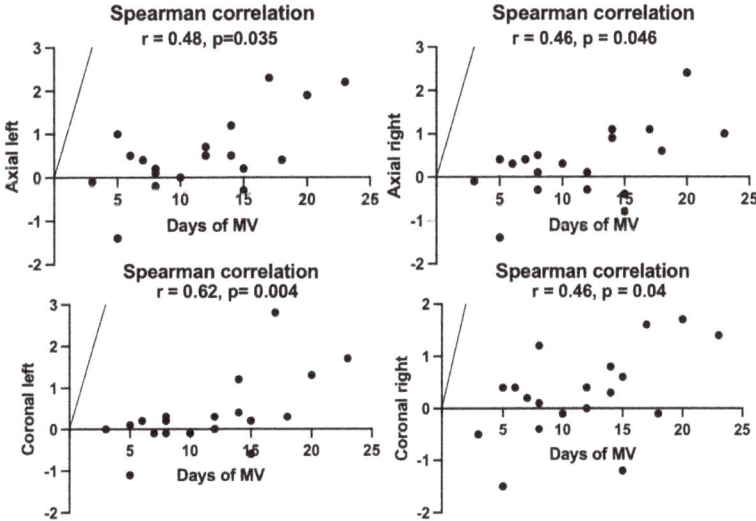

Figure 7. Correlation between the differences in the two diaphragmatic measurements and the duration of mechanical ventilation.

4. Discussion

The current study demonstrates that multiple trauma patients undergoing mechanical ventilation for more than 48 h may develop diaphragmatic dysfunction, characterized by a significant decrease in muscle thickness and a prolonged duration of mechanical ventilation.

Over the last decade, the management of multiple trauma patients benefited from continuous advances obtained in the fields of trauma life support or damage control resuscitation. However, less priority has been given to the impact of all implemented supportive measures [1,10]. It has already been proven that the occurrence of respiratory dysfunction after a traumatic injury and the need for invasive mechanical ventilation may be independent factors responsible for worsening the long-term outcome [4]. Trauma-related respiratory distress may be induced by a direct lung injury (e.g., chest trauma, aspiration of gastric content), as well as by the systemic inflammatory response secondary to traumatic shock or by extensive transfusions [11,12].

Although mechanical ventilation is undoubtedly a lifesaving therapy for many multiple trauma patients, excessive stress and strain applied to an injured lung during mechanical ventilation may cause an antithetical effect [13,14]. The use of elevated tidal volumes and driving pressures, as well as the inappropriate positive end-expiratory pressure values, are associated with exacerbated inflammatory responses (biotrauma) that generate additional detrimental effects on traumatic lung injuries [14,15].

In addition to VILI, secondary effects of mechanical ventilation on diaphragmatic muscle were also reported [8]. For patients undergoing invasive mechanical ventilation, several mechanisms of diaphragmatic myotrauma were described, such as excessive ventilatory support (over-assistance), inadequate diaphragmatic work unload (under-assistance), eccentric diaphragm contractions during patient-ventilator asynchrony or longitudinal atrophy caused by increased PEEP values [16]. All these mechanisms are finally translated into exacerbated inflammation, mitochondrial dysfunction, oxidative stress, autophagy, and protein catabolism [7,17]. Whether mechanical ventilation-related autophagy has a real detrimental effect is something that remains unknown, given that this process promotes the clearance of altered mitochondria and muscle function improvement [7]. Nevertheless, recent data suggest that calpain, a skeletal muscle protease, plays a central role in VIDD through the activation of the ubiquitin–proteasome system or caspase-3 [17].

Several diagnostic tools are proposed for diaphragmatic muscle dysfunction. However, in multiple trauma patients diaphragmatic, CT evaluation may be more advantageous, considering that it may provide data regarding diaphragmatic structural integrity and subdiaphragmatic processes that may influence respiratory mechanics [18,19]. Taking into account that CT scan has become a routine diagnostic tool, using the already acquired images for diaphragm muscle composition evaluation may be very time- and cost-efficient [20]. For all patients included in this current retrospective analysis, CT images ordered for different medical reasons were used.

In our study group, multiple trauma patients undergoing mechanical ventilation suffered a decrease in diaphragmatic muscle thickness after a relatively short duration of mechanical ventilation (6.08 days). Lee et al. reported that changes in diaphragmatic thickness were identified on CT scan examinations after a mean period of 18 days [21]. However, diaphragmatic ultrasound evaluation revealed that the thinning of the muscle might be detected even earlier, after only 48 h of mechanical ventilation [22]. A recent study by Gatti et al., who evaluated the thickness of the diaphragmatic muscle in six different areas, also revealed that the thickness of the left posterior pillar decreases with mechanical ventilation duration [23]. Moreover, it has also been demonstrated that diaphragm thickness correlates with the skeletal muscle index in patients undergoing mechanical ventilation, including multiple trauma patients [23,24].

Assuming that in the final study group, only multiple trauma patients were included, without any potential muscular dysfunction, the rate of the decrease of diaphragmatic thickness was remarkably high in comparison with similar research data.

Limitations

The main limitation of this study is the retrospective data evaluation. Considering that diaphragmatic dysfunction was evaluated only through a retrospective analysis of CT scans, no functional imaging was available.

Despite achieving a calculated sample size, one of the main limitations of this study is the limited sample size (n = 24).

At the moment, there is no recommended "reference" point for diaphragmatic measurements. In this context, the celiac axis was used as a reference point on both axial and coronal images based on previously published data [21]. However, recent data suggest that multiple reference points should be used considering the heterogeneous structure of the diaphragm [23].

Taking into account that the skeletal muscle index is considered an independent risk factor for prolonged mechanical ventilation, our current research lacks further data regarding body composition.

Further research may be needed in order to evaluate anatomical and functional diaphragmatic changes by combining CT scanning and ultrasonography.

5. Conclusions

Our current research suggests that diaphragmatic morphological changes may occur surprisingly faster after a relatively short duration of invasive mechanical ventilation in patients without any prior evidence of chronic comorbidities.

Evaluation of diaphragmatic dysfunction may be performed with a variety of imagistic tools. Computed tomography examination, routinely used for primary and secondary evaluation of multiple trauma patients, may also offer the advantage of diaphragmatic evaluation.

Author Contributions: Conceptualization, L.M. and C.C.; methodology, C.C. and A.-M.C.; software, A.B.; validation, R.T., O.A. and I.M.G.; formal analysis, A.B.; investigation, C.M. and S.C.; resources, R.D. and A.-M.C.; data curation, R.D.; writing—original draft preparation, C.C.; writing—review and editing, R.U.; visualization, L.M.; supervision, I.M.G.; project administration, S.C. All authors have read and agreed to the published version of the manuscript.

Funding: This research received no external funding.

Institutional Review Board Statement: The study was conducted in accordance with the Declaration of Helsinki and approved by the Clinical Emergency Hospital of Bucharest Ethics Committee (protocol code 11096/03.12.2019).

Informed Consent Statement: Patient consent was waived due to the retrospective analysis of the presented data.

Data Availability Statement: All presented data are available on demand.

Conflicts of Interest: The authors declare no conflict of interest.

References

1. Van Breugel, J.M.M.; Niemeyer, M.J.S.; Houwert, R.M.; Groenwold, R.H.H.; Leenen, L.P.H.; Van Wessem, K.J.P. Global changes in mortality rates in polytrauma patients admitted to the ICU—A systematic review. *World J. Emerg. Surg.* **2020**, *15*, 55. [CrossRef] [PubMed]
2. van Maarseveen, O.E.C.; Ham, W.H.W.; van de Ven, N.L.M.; Saris, T.F.F.; Leenen, L.P.H. Effects of the application of a checklist during trauma resuscitations on ATLS adherence, team performance, and patient-related outcomes: A systematic review. *Eur. J. Trauma Emerg. Surg.* **2020**, *46*, 65–72. [CrossRef] [PubMed]
3. Noorbakhsh, M.R.; Kriley, I.R. Management of severe respiratory failure in complex trauma patients. *J. Emerg. Crit. Care Med.* **2018**, *2*, 26. [CrossRef]
4. Ramin, S.; Charbit, J.; Jaber, S.; Capdevila, X. Acute respiratory distress syndrome after chest trauma: Epidemiology, specific physiopathology and ventilation strategies. *Anaesth. Crit. Care Pain Med.* **2018**, *38*, 265–276. [CrossRef]
5. Eman Shebl, R.; Samra, S.R.; Abderaboh, M.M.; Mousa, M.S. Continuous positive airway pressure ventilation versus Bi-level positive airway pressure ventilation in patients with blunt chest trauma. *Egypt. J. Chest Dis. Tuberc.* **2015**, *64*, 203–208. [CrossRef]
6. Hofman, M.; Andruszkow, H.; Kobbe, P.; Poeze, M.; Hildebrand, F. Incidence of post-traumatic pneumonia in poly-traumatized patients: Identifying the role of traumatic brain injury and chest trauma. *Eur. J. Trauma Emerg. Surg.* **2020**, *46*, 11–19. [CrossRef]
7. Peñuelas, O.; Keough, E.; López-rodríguez, L.; Carriedo, D.; Gonçalves, G. Ventilator-induced diaphragm dysfunction: Translational mechanisms lead to therapeutic alternatives in the critically ill. *Intensive Care Med. Exp.* **2019**, *7* (Suppl. S1), 48. [CrossRef]

8. Petrof, B.J. Diaphragm Weakness in the Critically Ill: Basic Mechanisms Reveal Therapeutic Opportunities. *Chest* **2018**, *154*, 1395–1403. [CrossRef]
9. Singer, P.; Blaser, A.R.; Berger, M.M.; Alhazzani, W.; Calder, P.C.; Casaer, M.P.; Hiesmayr, M.; Mayer, K.; Montejo, J.C.; Pichard, C.; et al. ESPEN guideline on clinical nutrition in the intensive care unit. *Clin. Nutr.* **2019**, *38*, 48–79. [CrossRef]
10. Supinski, G.S.; Morris, P.E.; Dhar, S.; Callahan, L.A. Diaphragm Dysfunction in Critical Illness. *Chest* **2018**, *153*, 1040–1051. [CrossRef]
11. Papadakos, P.J.; Karcz, M.; Lachmann, B. Mechanical ventilation in trauma. *Curr. Opin. Anaesthesiol.* **2010**, *23*, 228–232. [CrossRef] [PubMed]
12. Anderson, M.W.; Watson, G.A. Traumatic shock: The fifth shock. *J. Trauma Nurs.* **2013**, *20*, 37–43. [CrossRef]
13. Beitler, J.R.; Malhotra, A.; Thompson, B.T. Ventilator-induced Lung Injury. *Clin. Chest Med.* **2016**, *37*, 633–646. [CrossRef] [PubMed]
14. Cobilinschi, C.; Cotae, A.; Ungureanu, R.; Țincu, R.; Grințescu, I.M.; Mirea, L. Ventilation in critically ill obese patients—Why it should be done differently? *Signa Vitae* **2022**, 1–6. [CrossRef]
15. Gattinoni, L.; Marini, J.J.; Collino, F.; Maiolo, G.; Rapetti, F.; Tonetti, T.; Vasques, F.; Quintel, M. The future of mechanical ventilation: Lessons from the present and the past. *Crit. Care* **2017**, *21*, 183. [CrossRef]
16. Goligher, E.C.; Brochard, L.J.; Reid, W.D.; Fan, E.; Saarela, O.; Slutsky, A.S.; Kavanagh, B.P.; Rubenfeld, G.D.; Ferguson, N.D. Diaphragmatic myotrauma: A mediator of prolonged ventilation and poor patient outcomes in acute respiratory failure. *Lancet Respir. Med.* **2019**, *7*, 90–98. [CrossRef]
17. Hyatt, H.W.; Ozdemir, M.; Yoshihara, T.; Nguyen, B.L.; Deminice, R.; Powers, S.K. Calpains play an essential role in mechanical ventilation-induced diaphragmatic weakness and mitochondrial dysfunction. *Redox Biol.* **2021**, *38*, 101802. [CrossRef]
18. Kharma, N. Dysfunction of the diaphragm: Imaging as a diagnostic tool. *Curr. Opin. Pulm. Med.* **2013**, *19*, 394–398. [CrossRef]
19. Minami, T.; Manzoor, K.; McCool, F.D. Assessing Diaphragm Function in Chest Wall and Neuromuscular Diseases. *Clin. Chest Med.* **2018**, *39*, 335–344. [CrossRef]
20. Tolonen, A.; Pakarinen, T.; Sassi, A.; Kyttä, J.; Cancino, W.; Rinta-Kiikka, I.; Pertuz, S.; Arponen, O. Methodology, clinical applications, and future directions of body composition analysis using computed tomography (CT) images: A review. *Eur. J. Radiol.* **2021**, *145*, 109943. [CrossRef]
21. Lee, G.D.; Kim, H.C.; Yoo, J.W.; Lee, S.J.; Cho, Y.J.; Bae, K.; Lee, J.D. Computed tomography confirms a reduction in diaphragm thickness in mechanically ventilated patients. *J. Crit. Care* **2016**, *33*, 47–50. [CrossRef] [PubMed]
22. Grosu, H.B.; Lee, Y.I.; Lee, J.; Eden, E.; Eikermann, M.; Rose, K.M. Diaphragm Muscle Thinning in Patients Who Are Mechanically Ventilated. *Chest* **2012**, *142*, 1455–1460. [CrossRef] [PubMed]
23. Gatti, S.; Abbruzzese, C.; Ippolito, D.; Lombardi, S.; De Vito, A.; Gandola, D.; Meroni, V.; Sala, V.L.; Sironi, S.; Pesenti, A.; et al. Ultrasound Versus Computed Tomography for Diaphragmatic Thickness and Skeletal Muscle Index during Mechanical Ventilation. *Diagnostics* **2022**, *12*, 2890. [CrossRef] [PubMed]
24. Giani, M.; Rezoagli, E.; Grassi, A.; Porta, M.; Riva, L.; Famularo, S.; Barbaro, A.; Bernasconi, D.; Ippolito, D.; Bellani, G.; et al. Low skeletal muscle index and myosteatosis as predictors of mortality in critically ill surgical patients. *Nutrition* **2022**, *101*, 111687. [CrossRef] [PubMed]

Disclaimer/Publisher's Note: The statements, opinions and data contained in all publications are solely those of the individual author(s) and contributor(s) and not of MDPI and/or the editor(s). MDPI and/or the editor(s) disclaim responsibility for any injury to people or property resulting from any ideas, methods, instructions or products referred to in the content.

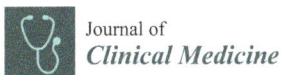

Systematic Review

Proadrenomedullin in the Management of COVID-19 Critically Ill Patients in Intensive Care Unit: A Systematic Review and Meta-Analysis of Evidence and Uncertainties in Existing Literature

Giorgia Montrucchio [1,2,*], Eleonora Balzani [1], Davide Lombardo [1], Alice Giaccone [1], Anna Vaninetti [1], Giulia D'Antonio [1], Francesca Rumbolo [3], Giulio Mengozzi [3] and Luca Brazzi [1,2]

1. Department of Surgical Sciences, University of Turin, 10126 Turin, Italy
2. Department of Anesthesia, Intensive Care and Emergency, Città della Salute e della Scienza Hospital, Corso Dogliotti 14, 10126 Turin, Italy
3. Clinical Biochemistry Laboratory, Città della Salute e della Scienza Hospital, University of Turin, 10126 Turin, Italy
* Correspondence: g.montrucchio@gmail.com

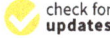

Citation: Montrucchio, G.; Balzani, E.; Lombardo, D.; Giaccone, A.; Vaninetti, A.; D'Antonio, G.; Rumbolo, F.; Mengozzi, G.; Brazzi, L. Proadrenomedullin in the Management of COVID-19 Critically Ill Patients in Intensive Care Unit: A Systematic Review and Meta-Analysis of Evidence and Uncertainties in Existing Literature. *J. Clin. Med.* **2022**, *11*, 4543. https://doi.org/10.3390/jcm11154543

Academic Editor: Spyros D. Mentzelopoulos

Received: 23 June 2022
Accepted: 2 August 2022
Published: 4 August 2022

Publisher's Note: MDPI stays neutral with regard to jurisdictional claims in published maps and institutional affiliations.

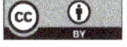

Copyright: © 2022 by the authors. Licensee MDPI, Basel, Switzerland. This article is an open access article distributed under the terms and conditions of the Creative Commons Attribution (CC BY) license (https://creativecommons.org/licenses/by/4.0/).

Abstract: Mid-regional proadrenomedullin (MR-proADM) is a new biomarker of endothelial damage and its clinical use is increasing in sepsis and respiratory infections and recently in SARS-CoV-2 infection. We conducted a systematic review and meta-analysis to clarify the use of MR-proADM in severe COVID-19 disease. After Pubmed, Embase, and Scopus search, registries, and gray literature, deduplication, and selection of full-texts, we found 21 studies addressing the use of proadrenomedullin in COVID-19. All the studies were published between 2020 and 2022 from European countries. A total of 9 studies enrolled Intensive Care Unit (ICU) patients, 4 were conducted in the Emergency Department, and 8 had mixed populations. Regarding the ICU critically ill patients, 4 studies evaluating survival as primary outcome were available, of which 3 reported completed data. Combining the selected studies in a meta-analysis, a total of 252 patients were enrolled; of these, 182 were survivors and 70 were non-survivors. At the admission to the ICU, the average MR-proADM level in survivor patients was 1.01 versus 1.64 in non-survivor patients. The mean differences of MR-proADM values in survivors vs. non-survivors was −0.96 (95% CI from −1.26, to −0.65). Test for overall effect: Z = 6.19 ($p < 0.00001$) and heterogeneity was $I^2 = 0\%$. MR-proADM ICU admission levels seem to predict mortality among the critical COVID-19 population. Further, prospective studies, focused on critically ill patients and investigating a reliable MR-proADM cut-off, are needed to provide adequate guidance to its use in severe COVID-19.

Keywords: proadrenomedullin; MR-proADM; SARS-CoV-2; COVID-19; biomarkers; intensive care; endothelitis

1. Introduction

Proadrenomedullin (pro-ADM) is a 52 multipotent regulatory amino acid peptide expressed in various tissues and organs, upregulated by hypoxia, inflammatory cytokines, bacterial products, and shear stress. Its precursor, mid-regional pro-ADM (MR-proADM), is currently considered an effective biomarker of endothelial damage as its increase in plasma seems to correlate with disease severity [1].

The mechanisms underlying this correlation are poorly defined even if associations with cardiovascular and thromboembolic complications, immunosuppression, and sepsis-like multiorgan dysfunction have been reported [2]. Regarding SARS-CoV-2, an association between MR-proADM levels and virus-induced endothelial damage is assumed. As endothelitis emerges as a prominent feature of the severe COVID-19 disease [3,4], an association between MR-proADM levels and virus-induced endothelial damage has been hypothesized as the pathophysiological mechanisms in COVID-19-induced critical illness seem related to an increased incidence of cardiovascular and thromboembolic complications, immune cell deactivation, and sepsis-like multiple organ failure. A rising number of studies has proposed that virus-induced endothelitis, resulting in impaired vascular blood flow, coagulation, and leakage, may partially explain the development of organ dysfunction and edema [5]. In this sense, since ADM has been shown to play a key role in reducing vascular hyper permeability and promoting endothelial stability and integrity following severe infections [3], MR-proADM might be a potential biomarker of COVID-19 severity and may be able to mimic disease progression, allowing the identification of patients most at risk of developing a severe form of SARS-CoV-2-related illness or multi-organ failure.

If the prognostic role of MR-proADM was demonstrated in the context of pneumonia, sepsis, and septic shock—currently the most studied areas evaluating the predictive capacity of this biomarker [3,6,7]—the pathological mechanism has not been fully clarified; nor is it in the case of severe COVID-19, where most of the studies have a limited size and were designed in the context of a pandemic emergency, with heterogeneity of objectives and study contexts.

To find an answer to uncertainties regarding the role of MR-proADM as a predictive marker of the severity of COVID-19 disease, we systematically present a review of the current literature. The possibility of constructing a meta-analysis capable of establishing the MR-proADM clinical severity cut-off in COVID-19 patients admitted to the Intensive Care Unit (ICU) was subsequently investigated.

2. Materials and Methods

This systematic review and meta-analysis followed the Preferred Reporting Items for Systematic Reviews and Meta-Analyses (PRISMA) statement [7]. The protocol was registered prospectively in OSF (DOI 10.17605/OSF.IO/V93EW, link https://osf.io/v93ew/ accessed on 1 May 2022). Since not all studies express values of pro-ADM levels by the same assessment technique, we refer to proADM when including results by all methods and to MR-proADM when levels were determined with the B.R.A.H.M.S. KRYPTOR compact PLUS (Thermo Fisher Scientific, Hennigsdorf, Germany) technique.

2.1. Eligibility Criteria

The research was conducted on 25 April 2022; randomized controlled trials (RCTs), non-randomized controlled trials (NRCTs), commentaries, letters, systematic reviews, and meta-analyses published in English and Italian were eligible for inclusion. The meta-analysis was then performed evaluating studies conducted only in the ICU setting to assess if MR-proADM levels may vary in survivors versus non survivors in critically ill patients with severe COVID-19 disease.

2.2. Information Sources

This systematic review was performed using Pubmed, Embase, and Scopus databases, and was implemented with the use of registries (clinicaltrials.gov, accessed on 25 April 2022) and gray literature searches.

2.3. Search Strategy

To perform the systematic review, the following search strategies were selected:
- PubMed: "proADM" [All Fields] AND ("COVID-19" [All Fields] OR "COVID-19" [MeSH Terms] OR "COVID-19 vaccines" [All Fields] OR "COVID-19 vaccines" [MeSH Terms] OR "COVID-19 serotherapy" [All Fields] OR "COVID-19 serotherapy" [Supplementary Concept] OR "COVID-19 nucleic acid testing" [All Fields] OR "COVID-19 nucleic acid testing" [MeSH Terms] OR "COVID-19 serological testing" [All Fields] OR "COVID-19 serological testing" [MeSH Terms] OR "COVID-19 testing" [All Fields] OR "COVID-19 testing" [MeSH Terms] OR "SARS-CoV-2" [All Fields] OR "SARS-CoV-2" [MeSH Terms] OR "severe acute respiratory syndrome coronavirus 2" [All Fields] OR

"ncov" [All Fields] OR "2019 ncov" [All Fields] OR (("coronavirus" [MeSH Terms] OR "coronavirus" [All Fields] OR "cov" [All Fields]) AND 1 November 2019:3000/12/31 [Date—Publication])); Embase, Scopus, clinicaltrials.gov, and greylit.org: ('proad-renomedullin'/exp OR proadrenomedullin) AND ('coronavirus disease 2019'/exp OR 'coronavirus disease 2019').

2.4. Selection and Data Collection Process

Search results were exported to EndNote V.X9 (Clarivate Analytics, Philadelphia, PA, USA). Duplicates were automatically removed. The review process was carried out in three steps consisting of title and abstract review process, full-text review process, and risk of bias assessment. For each level, four authors (G.M., E.B., D.L., and A.G.) independently screened the articles with conflicts resolved by a third author (L.B.).

2.5. Study Risk of Bias Assessment

To assess the risk of bias, the Risk Of Bias In Non-randomized Studies—of Interventions (ROBINS-i) tool [8] and the Rob 2.0 tool [9] were used for NRCTs and RCTs, respectively. Risk of bias assessment was carried out by four authors (G.M., E.B., D.L., and A.G.) independently; where discrepancies were noticed, a third author (L.B.) was involved to resolve them.

2.6. Synthesis Methods

The main outcome was the use of pro-ADM as a prognostic marker in patients with COVID-19. A planned Excel spreadsheet was used to extract data (patient's characteristics, type of surgery, follow-up periods, outcome measures, and main results). The results of the systematic review were reported in a summary table with the main features described for each study. All eligible studies were evaluated to collect data regarding MR-proADM levels among survivors and non-survivors in ICU population with severe COVID-19 disease. Given that the primary outcome was MR-proADM levels, data presented as median and interquartile range were converted into mean and standard deviation using validated online converters [10]. Estimates of effect were derived from quantitative analysis utilizing Review Manager 5.4 [11]. MR-proADM mean levels and standard deviations were used to evaluate mean differences (MD) with a 95% confidence interval (95% CI). Inverse variance method and random effects were used to assess overall MD. Statistical significance was set at $p < 0.05$. To evaluate the size of the effect of the MD, we considered levels of 0.2, 0.5, and 0.8 as small, medium, and large effects. Heterogeneity was assessed using the I^2 index, with values of 25%, 50%, and 75% taken to indicate low, moderate, and high levels of heterogeneity, respectively [12].

3. Results

3.1. Study Selection

The systematic literature search retrieved 65 results in databases and one in registers. A flow chart describing the complete literature search process is reported in Figure 1.

After de-duplication, 26 studies were selected for full-text review. Four papers were then excluded because they did not match the inclusion criteria. After an additional literature check, three papers were included in the systematic review [13–15]. A total of 20 articles were submitted to the systematic review.

In order to determine ICU-admitted patients' pro-ADM cut offs, a new revision of selected studies was made, with the aim to organize data in a meta-analysis. Only 4 studied satisfied meta-analysis inclusion criteria. The reasons for exclusion of the 17 papers were: 12 papers did not consider ICU population, 2 papers evaluated different outcomes (i.e., renal replacement therapy, superinfections) [15,16], 1 analyzed MR-proADM levels among children versus adults patients [17], 1 considered pro-ADM levels with a different technique (bioactive ADM) [18], and 1 was excluded because it presented a population already included in a previously published study [19].

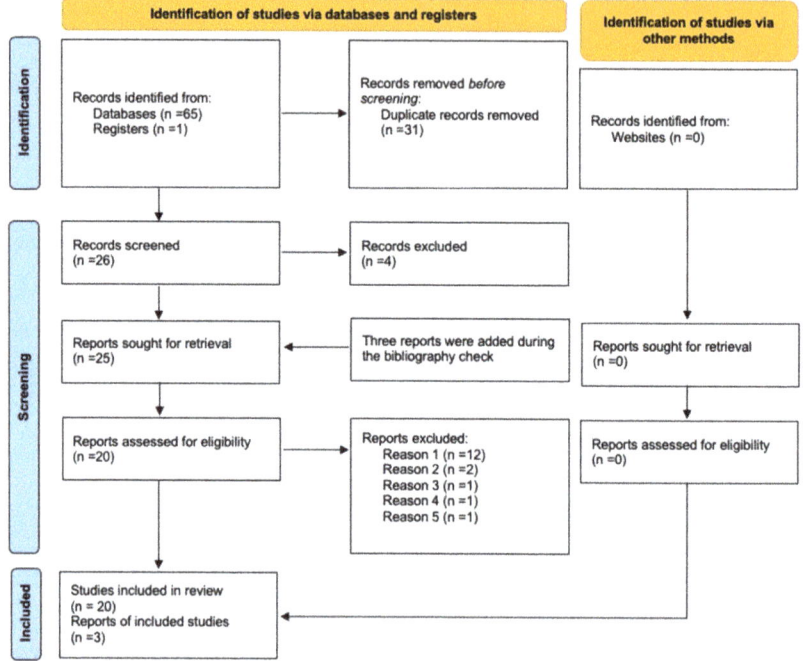

Figure 1. PRISMA flow-diagram. The reasons for exclusion: reason 1: papers which did not consider ICU population; reason 2: papers which evaluated different outcome (i.e., renal replacement therapy, superinfections); reason 3: analyzed MR-proADM levels among children versus adult patients; reason 4: considered pro-ADM levels with a different technique (bioactive ADM); reason 5: presented a population already included in a previously published study.

One of the four remaining studies included in the meta-analysis process did not report the standard deviation, and for this reason, was not included in calculation [20]. The meta-analysis was then performed with the three remaining studies.

3.2. Systematic Review

Study Characteristics

Characteristics of the individual studies are provided in Table 1.

The studies were published between 2020 and 2022. Of the 21 selected articles, 9 enrolled an ICU population, 4 were conducted in an Emergency Department (ED), and 8 had mixed populations. All studies were conducted in European countries except for 2, conducted in Russia: 8 studies were from Italy, 4 from Spain, 2 from the Netherlands, 2 from Germany, 1 from France, 1 from the UK, and 1 from Switzerland. The outcome most frequently considered was mortality. Of the 21 selected articles, 16 agree that the value of proADM predicts mortality or poor outcomes.

The enrollment period, as shown in Table 1, was similar for almost all the studies considered. Other data such as Area Under the Curve (AUC) and proADM considered cut-off are shown in Table 1. All studies considered used as MR-proADM determining levels the B.R.A.H.M.S. KRYPTOR compact PLUS (Thermo Fisher Scientific, Hennigsdorf, Germany) technique, except for one paper [18].

Table 1. Descriptive table of systematic review results, including the 20 full texts analyzed.

Author	Year	Type of Study	Country	Period	Number of Patient	Clinical Setting	Timing	Outcome	Findings	AUC	Cut Off
Benedetti et al. [21]	2021	prospective observational	Italy	March–April 2020	21	IMCU	admission (T0), 24 h (T1), T3 e 5	severe disease	• optimal MR-proADM cut-off point was 1.07 nmol/L (sensitivity 91% and specificity 71%) • strongest association with 30-days mortality	0.81	1.07 nmol/L
Garcia de Guadiana-Romualdo et al. [22]	2021	prospective observational	Spain	March–April 2021	99	ED	T0	mortality/severe disease progression	• highest performance for predicting 90-day mortality • low level shows high negative predictive value to rule-out mid-term mortality; • independent predictor for mid-term mortality; • highest prognostic accuracy for short-term mortality	0.871	0.80 nmol/L
Girona-Alarcon et al. [17]	2021	prospective observational cohort	Spain	March–June 2020	20	ICU	hospitalization	pediatric vs. adult population	• higher values in children than in adults		
Gregoriano et al. [23]	2021	prospective observational	Switzerland	February–April 2020	89	mixed population	T0, T1, T2, T3	in-hospital mortality	• increased 1.5-fold in patients with a fatal outcome • safe rule-out of in-hospital mortality in patients with low levels	0.78	0.93 nmol/L
Indirli et al. [24]	2022	retrospective	Italy	March–June 2020	116	IMCU	At admission	in-hospital mortality	• with copeptin, predicted in-hospital mortality, occurrence of sepsis or AKI	0.79	>1
Lhote et al. *	2021	prospective multicentric	France	July 2020 to February 2021	170	ICU	T0	SOFA at day 3	• insufficient data to confirm proADM validity	NA	NA
Lo Sasso et al. [25]	2021	retrospective observational	Italy	September–October 2020	110	mixed population	hospitalization	Inhospital mortality	• good accuracy for predicting mortality	0.95	1.73 nmol/L
Malinina et al. ** [15]	2020	retrospective observational	Russia		37	ICU		Bacterial superinfection	• predicts superinfections in patients with SARS-CoV-2 pneumonia		
Mendez et al. [26]	2021	longitudinal	Spain	March–June 2020	210	ED	T0	in-hospital mortality	• higher levels in COVID-19 patients associated with poor outcomes • a sustained increase is associated with altered DLCO	NA	1.16

Table 1. Cont.

Author	Year	Type of Study	Country	Period	Number of Patient	Clinical Setting	Timing	Outcome	Findings	AUC	Cut Off
Minieri et al. [27]	2021	not specified	Italy	not specified	321	ED	ED-triage	overall in-hospital mortality	• key role in the mortality risk stratification at the admission in ED	0.85	1.105
Montrucchio et al. [28]	2021	prospective observational	Italy	March–June 2020	57	ICU	T0–1, T3, T7, T14	ICU mortality—trend	• increased plasma levels indicate severity and worse prognosis in CAP, sepsis, ARDS, perioperative care • higher values in dying patients • predict mortality better than other biomarkers • repeated measurement may support a rapid decision-making	0.85	>1.8 nmol/L *
Moore et al. [29]	2022	prospective	UK	April–June 2020	135	ED	at the admission	30-days mortality	• predicts 30-day mortality	0.8441	1.54
Oblitas et al. [19]	2021	prospective	Spain	August–November 2020	95	ICU	once within 72 h of ICU admission	30-day mortality and 30-day combined event	• predicts 30-day mortality and 30-day poor outcomes	0.73 and 0.72	≥1
Popov et al. [30]	2021	prospective observational	Russia		97	mixed population		mortality	• most significant predictor of mortality compared to procalcitonin, saturation and NEWS score.	0.75	0.895 nmol/L
Roedl et al. [16]	2021	observational	Germany	March–September 2020	64	ICU	ICU admission	RRT versus no-RRT	• on ICU admission is a strong predictor for RRT • early prediction within 24 h after admission	0.69	
Simon et al. [18]	2021	prospective observational	Germany	March–April 2020	53	ICU	Daily, T1–7	ARDS, ECMO, MV, RRT	• associated with the severity of ARDS, • associated with need for organ support • correlation with 28-day mortality		bio-ADM: 70 pg/mL *
Sozio et al. [31]	2021	retrospective	Italy	March–May 2020	111	mixed population	ED admission	severe disease	• significantly higher in patients hospitalized with COVID-19 and with negative outcome	0.85	Mortality 0.895 nmol/L
Spoto et al. [32]	2020	prospective observational	Italy	April–June 2020	69	mixed population	hospitalization	endothelial damage, MOF, severe disease	• marker of organ damage, disease severity, and mortality • values ≥2 nmol/L were associated with a significantly higher mortality risk	0.78	ARDS 3.04; mortality 2 nmol/L

Table 1. Cont.

Author	Year	Type of Study	Country	Period	Number of Patient	Clinical Setting	Timing	Outcome	Findings	AUC	Cut Off
Van Oers et al. [33]	2021	prospective	the Netherlands	March–May 2020	105	ICU	on a daily basis, during the first 7 days	28-day mortalit	• with CT-proET-1 is able to identify patients with worst outcome • significantly higher levels of MR-proADM and CT-proET-1 in non-survivors persisted over time	0.84	1.57
Zaninotto et al. [34]	2021	retrospective	Italy	November	135	mixed population	7 days	clinical outcomes	• additional clinical value in stratifying risk and establishing the prognosis	0.900	1.50

List of abbreviations: Area Under the Curve, AUC; Emergency Department, ED; Intensive Care Unit, ICU; Intermediate Care Unit, IMCU; T: time express in days; Multiorgan Failure, MOF; Acute Respiratory Distress Syndrome, ARDS; Extracorporeal Membrane Oxygenation, ECMO; Diffusing capacity for carbon monoxide, DLCO; Mechanical Ventilation, MV; Renal Replacement Therapy, RRT; C-terminal proendothelin-1, CT-proET-1; MR-proadrenomedullin, MR-proADM; Sequential Organ Failure Assessment, SOFA. * *only abstract available.* ** *full-text article provided by the corresponding author.*

3.3. Meta-Analysis

Considering the four studies that were candidates for inclusion in the meta-analysis, one [20] could not be included due to lack of total population number. The other three studies reported MR-proADM admission values in ICU patient populations with critical COVID-19 disease divided by survivors and non-survivors. All studies considered were conducted in 2021. Regarding the country, one was conducted in Spain, one in Italy, and one in the Netherlands.

Among the selected studies, 252 patients were enrolled; of these, 182 were survivors and 70 non-survivors (Figure 2). At the admission to the ICU, the average MR-proADM level in survivor patients was 1.01 versus 1.64 in non-survivor patients. The MD of MR-proADM values in survivors vs. non-survivors was −0.96 (95% CI from −1.26, to −0.65). Test for overall effect: Z = 6.19 ($p < 0.00001$) and heterogeneity was $I^2 = 0\%$ (Figure 2).

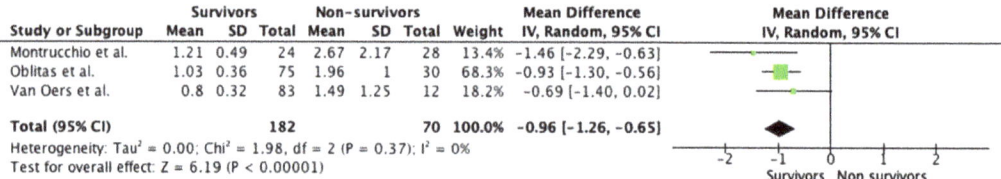

Study or Subgroup	Survivors Mean	SD	Total	Non-survivors Mean	SD	Total	Weight	Mean Difference IV, Random, 95% CI
Montrucchio et al.	1.21	0.49	24	2.67	2.17	28	13.4%	−1.46 [−2.29, −0.63]
Oblitas et al.	1.03	0.36	75	1.96	1	30	68.3%	−0.93 [−1.30, −0.56]
Van Oers et al.	0.8	0.32	83	1.49	1.25	12	18.2%	−0.69 [−1.40, 0.02]
Total (95% CI)			182			70	100.0%	−0.96 [−1.26, −0.65]

Heterogeneity: Tau² = 0.00; Chi² = 1.98, df = 2 (P = 0.37); I² = 0%
Test for overall effect: Z = 6.19 (P < 0.00001)

Figure 2. Forest plot of the hypothetical meta-analyzed results [14,28,33]. One of the four studies selected could not be included as it did not report the standard deviation. Analysis conducted with Review manager 5.4 [11].

All studies were prospective non-randomized clinical trials; therefore, the ROBINS-i tool was applied to assess the risk of bias. The overall risk of bias was low (Supplementary Table S1). Publication bias was not tested because of the small number of studies.

4. Discussion

This systematic review of the literature highlights the potential role of MR-proADM as a clinical prognostic biomarker in critically ill patients with COVID-19, although a lack of an unequivocal explanation regarding its mechanism of action remains. The growing interest in this promising biomarker and its potential role in the context of COVID-19 pandemic should be underlined. The meta-analysis evaluating only studies conducted in ICU seems to confirm the efficacy of the use of this biomarker, although it deserves further studies to increase the sample size and better define a reliable cut-off. The COVID-19 pandemic has renewed attention to the well-known need for a biomarker capable of differentiating the most critical patients to whom interventions and resources should be targeted. In addition, the characteristics of the new infection—especially at the beginning—highlighted the "weaknesses" of traditional biomarkers, such as procalcitonin and C-reactive protein, but also, d-dimer and cardiac enzymes, which were progressively used as "surrogates" for possible damage mechanisms.

Two and a half years after the onset of SARS-CoV2 pandemic, the importance of the mechanism of endothelial damage at the microvascular level has been widely demonstrated. In this regard, the application of the pro-ADM biomarker in this specific context seemed to be of great interest right from the start, to identify—as early as possible—those patients at greatest risk of poor prognosis. The lack of a univocal explanation for its mechanism of action has not discouraged various authors from considering it in the clinical setting, even if its applications remain varied. Overall, the studies included in our review agree in defining the validity of MR-proADM in the early stages of hospitalization as a prognostic biomarker. Elevated values were found in patients with more severe disease and correlated with statistical significance with patient mortality [35]. This aspect emerged both in the ICU setting and in the ED, opening important perspectives not only in terms of patient allocation but also in terms of possible discharge.

However, although the total number of patients involved in the studies is increasing, there is a huge variation in terms of population, outcome, and methods of assessing MR-proADM (Table 1). The prominent discrepancies that had already emerged in studies on proADM in patients with sepsis and septic shock [36] were further enhanced in the pandemic setting.

The reviewed studies focused on two different populations, represented by ED and ICU patients. Among them, different outcomes were considered, sometimes compromising inter-study comparability (i.e., the use of RRT [16], superinfections [15], children versus adult population [17]).

Another source of dissimilarity is the timing of biomarker testing. Most of the studies evaluated the baseline value of MR-proADM at the patient admission, with a single determination (Table 1). Among the articles considered, only six considered more than a single measurement, but with different intervals (i.e., 3 repeated measurements, daily measurements, etc.) [18,21,23,28,33,34]. However, the role of trend analysis of biomarker values over time is recently emerging in the COVID-19 [28] population, but also in sepsis and septic shock [37].

A clear heterogeneity is also reported on cut-off adopted by different authors, as it was in the more studied context of pneumonia, sepsis, and septic shock [3,6,7], where it seems reasonable to consider a difference within settings (ICU, ED, general wards) and the relative expected severity of patients. As the literature is not consistent in establishing a precise cut-off for increase mortality/severity risk, some authors refer to a value derived from their internal cohort, while others relate to literature-reported previous values.

Considering that establishing a cut-off is one of the most important clinical goals, particularly in the context of a pandemic where a reduction in available resources has been experienced, we propose the use of a meta-analytic approach to determine a clinical severity cut-off derived from available studies on MR-proADM in ICU admitted critically ill COVID-19 patients, excluding all studies involving a mixed population. Our aim was to achieve a possible threshold value for evaluation and access to the critical care area, based on defined endothelial damage and related likely organ failure. Considering cut-off values identified from the available scientific literature (Table 1), MR-proADM cut-off values proposed by Elke et al. among patients with severe sepsis or septic shock (namely 2.75 for low-severity patients and 10.9 nmol/for high-severity patients at baseline) [3] might not represent a useful reference for studies still in progress and/or about to be published. However, those values appear quite in line with the previous cut-offs proposed for respiratory infections, while it appears lower than those identified in sepsis or septic shock [22].

We suggest a cut-off evaluating the values expressed in Table 1 for the ICU population and considering the mean difference of the mean MR-proADM values in the two high and low-risk populations. It might be emphasized that this meta-analysis cannot be used to propose a MR-pro-ADM cut-off value for disease severity, as this would require an individual-patient meta-analysis followed by ROC curve construction and identification of the pro-ADM value corresponding to the best combination of sensitivity and specificity.

Furthermore, it is essential to note the significant difference between the values proposed in the meta-analysis concerning the ones expressed by Elke et al. (namely 0.96 in our meta-analysis vs. 2.5 in patients with sepsis and 10.9 in patients with septic shock in the manuscript by Elke et al. [3]). The reason for this discrepancy is currently not fully known. Although previous experience on the MR-proADM biomarker is related to sepsis and septic shock, the difference in the cut-offs underlines different physiopathological mechanisms. In septic shock, very high values refer to situations in which significant tissue hypoperfusion is present, with consequent organ failure. Otherwise, in the respiratory failure related to severe COVID-19 disease, the endothelial damage is likely to have a different origin, reflecting the need for specific cut-off values.

As discussed above, the overall number of articles on the subject is still limited. Furthermore, the studies considered show clinical heterogeneity concerning the type of population (ED versus ICU) and its severity, the outcomes, the timing of MR-proADM value(s), the cut-off considered, and the possible role of different confounders.

5. Conclusions

Despite the lack of randomized clinical trials and the clinical and methodological reported issues, an increased interest in the use of MRpro-ADM and its physiopathology implications in COVID-19 critically ill patients is emerging. In Europe, the current experience on the use of pro-ADM seems to highlight its validity in the early stages of hospitalization as a prognostic biomarker. High values have been found consistently in patients with more severe disease, both in ICUs and EDs, and correlated with statistical significance with patient mortality. Our meta-analysis confirms a significant difference in MR-proADM values at ICU admission between surviving and non-surviving patients.

Current evidence encourages further prospective and adequate studies on this promising predictive biomarker in the COVID-19 population, providing more specific guidance on its use and specific cut-offs. Other areas to be investigated in the next future are possibly confounding factors and the role of the biomarker trend during the time.

Supplementary Materials: The following supporting information can be downloaded at: https://www.mdpi.com/article/10.3390/jcm11154543/s1, Table S1: Adrenomedullin's definition and characteristics [38,39].

Author Contributions: Conceptualization, G.M. (Giorgia Montrucchioand), E.B. and L.B.; methodology, G.M. (Giorgia Montrucchioand) and E.B.; software, E.B.; validation, G.M. (Giorgia Montrucchioand) and L.B.; formal analysis, G.M. (Giorgia Montrucchioand), E.B., D.L., A.G., A.V. and G.D.; investigation, G.M. (Giorgia Montrucchioand), E.B., D.L., A.G., A.V. and G.D.; data curation, G.M. (Giorgia Montrucchioand), E.B., D.L., A.G., A.V. and G.D.; writing—original draft preparation, G.M. (Giorgia Montrucchioand) and E.B.; writing—review and editing, F.R., G.M. (Giulio Mengozzi) and L.B.; supervision, F.R. and G.M. (Giulio Mengozzi). All authors have read and agreed to the published version of the manuscript.

Funding: Funds required are provided by the Department of Surgical Sciences, University of Turin, 10126 Turin, Italy.

Informed Consent Statement: Patient consent was waived as this is a systematic review and meta-analysis, which therefore uses data already extracted from other studies. All studies considered collected informed consent from their patients.

Data Availability Statement: The datasets used and analyzed during the current meta-analysis are available from the corresponding author upon reasonable request.

Conflicts of Interest: All the authors declare that they have no conflict of interest in the field of the present article.

References

1. Saeed, K.; Legramante, J.M.; Angeletti, S.; Curcio, F.; Miguens, I.; Poole, S.; Tascini, C.; Sozio, E.; Del Castillo, J.G. Mid-regional pro-adrenomedullin as a supplementary tool to clinical parameters in cases of suspicion of infection in the emergency department. *Expert Rev. Mol. Diagn.* **2021**, *21*, 397–404. [CrossRef]
2. Saeed, K.; Wilson, D.C.; Bloos, F.; Schuetz, P.; van der Does, Y.; Melander, O.; Hausfater, P.; Legramante, J.M.; Claessens, Y.-E.; Amin, D.; et al. The early identification of disease progression in patients with suspected infection presenting to the emergency department: A multi-centre derivation and validation study. *Crit. Care* **2019**, *23*, 40. [CrossRef] [PubMed]
3. Elke, G.; Bloos, F.; Wilson, D.C.; Brunkhorst, F.M.; Briegel, J.; Reinhart, K.; Loeffler, M.; Kluge, S.; Nierhaus, A.; Jaschinski, U.; et al. The use of mid-regional proadrenomedullin to identify disease severity and treatment response to sepsis-a secondary analysis of a large randomised controlled trial. *Crit. Care* **2018**, *22*, 79. [CrossRef] [PubMed]
4. Wilson, D.C.; Schefold, J.C.; Baldirà, J.; Spinetti, T.; Saeed, K.; Elke, G. Adrenomedullin in COVID-19 induced endotheliitis. *Crit. Care* **2020**, *24*, 411. [CrossRef]
5. Varga, Z.; Flammer, A.J.; Steiger, P.; Haberecker, M.; Andermatt, R.; Zinkernagel, A.S.; Mehra, M.R.; Schuepbach, R.A.; Ruschitzka, F.; Moch, H. Endothelial cell infection and endotheliitis in COVID-19. *Lancet* **2020**, *395*, 1417–1418. [CrossRef]
6. Renaud, B.; Schuetz, P.; Claessens, Y.E.; Labarère, J.; Albrich, W.; Mueller, B. Proadrenomedullin improves Risk of Early Admission to ICU score for predicting early severe community-acquired pneumonia. *Chest* **2012**, *142*, 1447–1454. [CrossRef]

7. Van Paassen, J.; Van Dissel, J.T.; Hiemstra, P.S.; Zwaginga, J.J.; Cobbaert, C.M.; Juffermans, N.P.; De Wilde, R.B.; Stijnen, T.; De Jonge, E.; Klautz, R.J.; et al. Perioperative proADM-change is associated with the development of acute respiratory distress syndrome in critically ill cardiac surgery patients: A prospective cohort study. *Biomark. Med.* **2019**, *13*, 1081–1091. [CrossRef] [PubMed]
8. Sterne, J.A.; Hernán, M.A.; Reeves, B.C.; Savović, J.; Berkman, N.D.; Viswanathan, M.; Henry, D.; Altman, D.G.; Ansari, M.T.; Boutron, I.; et al. ROBINS-I: A tool for assessing risk of bias in non-randomised studies of interventions. *BMJ* **2016**, *355*, i4919. [CrossRef] [PubMed]
9. Sterne, J.A.C.; Savović, J.; Page, M.J.; Elbers, R.G.; Blencowe, N.S.; Boutron, I.; Cates, C.J.; Cheng, H.Y.; Corbett, M.S.; Eldridge, S.M.; et al. RoB 2: A revised tool for assessing risk of bias in randomized trials. *BMJ* **2019**, *366*, l4898. [CrossRef]
10. Luo, D.; Wan, X.; Liu, J.; Tong, T. Optimally estimating the sample mean from the sample size, median, mid-range, and/or mid-quartile range. *Stat. Methods Med. Res.* **2018**, *27*, 1785–1805. [CrossRef]
11. Revman Cp. Nordic Cochrane Centre, The Cochrane Collaboration. *Review Manager 5 (RevMan 5)*; Version 5.4; Nordic Cochrane Centre, The Cochrane Collaboration: Copenhagen, Denmark, 2020.
12. Higgins, J.P.T.; Thomas, J.; Chandler, J.; Cumpston, M.; Li, T.; Page, M.J.; Welch, V.A. *Cochrane Handbook for Systematic Reviews of Interventions*; John Wiley & Sons: Hoboken, NJ, USA, 2019.
13. Lippi, G.; Henry, B.M. Pooled analysis of mid-regional pro-adrenomedullin values in COVID-19 patients with critical illness. *Intern. Emerg. Med.* **2021**, *16*, 1723–1725. [CrossRef] [PubMed]
14. Oblitas, C.-M.; Galeano-Valle, F.; Ramírez-Navarro, J.; López-Cano, J.; Monterrubio-Manrique, Á.; García-Gámiz, M.; Sancho-González, M.; Arenal-López, S.; Walther, L.-A.-S.; Demelo-Rodríguez, P. Mid-Regional Pro-Adrenomedullin, Methemoglobin and Carboxyhemoglobin as Prognosis Biomarkers in Critically Ill Patients with COVID-19: An Observational Prospective Study. *Viruses* **2021**, *13*, 2445. [CrossRef]
15. Malinina, D.A.; Shlyk, I.V.; Polushin, Y.S.; Afanasiev, A.A.; Stanevich, O.V.; Bakin, E.A. The informative value of proadrenomedullin in patients with severe COVID-19. *Messenger Anesthesiol. Resusc.* **2020**, *17*, 31–38. [CrossRef]
16. Roedl, K.; Jarczak, D.; Fischer, M.; Haddad, M.; Boenisch, O.; de Heer, G.; Burdelski, C.; Frings, D.; Sensen, B.; Karakas, M.; et al. MR-proAdrenomedullin as a predictor of renal replacement therapy in a cohort of critically ill patients with COVID-19. *Biomarkers* **2021**, *26*, 417–424. [CrossRef]
17. Girona-Alarcon, M.; Bobillo-Perez, S.; Sole-Ribalta, A.; Hernandez, L.; Guitart, C.; Suarez, R.; Balaguer, M.; Cambra, F.J.; Jordan, I. The different manifestations of COVID-19 in adults and children: A cohort study in an intensive care unit. *BMC Infect. Dis.* **2021**, *21*, 87. [CrossRef]
18. Simon, T.P.; Stoppe, C.; Breuer, T.; Stiehler, L.; Dreher, M.; Kersten, A.; Kluge, S.; Karakas, M.; Zechendorf, E.; Marx, G.; et al. Prognostic Value of Bioactive Adrenomedullin in Critically Ill Patients with COVID-19 in Germany: An Observational Cohort Study. *J. Clin. Med.* **2021**, *10*, 1667. [CrossRef] [PubMed]
19. Oblitas, C.M.; Galeano-Valle, F.; Lopez-Cano, J.; Monterrubio-Manrique, A.; Garcia-Gamiz, M.; Ramirez-Navarro, J.; Sancho-Gonzalez, M.; Arenal-Lopez, S.; Alvarez-Sala Walther, L.; Demelo-Rodriguez, P. Potential prognostic biomarkers in COVID19: Role of mid-regional pro-adrenomedullin, methemoglobin and carboxyhemoglobin. *Intensive Care Med. Exp.* **2021**, *9*, 50. [CrossRef]
20. Lhote, S.; Van Grunderbeeck, N.; Colling, D.; Verchain, S.; Varillon, C.; Floch, P.; Vinsonneau, C.; Caulier, T.; Granier, M.; Mallat, J. Proadrenomedullin assessment of multi-organ failure in COVID-19 sepsis (PAMOCOS): A prospective, multicentric observational study. *Crit. Care* **2021**, *25*, 383. [CrossRef]
21. Benedetti, I.; Spinelli, D.; Callegari, T.; Bonometti, R.; Molinaro, E.; Novara, E.; Cassinari, M.; Frino, C.; Guaschino, R.; Boverio, R.; et al. High levels of mid-regional proadrenomedullin in ARDS COVID-19 patients: The experience of a single, italian center. *Eur. Rev. Med. Pharmacol. Sci.* **2021**, *25*, 1743–1751. [CrossRef]
22. García de Guadiana-Romualdo, L.; Martínez Martínez, M.; Rodríguez Mulero, M.D.; Esteban-Torrella, P.; Hernández Olivo, M.; Alcaraz García, M.J.; Campos-Rodríguez, V.; Sancho-Rodríguez, N.; Galindo Martínez, M.; Alcaraz, A.; et al. Circulating MR-proADM levels, as an indicator of endothelial dysfunction, for early risk stratification of mid-term mortality in COVID-19 patients. *Int. J. Infect. Dis.* **2021**, *111*, 211–218. [CrossRef] [PubMed]
23. Gregoriano, C.; Koch, D.; Kutz, A.; Haubitz, S.; Conen, A.; Bernasconi, L.; Hammerer-Lercher, A.; Saeed, K.; Mueller, B.; Schuetz, P. The vasoactive peptide MR-pro-adrenomedullin in COVID-19 patients: An observational study. *Clin. Chem. Lab. Med.* **2021**, *59*, 995–1004. [CrossRef] [PubMed]
24. Indirli, R.; Bandera, A.; Valenti, L.; Ceriotti, F.; Di Modugno, A.; Tettamanti, M.; Gualtierotti, R.; Peyvandi, F.; Montano, N.; Blasi, F.; et al. Prognostic value of copeptin and mid-regional proadrenomedullin in COVID-19-hospitalized patients. *Eur. J. Clin. Investig.* **2022**, *52*, e13753. [CrossRef] [PubMed]
25. Lo Sasso, B.; Gambino, C.M.; Scichilone, N.; Giglio, R.V.; Bivona, G.; Scazzone, C.; Muratore, R.; Milano, S.; Barbagallo, M.; Agnello, L.; et al. Clinical Utility of Midregional Proadrenomedullin in Patients with COVID-19. *Lab. Med.* **2021**, *52*, 493–498. [CrossRef]
26. Méndez, R.; González-Jiménez, P.; Latorre, A.; Piqueras, M.; Bouzas, L.; Yépez, K.; Ferrando, A.; Zaldívar-Olmeda, E.; Moscardó, A.; Alonso, R.; et al. Acute and sustained increase in endothelial biomarkers in COVID-19. *Thorax* **2022**, *77*, 400–403. [CrossRef] [PubMed]

27. Minieri, M.; Di Lecce, V.N.; Lia, M.S.; Maurici, M.; Bernardini, S.; Legramante, J.M. Role of MR-proADM in the risk stratification of COVID-19 patients assessed at the triage of the Emergency Department. *Crit. Care* **2021**, *25*, 407. [CrossRef] [PubMed]
28. Montrucchio, G.; Sales, G.; Rumbolo, F.; Palmesino, F.; Fanelli, V.; Urbino, R.; Filippini, C.; Mengozzi, G.; Brazzi, L. Effectiveness of mid-regional pro-adrenomedullin (MR-proADM) as prognostic marker in COVID-19 critically ill patients: An observational prospective study. *PLoS ONE* **2021**, *16*, e0246771. [CrossRef]
29. Moore, N.; Williams, R.; Mori, M.; Bertolusso, B.; Vernet, G.; Lynch, J.; Philipson, P.; Ledgerwood, T.; Kidd, S.P.; Thomas, C.; et al. Mid-regional proadrenomedullin (MR-proADM), C-reactive protein (CRP) and other biomarkers in the early identification of disease progression in patients with COVID-19 in the acute NHS setting. *J. Clin. Pathol.* **2022**; *in press*. [CrossRef]
30. Popov, D.A.; Borovkova, U.L.; Rybka, M.M.; Ramnenok, T.V.; Golukhova, E.Z. Predictive value of proadrenomedullin in patients with COVID-19. *Russ. J. Anesthesiol. Reanimatol.* **2020**, *6*, 6–12. [CrossRef]
31. Sozio, E.; Tascini, C.; Fabris, M.; D'Aurizio, F.; De Carlo, C.; Graziano, E.; Bassi, F.; Sbrana, F.; Ripoli, A.; Pagotto, A.; et al. MR-proADM as prognostic factor of outcome in COVID-19 patients. *Sci. Rep.* **2021**, *11*, 5121. [CrossRef] [PubMed]
32. Spoto, S.; Agrò, F.E.; Sambuco, F.; Travaglino, F.; Valeriani, E.; Fogolari, M.; Mangiacapra, F.; Costantino, S.; Ciccozzi, M.; Angeletti, S. High value of mid-regional proadrenomedullin in COVID-19: A marker of widespread endothelial damage, disease severity, and mortality. *J. Med. Virol.* **2021**, *93*, 2820–2827. [CrossRef]
33. van Oers, J.A.H.; Kluiters, Y.; Bons, J.A.P.; de Jongh, M.; Pouwels, S.; Ramnarain, D.; de Lange, D.W.; de Grooth, H.J.; Girbes, A.R.J. Endothelium-associated biomarkers mid-regional proadrenomedullin and C-terminal proendothelin-1 have good ability to predict 28-day mortality in critically ill patients with SARS-CoV-2 pneumonia: A prospective cohort study. *J. Crit. Care* **2021**, *66*, 173–180. [CrossRef]
34. Zaninotto, M.; Maria Mion, M.; Marchioro, L.; Padoan, A.; Plebani, M. Endothelial dysfunction and Mid-Regional proAdrenomedullin: What role in SARS-CoV-2 infected Patients? *Clin. Chim. Acta* **2021**, *523*, 185–190. [CrossRef]
35. Agnello, L.; Bellia, C.; Iacolino, G.; Gambino, C.M.; Petrancosta, R.; Lo Sasso, B.; Ciaccio, M. Mid-regional pro-adrenomedullin predicts poor outcome in non-selected patients admitted to intensive care unit. *Biochim. Clin.* **2018**, *42*, S171.
36. Piccioni, A.; Saviano, A.; Cicchinelli, S.; Valletta, F.; Santoro, M.C.; de Cunzo, T.; Zanza, C.; Longhitano, Y.; Tullo, G.; Tilli, P.; et al. Proadrenomedullin in Sepsis and Septic Shock: A Role in the Emergency Department. *Med. Kaunas* **2021**, *57*, 920. [CrossRef] [PubMed]
37. Bima, P.; Montrucchio, G.; Caramello, V.; Rumbolo, F.; Dutto, S.; Boasso, S.; Ferraro, A.; Brazzi, L.; Lupia, E.; Boccuzzi, A.; et al. Prognostic Value of Mid-Regional Proadrenomedullin Sampled at Presentation and after 72 Hours in Septic Patients Presenting to the Emergency Department: An Observational Two-Center Study. *Biomedicines* **2022**, *10*, 719. [CrossRef] [PubMed]
38. Marino, R.; Struck, J.; Maisel, A.S.; Magrini, L.; Bergmann, A.; Di Somma, S. Plasma adrenomedullin is associated with short-term mortality and vasopressor requirement in patients admitted with sepsis. *Crit. Care* **2014**, *18*, R34. [CrossRef]
39. Laterre, P.F.; Pickkers, P.; Marx, G.; Wittebole, X.; Meziani, F.; Dugernier, T.; Huberlant, V.; Schuerholz, T.; François, B.; Lascarrou, J.B.; et al. Safety and tolerability of non-neutralizing adrenomedullin antibody adrecizumab (HAM8101) in septic shock patients: The AdrenOSS-2 phase 2a biomarker-guided trial. *Intensive Care Med.* **2021**, *47*, 1284–1294. [CrossRef]

www.ingramcontent.com/pod-product-compliance
Lightning Source LLC
LaVergne TN
LVHW070453100526
838202LV00014B/1713

MDPI
St. Alban-Anlage 66
4052 Basel
Switzerland
www.mdpi.com

Journal of Clinical Medicine Editorial Office
E-mail: jcm@mdpi.com
www.mdpi.com/journal/jcm

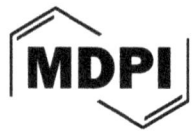

Disclaimer/Publisher's Note: The statements, opinions and data contained in all publications are solely those of the individual author(s) and contributor(s) and not of MDPI and/or the editor(s). MDPI and/or the editor(s) disclaim responsibility for any injury to people or property resulting from any ideas, methods, instructions or products referred to in the content.